Clinical Pathology of Soft-Tissue Tumors

Clinical Pathology of Soft-Tissue Tumors

edited by

Elizabeth Montgomery

*The Johns Hopkins University
Baltimore, Maryland*

Alan D. Aaron

*Georgetown University Hospital
Washington, DC, and
National Institutes of Health
Bethesda, Maryland*

MARCEL DEKKER, INC.   NEW YORK · BASEL

ISBN: 0-8247-0290-5

This book is printed on acid-free paper.

Headquarters
Marcel Dekker, Inc.
270 Madison Avenue, New York, NY 10016
tel: 212-696-9000; fax: 212-685-4540

Eastern Hemisphere Distribution
Marcel Dekker AG
Hutgasse 4, Postfach 812, CH-4001 Basel, Switzerland
tel: 41-61-261-8482; fax: 41-61-261-8896

World Wide Web
http://www.dekker.com

The publisher offers discounts on this book when ordered in bulk quantities. For more information, write to Special Sales/Professional Marketing at the headquarters address above.

Current printing (last digit):
10 9 8 7 6 5 4 3 2 1

PRINTED IN THE UNITED STATES OF AMERICA

Preface

When we were approached by Marcel Dekker, Inc., to create a text on soft-tissue sarcomas, our first question was whether there was a need for "yet another" volume on the subject. However, as a surgeon (ADA) and a pathologist (EM), sharing in the belief that proper management of soft-tissue sarcomas requires a multi-specialty approach, we realized that we each needed several tomes to cover the topic. Our primary goal in editing and contributing to this volume was therefore to provide a single and concise multidisciplinary reference for those entering this challenging field.

In pursuit of that goal, we have gathered a group of colleagues in a wide variety of relevant specialties whose contributions are as current and multidisciplinary as possible. In addition to chapters dealing with pathologic diagnosis of these tumors written with the depth necessary to supplement residents', fellows', and "front-line" practitioners' knowledge in a broad array of disciplines, the text outlines principles of surgical, oncologic, and radiation therapeutic approaches to these tumors and offers a section on rehabilitation.

No single text can serve as the complete guide to every area of medical practice involved in the management of soft-tissue tumors. However, we have attempted to create an effective teaching and reference tool for physicians and others who are involved in management of patients with soft-tissue tumors, and to provide a deeper understanding especially for those who do not treat these rare neoplasms on a regular basis.

We would like to thank our many colleagues who contributed a broad range of expertise as well as the editorial staff at Dekker, including Michele Sinoway, Kathleen Baldonado, Sandra Beberman, and Richard Johnson. We dedicate this book to our families and closest friends: Dr. Aaron to his lovely wife, Lynne, and two sons, Allister and Harrison, without whose support this work would not have been possible, Dr. Montgomery to her three children, Sasha, Peter, and Sean, who provided unflagging inspiration, and to Dr. Cyril Fisher for his tireless advice and patience.

Elizabeth Montgomery
Alan D. Aaron

Contents

Part Three   MANAGEMENT OF SOFT-TISSUE NEOPLASMS

Contributors

Alan D. Aaron, M.D.   Department of Orthopedic Surgery, Georgetown University Hospital, Washington, DC, and Clinical Consultant, National Institutes of Health, Bethesda, Maryland

Pedram Argani, M.D.   Department of Pathology, The Johns Hopkins Hospital, and Assistant Professor, The Johns Hopkins University, Baltimore, Maryland

Christopher A. Attinger, M.D.   Division of Plastic Surgery, Department of General Surgery, Georgetown University Hospital, Washington, DC

Kevin J. Cullen, M.D.   Lombardi Cancer Center, Georgetown University Medical Center, Washington, DC

Cyril Fisher, M.A., M.D., F.R.C.P.   Department of Histopathology, The Royal Marsden NHS Trust, London, England

Mary A. Furlong, M.D.   Department of Soft Tissue Pathology, Armed Forces Institute of Pathology, Washington, DC

Jay Greenberg, M.D.   Inova Fairfax Hospital for Children, Fairfax, Virginia

Christian H. Hansen, M.D.   Department of Pathology, St. Agnes Hospital, Baltimore, Maryland

Jeanne E. Hicks, M.D.   Rehabilitation Medicine Department, National Institutes of Health, Bethesda, Maryland; Department of Internal Medicine, George Washington Medical Center; and Department of Orthopedic Surgery, Georgetown University Medical Center, Washington, DC

Kalisha A. Hill, M.D.   Northwestern University Medical School and Northwestern Memorial Hospital, Chicago, Illinois

Andrea D. Johnson, M.D.   Department of Hematology/Oncology, Georgetown University Medical Center, Washington, DC

Michael R. Kuettel, M.D., Ph.D., M.B.A.   Department of Radiation Medicine, Roswell Park Cancer Institute, Buffalo, New York

William B. Laskin, M.D.   Northwestern University Medical School and Northwestern Memorial Hospital, Chicago, Illinois

John Lin, M.D.   Department of Radiology, University of Michigan Medical Center, Ann Arbor, Michigan

Elizabeth Montgomery, M.D.   Department of Pathology, The Johns Hopkins University, Baltimore, Maryland

G. Petur Nielson, M.D.   Department of Pathology, Massachusetts General Hospital, Boston, Massachusetts

John X. O'Connell, M.D., F.R.C.P.C.   Department of Pathology, Surrey Memorial Hospital, Surrey, British Columbia, Canada

David M. Parham, M.D.   Department of Pathology, University of Arkansas for Medical Sciences and Arkansas Children's Hospital Research Institute, Little Rock, Arkansas

Terrance D. Peabody, M.D.   Section of Orthopedic Surgery and Rehabilitation Medicine, Department of Surgery, University of Chicago, Chicago, Illinois

Anita A. Reddy, M.D.   Department of Radiation Oncology, Georgetown University Hospital, Washington, DC

Brian Shannon, M.D.   Department of Orthopedic Surgery, Georgetown University Hospital, Washington, DC

Salwa S. Sheikh, M.D.   Dhahran Health Center, Dhahran, Saudi Arabia

Sidney K. Suneja, M.D.   Walter Reed Army Medical Center, Washington, DC

Phyllis R. Vezza, M.D.   Department of Pathology, Our Lady of Fatima Hospital, North Providence, Rhode Island

Katherine E. Wolfe, M.D.   Department of Pathology, Georgetown University Medical Center, Washington, DC

James M. Woodruff, M.D.   Department of Pathology, Memorial Sloan-Kettering Cancer Center and Cornell University Medical College, New York, New York

Lawrence Yao, M.D.   Musculoskeletal Imaging, Georgetown University Medical Center, Washington, DC

Clinical Pathology of Soft-Tissue Tumors

1
Introduction to and Overview of Clinical Evaluation of Soft-Tissue Tumors

Alan D. Aaron
Georgetown University Hospital
Washington, DC, and
National Institutes of Health
Bethesda, Maryland

Elizabeth Montgomery
The Johns Hopkins University
Baltimore, Maryland

I. INCIDENCE

Cancer is the second leading cause of death in the United States, with more than 500,000 cases reported every year (1). Lung cancer is the most common cause of cancer-related death for both men and women, accounting for more than 140,000 deaths annually. On the other hand, there are only 6000 new cases of soft-tissue sarcoma reported each year, which compose approximately 1% of all malignant neoplasms (1). The incidence of adult soft-tissue sarcomas increases with age, with men having a slightly greater risk than women (1,2). With the annual clinical incidence of benign tumors at about 300/1,000,000 and the corresponding figure for soft-tissue sarcomas being 18/1,000,000, benign tumors are almost 200 times more common than sarcomas (3). For all cell types combined and most individual types, males are more commonly afflicted than females. Blood vessel sarcomas (primarily Kaposi's sarcoma) are more than 20 times more common among caucasian men than caucasian women, which is primarily due to the acquired immune deficiency syndrome (AIDS) epidemic among homosexual and bisexual men. Leiomyosarcoma is one of the few sarcomas more common among women, due especially to tumors of uterine origin. The rates of soft-tissue sarcoma are generally higher among African Americans than whites, with racial disparity especially great for leiomyosarcoma, particularly among women (4). Upon review of the incidence of soft-tissue sarcomas in both the United States and Canada, it is clear that there is an upward trend (5,6). In the 1980s, the overall increase in cases of soft-tissue sarcomas primarily reflected the dramatic increase in AIDS-related Kaposi's sarcoma in young and middle-aged men (7).

The rarity of soft-tissue sarcomas results in two problems relating to their diagnosis and treatment. Recognition of potentially malignant soft-tissue masses is problematic as the majority of primary care physicians and surgeons have had little exposure to sarcomas. The assumption that an asymptomatic mass is a lipoma can lead to significant delays in diagnosis. With regard to treatment, inexperience on the part of the surgeon or another member of the team may result in the undertreatment of primary or metastatic sites, potentially resulting in poorer outcome. Though lung cancer exacts a much greater risk of mortality, approximately 50% of patients diagnosed with soft-tissue sarcomas will die of their disease (3300 cases). Unlike bone sarcomas, in which great success has been demonstrated with chemotherapy over the past 30 years (20% vs. 58% 5-year survival), the mortality associated with soft-tissue sarcomas has remained relatively stable. Any measurable improvement related to survival in patients with soft-tissue sarcomas is best explained by improved methods of local rather than systemic treatment modalities. Because of unproven chemotherapeutic regiments, successful local control is paramount in providing patients with the best opportunity to achieve long-term survival.

II. DISTRIBUTION

Soft-tissue sarcomas can arise in any tissue of the musculoskeletal system. In a large series of 1685 adults with primary soft-tissue sarcomas, the most common location was the extremities (51%) (8). Of these 851 patients with extremity tumors, 40% had lesions in the lower extremity (672 patients) and 11% in the upper extremity (179 patients). Other sites included the retroperitoneum and abdomen (14%), trunk (14%), genitourinary sites (6%), viscera (5%), head and neck (5%), and other sites (5%). The most common histopathologic diagnosis was liposarcoma, followed by leiomyosarcoma and malignant fibrous histiocytoma. In the extremities and superficial trunk, liposarcoma and malignant fibrous histiocytoma were most common, whereas in the retroperitoneum and visceral tissues, leiomyosarcoma predominated. A similar distribution has been reported in other large series. In another 546 patients with soft-tissue sarcomas, 331 (60.6%) presented in the extremities, 39 (7.1%) in the head and neck, 114 (20.9%) in the thorax or abdominal wall, and 62 (11.4%) in the pelvis and intra-abdominal region (9). In reviews focusing on only extremity soft-tissue sarcomas, similar results are described, with approximately 70% occurring in the lower and 30% in the upper extremity (10). However, in the series by Markhede et al., 93.8% (91 of 97 patients) of soft-tissue sarcomas were located in the extremities (11). The most common location in the lower extremity is the thigh (60%), followed by the leg (13.3%) and the knee and popliteal region (11.4%) (12). The distribution of sarcomas may vary slightly depending on the specific histologic subtype. In a large series of 75 cases of myxofibrosarcoma, though a similar percentage arose in the upper extremity (34%), 70% of cases were localized in the dermal or subcutaneous tissue as opposed to myofascial regions (13). This is unusual as it is estimated that 30% of soft-tissue sarcomas present in the subcutaneous region (9,14). The anatomical distribution of sarcomas varies little between series, with 40% of lesions arising in the thigh, buttock, and groin region, 15–20% in the upper extremity, 10–15% in the head and neck region, 12–18% in the torso region, and approximately 12% in the retroperitoneal tissues (15,16).

III. ETIOLOGIC FACTORS

The cause of most soft-tissue tumors is unknown. Benign lesions have been associated with trauma and foreign materials; sarcomas have been linked to several chemical toxins and prior irradiation. The incidence of reported sarcomas following therapeutic irradiation is low, ranging from 0.03% to 0.3%. The latency period is between 5 and 10 years, although periods as short as 2 years have been reported, with the most common soft-tissue sarcoma subtype being malignant fibrous histiocytoma (17,18). The median reported total irradiation dose varies but is generally above 40 Gy, with sarcomas reported to develop after only 12 Gy. The number of reports documenting an association between soft-tissue sarcomas and prior radiation therapy is small. In a large review of 565 patients with sarcoma as a second malignancy, 160 (28%) were considered to have a radiation-associated sarcoma (19). The most common indication for radiation was breast cancer (26%), followed by lymphoma (25%) and carcinoma of the cervix (14%). The most common histologic types of radiation-associated sarcoma were osteosarcoma (21%), malignant fibrous histiocytoma (16%), and angiosarcoma/lymphangiosarcoma (15%). The majority of the tumors were high-grade (87%). In a review of a nationwide cancer registry, 33 cases of postradiation sarcoma were evaluated (20). The median interval from start of radiation therapy to detection of postradiation sarcoma was 13.2 years. Of 33 cases, 25 were soft tissue in origin. The most common histologic types were osteosarcoma (four extraskeletal osteosarcomas), malignant fibrous histiocytoma, and fibrosarcoma. The chest wall is the most commonly reported region, secondary to irradiation following mastectomy for breast cancer, with fibrosarcomas composing a large percentage of these cases (21,22). The incidence of chest wall soft-tissue sarcoma in patients receiving radiation therapy following mastectomy was recently reported in a large series 13,490 patients (23). Only 19 sarcomas were reported, with the relative risk of developing a radiation-induced sarcoma being only 2.2%. In a review of chest wall osteosarcomas, 29% (11/38) were radiation induced, compared with seven radiation associated soft-tissue sarcomas in a series of 149 chest wall soft-tissue sarcomas (24). Radiation-induced angiosarcomas are generally cutaneous in location and need to be differentiated from postmastectomy lymphedema angiosarcoma (25). Lymphangiosarcoma of the upper extremity following mastectomy and axillary lymph node resection, commonly known as Stewart-Treves syndrome, is indirectly related to longstanding lymphedema following surgery (26).

The cause of postradiation sarcomas is not clear. Recent studies have evaluated the effect of radiation on known sarcoma-associated gene mutations (27). Two such studies have demonstrated a link between p53 gene mutations and the incidence and prognosis of postradiation sarcomas. In a study of 24 patients with postradiation sarcomas, polymerase chain reaction sequencing confirmed a higher frequency of p53 gene mutations (58%) than reported in sporadic soft-tissue sarcomas (28). These results were confirmed in a smaller series of 11 patients with 9 patients demonstrating the presence of the p53 gene mutation (29). Of these 9 patients, 7 died during the follow-up period, whereas the 2 patients with tumor samples negative for the p53 gene mutation were still alive at the time of reporting. It is clearly documented that patients diagnosed with hereditary retinoblastoma demonstrate higher rates of specific cancers. In a study of 1604 patients with retinoblastoma, the cumulative incidence of a second cancer at 50 years after diagnosis was 51% for hereditary retinoblastoma and 5% for nonhereditary retinoblastoma (30). When these patients are irradiated, the relative risk of malignant transformation demonstrates a stepwise increase at all dose categories, with statistical significance being reported at 10–29.9 Gy and 30–59.9 Gy. This risk increases to 10.7-fold at doses of 60 Gy or greater. The type of radiation has not been demonstrated to affect the incidence of postirradiation sarcomas. In a study of 53 cases of postirradiation sarcoma, there was no difference between patients (39 patients) receiving megavoltage radiation and orthovoltage radiation (7 patients) with regard to type of sarcoma, location, or survival (31). Patients receiving megavoltage radiation demonstrated deeper tissue radiation changes and were associated with a shorter latency period. The clinical characteristics of patients diagnosed with postirradiation sarcomas were reported in a study of 344 cases (32). Characteristics common to these patients included the following: (a) diagnosis was made at an advanced stage and high grade; (b) tumor was located in areas where radical surgery could not be performed; (c) patient had a poor response to chemotherapy; (d) most patients with postirradiation sarcoma died from locally advanced and/or metastatic disease within a few months after diagnosis.

Benign and malignant soft-tissue tumors are a component of several familial disorders, including neurofibromatosis, Gardner's syndrome, familial retinoblastoma, and the Li-Fraumeni cancer family syndrome. Li-Fraumeni syndrome was originally reported in four families with a recognized autosomal dominant pattern of breast cancer, soft-tissue sarcoma, osteosarcoma, brain tumors, acute leukemia, adrenocortical carcinoma, and germ cell tumors (33–37). Studies document the greatest risk for family members to be in those in late childhood or adolescence, with an increased risk of breast cancer documented in mothers of children with soft-tissue sarcomas or bone sarcomas (38–41). In a review of 42 children with soft-tissue sarcoma or osteosarcoma, the incidence of Li-Fraumeni syndrome was investigated (42). Of these patients, 6 (7.1%) were reported to meet the diagnostic criteria for Li-Fraumeni syndrome. Germ line mutations of the p53 tumor-suppressor gene on chromosome 17 have been demonstrated in these families (43). Other studies have documented the impact of inherited p53 mutations on the incidence of cancer in families (44). An analysis of 475 tumors in 91 families with p53 germ line mutations demonstrated that breast carcinomas were most common (24.0%), followed by bone sarcomas (12.6%), brain tumors (12.0%), and soft-tissue sarcomas (11.6%). Soft-tissue sarcomas have also been associated with the hereditary form of retinoblastoma (45). Mutations of the retinoblastoma gene (*Rb-1*), located on the 13q14 chromosome, are closely linked to retinoblastoma as well as subsequent sarcomas (46). As with most series, soft-tissue sarcomas arising in patients with retinoblastoma generally occur in the lower extremities, though the risk is relatively high around the soft-tissues of the orbit following radiation therapy. Neurofibromatosis type 1, a dominantly inherited trait, is closely associated with an increased risk of malignant peripheral nerve sheath tumors (neurofibrosarcomas) in adults and rhabdomyosarcomas, fibrosarcomas, and liposarcomas in children (47,48). In an extensive review, approximately 5% of patients with neurofibromatosis developed malignant nerve sheath tumors (49). In another recent study of patients diagnosed with neurofibromatosis type 1, malignant tumors were reported 4 times as often as in the general population (50). Of 70 patients, 17 (24%) developed a total of 19 malignant tumors, including 5 sarcomas, 13 carcinomas, and 1 malignant melanoma. In addition, 4 pheochromocytomas, 2 adenomas, and 1 example of C-cell hyperplasia were diagnosed. In an attempt to determine the link between neurofibromatosis and sarcomas in children, a study of 157 patients with soft-tissue sarcomas was undertaken to reference the diagnostic features of neurofibromatosis in the group (51). Four children in the series were identified as having neurofibromatosis. Given this relatively high percentage, the authors suggested screening all children with sarcomas for neurofibromatosis.

Genetic links are also reported in the case of benign soft-tissue neoplasms. A high incidence of desmoid tumors (fibromatoses) is reported among patients with familial polyposis (Gardner's syndrome) (52–54).

Chemical agents implicated in the development of sarcomas include vinyl chloride (used industrially), thorium dioxide, and possibly the phenoxy herbicides

(55–57). Alkylating agents administered therapeutically for prior childhood malignancies have been implicated in adult sarcomas. A large meta-analysis of four Swedish case-control studies confirmed an increased incidence of soft-tissue sarcomas after occupational exposure to phenoxy herbicides and chlorinated phenols, irrespective of anatomical site or pathologic subtype (58). Additional studies from Sweden confirmed up to a sixfold increase risk of soft-tissue sarcoma associated with agricultural or forestry work involving exposure to phenoxyacetic acids or chlorophenols (59–63). Excess soft-tissue sarcomas were also observed among female rice weeders exposed to phenoxy herbicide 2,4,5-T in Italy (64). Agricultural workers in England and Wales, farmers exposed to phenoxyacetic herbicides and chlorophenols in New Zealand, and Danish gardeners have also been reported to be at increased risk for soft-tissue sarcomas (65–67). In a large study of soft-tissue sarcomas that included 21,183 workers from 11 countries, excess risk of soft-tissue sarcoma was associated with exposure to phenoxy herbicides, polychlorinated dibenzodioxin or furan, or tetrachlorodibenzo-*p*-dioxin (68).

Dioxin has been closely linked with an increased risk of soft-tissue sarcoma. In a study of more than 5000 workers, there was a threefold increased risk, increasing to ninefold among workers with more than 1 year of exposure and 20 or more years of latency (69). In a study of about 19,000 production workers and sprayers from 10 countries, a sixfold excess risk was observed 10–19 years after exposure (70). An excess risk of soft-tissue sarcoma has also been reported also among smaller cohorts exposed to dioxin in the manufacture of trichlorophenols and phenoxyacetic herbicides (71–75). The U.S. Environmental Protection Agency's Science Advisory Board classified dioxins as carcinogenic based on animal studies and the increased risk reported among dioxin-exposed workers; the increased risk of soft-tissue sarcomas was a key component of the report (76). Accidental environmental dioxin contamination has resulted in an increased incidence of soft-tissue sarcomas and other malignancies in other studies (77,78). Other insecticides have been linked to soft-tissue sarcomas. They include inorganic arsenical insecticides, hexachlorobenzene, and chlorinated hydrocarbon–based insecticides (79–81). Polyvinyl chloride has been associated with angiosarcomas of the liver and other soft-tissue sarcomas in several other studies (82,83).

Chronic lymphedema of the upper extremity in women secondary to radical mastectomy for breast cancer is closely associated with development of lymphangiosarcomas (Stewart-Treves syndrome) (84,85). Acquired lymphedema secondary to parasite-induced lymphedema (filaria) has also been associated with the development of lymphangiosarcoma (86). Families with lymphedema-distichiasis syndrome or other congenital or inherited syndromes resulting in lymphedema have a documented higher incidence of soft-tissue sarcomas (87).

IV. CLINICAL EVALUATION

The initial presenting sign of either benign or malignant soft-tissue neoplasms is almost invariably a previously unrecognized soft-tissue mass. Unfortunately, there are no symptoms or physical findings that are specific for soft-tissue sarcoma. This can result in delays in diagnosis and treatment for these patients. In a survey of approximately 5800 patients with sarcomas, at least half waited 4 months before being evaluated by a physician, with a 6-month or longer delay being reported by 20% of patients (88). Additional breaches of ideal care included the overuse of excisional biopsy as opposed to the generally preferred approach of incisional biopsy, low utilization of the American Joint Committee for Cancer Staging system, and a major reliance on computed tomography (CT) scans for pretreatment patient evaluation. In another study, Clasby et al. provides additional support for regionalization of patients (89). In this study, 377 patients with primary soft-tissue sarcoma were evaluated with respect to presentation, investigation, treatment, and outcome in comparison with defined criteria for optimal management. General surgeons (53.6%) treated most patients, regardless of tumor location. On the other hand, orthopedic surgeons treated only 27.1% of the total cases despite the high incidence of extremity tumors (60%). Overall, only 21.3% of patients were investigated optimally, with a wide variation among specialties. Only 60% were treated adequately with wide surgical resection and radiation therapy. Outcome was poorer in patients having a marginal excision and recurrence.

In an attempt to more clearly define those soft-tissue neoplasms that might be malignant on clinical grounds, Rydholm and colleagues reported a comparative evaluation of patients with lipomas vs. sarcomas in their patient population (90). Because lipoma is the most common soft-tissue tumor, Rydholm used lipomas as a representative benign soft-tissue tumor to compare with soft-tissue sarcomas regarding clinical presentation in an attempt to outline specific criteria suspicious for malignancy (90,91). During one year, 428 patients in a defined region were diagnosed with lipoma; only 4% (13 of 351 patients with solitary lipomas) of these tumors were located deep to the muscle fascia. Lipomas were found to be extremely rare in children, with the hand, thigh, lower leg, and foot being uncommon anatomical sites. The annual clinical incidence of lipoma was estimated to be 1/1000 persons. Similar results have been demonstrated in other studies of benign soft-tissue tumors, with only 1% being deep-seated and only 5% measuring greater than 5 cm (92). Review of presenting symptoms for patient with soft-tissue sarcomas demonstrated that only 10% of patients had had symptoms for more than a year. In addition to presentation and duration of symptoms, patient age beyond childhood was of no value in the differential diagnosis of a soft-tissue mass. Tumor size was also not predictive for malignancy, as similar results were found for both lipomas (3 cm for subcutaneous and 6 cm for deep-seated tumors) and soft-tissue sarcomas (4 cm for subcutaneous and 8 cm for deep-seated tumors). Based on these results, the Scandinavian criteria for patients at risk for a soft-tissue sarcoma include a tumor that is (a) larger than 5 cm, irrespective of depth and location; (b) located in the thigh, irrespective of depth and size; or (c) deep-seated, irrespective of location and size (90). Based on these criteria, about 10 patients with benign soft-tissue tumors would be referred for every sarcoma patient and 80% of sarcoma patients would be referred before surgery. This results in an excess referral rate of 10:1.

An issue that is central to the management of soft-tissue sarcomas is the need for tertiary centers to deliver this specialized care. Centralization of cancer patient care has been advocated in several studies. In a study of 502 pancreatico-duodenectomies carried out in 39 hospitals in the United States for pancreatic carcinoma, the authors reported that the hospital mortality was 6 times higher for patients treated in hospitals with low case numbers as compared with regional centers. Duration of stay and cost were lower in the large regional centers as well due to the lower complication rate (93). Similar results have been reported for patients with esophageal cancer requiring esophagectomies, with perioperative mortality being higher in those treated by inexperienced surgeons (94,95). Further support for the benefit of specialized cancer care is reflected in studies of hematologic malignancies. In Finland, a study of patients with multiple myeloma showed significantly better survival in areas utilizing randomized prospective trials (96). In a study of patients with Hodgkin's lymphoma, the results of 3607 patients who were managed in general hospitals was compared with the results of 2278 patients treated in comprehensive cancer centers (97). Patients treated in community hospitals were about 1.5 times more likely to die than those treated in comprehensive cancer centers. Differences in patient management are more apparent in studies of common neoplasms afflicting adults. In the case of breast cancer, several studies have supported the need for specialized cancer care in treating breast cancer patients. In a study of 3786 breast cancer patients, significant variations in 5-year survival were observed and related to the presence of a surgeon who specialized in breast cancer management (98). There was a 17% reduction in the risk of death for patients treated by specialist surgeons at 10 years. Patient survival was greater in patients treated by specialists (49.1%) than those treated by nonspecialists (41.5%).

Similar results have been demonstrated for the management of soft-tissue sarcomas. In a study by Gustafson et al., 375 patients with primary soft-tissue sarcomas of the extremity (329 patients) and chest wall (46 patients) were evaluated regarding the "quality" of care (99). Quality was measured as the total number of operations performed for the primary tumor, biopsy, excision, reexcision, and the local recurrence rate. A comparison was made between patients referred to a tumor center before surgery (195 patients), after surgery (102 patients), and not referred for management of the primary tumor (78 patients). The total number of operations for the primary tumor in patients not referred was 1.4 times higher and in patients referred after surgery 1.7 times higher than in patients referred before surgery. The local recurrence rate in patients not referred was 2.4 times higher and in patients referred after surgery 1.3 times higher than in patients referred before surgery. Given these results, patients clearly demonstrate better clinical outcomes when treated by physicians familiar with current clinical protocols.

However, this raises the question of whether patients can receive comparable care by cancer "specialists" in a community setting. With continued specialized training of physicians in academic or tertiary centers, the pool of cancer treatment expertise has increased in the community setting. This has resulted in improved communication between community hospitals and tertiary centers as well as enrollment of more patients into shared clinical protocols. Studies support the proposal that a network of specialized services in community hospitals and in cancer centers can produce results similar to those reported in academic centers. Community hospitals produced results similar to those of their counterparts in teaching institutions (100). Similar results have been reported by the U.S. Eastern Cooperative Oncology Group with regard to the treatment of leukemia (101). Due to the relative infrequency of patients presenting with soft-tissue sarcomas, surgeons need to be familiar with the current operative management of these patients. In addition, the concept and development of a cancer "team" composed of radiation oncologists, medical oncologists, radiologists, pathologists, and psychiatrists needs to be implemented to direct proper cancer care in these patients.

REFERENCES

1. Boring CC, Squires TS, Tong T, Montgomery S. Cancer statistics, 1994. CA Cancer J Clin 44(1):7–26, 1994.
2. Office of Population Censuses and Surveys. Cancer statistics and registrations, 1988, England and Wales. Series no. MB1(21). London: HMSO, 1994.
3. Rydholm A. Management of patients with soft-tissue tumors. Strategy developed at a regional oncology center. Acta Orthop Scand (Suppl 203):13–77, 1983.
4. Polednak AP. Incidence of soft-tissue cancers in blacks and whites in New York State. Int J Cancer 38(1):21–26, 1986.
5. Lynge E, Storm HH, Jensen OM. The evaluation of trends in soft-tissue sarcoma according to diagnostic criteria and consumption of phenoxy herbicides. Cancer 60(8): 1896–1901, 1987.
6. Ayiomamitis A. Epidemiology of cancer of the connective tissue in Canada during the period 1950–1985. Ca Detect Prev 13(3–4):149–156, 1988.
7. Ross JA, Severson RK, Davis S, Brooks JJ. Trends in the incidence of soft-tissue sarcomas in the United States from 1973 through 1987. Cancer 72(2):486–490, 1993.

8.   Brennan MF, Casper ES, Harrison L, Shiu MH, Gaynor J, Hajdu SI. The role of multi-
      modality therapy in soft-tissue sarcoma. Ann Surg 214(3):328–336, 1991.
9.   Coindre JM, Terrier P, Binh Bui N, Bonichon F, Collin F, Le Doussal V, Mandard
      AM, Vilain MA, Jacquemier J, Duplay H, Sastre X, Barlier C, Henry-Amar M, Mace-
      Lesechy J, Contesso G. Prognostic factors in adult patients with locally controlled
      soft-tissue sarcoma: a study of 546 patients from the French Federation of Cancer
      Centers sarcoma group. J Clin Oncol 14(3):869–877, 1996.
10. Potter DA, Kinsella T, Glatstein E, Wesley R, White DE, Seipp CA, Chang AE, Lack
      EE, Costa J, Rosenberg SA. High-grade soft-tissue sarcomas of the extremities. Can-
      cer 58(1):190–205, 1986.
11. Markhede G, Angervall L, Stener B. A multivariate analysis of the prognosis after
      surgical treatment of malignant soft-tissue tumors. Cancer 49(8):1721–1733, 1982.
12. Collin C, Hadju SI, Godbold J, Shiu MH, Hilaris BI, Brennan MF. Localized, oper-
      able soft-tissue sarcoma of the lower extremity. Arch Surg 121:1425–1433, 1986.
13. Mentzel T, Calonje E, Wadden C, Camplejohn RS, Beham A, Smith MA, Fletcher
      CD. Myxofibrosarcoma. Clinicopathological analysis of 75 cases with emphasis on
      the low grade variant. Am J Surg Pathol 20(4):391–405, 1996.
14. Rydholm A, Gustafson P, Rooser B, Willen H, Berg NO. Subcutaneous soft-tissue
      sarcoma. A population-based epidemiologic and prognostic study of 129 patients.
      J Bone Joint Surg 73B:662–667, 1991.
15. Rydholm A, Berg NO, Gullberg BO, Thorngren KG, Persson BM, Epidemiology of
      soft-tissue sarcoma in the locomotor system. Acta Pathol. Microbiol. Immunol Scand
      92(5):363–374, 1984.
16. Lindberg RD, Martin RG, Romsdahl MM, Barkley HT. Conservative surgery and
      post-operative radiotherapy in 300 adults with soft-tissue sarcomas. Cancer 47(10):
      2391–2397, 1981.
17. Robinson E, Neugut AI, Wylie P. Clinical aspects of portirradiation sarcomas. J Natl
      Cancer Inst 80(4):233–240, 1988.
18. Laskin WB, Silverman TA, Enzinger FM. Postradiation soft-tissue sarcomas. An
      analysis of 53 cases. Cancer 1988; 62(1):2330–2340.
19. Brady MS, Gaynor JJ, Brennan MF. Radiation-associated sarcoma of bone and soft-
      tissue. Arch Surg 127(12):1379–1385, 1992.
20. Wiklund TA, Blomqvist CP, Raty J, Elomaa I, Rissanen P, Miettinen M. Postirradia-
      tion sarcoma. Analysis of a nationwide cancer registry material. Cancer 68(3):524–
      531, 1991.
21. Adam YG, Reif R. Radiation-induced fibrosarcoma following treatment for breast
      cancer. Surgery 81:421–425, 1977.
22. O'Neil NB, Cocke W, Mason D, O'Neil MB Jr, Cocke W, Mason D, Hurley EJ.
      Radiation-induced soft-tissue fibrosarcoma: surgical therapy and salvage. Ann
      Thorac Surg 33(6):624–628, 1982.
23. Karlsson P, Holmberg E, Johansson KA, Kindblom LG, Carstensen J, Wallgren A.
      soft-tissue sarcoma after treatment for breast cancer. Radiother Oncol 38(1):25–31,
      1996.
24. Schwarz RE, Burt M. Radiation-associated malignant tumors of the chest wall. Ann
      Surg Oncol 3(4):387–392, 1996.
25. Cafiero F, Gipponi M, Peressini A, Queirolo P, Bertoglio S, Comandini D, Percivale P,
      Sertoli MR, Badelino F. Radiation-associated angiosarcoma; diagnostic and thera-

peutic implications. Two case reports and a review of the literature. Cancer 77(12): 2496–2502, 1996.

26. Stewart FW, Treves NP. Lymphangiosarcoma in postmastectomy lymphedema: a report of six cases in elephantiasis chirurgica. Cancer 1:64–81, 1948.

27. Brachman DG, Hallahan DE, Beckett MA, Yandell DW, Weichselbaum RR. p53 gene mutations and abnormal retinoblastoma protein in radiation-induced human sarcomas. Cancer Res 51(23 Pt 1):6393–6396, 1991.

28. Nakanishi H,Tomita Y, Myoui A, Yoshikawa H, Sakai K, Kato Y, Ochi T, Aozasa K. Mutation of the p53 gene in postradiation sarcoma. Lab Invest 78(6):727–733, 1998.

29. Taubert H, Meye A, Bache M, Hinze R, Holzhausen HJ, Schmidt H, Rath FW, Dunst J, Wurl P. p53 status in radiation-induced soft-tissue sarcomas. Strahlenther Onkol 174(8):427–430, 1998.

30. Wong FL, Boice JD Jr, Abramson DH, Tarone RE, Kleinerman RA, Stovall M, Goldman MB, Seddon JM, Tarbell N, Fraumeni JF Jr, Li FP. Cancer incidence after retinoblastoma. Radiation dose and sarcoma risk. JAMA 278(15):1262–1267, 1997.

31. Laskin WB, Silverman TA, Enzinger FM. Postradiation soft-tissue sarcomas. An analysis of 53 cases. Cancer 62(11):2330–2340, 1988.

32. Robinson E, Neugut AI, Wylie P. Clinical aspects of postirradiation sarcomas. J Natl Cancer Inst 80(4):233–240, 1988.

33. Li FP, Fraumeni JF Jr. Soft-tissue sarcomas, breast cancer, and other neoplasms. A familial syndrome? Ann Intern Med 71:747–752, 1969.

34. Li FP, Fraumeni JF, Mulvhill JJ, Blattner WA, Dreyfus MG, Tucker MA, Miller RW. A cancer family syndrome in 24 kindreds. Cancer Res 48(18):5358–5362, 1988.

35. Blattner WA, McGuire DB, Mulvihill JJ, Lampkin BC, Hananian J, Fraumeni JF. Genealogy of cancer in a family. JAMA 241(3):259–261, 1979.

36. Strong LC, Stine M, Norsted TL. Cancer in survivors of childhood soft-tissue sarcoma in their relatives. J Natl Cancer Inst 79(6):1213–1220, 1987.

37. Hartley, AL, Birch JM, Kelsey AM, Marsden HB, Harris M, Tearre MD. Are germ cell tumors part of the Li-Fraumeni cancer family syndrome? Cancer Genet Cytogenet 42(2):221–226, 1989.

38. Li FP, Fraumeni JF Jr. Prospective study of a family cancer syndrome. JAMA 247(19):2692–2694, 1982.

39. Garber JE, Goldstein AM, Kantor AF, Dreyfus MG, Fraumeni JF Jr, Li FP. Follow-up study of twenty-four families with Li-Fraumeni syndrome. Cancer Res 51(22): 6094–6097, 1991.

40. Birch JM, Hartley AL, Blair V, Kelsey AM, Harris M, Teare MD, Jones PH. Identification of factors associated with high breast cancer risk in the mothers of children with soft-tissue sarcoma. J Clin Oncol 8(4):583–590, 1990.

41. Hartley AL, Birch JM, Marsden HB, Harris M. Breast cancer risk in mothers of children with osteosarcoma and chondrosarcoma. Br J Cancer 54(5):819–823, 1986.

42. Carnevale A, Lieberman E, Cardenas R. Li-Fraumeni syndrome in pediatric patients with soft-tissue sarcoma or osteosarcoma. Arch Med Res 28(3):383–386, 1997.

43. Malkin D, Li FP, Strong LC, Fraumeni JF Jr, Nelson CE, Kim DH, Kassel J, Gryka MA, Bischoff FZ, Tainsky MA. Germ line p53 mutations in a familial syndrome of breast cancer, sarcomas, and other neoplasms. Science 250(4985):1233–1238, 1990.

44. Kleihues P, Schauble B, zur Hausen A, Esteve J, Ohgaki H. Tumors associated with p53 germline mutations: a synopsis of 91 families. Am J Pathol 150(1):1–13, 1997.

45. Sanders BM, Jay M, Draper GJ, Roberts EM. Non-ocular cancer in relatives of retinoblastoma patients. Br J Cancer 60(3):358–365, 1989.
46. Hansen MR, Koufos A, Gallie BL, Phillips RA, Fodstad O, Brogger A Gedde-Dahl T, Cavenee WK. Osteosarcoma and retinoblastoma: a shared chromosomal mechanism revealing recessive predisposition. Proc Natl Acad Sci USA 82(18):6216–6220, 1985.
47. Bader JL. Neurofibromatosis and cancer: an overview. Dysmorph Clin Gen 1:43–48, 1987.
48. McKeen EA, Bodurtha J, Meadows AT, Douglas EC, Mulvihill JJ. Rhabdomyosarcoma complicating multiple neurofibromatosis. J Pediatr 93(6):992–993, 1978.
49. Sorensen SA, Mulvihill JJ, Nielsen A. Long-term follow-up of von Recklinghausen neurofibromatosis. N Engl J Med 314(16):1010–1015, 1986.
50. Zoller ME, Rembeck B, Oden A, Samuelsson M, Angervall L. Malignant and benign tumors in patients with neurofibromatosis type 1 in a defined Swedish population. Cancer 79(11):2125–2131, 1997.
51. Hartley AL, Birch JM, Marsden HB, Harris M, Blair V. Neurofibromatosis in children with soft-tissue sarcoma. Pediatr Hematol Oncol 5(1):7–16, 1988.
52. McAdam, WA, Goligher, JC. The occurrence of desmoids in patients with familial polyposis coli. Br J Surg 57(8):618–631, 1970.
53. Rustgi AK. Hereditary gastrointestinal polyposis and nonpolyposis syndromes. N Engl J Med 331(25):1694–1702, 1994.
54. Posner MC, Shiu MH, Newsome JL, Hajdu SI, Gaynor JJ, Brennan MF. The desmoid tumor: not a benign disease. Arch Surg 124(2):191–196, 1989.
55. Hoar SK, Blair A, Holmes FF, Boysen CD, Robel RJ, Hoover R, Fraumeni JF. Agricultural herbicide use and risk of lymphoma and soft-tissue sarcoma. JAMA 256(9):1141–1147, 1986.
56. Sarma PR, Jacobs J. Thoracic soft-tissue sarcoma in Vietnam veterans exposed to agent orange. N Engl J Med 306:1109, 1986.
57. Tucker MA, D'Angio G, Boice JD, Strong LC, Li FP, Stovall M, Stone BJ, Green DM, Lombardi F, Newton W. Bone sarcomas linked to radiotherapy and chemotherapy in children. N Engl J Med 317:588–593, 1987.
58. Hardell L, Eriksson M, Degerman A. Meta-analysis of four Swedish case-control studies on exposure to pesticides as risk-factor for soft-tissue sarcoma including the relation to tumour localization and histological type. Int J Oncol 6:847–851, 1995.
59. Hardell L, Sandstrom A. Case-control study: soft-tissue sarcomas and exposure to phenoxyacetic acids or chlorophenols. Br J Cancer 39(6):711–717, 1979.
60. Hardell L, Axelson O. Soft-tissue sarcoma, malignant lymphoma, and exposure to phenoxyacids or chlorophenols. Lancet 1(8286):1408–1409, 1982.
61. Eriksson M, Hardell L, Adami HO. Exposure to dioxins as a risk factor for soft-tissue sarcoma: a population-based case-control study. J Natl Cancer Inst 82(6):486–490, 1990.
62. Eriksson M, Hardell L, Berg NO, Moller T, Axelson O. Soft-tissue sarcomas and exposure to chemical substances: a case-reference study. Br J Ind Med 38(1):27–33, 1981.
63. Wingren G, Fredrikson M, Brage HN, Nordenskjold B, Axelson O. Soft tissue sarcoma and occupational exposures. Cancer 66(4):806–811, 1990.

64. Vineis P, Terracini B, Ciccone G, Cignetti A, Colombo E, Donna A, Maffi L, Pisa R, Ricci P, Zanini E. Phenoxyherbicides and soft-tissue sarcomas in female rice weeders: a population-based case-referent study. Scand J Work Environ Health 13(1): 9–17, 1987.
65. Balarajan R, Acheson ED. Soft tissue sarcomas in agriculture and forestry workers. J Epidemiol Comm Health 38(2):113–116, 1984.
66. Smith AH, Pearce NE, Fisher DO, Giles HJ, Teague CA, Howard JK. Soft tissue sarcoma and exposure to phenoxyherbicides and chlorophenols in New Zealand. J Natl Cancer Inst 73(5):1111–1117, 1984.
67. Hansen ES, Hasle H, Lander F. A cohort study of cancer incidence among Danish gardeners. Am J Ind Med 21(5):651–660, 1992.
68. Kogevinas M, Kauppinen T, Winkelmann R, Becher H, Bertazzi PA, Bueno-de-Mesquita HB, Coggon D, Green L, Johnson E, Littorin M, Lynge E, Marlow DA, Mathews JD, Neuberger M, Benn T, Pannett B,, Pearce N, Saracci R. Soft tissue sarcoma and non-Hodgkin's lymphoma in workers exposed to phenoxy herbicides, chlorophenols, and dioxins: two nested case-control studies. Epidemiology 6(9):396–402, 1995.
69. Fingerhut MA, Halperin WE, Marlow DA, Piacitelli LA, Honchan PA, Sweeney MH, Greife AL, Dill PA, Steenland K, Suruda AJ. Cancer mortality in workers exposed to 2,3,7,8-tetrachlorodibenzo-p-dioxin. N Engl J Med 324(4):212–218, 1991.
70. Saracci R, Kogevinas M, Bertazzi PA, Bueno de Mesquita BH, Coggon D, Green LM, Kauppinen T, L'Abbe KA, Littorin M, Lynge E. Cancer mortality in workers exposed to chlorophenoxy herbicides and chlorophenols. Lancet 338(8774):1027–1032, 1991.
71. Zack JA, Suskind RR. The mortality experience of workers exposed workers to tetrachlorodibenzodioxin in a trichlorophenol process accident. J Occup Med 22(1):11–14, 1980.
72. Cook RR, Townsend JC, Ott MG, Silverstein LG. Mortality experience of employees exposed to 2,3,7,8-tetrachlorodibenzo-p-dioxin (TCDD). J Occup Med 22(8):530–532, 1980.
73. Cook RR. Dioxin, chloracne, and soft-tissue sarcoma. Lancet 1(8220):618–619, 1981.
74. Johnson FE, Kugler AM, Brown SM. Soft tissue sarcomas and chlorinated phenols. Lancet 2(8236):40, 1981.
75. Lynge E. Cancer in phenoxy herbicide manufacturing workers in Denmark, 1947–87: An update. Cancer Causes Control 4(3):261–272, 1993.
76. US Environmental Protection Agency, Scientific Advisory Board: Re-evaluating dioxin. Science Advisory Board's review of EPA's reassessment of dioxin and dioxin-like compounds. Washington, DC: US Government Printing Office, Report No. EPA-SAB-EC-95-021, 1995.
77. Bertazzi P, Pesatori A, Consonni D, Tironi A, Landi MT, Zocchetti C. Cancer incidence in a population accidentally exposed to 2,3,7,8-tetrachlorodibenzo-para-dioxin. Epidemiology 4(5):398–406, 1993.
78. McConnell R, Anderson D, Russell W, Anderson KE, Clapp R, Silbergeld EK, Landrigan PJ. Angiosarcoma, porphyria cutanea tarda, and probably chloracne in a worker exposed to waste oil contaminated with 2,3,7,8-tetrachlorodibenzo-p-dioxin. Br J Ind Med 50(8):699–703, 1993.

79. Popper H, Thomas LB, Telles NC, Falk H, Selikoff IJ. Development of hepatic angiosarcoma in man induced by vinyl chloride, thorotrast, and arsenic. Am J Pathol 92(2):349–369, 1978.
80. Zahm SH, Blair A, Holmes FF, Boyson CD, Robel RJ. A case-referent study of soft-tissue sarcoma and Hodgkin's disease: farming and insecticide use. Scand J Work Environ Health 14(4):224–230, 1988.
81. Grimalt JO, Sunyer J, Moreno V, Amaral OC, Sala M, Rosell A, Anto JM, Albaiges J. Risk excess of soft-tissue sarcoma and thyroid cancer in a community exposed to airborne organochlorinated compound mixtures with a high hexachlorobenzene content. Int J Cancer 56(2):200–203, 1994.
82. Falk H, Thomas LB, Popper H, Ishak KG. Hepatic angiosarcoma associated with androgenic-anabolic steroids. Lancet 2(8152):1120–1123, 1979.
83. Pearce N, Smith AH, Reif JS. Increased risks of soft-tissue sarcoma, malignant lymphoma, and acute myeloid leukemia in abattoir workers. Am J Ind Med 14(1):63–72, 1988.
84. Stewart FW, Treves N. Lymphangiosarcoma in post-mastectomy lymphedema. Cancer 1:64, 1948.
85. Dubin HV, Creehan EP, Headington JT. Lymphangiosarcoma and congenital lymphedema of the extremity. Arch Dermatol 110(4):608–614, 1974.
86. Muller R, Hajdu SI, Brennan MF. Lymphangiosarcoma associated with chronic filarial lymphedema. Cancer 59(1):179–183, 1987.
87. Falls HF, Kerlesz ED. A new syndrome combining pterygium colli with developmental anomalies of the eyelids and lymphatic of the lower extremities. Trans Am Ophth Soc 62:248–275, 1964.
88. Lawrence W Jr, Donegan WL, Natarajan N, Mettlin C, Beart R, Winchester D. Adult soft-tissue sarcomas. A pattern of care survey of the American College of Surgeons. Ann Surg 205(4):349–359, 1987.
89. Clasby R, Tilling K, Smith MA, Fletcher CDM. Variable management of soft-tissue sarcoma: regional audit with implications for specialist care. Br J Surg 84(12):1692–1696, 1997.
90. Rydholm A. Centralization of soft-tissue sarcoma. The southern Sweden experience. Acta Orthop Scand (Suppl 273) 68:4–8, 1997.
91. Rydholm A, Berg NO. Size, site and clinical incidence of lipoma. Factors in the differential diagnosis of lipoma and sarcoma. Acta Orthop Scand 54(6):929–934, 1983.
92. Myhre-Jensen, O A consecutive 7-year series of 1331 benign and soft-tissue tumors. Acta Orthop Scand 52(3):287–293, 1981.
93. Gordon TA, Burleyson GP, Tielsch JM, Cameron JL. The effects of regionalization on cost and outcome for one general high-risk surgical procedure. Ann Surg 221(1):43–49, 1995.
94. Matthews HR, Powell DJ, McConkey CC. Effects of surgical experience of the results of resection for oesophageal carcinoma. Br J Surg 73(8):621–623, 1986.
95. Gulliford MC, Barton JR, Bourne HM. Selection for oesophagectomy and postoperative outcome in a defined population. Qual Health Care 2:17–20, 1993.
96. Karjalainen S, Palva I. Do treatment protocols improve end results? A study of survival of patients with multiple myeloma in Finland. Br Med J 299(6707):1069–1072, 1989.

97. Davis S, Dahlberg S, Myers M, Chen A, Steinhorn SC. Hodgkin's disease in the United States: a comparison of patient characteristics and survival in the centralized cancer patient data system and the surveillance, epidemiology and end results program. J Natl Cancer Inst 78(3):471–478, 1987.
98. Gillis CR, Hole DJ. Survival outcome of care by specialist surgeons in breast cancer: a study of 3786 patients in the west of Scotland. Br Med J 312(7024):145–148, 1996.
99. Gustafson P, Dreinhofer KE, Rydholm A. Soft tissue sarcoma should be treated at a tumor center. A comparison of quality of surgery in 375 patients. Acta Orthop Scand 65(1):47–50, 1994.
100. Kingston RD, Walsh S, Jeacock J. Colorectal surgeons in district general hospitals produce similar survival outcomes to their teaching hospital colleagues: review of 5 year survivals in Manchester. J R Coll Surg Edin 37(4):235–237, 1992.
101. Begg CB, Carbone PP, Elson PJ, Zelen M. Participation of community hospitals in clinical trials: analysis of five years of experience in the Eastern Cooperative Oncology Group. N Engl J Med 306(18):1076–1080, 1982.

2

Radiologic Imaging of Soft-Tissue Tumors

John Lin
University of Michigan Medical Center
Ann Arbor, Michigan

Sidney K. Suneja
Walter Reed Army Medical Center
Washington, DC

Lawrence Yao
Georgetown University Medical Center
Washington, DC

I. INTRODUCTION

The imaging evaluation of soft-tissue tumors has been advanced dramatically by cross-sectional imaging, which includes computed tomography (CT), magnetic resonance imaging (MRI), position emission tomography (PET), single photon emission computed tomography (SPECT), and ultrasonography. Accurate imaging evaluation becomes more important with recent advances in treatment, such as limb salvage surgery (1–4). The imaging evaluation serves to detect suspected lesions, formulate an appropriate differential diagnosis, and assist in the staging of tumors. Imaging studies are also useful for surgical planning, biopsy guidance, and posttreatment follow-up. Certain imaging features may aid in the differentiation of benign from malignant lesions, and these will be emphasized in the following discussion.

Many soft-tissue lesions have a nonspecific appearance on imaging studies, and correlation with clinical history is important. Patient age at presentation, location of the lesion, duration of symptoms, rate of lesion growth, and history of relevant trauma all influence a thoughtful differential diagnosis. Kransdorf summarized a retrospective analysis of more than 31,000 soft-tissue tumors in which an imaging workup had been performed. Benign and malignant lesions were analyzed separately (5,6). Tabulated data included prevalence, patient age at presentation, sex, and anatomical site.

The majority of soft-tissue tumors could be classified into eight benign and seven malignant categories (5,6). The most common benign lesions, in descending order, were lipoma and lipoma variants, fibrous histiocytoma, nodular fasciitis, hemangioma, fibromatosis, neurofibroma, schwannoma, and giant cell tumor of tendon sheath. The most common malignant lesions, in descending order, were malignant fibrous histiocytoma, liposarcoma, leiomyosarcoma, malignant peripheral nerve sheath tumor, dermatofibrosarcoma protuberans, synovial sarcoma, and fibrosarcoma. Because imaging and clinical features are often nonspecific, lesion prevalence, anatomical location, and patient age should all be considered in formulating a meaningful differential diagnosis.

The workup of a suspected soft-tissue tumor usually includes one or more imaging tests. Knowledge of the advantages and disadvantages of each modality facilitates a more cost-effective imaging evaluation. The radiologist should be a consultant to the clinician in formulating the most effective workup, and the MRI or CT examinations for suspected mass lesions should be tailored and monitored appropriately. Direct involvement of the radiologist in the sonographic examination is particularly critical.

II. THE ROLE OF THE IMAGING EVALUATION

The imaging evaluation of suspected soft-tissue tumors should be approached in a purposeful manner. Imaging may be performed to address the following specific questions.

1. *Detection*: Imaging can determine whether a clinically suspected soft-tissue mass is truly present. On occasion, clinical presentation and physical examination may falsely suggest the presence of a soft-tissue mass when hypertrophy or atrophy of supporting structures distorts the anatomy and creates a "pseudomass" (Fig. 1) (7,8). Alternatively, a patient may have nonspecific complaints of pain and/or swelling, without a palpable mass. In particular, this may be more worrisome within deep tissues, such as in the thigh or pelvis. Imaging can often clarify these situations and obviate the need for biopsy.

2. *Localization*: Precise anatomical localization of a soft-tissue lesion aids diagnosis and management. When the origin of the lesion can be accurately determined, the differential diagnosis can be narrowed. MRI is the modality of choice in this role (8–15). Whether the lesion arises in the muscle or represents a primary osseous lesion with an associated soft-tissue mass (Fig. 2) has important

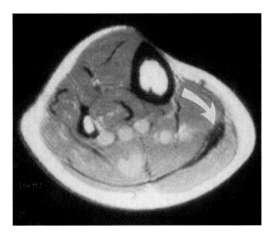

FIG. 1 Axial-balanced MRI of the calf shows a low-signal area of thickening, consistent with scar formation around a rupture of the plantaris tendon (*arrow*), characteristically interposed between gastrocnemius and soleus. The injury was likely sustained but not recognized at the time of a car accident, and the patient presented 6 months later with this "pseudomass."

implications for diagnosis and treatment. Articular processes (Fig. 3) must be distinguished from primary soft-tissue lesions.

    3. *Characterization*: The size and shape of a lesion can be accurately determined with cross-sectional imaging. Although lesion size is not a reliable criteria for differentiating between benign and malignant lesions, it may be relevant to prognosis (3,16,17). The accurate documentation of lesion growth or stability on follow-up studies also relays important information about potential malignancy. The shape or morphology of a soft-tissue mass can aid differential diagnosis, as does the detection of lesion mineralization, necrosis, and vascularity (3,18–28).

    4. *Diagnosis*: A specific and confident diagnosis can be made based on the imaging findings in certain situations, particularly with fat containing or vascular masses. In other cases, a limited differential diagnosis can be offered, and particularly when a sarcoma is excluded, diagnostic thinking and management are greatly influenced. Examples would include imaging diagnoses of a normal variant, such as an accessory muscle, or the strongly suggestive findings of abscess (Fig. 4), hematoma (Fig. 5), myositis ossificans (Fig. 6), or masses secondary to articular disease (Fig. 3).

    5. *Biopsy planning and guidance*: The workup of suspected soft-tissue masses often requires biopsy, which may be performed percutaneously (with or without imaging guidance) or by open surgical technique. The imaging workup contributes to a working diagnosis, and aids in the choice of biopsy approach.

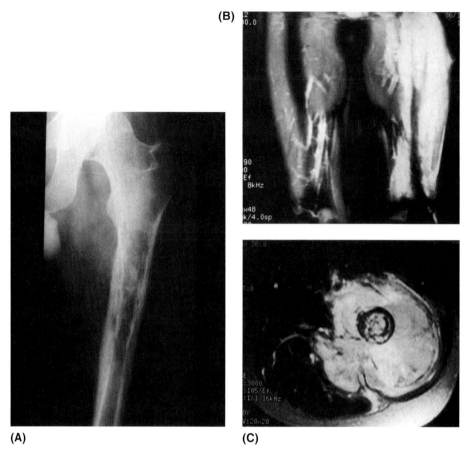

FIG. 2 Ewing's sarcoma of the left thigh in a 29-year-old man with a large associated soft-tissue mass. (A) Radiograph shows a destructive, permeative lesion within the left femur with lamellated periosteal reaction. Coronal STIR (B) and axial fat-saturated, T2-weighted (C) MR images show the large extrasosseous component of the tumor resulting in a soft-tissue mass.

Biopsy planning should be done in communication with the treating surgeon; ideally, the biopsy approach should parallel the surgical approach so that the biopsy tract can be resected (1,3,4,19,29). Intermuscular, intracompartmental needle trajectories are generally preferable. Imaging (Fig. 7) can help distinguish viable regions of tumors, thereby facilitating a greater diagnostic yield. Diagnostic imaging studies should be obtained prior to biopsy to avoid confusion caused by local tissue changes related to the procedure (10,11,29,30).

6. *Preoperative planning and staging*: The staging of soft-tissue tumors relies on accurate assessment of the extent of disease (3,4,31–33). The lesion size,

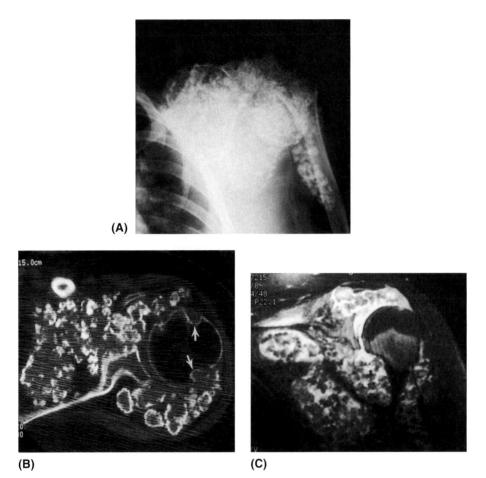

FIG. 3 Synovial osteochondromatosis of the left shoulder in a 17-year-old girl. (A) Radiograph demonstrates extensive calcified/ossified masses present in a juxta-articular location about the left shoulder. (B) CT scan confirms the articular involvement with innumerable ossified bodies with associated erosions (*arrows*) present. (C) Coronal fat-saturated, T2-weighted MR image shows the extent of the joint distention with densely packed ossified intra-articular bodies.

location, presence of neurovascular or articular involvement, compartmental extent, and presence of metastasis all influence the treatment plan. In general, MRI is superior to CT in this role (13,14,34–38). Because the lungs are the predilected site for distant metastases from soft-tissue tumors, CT of the chest should be part of the staging workup of a patient with a high-grade soft-tissue sarcoma (4,10,39).

    7. *Postoperative evaluation*: The level of clinical concern over residual tumor or local recurrence of tumor determines the frequency of imaging surveil-

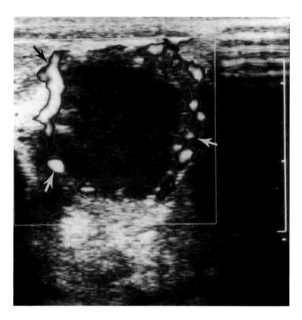

FIG. 4   Abscess of the left anterior thigh in a 22-year-old man. Ultrasonography with power Doppler imaging shows a hypoechoic complex fluid collection with marked increased flow in a peripheral rim pattern (*arrows*) consistent with an abscess, confirmed at surgery.

lance in the postoperative patient. Relevant factors include tumor histology, size, location, histologic grade, response to chemotherapy, and adequacy of surgical margins. Accurate imaging assessment is complicated in postoperative cases by tissue changes caused by surgery and/or radiation therapy. A baseline posttreatment examination is best obtained at 2–3 months after surgery, when imaging changes related to postsurgical edema and wound healing have stabilized (7,19). This baseline exam serves as an important reference or comparison for follow-up studies in assessing for interval changes (40,41).

III.   IMAGING MODALITIES AND APPLICATIONS

A.   Radiography

The utility of radiographs for evaluation of soft-tissue masses is limited. However, since radiography is widely available and relatively inexpensive, a radiographic evaluation is probably indicated in the case of soft-tissue masses that are either close to joints or relatively large (greater than 3 cm). In the case of periarticular masses, radiographs may reveal that the mass is related to an underlying arthropa-

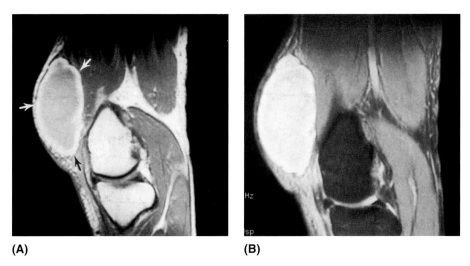

(A)   **(B)**

FIG. 5   Hematoma of the distal thigh in a 24-year-old man. Sagittal T1-weighted (A) and
sagittal fat-saturated, T2-weighted (B) MRI images show a large subcutaneous mass anteriorly. The signal intensity is increased on the T2-weighted sequence and predominantly
slightly increased signal to muscle with a rim of hyperintensity on T1-weighted sequence
compatible with hemorrhage (*arrows*).

thy. Synovial cysts are common in rheumatoid arthritis, and periarticular masses
may also be a presenting finding of gout or pigmented villonodular synovitis.

Radiographs confer valuable differential diagnostic information if they reveal calcification or ossification. Ossification is distinguished by the presence
of identifiable bony trabecula or cortical bone formation. Ossification may herald
myositis ossificans (Fig. 6) or, less commonly, an extraskeletal osteosarcoma. Calcification, on the other hand, may indicate a chondroid lesion, synovial sarcoma,
or tumoral calcinosis (Fig. 8). Finally, discrete calcification in venous thrombosis
or "phlebolith" formation is a reliable indicator of a hemangioma (Figs. 9 and 10).

Less commonly, in the case of large tumors, fatty elements may be identified
on plain radiographs and may aid in differential diagnosis, indicating the presence
of a lipoma, lipoma variant, or liposarcoma (Fig. 11). In the case of large or deep
masses, radiographs may help detect underlying bony involvement or, in some
cases, may suggest a periosteal or surface bony origin to the lesion. A common example is exostosis or osteochondroma (Fig. 12). In the case of bony erosion, the
nature of the underlying bony involvement may also provide information about
the rate of lesion growth. For instance, smooth and well-defined bony erosion is
a good indication of nonaggressive tumor behavior. In most cases, however, the
radiographic evaluation of a soft-tissue mass will be nonspecific, and more advanced imaging or biopsy will be required.

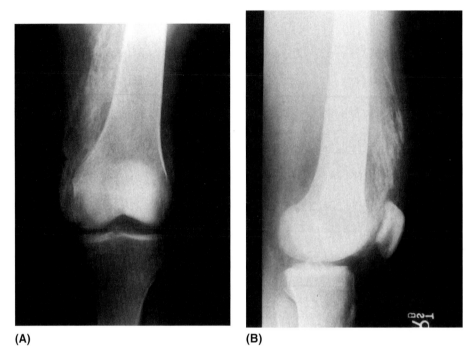

(A) **(B)**

FIG. 6 Myositis ossificans of the right thigh in a 22-year-old woman. Anteroposterior (A) and lateral (B) radiographs reveals a calcified and ossified mass in the distal thigh anteriorly which developed over a period of 1 month, following trauma.

B. Computed Tomography

Although MRI has higher sensitivity for soft-tissue lesion detection, CT remains a useful, fast, and relatively accessible technique for the general evaluation of soft-tissue masses. In addition, patients who are claustrophobic can better tolerate CT scanning because the gantry is less confining than that in MRI. Masses that involve the abdomen or pelvis, such as retroperitoneal liposarcomas or leiomyosarcomas of the stomach or inferior vena cava, are perhaps optimally evaluated by CT, with both intravenous and oral contrast. For evaluation of lesions in the chest or chest wall, CT may also be preferable to MRI because CT is less severely degraded by respiratory and cardiac motion. Furthermore, with the advent of helical CT, large body areas can be scanned at high resolution during a single breath-hold, nearly eliminating the problem of respiratory motion.

CT, particularly after intravenous contrast administration, can define the extent of many soft-tissue lesions, as well as their relationship to neighboring neurovascular and skeletal structures. Definition of the exact margin of lesions can be

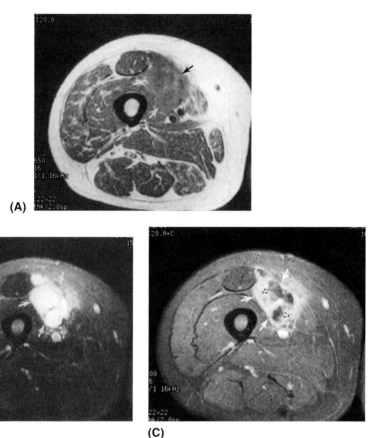

FIG. 7 Synovial cell sarcoma of the right thigh in a 54-year-old man. Axial T1-weighted (A) and axial fat-saturated, T2-weighted (B) MR images demonstrate a lobulated soft-tissue mass (*arrows*) within the vastus medialis muscle. The lesion is poorly defined and hypo- to isointense to muscle on T1-weighted sequence and homogeneously hyper-intense with mild peritumoral edema superficially on T2-weighted sequence. (C) Axial fat-saturated, T1-weighted postcontrast MR image shows inhomogeneous enhancement of the lesion (*white arrows*) with irregular central regions of nonenhancement consistent with necrotic tumor (*open arrows*).

more difficult on CT than on MRI (9) because lesional attenuation characteristics on CT may often closely approximate that of muscle or may be poorly distin-guishable from surrounding soft-tissue edema. After the administration of intra-venous contrast, cystic or necrotic portions of lesions can be better defined. The optimal timing of the intravenous injection has not been closely studied, but ve-nous phase or even more delayed scanning is usually preferred.

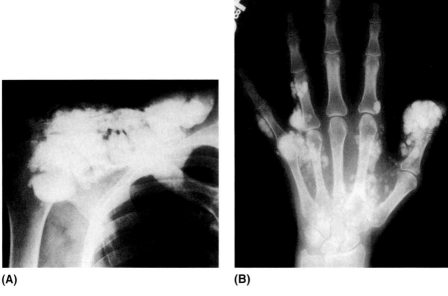

(A)   **(B)**

FIG. 8 Tumoral calcinosis of the right shoulder and left hand in a 58-year-old man. (A) Anteroposterior (AP) view of the right shoulder demonstrates massive, lobulated dense calcifications obscuring the underlying bone. (B) AP view of the left hand in the same patient shows widespread, multifocal, lobulated dense calcifications within the soft tissues.

The attenuation values of lesions on CT allow accurate identification of fat within lesions and may help differentiate lipomas from liposarcomas or lipoma variants (Fig. 11). CT also permits reliable diagnosis of vascular tumors. In this way, CT, like MRI, has some degree of histologic specificity in the classification of a soft-tissue mass (34,44). One major advantage of CT imaging over MR evaluation is in the assessment of soft-tissue calcification or ossification, which also aids differential diagnosis (3,9,13–15,42,43). The presence and pattern of mineralization is accurately determined by CT but is poorly depicted by MRI (45).

General morphologic guidelines for determining the aggressiveness and potential malignant nature of a mass apply to CT as well as MRI. Features of a non-aggressive mass include a smooth, well-defined margin, homogeneous attenuation, lack of invasion of adjacent structures, preservation of surrounding fat planes, and smaller size. CT features of an aggressive process include a poorly defined border, heterogeneity in density, invasion of adjacent structures, blurring of surrounding fat planes, and larger size.

CT scanning of the chest is a standard part of staging high- and intermediate-grade soft-tissue sarcomas because hematogenous spread to the lungs

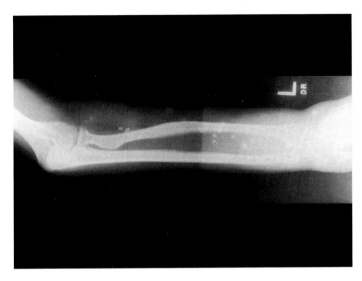

FIG. 9 Congenital venous malformation of the left forearm in a 21-year-old woman. Anteroposterior radiograph of the left forearm demonstrates multiple, small, rounded calcifications with central lucencies consistent with phleboliths.

(Fig. 13) is the most common manifestation of metastatic disease (10,19,39). An abdominal and pelvic CT with intravenous and oral contrast to assess for multifocal disease or satellite lesions may be indicated in the case of liposarcomas of the thigh and buttock regions.

CT is well suited for the guidance of percutaneous needle biopsy (Fig. 14) for either primary diagnosis or assessment of possible recurrent/residual disease (46,47). Neurovascualar structures can be visualized and avoided, resulting in fewer complications than a blind biopsy, and even deep lesions can be approached safely and quickly. An approach that does not compromise a subsequent surgical approach can also be more easily defined with CT, which nicely depicts compartmental anatomy, something that is more difficult to establish with ultrasonography. CT can target viable, enhancing portions of necrotic lesions precisely, which can increase the success rate of biopsy. Multiple biopsy specimens can be obtained through a single needle puncture utilizing a coaxial system, where sampling of different regions of the mass is done by redirection of the outer sheath (16,47). This facilitates more accurate grading of the lesion without increasing procedural morbidity. Several studies suggest that CT-guided core biopsy, when done with sufficient yield, is an effective primary strategy for definitive diagnosis of mesenchymal neoplasms. When the results of core biopsy are inconsistent with the clinical or imaging presentation, or when specimen quality is poor, open biopsy is warranted.

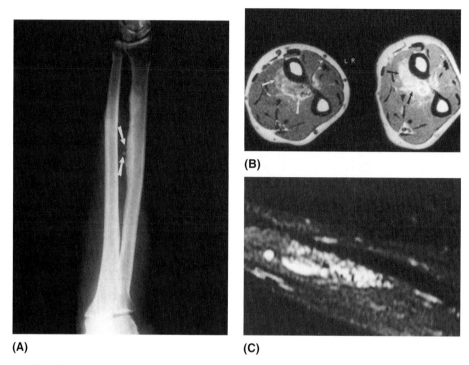

FIG. 10 Hemangioma of the left forearm in a 43-year-old man. (A) Anteroposterior radiograph of the left forearm demonstrates a focal region of benign appearing cortical thickening of the radius adjacent to a couple phleboliths (*arrows*). (B) Axial T1-weighted and corresponding axial T1-weighted postcontrast MR images demonstrate poorly marginated lesion with irregular foci of increased signal likely representing fat on precontrast study (*white arrows*) and marked enhancement following contrast injection (*black arrows*). (C) Coronal STIR sequence shows typical striated-septated appearance of a hemangioma.

C. Magnetic Resonance Imaging

MRI is the imaging modality of choice for evaluation of suspected soft-tissue masses. Practical advantages of MRI include its ability to obtain images in multiple and various imaging planes, and its lack of ionizing radiation exposure. More importantly, MRI has exquisite soft-tissue contrast, which increases its sensitivity to detect lesions and define lesion margins. For this reason, MRI is superior to CT in most diagnostic respects, with the exceptions that MRI is less effective in the detection of calcification, ossification, or gas formation (9,12–15,34–38,44,48). Finally, MRI is quite limited where implanted hardware is present, whereas CT may still provide some diagnostic information in such settings.

With CT, the attenuation of a soft-tissue lesion can often be similar to that of the adjacent tissues, particularly muscle. This is rarely a problem with MRI,

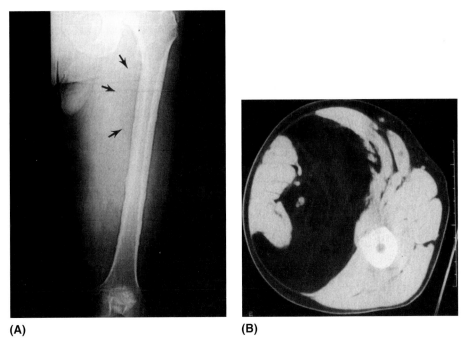

(A)   **(B)**

FIG. 11   Low-grade liposarcoma of the left thigh in a 70-year-old man. (A) Scout view demonstrates a large lucency (*arrows*) in the medial soft-tissues of the thigh adjacent to the medial cortex of the proximal femur. (B) CT scan shows a large fat-density mass occupying the majority of the medial thigh, displacing the adjacent muscles. Minimal stranding with soft-tissue density is present the lesion.

where modifying imaging parameters usually allow distinction between lesion and adjacent tissues. Thus, MRI better defines the extent of involvement of anatomical compartments and specific muscles. Establishment of the extent of a soft-tissue tumor is also facilitated by the multiplanar imaging capability of MRI. For similar reasons, MRI may also hold an advantage over CT in the evaluation of neurovascular structures (13,34–38). As with CT, peritumoral edema can be difficult to distinguish from tumor on MRI.

The major determinants of tissue signal on MRI are proton T1 relaxation, T2 relaxation, and the density of mobile protons. On T1-weighted MR images, soft-tissue tumors are typically low in signal intensity, given their longer T1 relaxation compared to muscle (10,11,30,49,50). Short T1 components of lesions that may have higher signal on T1-weighted images include fat, subacute hemorrhage, melanin, and certain proteins. Most soft-tissue tumors are high in signal intensity on T2-weighted images, possessing a longer T2 relaxation than muscle (10,11,30,49,50). Exceptions include hemosiderin-laden lesions, such as

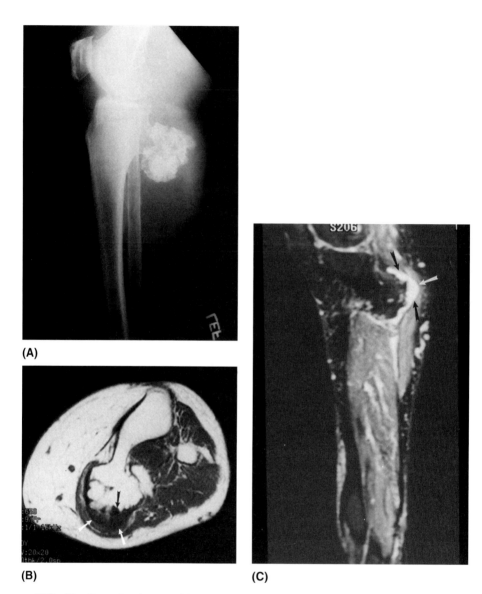

(A)

(B)   **(C)**

FIG. 12 Osteochondroma with secondary chondrosarcoma in a 70-year-old woman. (A) Lateral radiograph of the knee shows a large calcified/ossified mass connected to the posterior tibia via a stalk of bone. Axial T1-weighted (B) and sagittal STIR (C) MR images demonstrate the continuity of the medullary and cortical portions of the tibia with the mass characteristic for osteochondromas. In addition, the cartilaginous cap (*arrows*) of the exostosis is thicker than 2 cm, raising the suspicion for secondary malignancy. Biopsy confirmed the presence of chondrosarcoma in this region.

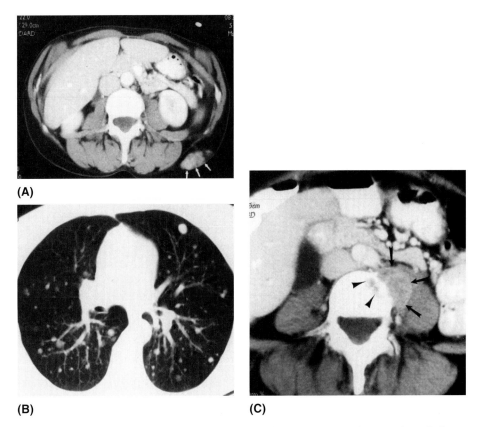

FIG. 13 Metastatic leiomyosarcoma in a 63-year-old woman. (A) CT scan through the abdomen shows a soft-tissue density mass (*arrows*) present in the subcutaneous tissues of the left back region proven to be leiomyosarcoma. (B) CT scan of the chest reveals numerous variable-size pulmonary nodules consistent with metastases. (C) CT scan focused on lumbar spine shows a destructive bone lesion (*arrowheads*) in the L4 vertebral body and associated paraspinal soft-tissue mass (*arrows*).

pigmented villonodular synovitis (Fig. 15), and heavily calcified lesions. Finally, some lesions with a low mobile proton density will exhibit a relatively low signal on all sequences, such as very hypocellular, fibrous lesions like plantar fibroma and certain desmoid tumors (30,43,49,51). Unfortunately, the overall specificity of MRI for soft-tissue tumor type is relatively low based merely on signal intensity and spin characteristics.

Using both signal and morphologic characteristics, MRI can be slightly more helpful in differentiating benign from malignant lesions than CT. Characteristic features of a benign tumor include small size, well-defined margins, and homogeneous signal intensity. Malignant tumors are typically larger, poorly

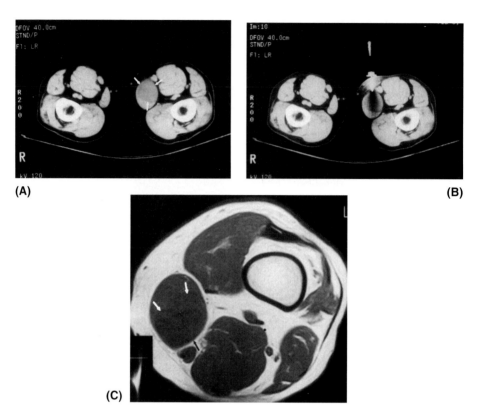

FIG. 14 Myxoid liposarcoma of the left thigh in a 53-year-old man. (A) CT scan in the prone position shows a large, homogeneous, well-defined, intramuscular mass (*arrows*) involving the sartorius, which is lower density than muscle. (B) CT scan during core needle biopsy, again in the prone position, showing introducer/cannula in position. Axial T1-weighted (C) and sagittal T2-weighted (D) MR images show the mass (*arrows*) to be iso-intense to muscle on the T1-weighted sequence and hyperintense on the T2-weighted sequence. These findings could be confused with a cystic mass. (E) Axial T1-weighted postcontrast image demonstrates diffuse, slightly heterogeneous contrast enhancement consistent with a solid tumor (*arrows*).

marginated, heterogeneous in signal intensity, and may exhibit peritumoral edema, or invasion or encasement of adjacent structures (Fig. 16). Unfortunately, exceptions are not uncommon (Fig. 14). Biopsy is usually required unless the MRI image can definitively show a lipoma, vascular lesion, or simple cyst. The correct diagnosis can often be strongly suggested based on MRI features in the case of liposarcoma, desmoid tumor, and peripheral nerve sheath tumor.

The importance of short inversion time inversion-recovery (STIR) imaging sequences in the evaluation of soft-tissue tumors has been recognized for some

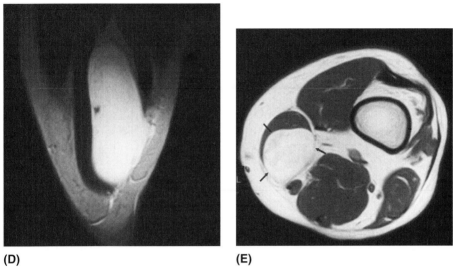

(D)   (E)

FIG. 14 (*Continued*)

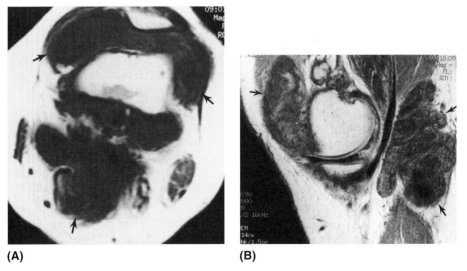

(A)   (B)

FIG. 15 Pigmented villonodular synovitis (PVNS) of the left knee in a 26-year-old woman. Axial T1-weighted (A) and sagittal T2-weighted (B) MR images demonstrate extensive lobulated masses (*arrows*) surrounding the knee distending the suprapatellar bursa and posteriorly into a Baker's cyst. Low signal intensity is seen on both sequences characteristic of hemosiderin deposition seen with PVNS.

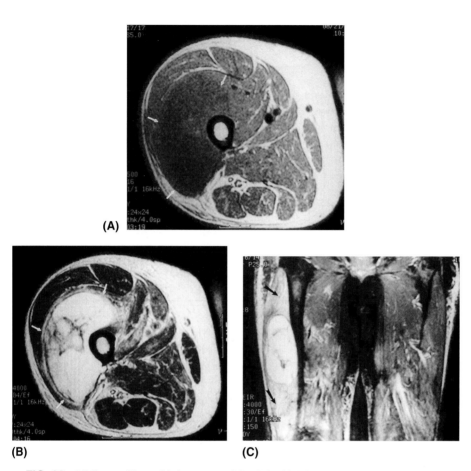

FIG. 16 Malignant fibrous histiocytoma of the right thigh in a 69-year-old man. (A) Axial T1-weighted MR image shows an indistinct mass (*arrows*) involving the quadriceps (primarily the vastus intermedius and vastus lateralis muscles), which is slightly hypointense to muscle. (B) Axial T2-weighted MR image shows a large hyperintense lesion (*arrows*) that better defines the margins of the mass and reveals a heterogeneous pattern. (C) Coronal STIR sequence demonstrates the heterogeneous hyperintense mass and extensive associated peritumoral edema (*arrows*).

time. Normal fat is selectively suppressed on STIR images, and both prolongations in T1 and T2 relaxation contribute to the conspicuity of tissues on STIR. Investigators have noted greater conspicuity of both tumor and infectious processes with STIR imaging as compared to routine spin echo sequences (10,19,52,53). In addition, STIR imaging has proved to be superior to spin-echo MRI in the delineation of peritumoral edema and peripheral microscopic tumor infiltration (10,19).

MRI evaluations of the central nervous system are routinely performed with the administration of paramagnetic intravenous contrast, usually a chelate of gadolinium. However, the indications for intravenous administration of gadolinium contrast for soft-tissue evaluation are not agreed upon. Contrast enhancement does aid differentiation of viable from necrotic regions within a mass (10,18,20–23,54,55). It can also be helpful in distinguishing a cystic lesion from a solid lesion, particularly in the case of small lesions (Fig. 17). Finally, contrast administration is likely of some benefit in making the often very difficult distinction between recurrence of tumor and posttreatment scar tissue. However, scar tissue will enhance for a variable period of time, and irradiated tissue may exhibit increased contrast enhancement indefinitely (18,22,56). Often, changes in the pattern of enhancement may be telling in the surveillance for recurrent disease (19,23,56,57).

Dynamic contrast-enhanced MRI has been investigated as a potential method of distinguishing benign from malignant soft-tissue tumors (10,18,20–23,54,55). With this technique, fast MRI sequences are serially acquired during and immediately after the intravenous administration of gadolinium, and the degree of enhancement is analyzed as a function of time. This kind of analysis gives information about perfusion and local tissue blood volume, which may confer greater diagnostic information than late, postcontrast enhancement imaging, which largely reflects capillary permeability. In general, malignant lesions show a higher rate of perfusion than benign lesions (18,22,56). Early studies show a significant overlap in these dynamic characteristics for benign and malignant lesions, limiting the primary diagnostic utility of this method (19,23,56,57). It may be of greater value in distinguishing recurrent disease from scar and for gauging the efficacy of chemotherapy. Meanwhile, scanner hardware continues to improve, and the efficacy of more quantitative perfusion imaging remains to be established.

MR spectroscopy (MRS) has been widely applied to the study of CNS tumors, but there has been considerably little experience with soft-tissue tumors, despite the exciting potential of this technology to assess treatment response. More experience exists with ^{31}P-MRS than with ^{1}H-MRS, and preliminary results suggest that changes in intracellular pH and phosphometabolite concentrations, in particular decreases in inorganic phosphate or in the phosphomonoester/phosphocreatine ratio, may be indicators of treatment efficacy. Other functional MRI techniques, such as diffusion-weighted imaging, may also eventually prove useful in this application.

D. Ultrasonography

Ultrasonography possesses several advantages over other modalities. These include greater accessibility, portability, short scan times, and lower costs. The capabilities to perform dynamic real-time imaging, contralateral imaging for pur-

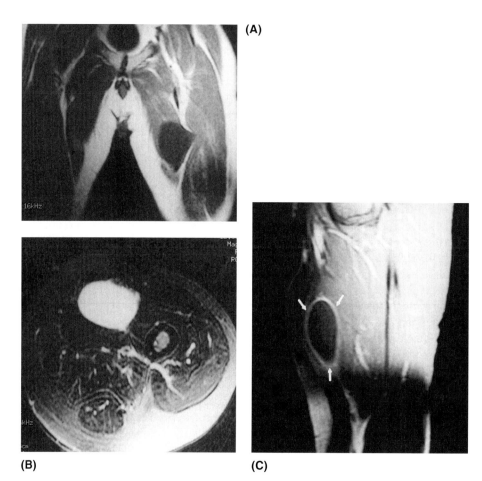

FIG. 17 Lymphocele of the left thigh in a 37-year-old man. Coronal T1-weighted (A) and axial fat-saturated, T2-weighted (B) MR images show a well-defined, homogeneous lesion in the medial thigh, hypointense (A) and hyperintense (B) respectively. (C) Sagittal fat-saturated, T1-weighted postcontrast MR image demonstrates thin, peripheral rim enhancement (arrows) consistent with a simple cystic lesion.

poses of comparison, and fast multiplanar imaging are also general, practical advantages of ultrasonography (19,24,25,27). Advances in color flow and power Doppler have further improved the diagnostic value of ultrasonography. By virtue of real-time, multiplanar imaging, ultrasonography is also a nearly ideal technique to guide percutaneous biopsy (40,46,48).

With the continued improvement of high-resolution linear array transducers, ultrasonography can produce highly detailed images with a resolution that surpasses that of MRI and CT (27,59). Higher frequency probes (9–13 MHz) are indicated for evaluation of superficial structures or subcutaneous masses, whereas deeper lesions require a lower frequency transducer (3.5–7 MHz). Ultrasonography is limited in its capability to depict large anatomical segments or lesions as compared with other cross-sectional imaging modalities due to the smaller field of view. The split-screen feature available on most units allows visualization of larger lesions by doubling the field of view. An extended-field-of-view imaging feature was recently introduced (SieScape, Siemens Medical Systems) which synthesizes panoramic images of large anatomical areas using continuous transducer motion across the area of interest (Fig. 18) (60,61). This technology allows for a more complete depiction of the lesion and its relationship to adjacent structures, which is especially valuable with larger masses.

A standoff pad may be helpful in the assessment of very superficial structures to limit reverberation artifacts, although the use of copious coupling gel is usually adequate. It is important to ensure that the region of interest is within the focal zone of the transducer to maintain the highest image resolution. Multiple focal zones can be used to provide more uniform resolution over a larger region, although there will be a corresponding reduction in image frame rate.

Both static and dynamic techniques are useful during sonographic examination of soft-tissue lesions. Standard characteristics, such as size, shape, location, and echogenicity, can be determined with static evaluation. The dynamic evaluation uses different manual maneuvers or compression to better define the relationship of the lesion to adjacent structures and to reproduce symptoms in certain situations. For example, standing the patient up may help to distend a vascular

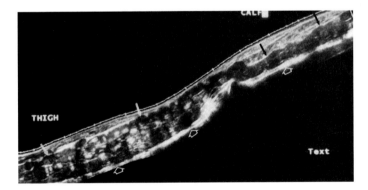

FIG. 18 Plexiform neurofibroma of the right leg in a 19-year-old man with neurofibromatosis. Extended field-of-view sagittal sonogram shows a massive multilobulated lesion (*arrows*) occupying nearly the entire posterior aspect of the leg abutting the posterior cortex (*open arrows*) of the femur and tibia in the distribution of the sciatic nerve and tibial nerve, respectively. Similar findings were noted in the left leg.

lesion in the lower extremities, while muscle contraction can accentuate muscle herniation, a finding that can clinically mimic a mass. The compressibility of a lesion further characterizes the consistency of a mass. Correlation with the contralateral, unaffected side of the body is a convenient maneuver in musculoskeletal ultrasonography that often clarifies confusing anatomy, and may better demonstrate a subtle abnormality from surrounding normal structures.

Color flow Doppler is a powerful innovation whereby the individual Doppler frequency shifts of reflected sound are mapped onto the gray-scale ultrasonographic image using a color-based code. The Doppler shift, when corrected for the angle of insonification, is related to flow velocity. This mapping of frequency shifts is performed over a sensitive area that the user can tailor in terms of size and location within the gray-scale image. The same limitations exist for color Doppler that exist for conventional continuous wave Doppler techniques; sensitivity to the angle of insonification and frequency aliasing.

Power Doppler ultrasonography overcomes the limitations of conventional color Doppler to a large degree by integrating the power spectrum of the Doppler shift. In this way, power Doppler maps the mere presence of flow and color-codes what is more closely analogous to a perfusion or circulatory fraction. Power Doppler is more sensitive for the detection of low-flow states and is less dependent on the angle of insonification. Power Doppler does not provide information about flow direction or velocity and is highly sensitive to patient motion. Color and power Doppler imaging are both useful in assessing the vascularity of lesions (19,24). Absence of blood flow is suggestive but not diagnostic of benignity (25,28). These techniques may also be useful in identifying inflammatory and infectious lesions (Fig. 4), and distinguishing them from nonhyperemic processes (26).

Ultrasonography is a useful technique for guiding the biopsy or aspiration of soft-tissue masses (Fig. 19). Special biopsy ultrasonographic probes are available that facilitate needle targeting and mechanical needle guidance. Experienced sonographers are usually comfortable with "free-hand" biopsy technique. With experience, procedures can be performed rapidly, and patient positioning is not limited by the design restraints of the imaging device. Ultrasonography permits continuous imaging of the target mass and adjacent structures, including vessels and nerves, and continuous real-time visualization of the needle as it is advanced into the appropriate portion of the lesion. Color and power Doppler can help identify the viable portion of a necrotic or hemorrhagic lesion during biopsy, resulting in a higher diagnostic yield. Large vessels can also be more easily identified and thus avoided.

Ultrasonography has been shown to be effective for the assessment of recurrent soft-tissue sarcoma (40,41), and it has cost advantages over CT or MRI. Ultrasonography is not widely used for this purpose because it is more operator-dependent, and longitudinal follow-up studies are not as easily compared with prior exams.

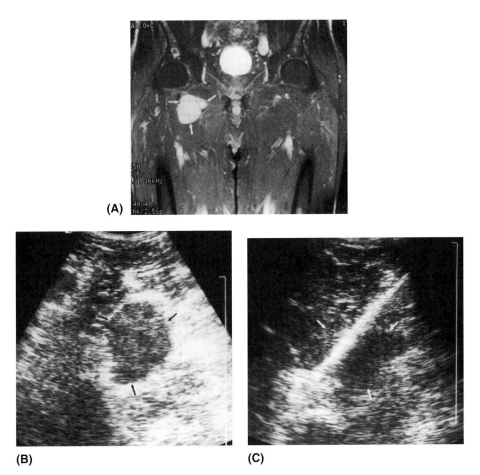

FIG. 19   Hemangiopericytoma of the right thigh in a 69-year-old man. (A) Coronal fat-saturated, T1-weighted postcontrast MR image reveals a markedly enhancing mass (*arrows*) within the medial thigh musculature. Transverse sonograms before (B) and during (C) biopsy of the medial thigh demonstrates a fairly well-defined hypoechoic mass (*arrows*) corresponding to the finding seen on MRI and illustrates needle localization within the tumor (C).

E.   Conventional Contrast Angiography

Since the advent of CT and MRI, the role of conventional angiography in the evaluation of soft-tissue tumors has decreased markedly. Most angiographic findings of soft-tissue tumors do not distinguish between benign and malignant lesions reliably (62–66), angiography alone is less effective at defining disease extent than cross-sectional imaging (67). Assessment of tumor vascularity can now be accomplished with a variety of noninvasive methods, such as contrast-enhanced CT or MRI, or color and power Doppler–assisted ultrasonography. Identification of major feeding or draining vessels may be important for surgical planning, but this can be done effectively with CT angiography or MR angiography techniques.

Arteriography may be helpful for the preoperative evaluation of vascular lesions, such as hemangiomas and arteriovenous malformations, especially when preoperative and therapeutic embolization is anticipated (68,69). Embolization of hypervascular tumors prior to surgical therapy substantially decreases intraoperative and postoperative bleeding complications. Intravascular access may also occasionally be needed for the targeted, arterial delivery of chemotherapeutic agents, or for isolated limb perfusion therapy, which have been used successfully in selected clinical settings.

F. Nuclear Scintigraphy

The role of scintigraphy in the evaluation of soft-tissue masses is less well established than that of CT and MRI, and it may be correspondingly underutilized. Radionuclide imaging depicts biochemical events in tissue, and this functional aspect of scintigraphy may pose an advantage over anatomical imaging techniques. However, our knowledge of scintigraphic tumor imaging comes predominantly from experience with tumors of the CNS and carcinomas. Furthermore, soft-tissue sarcomas are widely variegated in their biology, and conclusions about scintigraphy with regard to particular histologic types of soft-tissue tumors are likely not generalizable to all sarcomas.

The utility of scintigraphy in primary evaluation of soft-tissue masses is limited. Scintigraphic techniques may shed light on the likelihood of malignancy vs. benignity of masses, and the intensity of tracer uptake may also correlate with tumor grade in cases of malignancy. Scintigraphy holds greater promise for tumor staging by virtue of the larger imaging "window" provided by these techniques as compared with MRI, CT, and ultrasonography. For example, lymph node and more distant metastases, as well as bony involvement, may theoretically be assessed with one comprehensive whole-body exam.

1. Techniques and Radiopharmaceuticals

Nuclear medicine imaging techniques that are currently used for the evaluation of sarcomas include gamma camera imaging or SPECT with 201-thallium chloride and 99m-technetium-sesta-MIBI (methoxyisobutylisonitrile), and PET imaging with 18F-fluoro-2-deoxy-D-glucose (FDG). Gallium-67 citrate has a limited role in soft-tissue sarcoma imaging but is effective for evaluation of lymphoma and melanoma.

The efficacy of PET imaging is increasingly recognized for staging patients with cancer, particularly since the development of whole body scan implementations (70). PET scanners acquire volumetric datasets and can generate tomographic images that have a 10-fold greater contrast than planar images, increasing the sensitivity for smaller lesions. PET data can also be obtained dynamically, generating kinetic information. However, PET imaging is technology-intensive, expensive, and not widely available. The cost of cyclotrons for positron tracer generation further limits the accessibilty of PET. This limitation has been partially overcome by the emergence of commercial distributors of positron-emitting nuclides, particularly [18]F.

Gamma camera imaging with positron-emitting tracers has been implemented using high-energy collimation and dual-head equipment, but the sensitivity is still 15-fold less than with conventional coincidence detection–based collimated PET scanners, and spatial resolution is significantly poorer.

^{99}Tc-MIBI, thallium, and FDG can all be considered general-purpose tumor imaging agents. Their mechanisms of localization are multifactorial and not histology-specific, and are related to increased blood flow and permeability of endothelium as well as increases in cell proliferation and metabolism. Thallium-201 chloride uptake is dependent on the function of the cellular sodium-potassium pump and ATPase activity, which tends to be higher in malignant tissue. [99m]-Tc-sesta-MIBI is a lipophilic cationic compound whose uptake is proportional to blood flow, mitochondrial activity, and plasma membrane potential. FDG uptake is dependent on blood flow, blood glucose and insulin levels, and tissue hexokinase and phosphatase activity. ^{18}F-FDG is phosphorylated by hexokinase to ^{18}F-FDG-6-phosphate, which is metabolically inert, not being a substrate for glycolysis. However, FDG is taken up in tissues in proportion to cellular glucose metabolism.

Other metabolically active tracers have been developed for PET imaging. ^{18}F-Fluoromisonidazole (FMISO) is an imidazole compound that is trapped in hypoxic cells (71). Since many malignant tumors outgrow their blood supply, cell hypoxia in tumors is common, and hypoxia decreases the sensitivity of tumor tissues to radiation and thus lessens the efficiency of radiotherapy. Hence, PET with FMISO may help plan adjuvant treatment for tumors. Amino acids that have been labeled for PET imaging include L-methyl-^{11}C-methionine and L-1-^{11}C-tyrosine. Uptake of these tracers is related to cell proliferation and mitotic rate.

Localization of these radiopharmaceuticals is not specific for malignancy. For example, certain benign lesions can localize thallium, including granulomatous disease, Paget's disease, myositis ossificans, fibrous dysplasia, and ossifying fibroma. Similarly, MIBI also shows uptake in benign and malignant disease. Infections exhibit increased uptake on FDG PET, and this technique may actually hold promise for diagnosis of acute and chronic osteomyelitis.

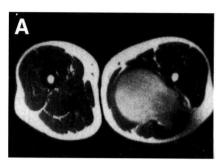 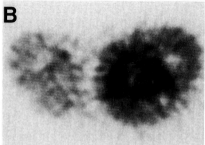

FIG. 20 Low-grade myxoid liposarcoma: On the left (A), axial MRI shows a large, well-defined mass in left adductor magnus. Axial FDG PET image on the right (B), while resolution limited, shows heterogeneous increased uptake in this low-grade lesion. The magnitude of tracer uptake can be quantified relative to the injected dose, if appropriate corrections are made for attenuation and decay. (Reprinted with permission of the Society of Nuclear Medicine from Adler LP, Blair HF, Makley JT, et al. Noninvasive grading of musculoskeletal tumors using PET. J Nucl Med 1991; 32:1508–1511.)

2. Scintigraphy, Tumor Biology, and Clinical Applications

Increased regional glucose metabolism and energy consumption characterize malignancy, especially poorly differentiated and high-grade neoplasia. Tumor grade has been shown to correlate with increased FDG uptake due to elevated glycolytic metabolism in tumor cells (Fig. 20) (72,73). Tumor grade is also correlated with intensity of thallium uptake and the proliferative activity of tumor cells (74). Heterogeneity in tumor grade and viability may be depicted by thallium and FDG scans (Fig. 21).

Tumors that respond to treatment show decreased tracer uptake on FDG PET studies (75). Amino acid imaging may prove to be more specific than FDG for showing a treatment response by more directly reflecting changes in cell proliferation. Necrosis after preoperative chemotherapy in sarcomas can be identified as a reduction of thallium uptake. Thallium scan conversion from positive to negative after chemotherapy is predictive of 95% tumor necrosis. MIBI uptake patterns parallel that of thallium. However, decreased MIBI uptake may also indicate development of multidrug resistance (MDR) conferred by p-glycoprotein expression by tumor cells.

Response or nonresponse to chemotherapy as reflected by intensity of thallium, MIBI, or FDG uptake may be used to tailor chemotherapy. Scintigraphic information about chemotherapy's effect may also influence surgical management by better indicating which soft-tissue sarcomas can be managed by wide resection rather than radical excision or amputation. The precise roles for scintigraphy

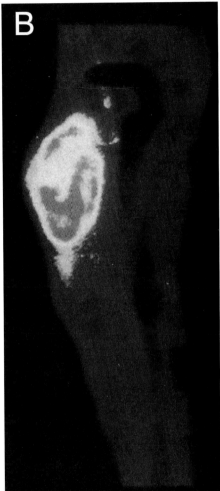

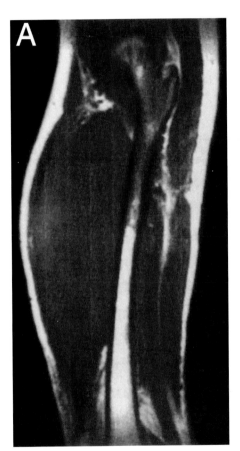

FIG. 21   High-grade fibrosarcoma. Sagittal MRI of the thigh shows a large anterior mass abutting the femur (A). Corresponding sagittal image (B, right) from FDG PET study shows inhomogeneous intense uptake. Specific uptake values correlate with tumor grade but do not distinguish benign from low-grade lesions. (Reprinted with permission, from Society of Nuclear Medicine from Nieweg OE, Pruim J, van Ginkel RJ, et al. Fluorine-18-fluorodeoxyglucose PET imaging of soft-tissue sarcoma. J Nucl Med 1996; 37:257–261.)

and the added value of quantitative vs. visual analysis in decision making is still evolving.

Scar tissue that forms after surgery or radiation therapy typically has decreased metabolic activity compared with tumor, which may allow differentiation of scar from residual tumor with scintigraphy. Unfortunately, few studies exist that compare scintigraphy to MRI for sarcoma evaluation. Again, there is more experience with the scintigraphic detection of recurrent carcinomas than that of recurrent sarcomas. In one study, thallium scanning had greater sensitivity and specificity for recurrent sarcoma than CT or MRI (76). FDG PET should theoretically have a greater efficacy than thallium or MIBI by virtue of higher spatial resolution and detection sensitivity, but this remains to be proven.

The efficacy of these scintigraphic techniques likely depends on the biological aggressiveness of the tumors, so they may be more appropriate for surveillance after treatment of high-grade tumors. Currently, scintigraphy has achieved only broad use in the surveillance of lymphomas and is not routinely used after treatment of other sarcomas.

IV. CENTRAL ISSUES IN IMAGING OF SOFT-TISSUE MASSES: OVERVIEW

A. Histologic Characterization by Imaging

The histologic characteristics of a soft-tissue mass can be suggested by imaging criteria in certain cases. For example, fat-containing lesions are accurately identified by CT or MRI (Figs. 11 and 22). Simple cystic lesions, such as ganglionic lesions, have a characteristic appearance on ultrasonography (Fig. 23) and can usually be accurately identified on CT or MRI, especially when intravenous contrast enhancement is given (Fig. 17). Some fibrous tumors and most hemosiderin-laden lesions demonstrate characteristic regions of low signal intensity on both T1-weighted and T2-weighted MRI sequences (Fig. 15). Vascular tumors can be identified by their morphology and by the presence of large feeding or draining vessels. Larger, high-flow vessels appear as serpiginous flow voids on MRI studies (Fig. 10). Low-flow lesions, such as hemangiomata, can be accurately diagnosed based largely on their morphology and fat content. Neurogenic tumors may demonstrate a fusiform shape and may be shown to be contiguous with the parent nerve itself. Calcification patterns within a soft-tissue mass can be fairly characteristic. Peripheral calcification, with centripetal progression of calcification over time, is characteristic of myositis ossificans (Fig. 6). Flocculent or stripped calcification is typical of chondroid lesions. When imaging features are analyzed collectively, the differential diagnosis can often be significantly narrowed and, in some cases, a very specific diagnosis can be made.

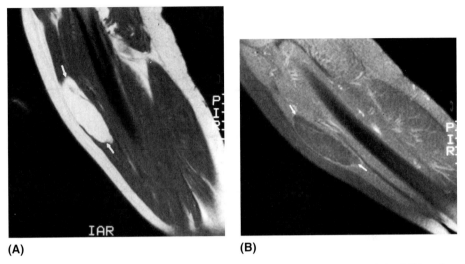

(A) **(B)**

FIG. 22 Lipoma of the left thigh in a 42-year-old woman. Sagittal T1-weighted (A) and fat-saturated, T1-weighted (B) MR images shows a nearly homogeneous, well-defined intramuscular lesion isointense to the subcutaneous tissues and demonstrating fat saturation consistent with a lipoma (*arrows*). A single, thin, low-intensity, linear structure representing a fibrous septation is not uncommon and remains consistent with a lipoma.

B. Benign or Malignant?

Currently, no imaging modality consistently distinguishes benign from malignant soft-tissue masses (10,14,15,21,43,49,50,77,78,79). Studies report variable accuracies for CT or MRI in separating benign from malignant lesions, and this likely reflects variances and bias in patient selection. Some soft-tissue masses have characteristic imaging features that are sufficiently specific to obviate surgery or biopsy. These entities include lipomas (Fig. 22), simple cystic lesions (Fig. 23), benign vascular tumors (Figs. 9 and 10), pigmented villonodular synovitis (Fig. 15), and synovial osteochondromatosis (Fig. 3). Less common lesions, such as elastofibroma dorsi (Fig. 24), lipoma arborescens (Fig. 25), and fibrolipomatous hamartoma of peripheral nerves, can also be diagnosed by pathognomonic imaging criteria.

General imaging criteria for benign lesions include small size, smooth margins, superficial location, homogeneous internal signal or architecture, absence of associated edema, and lack of involvement or infiltration of adjacent structures. Malignant features include large size, poorly defined margins, deep location, heterogeneous signal or complex architecture (including rarefaction or necrosis), associated edema, and invasion of adjacent structures. However, exceptions to each of these signs are not unusual.

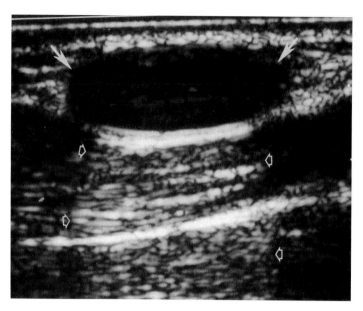

FIG. 23   Ganglion cyst of the wrist in a 48-year-old woman. Sagittal sonogram of the dorsal aspect of the base of the thumb reveals a simple cystic structure (*arrows*) adjacent to the extensor pollicis longus tendon. Note the well-defined margins and the posterior acoustic enhancement (*open arrows*).

Soft-tissue sarcomas can appear well marginated (15,43,79) (Fig. 11). Typically, sarcomas develop as intramuscular lesions, respecting fascial boundaries, remaining within the anatomical compartment of origin until they become quite large. As they grow, a pseudocapsule consisting of compressed adjacent normal tissue can result in a relatively well-defined border.

Homogeneity of signal intensity on MRI is only a relative indicator of benignity. This is particularly true for small lesions, and myxoid-containing soft-tissue sarcomas can appear quite homogeneous or cystic on routine MRI (43,79) (Fig. 14). Administration of intravenous contrast permits more accurate differentiation of these entities, as does ultrasonographic examination (16,17,32).

Perilesional edema is seen more often with a malignant lesion (10,49,50, 80,81) (Fig. 16). Exceptions include inflammatory or infectious processes and posttraumatic lesions, such as hematomas. This sign is of limited value if the lesion has been previously biopsied. Because only a minority of soft-tissue sarcomas demonstrate perilesional edema, the absence of this sign is not particularly valuable.

Invasion or infiltration of adjacent structures may be the imaging feature most predictive of malignancy. This finding is present in only a minority of

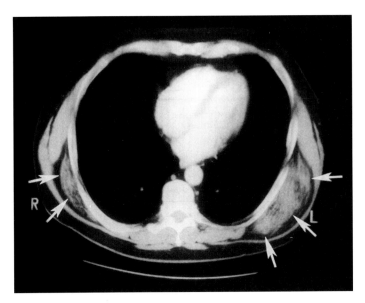

FIG. 24 Elastofibroma dorsi. CT scan shows bilateral masses (*arrows*) with slightly irregular margins characteristically located deep to the serratus anterior muscles, which are displaced but not invaded.

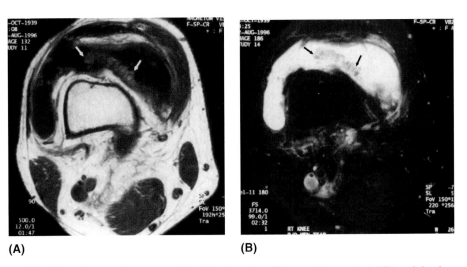

(A)   (B)

FIG. 25 Lipoma arborescens of the right knee in a 57-year-old man. Axial T1-weighted (A) and axial fat-saturated, T2-weighted (B) MR images show the presence of a large joint effusion and small frond-like synovial masses (*arrows*) with signal intensity consistent with fat, characteristic for this disorder.

malignant soft-tissue tumors; thus, it also has a low negative predictive value. Again, some aggressive benign lesions, such as fibromatosis, can also encase or infiltrate adjacent structures.

C. Follow-up Imaging After Treatment

Imaging is routinely performed to detect recurrent or residual tumor after surgery. For this application, the most effective modality is MRI (38,77). Ultrasonography has also been shown to be accurate in the detection of local recurrence, but may be less reproducible for longitudinal follow-up evaluations (40,41).

Direct comparison of current imaging studies should be made with prior studies. Usually, the first exam performed after treatment is the most useful single baseline reference. Ideally, the same sequences and imaging parameters should be performed at each imaging evaluation to facilitate accurate comparison between studies.

Imaging may also be used to assess response to therapy during treatment or before definitive surgery. Response to therapy is usually manifested by a reduction in tumor bulk, or by an increase in necrosis, manifested by greater tumor rarefaction or diminished contrast enhancement. Physiologic imaging techniques (such as FDG-PET, thallium, MR spectroscopy) may emerge as better gauges of treatment efficacy than simple assessment of changes in tumor size on anatomical imaging.

Following surgical resection, MRI or CT exams are probably more sensitive if performed with intravenous contrast administration. Because postoperative tissue changes enhance for variable periods, and radiated tissue and denervated muscle may exhibit abnormal and increased enhancement indefinitely, the presence of enhancement is nonspecific (7,19). The morphology, magnitude, and change in pattern of enhancement, then, must all be analyzed carefully in the assessment for recurrent disease (19,21,39,77). Newer imaging techniques, such as FDG-PET and diffusion-weighted MRI, may eventually improve diagnosis in this challenging setting.

The definitive differentiation of recurrent tumor from postsurgical scar usually requires biopsy. Percutaneous needle biopsy is the procedure of choice when performed under cross-sectional imaging guidance and with careful correlation with the preprocedural imaging studies that prompt the biopsy.

V. SUMMARY

Imaging plays an essential role in the assessment of suspected soft-tissue tumors and tumorlike processes. Imaging studies are useful to confirm the presence of suspected lesions and establish a working diagnosis. For soft-tissue tumors, imaging plays an important role in staging, biopsy guidance, surgical planning, and posttreatment surveillance. In general, MRI is the most powerful and versatile modality for noninvasive evaluation of soft-tissue masses. CT is the most practical modality for biopsy guidance. It is still difficult to consistently distinguish benign from malignant soft-tissue lesions based on imaging, but greater diagnostic specificity may be rendered by innovations in functional imaging.

REFERENCES

1. McDonald DJ. Limb-salvage surgery for treatment of sarcomas of the extremities. AJR 163:509–513, 1994.
2. Smith DK, Parsons YW. Re: Limb-salvage surgery for treatment of sarcomas of the extremities. AJR 163:514–516, 1994.
3. Moreau G, Bush CH, Scarborough MT, Enneking WF. Surgical considerations in a diagnostic imaging evaluation of musculoskeletal masses. MRI Clin North Am 3:577–590, 1995.
4. Peabody TD, Gibbs CP, Simon MA. Evaluation and staging of musculoskeletal neoplasm. J Bone Joint Surg Am 80:1204–1218, 1998.
5. Kransdorf MJ. Benign soft-tissue tumors in a large referral population: Distribution of diagnoses by age, sex and location. AJR 164:395–402, 1995.
6. Kransdorf MJ. Malignant soft-tissue tumors in a large referral population: Distribution of diagnoses by age, sex and location. AJR 164:129–134, 1995.
7. Marcantonio DR, Weatherall PT, Hudson BH. Practical considerations in the imaging of soft-tissue tumors. Orthop Clin North Am 29:1–17, 1988.
8. Jelinek J, Kransdorf MJ. MR imaging of soft-tissue masses. Mass-like lesions that simulate neoplasms. MRI Clin North Am 3:727–741, 1995.
9. Berquist TH. Magnetic resonance imaging of musculoskeletal neoplasms. Clin Orthop 244:101–108, 1989.
10. Hanna SL, Fletcher BD. MR imaging of malignant soft-tissue tumors. MRI Clin North Am 3:629–650, 1995.
11. Massengill AD, Seeger LL, Eckardt JJ. The role of plain radiograph, computed tomography, and magnetic resonance imaging in sarcoma evaluation. Hematoloncol Clin North Am 9:571–604, 1995.
12. Beyers GE, Berquist TH. MR imaging techniques for soft-tissue lesions. MRI Clin North Am 3:563–576, 1995.
13. Pettersson H, Gillespy T, Hamlin DJ, Enneking WG, Springfield DS, Andrew ER, Spanier S, Slone R. Primary musculoskeletal tumors: examination with MR imaging compared with conventional modalities. Radiology 164:237–241, 1987
14. Sundaram M, McGuire MH, Herbold DR. Magnetic resonance imaging of soft-tissue masses: an evaluation of fifty-three histologically proven tumors. Magn Reson Imaging 6:237–248, 1988.
15. Totty WG, Murphey WA, Lee JKT. Soft-tissue tumors: MR imaging. Radiology 160:135–141, 1986.
16. Myhre-Jensen O. A consecutive 7-year series of 1331 benign soft-tissue tumors. Acta Orthop Scand 52:287–293, 1981.
17. Rydholm A. Management of patients with soft-tissue tumors. Strategy developed at a regional oncology center. Acta Orthop (Suppl 203) 54:1–77, 1983.

18. Erlemann R, Reiser MF, Peters PE, Vassallo P, Nommensen B, Kusnierz-Glaz CR, Ritter J, Roessner A. Musculoskeletal neoplasms: static and dynamic Gd-DTPA-enhanced MR imaging. Radiology 171:767–773, 1989.

19. Munk PL, Poon PY, Chhem RK, Janzen DL. Imaging of soft-tissue sarcomas. Can Assoc Radiol J 45:438–446, 1994.

20. Pettersson H, Eliasson J, Egund N, Rooser B, Willen H, Rydholm A, Berg NO, Holtas S. Gadolinium-DTPA enhancement of soft-tissue tumors in magnetic imaging—preliminary clinical experience in five patients. Skeletal Radiol 17:319–323, 1988.

21. Beltran J, Chandnani V, McGhee RA, Kursungoglu-Brahme S. Gadopentetate Dimeglumine-enhanced MR imaging of the musculoskeletal system. AJR 156:457–466, 1991.

22. Vestraete KL, De Deene Y, Roels H, Dierick A, Uyttendaele D, Kunnen M. Benign and malignant musculoskeletal lesions: dynamic contrast-enhanced MR imaging—parametric "first pass" images depict tissue vascularization and perfusion. Radiology 192:835–843, 1994.

23. Benedikt RA, Jelinek JS, Kransdorf MJ, Moser RP, Berrey BH. MR imaging of soft-tissue masses: role of gadopentetate dimeglumine. J Magn Reson Imaging 4:485–490, 1994.

24. Taylor GA, Perlman EJ, Scherer LR, Gearhart JP, Leventhal BG, Wiley J. Vascularity of tumors in children: Evaluation with color Doppler imaging. AJR 157:1267–1271, 1991.

25. Newman JS, Adler RS, Bude RO, Rubin JM. Detection of soft-tissue hyperemia: value of power Doppler sonography. AJR 163:385–389, 1994.

26. Latifi HR, Siegel MJ. Color Doppler flow imaging of pediatric soft-tissue masses. J Ultrasound Med 13:165–169, 1994.

27. van Hoslbeeck M, Introcaso JH. Musculoskeletal ultrasonography. Radiol Clin North Am 30:907–925, 1992.

28. Rubin JM, Bude RO, Carson PL, Bree RL, Adler RS. Power Doppler US: a potentially useful alternative to mean frequency-based color Doppler US. Radiology 190:853–856, 1994.

29. Shives TC. Biopsy of soft-tissue tumors. Clin Orthop 289:32–35, 1993.

30. Sundaram M, McLeod RA. MR imaging of tumor and tumor like lesions of bone and soft-tissue. AJR 155:817–824, 1990.

31. Enneking WF, Spanier SS, Goodman MA. A system for the surgical staging of musculoskeletal sarcoma. Clin Orthop 153:106–120, 1980.

32. Peabody TD, Simon MA. Principles of staging of soft-tissue sarcomas. Clin Orthop 289:19–31, 1993.

33. Russell WO, Cohen J, Edmonson JH, Enzinger F, Hadju SI, Heise H, Martin RG, Miller W, Schmitz RL, Suit HD. Staging system for soft-tissue sarcoma. Semin Oncol 8:156–159, 1981.

34. Tehranzadeh J, Manymneh W, Ghavan C, Morillo G, Murphy BJ. Comparison of CT and MR imaging in musculoskeletal neoplasms. J Comput Assist Tomogr 13:466–472, 1989.

35. Aisen AM, Martel W, Braunstein EM, McMillin KI, Phillips WA, Kling TF. MRI and CT evaluation of primary bone and soft-tissue tumors. AJR 146:749–756, 1984.

36. Chang AE, Matory YL, Dwyer AJ, Hill SC, Girton ME, Steinberg SM, Knop RH, Frank JA, Hyams D, Doppman JL. Magnetic resonance imaging versus computed tomography in the evaluation of soft-tissue tumors of the extremity. Ann Surg 205: 340–348, 1987.

37. Demas BE, Heelan RT, Lane J, Marcove R, Hajdu S, Brennan MF. Soft-tissue masses of the locomotor system: comparison of MR and CT in determining extent of disease. AJR 150:615–620, 1988.

38. Petasnick JP, Turner DA, Charters JR, Gitelis S, Zacharias CE. Soft-tissue masses of the locomotor system: comparison of MR imaging with CT. Radiology 160:125–133, 1986.

39. Varma DGK, Jackson EF, Pollock RE, Benjamin RS. Soft-tissue sarcoma: MR imaging vs. sonography for detection of local recurrences. MRI Clin North Am 3:695–712, 1995.

40. Choi H, Varma DGK, Fornage BD, Kim EE, Johnston DA. Soft-tissue sarcoma: MR imaging vs.sonography for detection of local recurrence after surgery. AJR 157: 353–358, 1991.

41. Pino G, Conzi GF, Murolo C, Schenone F, Magliani L, Imperiale A, Dato G, Panetta M, Toma S. Sonographic evaluation of local recurrences of soft-tissue sarcomas. J Ultrasound Med 12:23–26, 1993.

42. Cohen MD, Weetman RM, Proviser AJ, Grosfeld JL, West KW, Cory DA, Smith JA, McGuire W. Efficacy of magnetic resonance imaging in 139 children with tumors. Arch Surg 121:522–529, 1986.

43. Kransdorf MJ, Jelinek JS, Moser RP, Utz JA, Brower AC, Hudson TM, Berry BH. Soft-tissue masses: diagnosis using MR imaging. AJR 153:541–547, 1989.

44. Weekes RG, Berquist TH, McLeod RA, Zimmer WD. Magnetic resonance imaging of soft-tissue tumors: comparison with computed tomography. Magn Reson Imaging 3:345–352, 1985.

45. Bloem JL, Taminiau AHM, Eulderink F, Hermans J, Pauwels EK. Radiologic staging of primary bone sarcoma: MR imaging, scintigraphy, angiography, and CT correlated with pathologic examination. Radiology 169:805–810, 1988.

46. Charboneau JW, Reading CC, Welch TJ. CT and sonographically guided needle biopsy: current techniques and new innovations. AJR 154:1–10, 1990.

47. Dupuy DE, Rosenberg AE, Punyaratabandhu T, Tan MH, Mankin HJ. Accuracy of CT-guided needle biopsy of musculoskeletal neoplasms. AJR 171:759–762, 1998.

48. Hudson TM, Hamlin DJ, Enneking MD, Petterson H. Magnetic resonance imaging of bone and soft-tissue tumors: early experience in 31 patients compared with computed tomography. Skeletal Radiol 13:134–146, 1985.

49. Crim JR, Seeger LL, Yao L, Chandnani V, Eckardt JJ. Diagnosis of soft-tissue masses with MR imaging: can benign masses be differentiated from malignant ones? Radiology 185:581–586, 1992.

50. Moulton JS, Blebea JS, Dunco DM, Braley SE, Bisset GS, Emery KH. MR imaging of soft-tissue masses: diagnostic efficacy and value of distinguishing between benign and malignant lesions. AJR 164:1191–1199, 1995.

51. Berquist TH, Ehman RL, King BF, Hodgman CG, Iistrup DM. Value of MR imaging in differentiating benign from malignant soft-tissue masses: study of 95 lesions. AJR 155:1251–1255, 1990.

52. Shuman WP, Baron RL, Peters MJ, Tazioli PK. Comparison of STIR and spin-echo MR imaging at 1.5T in 90 lesions of the chest, liver, and pelvis. AJR 152:853–859, 1989.

53. Dwyer AJ, Frank JA, Sank VJ, Reinig JW, Hickey AM, Doppman JL. Short-TI inversion recovery pulse sequence: analysis and initial experience in cancer imaging. Radiology 168:827–836, 1988.

54. Erlemann R, Vassallo P, Bongartz G., Muller-Miny H, Rummeny E, Stober U, Peters PE. Musculoskeletal neoplasms: fast low-angle shot imaging with and without Gd-DTPA. Radiology 176:489–495, 1990.

55. Vanel D, Shapeero LG, Tardivon A, Western A, Guinebretiere JM. Dynamic contrast-enhanced MRI with subtraction of aggressive soft-tissue tumors after resection. Skeletal Radiol 27:505–510, 1998.

56. Mirowitz SA, Totty WG, Lee JKT. Characterization of musculoskeletal masses using dynamic GdDTPA enhanced spin-echo MRI. J Comput Assist Tomogr 16:120–125, 1992.

57. Fletcher BD, Hanna SL. Musculoskeletal neoplasms: dynamic Gd-DTPA enhanced imaging (letter). Radiology 177:287–288, 1990.

58. Christensen RA, Van Sonnenberg E, Casola G, Wittich GR. Interventional ultrasound in the musculoskeletal system. Radiol Clin North Am 26:145–146, 1988.

59. Fornage BD. Soft-tissue masses. In Fornage BD, ed. Clinics in diagnostic ultrasound. Volume 30. Musculoskeletal ultrasound. New York: Churchill Livingstone, 1995: 21–42.

60. Weng L, Tirumalai AP, Lowery CM, Nock LF, Gustafson DE, Von Behren PL, Kim JH. US extended-field-of-view imaging technology. Radiology 203:877–880, 1997.

61. Barberie JE, Wong AD, Cooperberg PL, Carson BW. Extended field-of-view sonography in musculoskeletal disorders. AJR 171:751–757, 1998.

62. Martel W, Abell MR. Radiologic evaluation of soft-tissue tumors. Cancer 32:352–366, 1973.

63. Viamonte MM, Roen S, Le Page J. Nonspecificity of abnormal vascularity in the angiographic diagnosis of malignant neoplasms. Radiology 106:59–63, 1973.

64. Lois JF, Fischer HJ, Deutsh LS, Stambuck EC, Gomes AS. Angiography in soft-tissue sarcomas. Cardiovasc Interv Radiol 7:309–316, 1984.

65. Herzberg DL, Schreiber MH. Angiography in mass lesion of the extremities. AJR 111:541–546, 1971.

66. Halpern M, Freiberger RH. Arteriography in orthopedics. AJR 4:194–206, 1965.

67. Ekelund L, Herrlin K, Rydholm A. Comparison of computed topography and angiography of the extremities. Acta Radiol Diagn 23:15–28, 1982.

68. Widlus DM, Murray RR, White RI, Osterman FA, Schreiber ER, Satre RW, Mitchell SE, Kaufman SL, Williams GM, Weiland AJ. Congenital arteriovenous malformations: tailored embolotherapy. Radiology 169:511–516, 1988.

69. Yakes WF, Pevsner R, Reed M, Donohue HJ. Serial embolizations of an extremity arteriovenous malformation with alcohol via direct percutaneous puncture. AJR 146:1038–1040, 1986.

70. Dalboom M, Hoffman EJ, Hoh CK, et al. Evaluation of a PET scanner for whole body imaging. J Nucl Med 33:1191–1199, 1992.

71. Koh WJ, Rasay JS, Evans ML, et al. Imaging tumor hypoxia in human tumors with [F-18] fluromisonidazole. Int J Radiat Oncol Biol Phys 22:199–212, 1992.
72. Kern KA, Brunetti A, Norton JA, et al. Metabolic imaging of human extremity musculo-skeletal tumors by PET. J Nucl Med 29:181–186, 1988.
73. Adler LP, Blair HF, Makley JT, et al. Noninvasive grading of musculoskeletal tumors using PET. J Nucl Med 32:1508–1512, 1991.
74. Arbab AS, Koizumi K, Araki T. Uptake of Tc99m-tetrofosmin, TcMIBI and T1201C1 in tumor cell lines. J Nucl Med 37:1551–1556, 1996.
75. Ichiya Y, Kuwabara Y, Otsuka M, et al. Assessment of response to cancer treatment using FDG and PET. J Nucl Med 32:1655–1660, 1991.
76. Kostakoglu L, Panicek DM, Divgi CR, et al: Correlation of localization of thallium chloride scans with those of other imaging modalities and histology following treatment in patients with bone and soft-tissue sarcomas. Eur J Nucl Med 22:1233–1237, 1995.
77. Vanel D, Shapeero LG, DeBaere T, Gilles R, Tardivon A, Genin J, Guinebretire JM. MR imaging in the follow-up of malignant and aggressive soft-tissue tumors: results of 511 examinations. Radiology 190:263–268, 1994.
78. Ma LD, Frassica FJ, Scott VW, Fishman EK, Zerhouni EA. Differentiation of benign and malignant musculoskeletal tumors: potential pitfalls with MR imaging. Radiographics 15:349–366, 1995.
79. Weatherall PT. Benign and malignant masses: MR imaging differentiation. MRI Clin North Am 3:672–673, 1995.
80. Beltran J, Simon DC, Katz W, Weis LD. Increased MR signal intensity in skeletal muscle adjacent to malignant tumors: pathologic correlation and clinical relevance. Radiology 162:251–255, 1987.
81. Hanna SL, Fletcher BD, Parham DM, Bugg MF. Muscle edema in musculoskeletal tumors: MR imaging characteristics and clinical significance. J Magn Reson Imaging 1:441–449, 1991.

3
Biopsy: Indications and Techniques for Soft-Tissue Masses

Terrance D. Peabody
University of Chicago
Chicago, Illinois

I. INTRODUCTION

Ideally, the evaluation and treatment of a patient with a soft-tissue mass would involve a systematic approach, including a thorough history, careful physical examination, and useful imaging studies. Such an approach would yield a short list of potential diagnoses, and the performance of a biopsy would lead to an accurate diagnosis. The result of the cytologic and histologic analysis, when combined with knowledge of both the local and distant extent of the tumor, would allow an estimation of the patient's prognosis, determine the nature and scope of the operative intervention, and define the role of additional therapies, such as chemotherapy and radiation therapy [1,2].

Unfortunately, however, in practice, the clinical evaluation of a patient with a soft-tissue mass is often inaccurate [3]. This is especially true of small masses, asymptomatic masses, or masses that have been present for a long time. The patient often has a poor recollection of events, such as the duration of the mass, and is often unable to report reliably any changes in size. In many cases, a vague and misleading history of trauma is given. More worrisome, some malignant tumors are present for a long period, often many years, without causing symptoms that would prompt medical attention. For the physician, palpation of a soft-tissue mass is an inaccurate indicator of tumor size and depth. In addition, unlike the situation with bone tumors, imaging tests are often nonspecific [4]. Finally, the majority of soft-tissue tumors are posttraumatic, inflammatory, or benign and require no intervention. The difficulty, then, is in differentiating these masses from the relatively rare, but potentially lethal, malignant tumors, such as soft-tissue sarcomas and lymphomas.

Given the problems with clinical evaluation, often the only manner in which to differentiate a benign from a malignant soft-tissue tumor is to perform a biopsy. This means that in many cases biopsies will be performed by practitioners who have little or no experience in the management of soft-tissue malignancies and who will not ultimately be responsible for the care of the patient. Similarly, the interpreting pathologist, who may only see one musculoskeletal sarcoma per year, will often be called on to give an opinion (5). It is obvious that a directed and focused discussion regarding the biopsy of soft-tissue masses is important (6,7).

II. GENERAL CONSIDERATIONS AND INDICATIONS FOR BIOPSY

Technically speaking, a biopsy is a deceptively simple procedure (3). However, an understanding of the indications for biopsy, the specific technique recommended, the anatomical site selected, and the interpretation of the result have serious implications and require extensive training and experience. A biopsy is necessary when a soft-tissue mass is suspected of being a malignant tumor. Biopsies may be open procedures or closed percutaneous procedures. Open biopsies may be incisional (removal of part of the tumor) or excisional (removal of the entire tumor). Closed biopsies may include fine-needle aspiration cytology and trephine procedures.

Currently, there is an emphasis on limb-preserving surgery for malignant soft-tissue tumors of the extremities. This involves a multidisciplinary approach in which diagnostic radiologists, pathologists, surgeons, radiation oncologists, and medical oncologists participate (8). Communication among these specialists is important prior to the biopsy for outlining of the differential diagnosis, improving the interpretation of the biopsy, and outlining a treatment strategy (1).

It is important to note that the biopsy should be performed as a final step in patient evaluation. All local imaging studies should be performed prior to the biopsy (1,5). The reasons for this are that the clinical and radiographic features will narrow the list of possible diagnoses and facilitate a more accurate pathologic interpretation of the biopsy material. In addition, an accurate measurement of tumor size and depth can be made based on preoperative imaging. Imaging will also assist the person performing the biopsy to identify the most accessible site for the procedure. More importantly, the biopsy may degrade local imaging by superimposing postprocedural artifact in the form of local trauma, inflammation, and hematoma formation (Fig. 1). Finally, imaging prior to the biopsy may reveal the diagnosis, as is the case with many lipomas, and a biopsy may prove unnecessary (Fig. 2A, B).

Tumors larger than a few centimeters or located below the fascia should be considered malignant until proven otherwise (4). Because of the rarity of soft-

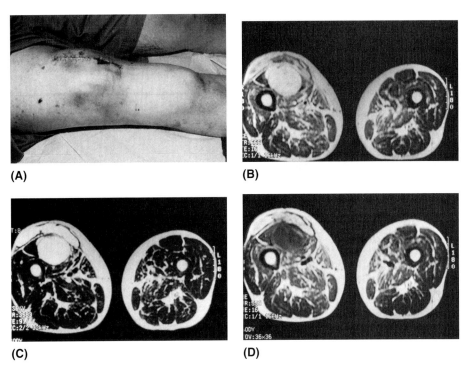

FIG. 1 Postoperative photograph (A) following a large incisional biopsy of an anterior thigh mass complicated by significant hematoma formation and contamination of the subcutaneous tissue of the anterior and distal thigh. (B–D) Photographs taken of magnetic resonance images performed after in-office incisional biopsy of a soft-tissue mass. The T1'- (B), T2'- (C), and T1-weighted gadolinium-enhanced (D) images demonstrate remaining tumor in the vastus medialis, with more superficial extensive hematoma formation involving the subcutaneous tissue of the anterior and lateral thigh. The value of this imaging test in determining the precise extent of the tumor is degraded by postprocedural artifact.

tissue sarcomas and the emphasis on limb-sparing surgery requiring a multidisciplinary approach, it is recommended that patients with large or deep tumors be referred to a tertiary center prior to biopsy (4). However, given the large number of benign tumors, it is inevitable that most tumors will be biopsied outside tertiary centers. In order to prevent biopsy-related complications and possible adverse effects on limb salvage or survival, physicians must follow certain principles.

Although there is no consensus on what type of biopsy is best (3,9), an open incisional biopsy is a common method of obtaining tissue for histologic evaluation and is recommended over excision for any suspicious masses in the retroperitoneum or extremities (10). The risks and problems encountered in a second operation for removal of the tumor are outweighed by the difficulties posed by an

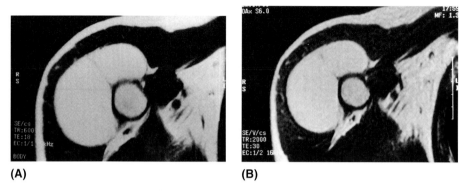

(A)   **(B)**

FIG. 2 (A) Photograph of a T1-weighted magnetic resonance image of a large shoulder mass in a 60-year-old man. The mass is homogeneous and has signal characteristics identical to those of normal subcutaneous fat. (B) Photograph of a T2-weighted image from the same individual. The mass, similarly, is homogeneous and has signal characteristics identical to those of surrounding subcutaneous fat as well as axillary fat. This was considered to be characteristic of a benign intramuscular lipoma, and no further intervention was required.

inadequate marginal excision of a deep soft-tissue sarcoma (11). An incisional biopsy allows for removal of sufficient tissue, not only for histologic evaluation but for related studies such as cytogenetics, molecular genetics, immunohistochemistry, electron microscopy, and flow cytometry (12). An open incisional biopsy is superior to needle aspiration cytology or trephine biopsy in determining tumor grade and histology (12). Tumor grade, a histologic estimate of metastatic potential based on cellular atypia, frequency of mitoses, extent of necrosis, and differentiation, will determine, in many treatment centers, whether patients receive preoperative radiation and/or chemotherapy (8). An open incisional biopsy is also recommended when the differential diagnosis is wide and varied because, in most cases, it will obtain representative tissue thus minimizing the sampling errors seen with more limited biopsy techniques (7). The accuracy rate of open incisional biopsy is reported to be 96% (13).

Open excisional biopsy, also known as marginal excision, is an operative procedure best reserved for patients in whom preoperative clinical evaluation and imaging show the tumor to be benign, such as a lipoma, or very small (less than 3 cm) (Fig. 3A–F). Additional treatment in the form of reoperation or radiation therapy may be necessary when the pathologic evaluation of these excised tumors reveals evidence of malignancy. An excisional biopsy carries the highest accuracy. However, it is not recommended in the management of most soft-tissue masses because, except for lipomas, preoperative imaging cannot differentiate benign from malignant tumors.

Of increasing popularity are more limited biopsy techniques performed percutaneously in the form of fine-needle aspiration cytology or trephine biopsy (Tru-cut, Baxter Healthcare, Valencia, CA). The advantages of these techniques are the low risk of complications (hematoma and infection), little or no need for anesthesia or analgesia, avoidance of hospitalization, cost reduction, minimal tumor contamination, and rapid interpretation of the results (14). In addition, closed biopsy techniques can be combined with imaging techniques for accurate biopsy of deep-seated tumors, such as those in the pelvis or about the spine (7) (Fig. 4). However, an accurate interpretation of a limited biopsy sample is more difficult than that of one obtained from an open procedure and requires extensive training and experience. These techniques are not recommended in centers that only occasionally encounter these types of tumors.

Trephine biopsies use a cannulated needle with an inner trocar and specimen notch obtaining a core of tissue, which in many cases preserves not only the cell type but also the cellular architecture. This allows a determination of histology and tumor grade. This determination would obviously be most important in those treatment centers where preoperative chemotherapy or radiation might be used. Core biopsies were noted to have greater than 80% accuracy in the few studies investigating soft-tissue tumors (2,13). As with any limited biopsy technique, caution should be exercised in the interpretation of cystic or myxomatous tumors. In two studies, only one complication—an infection—was noted. The cost related to a core biopsy was $1106, compared with $7234 for an incisional biopsy performed in the operating room (13).

First developed in a musculoskeletal center that did not alter its operative or adjuvant management based on tumor histology or grade, aspiration cytology from fine-needle biopsies became important in the diagnosis and management of soft-tissue tumors (14). Fine-needle aspiration cytology is at least 90% accurate in differentiating benign from malignant soft-tissue tumors (15). It is a minimally invasive procedure with very few complications. In one large study, fine-needle aspiration was found correctly to diagnose malignancy in 66 of 74 patients and to diagnose benign tumors correctly in 260 of 271 patients. It was nondiagnostic in 4 sarcomas and 16 benign tumors. In only two instances did a false diagnosis lead to an altered outcome. In addition, fine-needle aspiration cytology is a reliable method for diagnosing local recurrence or metastasis and is especially helpful in the evaluation of aspirated fluid from cystic masses when combined with diagnostic ultrasound (16). The limitation of fine-needle aspiration, in addition to lack of familiarity on the part of many interpreting physicians dealing with soft-tissue masses, has to do with the inability to sample small and deep-seated tumors (14). Also, malignant vascular tumors, spindle cell tumors, and benign lipoma variants, such as pleomorphic lipomas, spindle cell lipomas, hibernomas, and lipoblastomas, pose diagnostic difficulties. In approximately 75% of cases, grade can be estimated, but grade and a reliable histologic diagnosis are better obtained

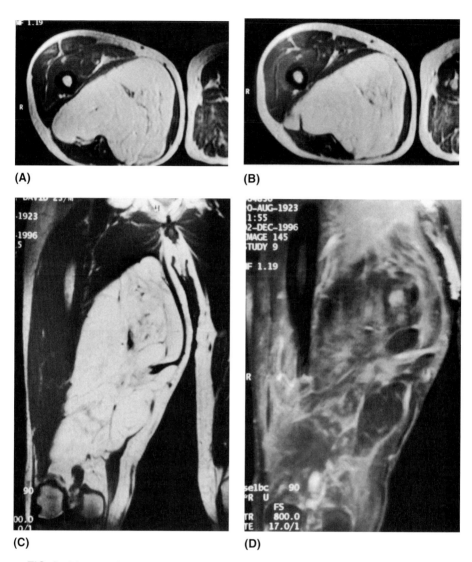

FIG. 3 Photographs of T1- (A) and T2- (B) weighted magnetic resonance images through the thigh of a 65-year-old man with a very large adductor mass of the thigh. The mass is homogeneous, and signals are identical to those of surrounding subcutaneous fat. Photographs in coronal section of T1-weighted (C) and fat suppression (D) images of the same large intramuscular mass, showing that the mass remains essentially homogeneous with a few fine septations and trapped muscle. This uniformly suppresses the fat suppression image. (E) Intraoperative photograph showing the large encapsulated mass as it is being marginally excised from the thigh. (F) Photograph of the gross specimen of the marginally resected intramuscular lipoma of the thigh. A few muscle fibers can be seen on the surface; however, because the preoperative imaging studies are consistent with a benign lipoma, the lesion was resected in the plane of its capsule.

60

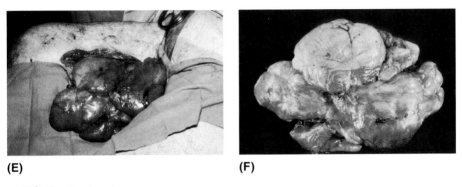

(E) **(F)**

FIG. 3 *Continued*

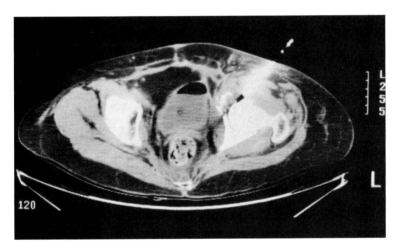

FIG. 4 Photograph of a CT scan showing the placement of a core needle into a soft-tissue mass about the anterior hip for diagnostic biopsy.

with trephine or open biopsies. An additional limitation historically, but one that is becoming less problematic as new techniques evolve, is the performance of pathologic studies such as flow cytometry, electron microscopy, and immuno-histochemistry.

Because of the sample size, a positive report of a fine-needle aspiration is more valuable than a negative report. When a negative report is received but the mass appears suspicious, an open procedure can subsequently be performed in most cases without difficulty. For that reason, in many centers fine-needle aspiration or trephine biopsy is performed often on the first visit, with open procedures scheduled at a later time if the closed procedure is nondiagnostic.

III. SPECIFIC BIOPSY TECHNIQUES

Regardless of the type of biopsy selected, certain principles must be followed so that representative tissue is obtained and complications that would threaten a patient's limb or life are avoided. First, the procedure must be performed with an aseptic technique to prevent infection. Second, the site of the biopsy must be in a tumor region that can later be excised en bloc with the underlying tumor (Fig. 5A–C). The surgeon must have knowledge of various soft-tissue flaps utilized in both limb-sparing and amputation procedures to avoid contamination of these flaps with tumor. If a pathologist or radiologist is performing the procedure, the surgeon must communicate the preferred biopsy site to those individuals.

Most often, based on preoperative imaging, the biopsy should be placed at the vertex of the tumor, away from vital nerve or vascular structures of the limb. In the upper extremity, the medial neurovascular bundle consisting of the brachial artery, vein, ulnar nerve, and median nerve should be avoided. In the lower ex-

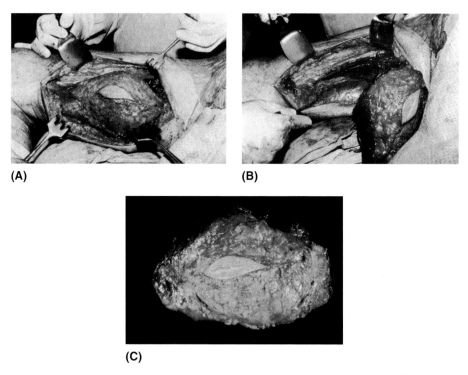

(A)   **(B)**

(C)

FIG. 5   Intraoperative photographs (A, B) and postoperative gross photograph (C) of a resected soft-tissue sarcoma from the right groin. The biopsy tract, including subcutaneous fat and fascia, was resected en bloc with the underlying tumor specimen.

tremity, the biopsy site should be located at a distance from the sciatic nerve posteriorly and the superficial femoral artery and vein anteriorly. In addition, the biopsy site should not be placed over major tendon insertions (tibial tuberosity) and should not pass through a joint (Fig. 6A–D). It should proceed directly through skin, fascia, and muscle. The deep surface of the tumor should not be violated. In cases where an open biopsy is necessary, the incision should be oriented longitudinally in the limb, as this will facilitate en bloc excision of the biopsy site with the underlying tumor. Transverse incisions on the extremities are to be avoided (Fig. 7). In addition, contamination of anatomical compartments not involved by the tumor should be avoided either by direct surgical intervention or by hematoma formation (Fig. 8). This means that hematomas must be prevented either by pressure or cauterization in an open technique. If a drain is to be used, it should be placed in line with and close to the operative incision (Fig. 9).

The use of tourniquets is controversial largely for theoretical reasons. A tourniquet facilitates the biopsy procedure and allows visualization of the muscle because it turns from red to a salmon color as the tumor pseudocapsule is approached. However, if a tourniquet is used, it must be deflated prior to wound closure to ensure hemostasis and to prevent hematoma formation.

A. Open Incisional Biopsy

Open incisional biopsy is the safest and most reliable means of making the diagnosis in both benign and malignant soft-tissue tumors. The incision should be as small as is compatible with obtaining an adequate tumor specimen. After the incision, dissection should be sharp, proceeding through muscle directly without developing skin or fascial flaps (9,17). Often, a color change from red to salmon heralds the approach of the tumor pseudocapsule. Malignant tumors are usually gray or white. The best tissue to be sampled lies in the area of the pseudocapsule–tumor interface because the periphery of the tumor is the most viable section. It is best to avoid the central, more necrotic areas in malignant tumors.

Sharp techniques are used to avoid crushing of the tumor specimen. Frozen section should be performed in all cases if possible. This allows confirmation of representative and adequate pathologic material, even if definitive surgery is not planned. Meticulous hemostasis is essential for the prevention of tumor spread by hematoma. This requires careful use of electrocautery and physical adjuvants. The wound should be closed in multiple layers so that hemorrhage is contained. Drains may be used but must be placed close to and in line with the incision to allow future excision of the drain site along with the tumor bed. An outside-in technique for placement of the drain is preferable. A stab wound is made in line with the incision, and the drain is introduced into the biopsy site in a retrograde manner with a hemostat. Widespread infiltration of a local anesthetic agent or sutures placed some distance from the wound increase contamination and should not be used.

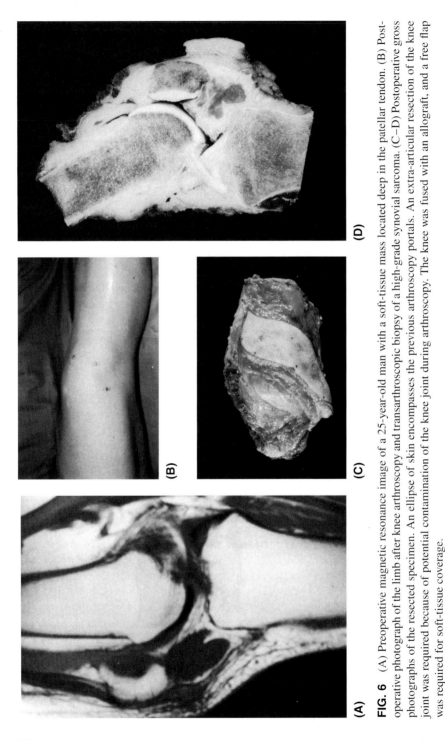

FIG. 6 (A) Preoperative magnetic resonance image of a 25-year-old man with a soft-tissue mass located deep in the patellar tendon. (B) Post-operative photograph of the limb after knee arthroscopy and transarthroscopic biopsy of a high-grade synovial sarcoma. (C–D) Postoperative gross photographs of the resected specimen. An ellipse of skin encompasses the previous arthroscopy portals. An extra-articular resection of the knee joint was required because of potential contamination of the knee joint during arthroscopy. The knee was fused with an allograft, and a free flap was required for soft-tissue coverage.

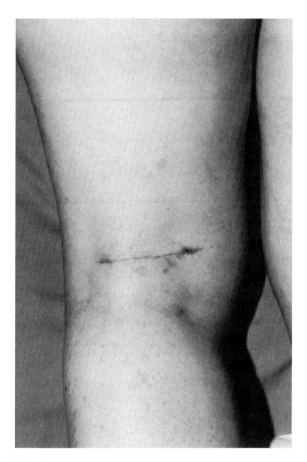

FIG. 7 Postoperative photograph after a myxoid liposarcoma was excisionally biopsied through a transverse incision of the popliteal fossa. This biopsy site is difficult to resect. Longitudinal incisions are recommended in the biopsy of extremity tumors.

Antibiotic therapy may be administered after the collection of pathologic specimens for bacterial, fungal, and acid-fast culture if infection is suspected. The use of a tourniquet during the biopsy procedure allows better visualization and minimizes intraoperative blood loss. The limb must not be forcibly exsanguinated prior to the biopsy. The tourniquet should be released prior to wound closure.

Surgery may proceed immediately if the clinical, radiographic, and pathologic diagnoses coincide and the patient and surgeon are prepared. Any discrepancies should prompt the surgeon to await a final pathology report. In benign soft-tissue tumors that require only a marginal excision, such as lipomas or hemangiomas, the excision may be performed through the biopsy incision after closure

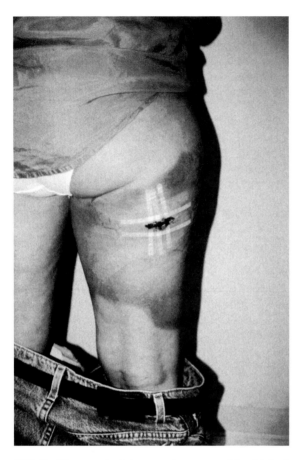

FIG. 8   Photograph of the posterior aspect of the thigh of a woman who, one week prior, underwent an open excisional biopsy of a malignant mesenchymoma from the soft tissues of the posterior thigh. The biopsy was performed in an office through a transverse incision and without the availability of electrocautery. This resulted in a significant hematoma occupying the entire posterior and medial aspect of the thigh, as well as resulting in an open wound as this hematoma liquefied. A wide local excision was performed with a free flap, and radiation therapy was advised because of potential contamination of the surrounding soft tissues.

of what is available of the pseudocapsule of the tumor. This minimizes any potential contamination of the incision bed. If immediate surgery is to be performed for a malignant tumor, it is important to close the wound carefully and to seal the incision with an adhesive barrier. The extremity is then reprepped and draped, and gowns and gloves, as well as instruments, are changed (3).

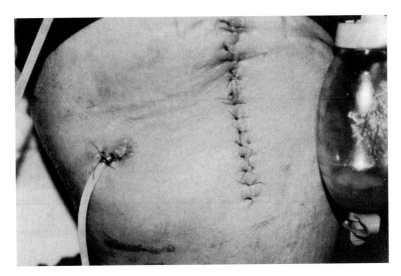

FIG. 9 Photograph of the right thigh of a 56-year-old woman after an excisional biopsy of an unsuspected myxoid liposarcoma. The operative drain is placed well away from the biopsy site. The drain site was included in the reresection, which required a transabdominal flap for adequate coverage. It is recommended that drains be placed in line and close to the biopsy incision.

B. Excisional Biopsy

An open excisional biopsy is recommended only for very small tumors (less than 3 cm) or in cases where the preoperative MRI is diagnostic of a lipoma. In these cases, again, a longitudinal incision is made that is long enough to facilitate removal of the tumor. The mass is then dissected in the interface between the tumor capsule and the surrounding normal soft tissue. After the mass is mobilized from the surrounding soft tissue and removed, careful hemostasis is maintained. Radiopaque markers, such as metallic vascular clips, are often used to mark the intraoperative margins of the resection. In a fashion similar to that of the incisional biopsy, the wound should be closed in multiple layers and drains kept in line with the incision and close to the operative wound. If pathologic evaluation shows evidence of a malignancy, then additional treatment in the form of reoperation or radiation may be necessary.

C. Trephine Core Biopsy

The trephine core biopsy procedure utilizes a cannulated trocar system that allows cores of tissue to be obtained with preservation of the architecture of the specimen. Because of the heterogeneity of many soft-tissue tumors, this can be especially helpful in making a diagnosis. The system includes a 14-gauge cannulated needle with an inner trocar and specimen notch (Fig. 10A–F). After preparation of the skin and infiltration of a local anesthetic agent, a no. 11 blade is used to incise the skin 2–3 mm in length (Figs. 11–13). The Tru-cut is then placed in the tumor bed. There are markings on the sheath of the cannulated needle to allow the person performing the biopsy to place it at the correct depth based on preprocedural imaging. The outer cannula sheath is then retracted, exposing the inner trocar tip in the specimen notch (Fig. 14). The outer cannula is then sharply advanced, trapping an inner core of tissue (Fig. 15). This procedure is repeated, with approximately three cores of tissue made available for pathologic review (Fig. 16). The specimens are processed in formalin or in glutaraldehyde. Frozen sections may be performed (Fig. 17). Pressure is maintained over the biopsy site for several minutes to minimize hematoma formation. A sterile strip or bandage is applied. In our institution, we have obtained good results with a slight modification of this technique. The modification is to enter the tumor with the outer cannula retracted, perforating it only with the sharp tip of the needle and the exposed specimen notch. The outer cannula is then advanced, trapping the tissue. The rest of the procedure is as described.

D. Fine-Needle Aspiration

Fine-needle aspiration cytologic analysis is most valuable in superficial soft-tissue masses. It is also valuable in the evaluation of local recurrence or lymphatic extension of a soft-tissue tumor. The pathologist or cytologist relies on clumps of cells or single cells to make a diagnosis. Obviously, accuracy is greater in homogeneous than in inhomogeneous tumors. The interpreting physician must be experienced in bone and soft-tissue cytology. Despite the limited nature of the procedure, the importance of biopsy site and of potential contamination are as serious a consideration with fine-needle aspiration as with any other biopsy procedure.

After preparation of the skin, a 0.8-mm-diameter needle (22-gauge) is used to make serial aspirations of the tumor bed through a single entry site. This is performed under aseptic technique and usually at the palpable vertex of the lesion. The deep tumor border is avoided (18). A specimen is prepared immediately by the cytology technician in attendance, and the tissues are fixed according to the preference of the cytologist. This may involve placing aspirates in ethanol for hematoxylin-eosin examination or air-drying and staining the specimens with Grunwald-Giemsa stain. Pressure is maintained at the biopsy site to minimize hematoma formation.

E. Tissue Preparation and Postbiopsy Care

Regardless of the specific biopsy technique used, communication between the person performing the biopsy and the pathologist is essential. The pathologist must

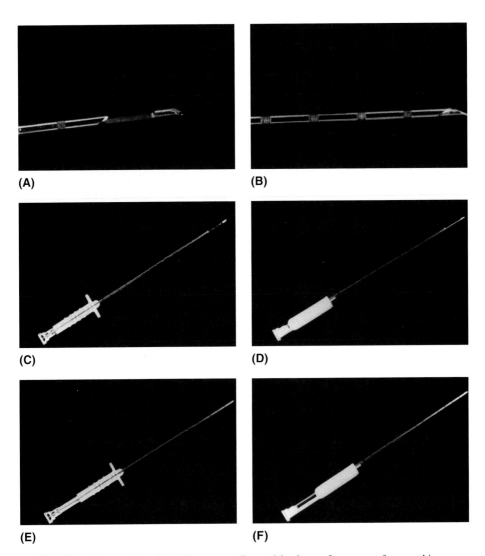

(A)   (B)

(C)   (D)

(E)   (F)

FIG. 10 Photographs of the Tru-cut needle used in the performance of a core biopsy. Parts A and B demonstrate the markings on the sheath to determine depth of penetration. Part A demonstrates the outer sheath in a retracted position, and Part B the outer sheath in a closed position. Parts C–F are photographs of the Tru-cut needle in frontal and lateral planes with the outer cannula retracted (C, D) exposing the underlying specimen notch, and then advanced, closing (E, F) that specimen notch.

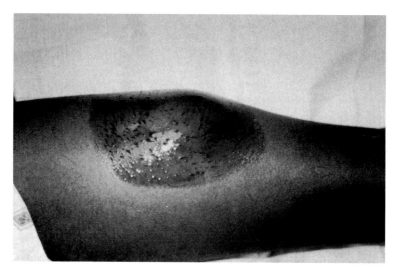

FIG. 11 Gross photograph of a thigh mass in a 21-year-old man after the skin was pre-pared with Betadine.

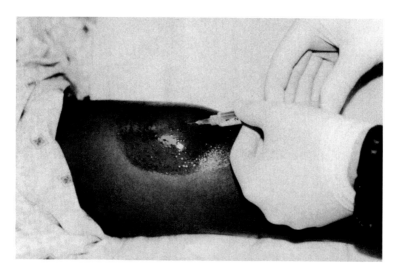

FIG. 12 The skin and region to be biopsied are infiltrated with local anesthetic under ster-ile conditions.

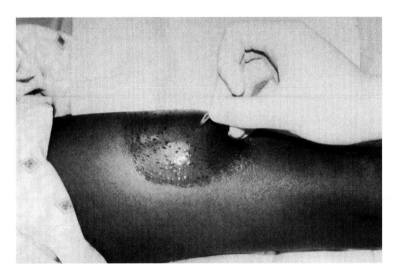

FIG. 13 The site is incised longitudinally 2–3 mm to allow passage of the Tru-cut needle.

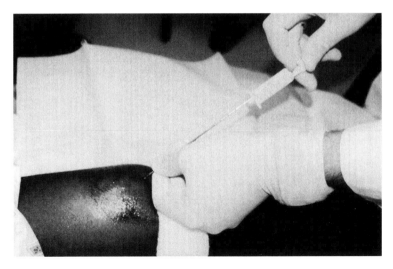

FIG. 14 The Tru-cut needle is then placed within the tumor bed with the outer cannula retracted to expose the inner specimen notch.

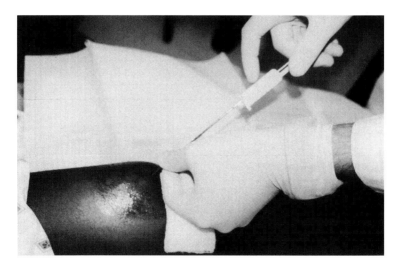

FIG. 15 The cannula is then advanced, trapping tissue within the specimen notch.

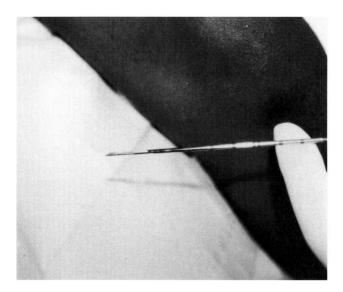

FIG. 16 Removing the Tru-cut needle in a closed position and then retracting the outer cannula, exposing the tissue which has been trapped in the specimen notch.

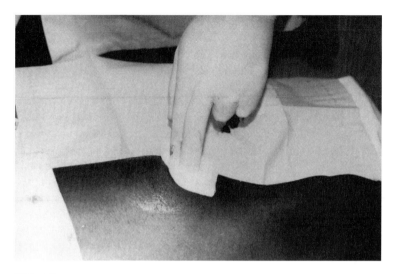

FIG. 17 Pressure is applied to the site for several minutes to minimize hematoma formation.

be aware of the most likely diagnosis based on the clinical and radiographic findings. This allows useful interpretation of frozen sections and ensures that tissue is preserved for future testing. In addition to paraffin fixation, tissue may be frozen or placed in glutaraldehyde for electron microscopy, cytogenetic study, and cell culture. Because infection is often misinterpreted as tumor or vice versa, biopsy specimens should also be examined for aerobic, anaerobic, fungal, and acid-fast bacillus culture in cases where the cause is indeterminate.

After the biopsy, as with all invasive procedures, limb swelling, edema, and bleeding must be minimized. In procedures requiring an open approach, a sterile compressive dressing is applied with the involved portion of the limb immobilized to allow soft-tissue healing and to minimize hematoma formation. The limb is elevated to minimize edema. The weight bearing status or activity status is usually determined based on the amount of soft tissue resected. After a fine-needle aspiration or Tru-cut biopsy, activity is generally allowed as the patient tolerates it. After an open biopsy, activity is commonly restricted to no active or passive motion of the underlying muscle for 1–2 weeks. Good nutrition is encouraged. Adjuvant therapy in the form of chemotherapy or radiation therapy can be administered immediately to patients who have percutaneous biopsies but must await wound healing in those having an open biopsy.

IV. HAZARDS OF BIOPSY

As stated earlier, a biopsy is a technically simple procedure, but one that requires a great deal of thought, knowledge, and experience. Poorly placed or poorly performed biopsy, or postbiopsy complications, may risk the surgeon's ability to preserve a limb and possibly may compromise survival (19). Complications include hematoma, infection, wound dehiscence, tumor contamination of vital anatomical structures, and tumor fungation through the biopsy site (2). An open biopsy, be it incisional or excisional, has a higher risk of these complications than does a closed biopsy (3) (Fig. 18A, B). One must also consider the scheduling, time, and cost of an open biopsy as compared to a closed biopsy and the delay that an open biopsy presents in receiving adjuvant therapy if that is necessary. Closed biopsy has a small risk of biopsy-related complications. The main hazard with closed biopsy is insufficient tissue to make a diagnosis or sampling error resulting in an inaccurate diagnosis.

Several studies have shown that there is an increased risk of biopsy-related complications affecting patient outcome if biopsies are done for malignant soft-tissue tumors outside tertiary referral centers. In one study, major diagnostic errors, defined as errors that alter patient management, were reported in 18% of patients (6). Those requiring an alteration in the type of operative procedure that the patient underwent or the use of adjuvant therapy occurred in 19% of patients. A change in the type of operation resulting in increased disability, local recurrence, and death was reported in 17% of patients with soft-tissue malignancies. There

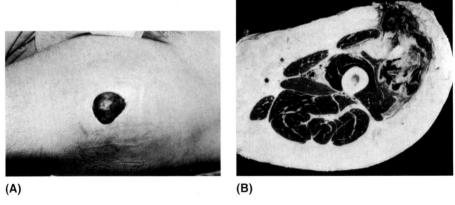

(A)   **(B)**

FIG. 18 (A) Postoperative photograph taken one week after open biopsy of a high-grade synovial sarcoma of the thigh in a 34-year-old man, demonstrating that the wound is separated and tumor is fungating through it. (B) Gross photograph of the amputated limb, demonstrating that the tumor has grown through the biopsy site, exiting the skin.

were 18 "unnecessary" amputations because of biopsy-related complications. There was a 2–12 times greater rate of error, complications, and changes in patient treatment course and outcome when biopsies were done outside the referral center. Although this study included both bone and soft-tissue malignancies, 40% of cases involved soft-tissue tumors, and the authors noted that soft-tissue tumors were more problematic than bone lesions. In patients biopsied largely in community hospitals, there was a closed biopsy error rate, including incorrect diagnosis and nondiagnostic tissue, in 40% of patients. This was contrasted with 24% of patients who had open biopsies. The authors noted, however, that the rate of altered outcomes was lower for those with closed biopsies, indicating that open biopsies and their related complications had a greater impact on the functional outcome and on the management of the patient. Interestingly, this study was compared to the same study done 10 years earlier by the same authors, and no change had been seen after 10 years of fairly intensive education (19). An additional study showed an increased rate of local recurrence in patients who were biopsied prior to referral to a tertiary center of 35% compared to 13% in those who did not have a biopsy. Therefore, not only may the initial management be altered (in many cases amputations are performed that may not be necessary without a biopsy-related problem), but also patients with sarcomas who undergo intervention prior to referral are at high risk of local recurrence (20).

It is obvious, then, that biopsy of soft-tissue masses is difficult and is associated with complications that at times may affect both the ability to preserve a limb or save a life. Biopsies should be performed by experienced physicians, and if the physician suspects that a soft-tissue mass represents an underlying malignancy, the patient should be referred to a tertiary center prior to biopsy.

V. CONCLUSION

In conclusion, biopsy of a soft-tissue lesion, although a technically simple procedure, requires preoperative planning and preparation as well as knowledge regarding the behavior and management of musculoskeletal neoplasms. The biopsy is as important as any other procedure that the patient is to undergo, and it is important to plan the biopsy as carefully as the resection. Careful anatomical site selection, hemostasis, and wound closure are imperative.

The goal in performing a biopsy is to obtain adequate tissue with minimal trauma. Percutaneous techniques, such as trephine or fine-needle aspiration, are increasingly popular and in some centers are associated with a high rate of diagnostic accuracy. Communication is essential among the surgeon, pathologist, radiologist, radiation therapist, and medical oncologist involved in the multidisciplinary management of these patients.

If the treating physician lacks experience in the diagnosis and management of soft-tissue tumors, it is recommended that prompt consultation with an experienced physician be undertaken. If a center is unequipped to perform the diagnostic studies, adjuvant treatment, and definitive surgery, it is best to refer that patient prior to the biopsy to avoid complications that may impact the ability to preserve life and limb (19). It is recommended that patients with large (more than 5 cm) or deep soft-tissue tumors having malignant characteristics should be referred to a physician competent in musculoskeletal oncology.

REFERENCES

1. Peabody TD, Gibbs CP, Jr, Simon MA. Evaluation and staging of musculoskeletal neoplasms. J Bone Joint Surg 80A:1204–1218, 1998.
2. Serpell JW, Pitcher ME. Pre-operative core biopsy of soft-tissue tumours facilitates their surgical management. Aust NZ J Surg 68:345–349, 1998.
3. Simon MA. Biopsy of musculoskeletal tumors. J Bone Joint Surg Am 64:1253–1257, 1982.
4. Simon MA, Biermann JS. Biopsy of bone and soft-tissue lesions. J Bone Joint Surg 75A:616–621, 1993.
5. Van Geel AN, Van Unnik JAM, Keus RB. Diagnosis and treatment of soft tissue tumours: the Dutch nationwide-accepted consensus. Sarcoma 2:183–191, 1998.
6. Mankin HJ, Lange TA, Spanier SS. The hazards of biopsy in patients with malignant primary bone and soft-tissue tumors. J Bone Joint Surg Am 64:1121–1127, 1982.
7. Springfield DS, Rosenberg A. Editorial: Biopsy: complicated and risky. J Bone Joint Surg Am 78:639–643, 1996.
8. Peabody TD, Simon MA. Principles of staging of soft-tissue sarcomas. Clin Orthop Rel Res 289:19–31, 1993.
9. Shives TC. Biopsy of soft-tissue tumors. Clin Orthop Rel Res 289:32–35, 1993.
10. Lawrence W Jr. Operative management of soft tissue sarcomas: impact of anatomic site. Semin Surg Oncol 10:340–346, 1994.
11. Temple WJ, Bramwell V, Eisenhauer E, Jenkin RDT, Langer F, Worth AJ. Guidelines for the surgical management of soft-tissue sarcoma. Report of the Canadian sarcoma group. Can J Surg 31:410–412, 1988.
12. Huvos AG. The importance of the open surgical biopsy in the diagnosis and treatment of bone and soft-tissue tumors. Hematol Oncol Clin North Am 9:541–544, 1995.
13. Skrzynski MC, Biermann JS, Montag A, Simon MA. Diagnostic accuracy and charge-savings of outpatient core needle biopsy compared with open biopsy of musculoskeletal tumors. J Bone Joint Surg Am 78:644–649, 1996.
14. Akerman M. Fine-needle aspiration cytology of soft tissue sarcoma: benefits and limitations. Sarcoma 2:155–161, 1998.
15. Rydholm A. Soft tissue lesions in adults: Biopsy—yes or no? Ann Oncol 3:S57–S58, 1992.

16. Lange TA, Austin CW, Seibert JJ, Angtuaco TL, Yandow DR. Ultrasound imaging as a screening study for malignant soft-tissue tumors. J Bone Joint Surg Am 69:100–105, 1987.

17. Peabody TD, Simon MA. Making the diagnosis: keys to a susccessful biopsy in children with bone and soft-tissue tumors. Orthop Clin North Am 27:453–460, 1996.

18. Rydholm A. Management of patients with soft-tissue tumors. Strategy developed at a regional oncology center. Acta Orthop Scand 54(Suppl 203):54:1–77, 1983.

19. Mankin HJ, Mankin CJ, Simon MA. The hazards of biopsy, revisited. J Bone Joint Surg Am 78:656–663, 1996.

20. Thompson RC, Hartman R, Swanson P, Dusenbury K. Local recurrence and survival in soft tissue sarcomas: the relation of biopsy. Chir Organi Mov 75(Suppl N1):131–133, 1990.

4
Classification and Histologic Grading of Soft-Tissue Tumors

Mary A. Furlong
Armed Forces Institute of Pathology
Washington, DC

Elizabeth Montgomery
The Johns Hopkins University
Baltimore, Maryland

I. CLASSIFICATION

Soft-tissue tumors represent a unique and heterogeneous group of neoplastic and nonneoplastic entities with a broad range of differentiation and clinical behavior. Historically, their classification into a logical and understandable system has been difficult and remains so. In general, soft-tissue tumors arise mainly form embryologic mesoderm, which includes muscle, adipose tissue, fibrous connective tissue, and vascular structures. Neuroectodermally derived components in the peripheral nervous system have also been traditionally included under the heading of soft-tissue tumors (1–3).

Stout, a pioneer in the world of soft tissue, was one of the first to classify these tumors based on their presumed histogenesis (2,3), recognizing at the time the complexity of such lesions: "If the various tumors developing from these tissues reproduced their prototypic tissues in pure form, albeit in various stages of differentiation, recognition [and possibly classification] would be relatively simple" (3). Stout's classification is somewhat of a prototype for modern schemes. His original classification has changed significantly with the addition of new categories and the refinement of others (Table 1).

The difficulty in classifying soft-tissue tumors, then and now, arises mainly from the fact that the cell of origin for many of these lesions remains unknown. The debate as to whether they arise from a pleuripotent primitive mesenchymal cell or from mature adult counterparts or neither is beyond the scope of this dis-

Table 1 Original Classification Headings of Soft-Tissue Tumors

Benign tumors
Fibroblastic tumors
Myxomatoses
Fibrous histiocytomas
Lipomatoses
Myomatoses
Angiomatoses
Other

Malignant tumors
Mesenchymal tumors
Tumors of muscle
Angiosarcomatoses
Lymphoid and reticuloid tumors
Other

Source: Modified from Stout. Atlas of tumor pathology, Fascicle 1. Armed Forces Institute of Pathology, 1967.

cussion. Suffice it to say that many authors deem it inappropriate to assign histogenesis (4,5). Furthermore, previous methods of grouping soft-tissue tumors have frequently been based on specific gross or microscopic features, thus producing a largely descriptive classification scheme (1). Such a descriptive classification is not directly useful to the clinician regarding biological behavior and prognosis. In addition, there are benign reactive and neoplastic processes that morphologically "look" malignant—another discrepancy that makes a descriptive classification scheme problematic. Some authors have categorized soft-tissue tumors according to aggressiveness or malignant potential as a guide to clinical management (6). Most current classifications are based on adult histologic differentiation or presumed histologic differentiation. A commonly used phrase is "line of differentiation," which implies the adult tissue or embryologic counterpart that the tumor mimics rather than implicating a specific cell of origin (1,4,7,10).

In addition to early classification schemes by Stout in 1952 (2), 1967 (3), and later revised in 1983 (8), the World Health Organization (WHO) published its first edition of Histological Typing of Soft Tissue Tumors in 1969 (9) under the auspices of the International Reference/Collaborating Center for the Histological Classification of Soft Tissue Tumors at the Armed Forces Institute of Pathology. This collaborative international effort, revised in 1994 (10), has devised a classification based primarily on microscopic features and line of differentiation. The above classification utilizes knowledge gained over the past decades through mod-

Table 2 Fibrous Tissue Tumors

Benign
- Fibroma
- Keloid
- Nodular fascitis
- Proliferative fascitis
- Proliferative myositis
- Elastofibroma
- Fibrous hamartoma of infancy
- Myofibromatosis
    Solitary
    Multicentric
- Fibromatosis colli
- Calcifying aponeurotic fibroma
- Hyalin fibromatosis

Fibromatosis
- Superficial
    Palmar and plantar
    Infantile digital
- Deep
    Abdominal (desmoid)
    Extra-abdominal
    Intra-abdominal and Mesenteric
    Infantile

Malignant
- Fibrosarcoma
    Adult
    Congenital or infantile

Source: Modified from Weiss SW. Histological typing of soft tissue tumours, 1994.

ern, ancillary techniques, such as immunohistochemistry. The degree to which these histochemical and cellular applications will aid in the diagnosis and hence the classification of soft-tissue tumors remains to be seen. Classification schemes will undoubtedly expand with new entities and will be redefined with emerging cellular characteristics. The WHO classification has 15 separate histologic soft-tissue categories, which will be referred to and briefly commented on in the following sections.

The first category of soft-tissue tumors includes lesions of fibrous tissue (Table 2), subcategorized into benign lesions, fibromatoses, and malignant lesions. Histologically, lesions in this category are variably composed of fibroblasts

Table 3   Fibrohistiocytic Tumours

Benign
- Fibrous histiocytoma
- Cutaneous histiocytoma
- Deep histiocytoma
- Juvenile xanthogranuloma
- Reticulohistiocytoma
- Xanthoma

Intermediate
- Atypical fibroxanthoma
- Dermatofibrosarcoma protuberans and Bednar tumour
- Giant cell fibroblastoma
- Plexiform fibrohistiocytic tumor
- Angiomatoid fibrous histiocytoma

Malignant
- Malignant fibrous histiocytoma
    Storiform/pleomorphic
    Myxoid
    Giant cell
    Xanthomatous/inflammatory

Source: Modified from Weiss SW. Histological typing of soft tissue tumours, 1994.

and myofibroblasts (5). Within the benign category are reactive, hamartomatous, and tumor-like lesions as well as benign fibrous tumors. The fibromatoses form a separate subcategory in the above classification, referring specifically to lesions that may recur but do not metastasize (10). Finally, malignant lesions include three fibrosarcomatous distinctions.

Fibrohistiocytic lesions head the second category (Table 3), and although possibly a misnomer (5,10) in reference to the line of differentiation, this category has been generally accepted by most pathologists. Along with benign lesions, an intermediate subcategory exists in regard to clinical behavior and includes such lesions as dermatofibrosarcoma protuberans and atypical fibroxanthoma. Malignant fibrous histiocytoma is listed along with its variants.

The classification of lipomatous tumors among pathologists is controversial. The above classification subcategorizes lipomatous tumors into benign and malignant entities (Table 4). However, terminology and categorization regarding atypical lipomatous tumors are the subject of much debate (6,10), and are not fully considered here. In addition, two relatively recently recognized lipoma variants,

Table 4 Lipomatous Tumors

Benign
- Lipoma
- Lipoblastoma (fetal lipoma)
- Lipomatosis
- Angiolipoma
- Spindle cell lipoma
- Pleomorphic lipoma
- Angiomyolipoma
- Myelolipoma
- Hibernoma
- Atypical lipoma

Malignant
- Well-differentiated liposarcoma
    Lipoma-like
    Sclerosing
    Inflammatory
- Myxoid liposarcoma
- Round cell liposarcoma
- Pleomorphic liposarcoma
- Differentiated liposarcoma

Source: Modified from Weiss SW. Histological typing of soft tissue tumours, 1994.

chondroid lipoma (11) and myolipoma (12), are not as yet considered in the WHO classification. It is worth mentioning that dedifferentiated liposarcoma has been added as a subtype of liposarcoma in view of its clinical aggressiveness and ability to metastasize (6,10). Also, some authors recognize spindle cell liposarcoma as a specific histologic variant (13).

It is interesting to note that in Stout's first classification (5) a single "myomatoses" category was implemented. Since then, muscle tumors have been categorized into smooth and skeletal types (Tables 5 and 6). Among the smooth muscle group, benign tumors include leiomyoma, which can occur in deep and superficial soft tissues (14), epithelioid leiomyoma, and angioleiomyoma (vascular leiomyoma). Angioleiomyoma has been further histologically classified as capillary or solid, cavernous, and venous by some authors (15). The last in the benign category is leiomyomatosis peritonealis disseminata (LPD), a tumor-like condition occurring in women. Leiomyosarcoma, a rare tumor of the soft tissues, is listed in the above classification with its epithelioid variant.

Table 5 Smooth Muscle Tumors

Benign
- Leiomyoma
- Angiomyoma
- Epithelioid leiomyoma
- Leiomyomatosis peritonealis disseminata

Malignant
- Leiomyosarcoma
- Epithelioid leiomyosarcoma

Source: Modified from Weiss SW. Histiological typing of soft tissue tumours, 1994.

Table 6 Skeletal Muscle Tumours

Benign
- Rhabdomyoma
  Adult
    Genital
  Fetal

Malignant
- Rhabdomyosarcoma
- Embryonal rhabdomyosarcoma
- Botryoid rhabdomyosarcoma
- Spindle cell rhabdomyosarcoma
- Alveolar rhabdomyosarcoma
- Pleomorphic rhabdomyosarcoma
- Rhabdomyosarcoma with ganglionic differentiation

Source: Modified from Weiss SW. Histological typing of soft tissue tumours, 1994.

Tumors of skeletal muscle compose the next category, including the benign rhabdomyoma and its variants as well as the malignant counterpart, rhabdomyosarcoma. Several histologic subtypes of the latter are listed in the WHO classification (Table 6). Further classification of these tumors with clinical and prognostic significance, especially in childhood, has been the goal of the Intergroup Rhabdomyosarcoma Study for many years (16). The reader is referred to the chapter on pediatric tumors for a more detailed description of these clinical and histologic entities.

Continuing to refer to the WHO classification, endothelial tumors of blood and lymph vessels are an extensive group of lesions ranging from the benign papillary endothelial hyperplasia to the malignant Kaposi's sarcoma and angiosarcoma

Table 7   Endothelial Tumors of Blood and Lymph Vessels

Benign
- Papillary endothelial hyperplasia
- Hemangioma
- Capillary hemangioma
- Cavernous hemangioma
- Venous hemangioma
- Epithelioid hemangioma
- Pyogenic granuloma
- Acquired tufted hemangioma
- Lymphangioma
- Lymphangiomyoma
- Lymphangiomyomatosis
- Angiomatosis
- Lymphangiomatosis

Intermediate
- Spindle cell hemangioendothelioma
- Endovascular papillary angioendothelioma (Dabska tumor)
- Epithelioid hemangioendothelioma

Malignant
- Angiosarcoma
- Lymphangiosarcoma
- Kaposi sarcoma

Source: Modified from Weiss SW. Histological typing of soft tissue tumours, 1994.

(Table 7). An intermediate group has been recently recognized (10) to include spindle cell hemangioendothelioma, endovascular papillary angioendothelioma, and epithelioid hemangioendothelioma, all entities behaving in a borderline to malignant fashion. Most observers believe that epithelioid hemangioendothelioma is frankly malignant, but recent series show that spindle cell hemangioendothelioma behaves in a benign fashion and thus this entity will probably ultimately be reclassified as "spindle cell hemangioma."

Perivascular tumors form their own category (Table 8) with benign and malignant varieties of hemangiopericytoma and glomus tumor.

Only the tenosynovial giant cell tumor is listed under the synovial tumor category in its benign and malignant subtypes (Table 9). "Synovial" sarcoma, a common adult soft-tissue tumor, is a misnomer (17) and classified under miscellaneous in the above classification scheme.

Table 10 lists tumors both of mesothelial origin and of submesothelial connective, tissue including solitary fibrous tumor of pleura and peritoneum as well

Table 8 Perivascular Tumors

Benign
- Benign hemangiopericytoma
- Glomus tumor

Malignant
- Malignant hemangiopericytoma
- Malignant glomus tumor

Source: Modified from Weiss SW. Histological typing of soft tissue tumours, 1994.

Table 9 Synovial Tumors

Benign
- Tenosynovial giant cell tumor
    Localized
    Diffuse

Malignant
- Malignant tenosynovial giant cell tumor

Source: Modified from Weiss SW. Histological typing of soft tissue tumours, 1994.

Table 10 Mesothelial Tumors

Benign
- Solitary fibrous tumor of pleura and peritoneum
- Multicystic mesothelioma
- Adenomatoid tumor
- Well-differentiated papillary mesothelioma

Malignant
- Malignant solitary fibrous tumor of pleura and peritoneum
- Diffuse mesothelioma
    Epithelial
    Spindle
    Biphasic

Source: Modified from Weiss SW. Histological typing of soft tissue tumours, 1994.

as benign and malignant variants of mesothelioma. Both benign and malignant forms of solitary fibrous tumor can occur in the soft tissues (18,19). The reader is referred to the appropriate chapter for a more comprehensive discussion of these interesting entities.

Table 11   Neural Tumors

Benign
- Traumatic neuroma
- Morton's neuroma
- Neuromuscular hamartoma
- Nerve sheath ganglion
- Schwannoma
- Plexiform schwannoma
- Cellular schwannoma
- Degenerated schwannoma
- Neurofibroma
    Diffuse
    Plexiform
    Pacinian
    Epithelioid
- Granular cell tumor
- Melanocytic schwannoma
- Neurothekeoma
- Ectopic meningioma
- Ectopic ependymoma
- Pigmented neuroectodermal tumor of infancy

Malignant
- Malignant peripheral nerve sheath tumor
- Malignant peripheral nerve sheath tumor with rhabdomyosarcoma
- Epithelioid malignant peripheral nerve sheath tumor
- Malignant granular cell tumor
- Clear cell sarcoma
- Malignant melanotic schwannoma
- Neuroblastoma
- Ganglioneuroblastoma

Source: Modified from Weiss SW. Histological typing of soft tissue tumours, 1994.

Neural tumors form a wide variety of hamartomatous, benign and malignant lesions listed in Table 11. Paraganglioma of soft tissues is recognized in the WHO classification, as are bony and chondroid lesions (Tables 12 and 13).

Pleuripotent mesenchymal tumors have been recognized since Stout's first description in 1948 (20). They form an interesting group of benign and malignant lesions having more than one line of differentiation, usually of lipomatous, myogenous, and osteocartilaginous origins (Table 14).

Finally, miscellaneous and unclassified tumors form the final categories of the WHO classification. Table 15 includes a diverse group of histologic entities as yet to be further classified.

Table 12   Paraganglionic Tumors

Benign
• Paraganglioma

Malignant
• Malignant paraganglioma

Source: Modified from Weiss SW. Histological typing of soft tissue tumours, 1994.

Table 13   Cartilage and Bone Tumors

Benign
• Panniculitis ossificans
• Myositis ossificans
• Fibrodysplasia ossificans progressiva
• Extraskeletal chondroma
• Extraskeletal osteochondroma
• Extraskeletal osteoma

Malignant
• Extraskeletal chondrosarcoma
• Well-differentiated chondrosarcoma
• Myxoid chondrosarcoma
• Mesenchymal chondrosarcoma
• Extraskeletal osteosarcoma

Source: Modified from Weiss SW. Histological typing of soft tissue tumours, 1994.

Table 14   Pluripotential Mesenchymal Tumors

Benign
• Mesenchymoma

Malignant
• Malignant mesenchymoma

Source: Modified from Weiss SW. Histological typing of soft tissue tumours, 1994.

II.   GRADING

Some of the same inherent, often controversial problems of classifying soft-tissue tumors are also problematic in devising a practical, useful, and reproducible grading system. Such a system is necessary and clinically applicable in terms of selecting patients for appropriate surgery and/or adjuvant therapy. Again, some

Table 15 Miscellaneous Tumors

Benign
• Congenital granular cell tumor
• Tumoral calcinosis
• Myxoma
    Cutaneous
    Intramuscular
• Angiomyxoma
• Amyloid tumor
• Parachordoma
• Ossifying fibromyxoid tumor
• Juvenile angiofibroma
• Inflammatory myofibroblastic tumor

Malignant
• Alveolar soft part sarcoma
• Epithelioid sarcoma
• Extraskeletal Ewing sarcoma
• Synovial sarcoma monophasic fibrous type
• Malignant extrarenal rhabdoid tumor
• Desmoplastic small cell tumor

Source: Modified from Weiss SW. Histological typing of soft tissue tumours, 1994.

authors do not advocate the grading of soft-tissue tumors (6). However, it is generally accepted that histologic grade is an important, significant prognostic parameter in regard to soft-tissue neoplasms (21–25). Most pathologists attempt to accurately diagnose and grade soft-tissue tumors based on regionally accepted histologic criteria. As previously mentioned, many soft-tissue tumor subtypes by definition are assigned a grade a priori. Overall, the rarity of soft-tissue tumors does not practically allow for separate grading criteria for each histologic soft-tissue subtype. Therefore, general grading systems have been devised and studied over the past two decades in order to establish histologic parameters as well as to correlate these parameters with prognosis, recurrence, metastasis-free and overall survival.

Markhede et al., using a four-grade system (21), found that histologic grade had a significant effect on risk of metastasis and survival. They also found that grade had a significant influence on local recurrence, although the most important factor relating to this issue was adequacy of the surgical procedure (21).

Myhre-Jensen followed with a study in 1983 correlating grade with survival using a three-tier grading system based primarily on mitotic index (22). Other factors considered as part of a mean score were cellularity, anaplasia, and necrosis. Overall survival rates for grades I, II, and III were 97%, 67%, and 38%, respectively (22). In 1990, Myhre-Jensen presented a second series of 278 patients with soft-tissue sarcomas, again supporting the significance of histologic grade as a strong prognostic factor (26).

Further studies in 1984 by Costa et al. at the National Cancer Institute (NCI) showed necrosis as the most important prognostic indicator for tumors grades II and III. Furthermore, necrosis was predictive of survival after the first recurrence (23). Prognostic factors included in the grading system are presented in Table 16. The three-grade system is based on absent (I), minimal (II), and moderate to massive (III) necrosis (Table 17). Overall survival rates were 100%, 73%, and 46%,

Table 16 National Cancer Institute Histopathologic Grading of Soft-Tissue Tumors

Histologic parameters
- Necrosis
- Cellularity
- Pleomorphism
- Mitosis

Grade
- I—Well-differentiated
- II—<15% necrosis (none or minimal)
- III—>15% necrosis (moderate or marked)

Source: Modified from Costa J, et al. *Cancer* 53:530–541, 1994.

Table 17 National Cancer Institute Three-Grade System

Grade I	Grade I–III
• Well-differentiated liposarcoma	• Leiomyosarcoma
• Myxoid liposarcoma	• Chondrosarcoma
• Dermatofibrosarcoma protuberans	• Malignant peripheral nerve sheath tumor
	• Hemangiopericytoma
Grade II–III	**Grade III**
• Round cell liposarcoma	• Ewing sarcoma
• Malignant fibrous histocytoma	• Rhabdomyosarcoma
• Clear cell sarcoma	• Osteosarcoma
• Angiosarcoma	• Alveolar soft part sarcoma
• Epithelioid sarcoma	• Synovial sarcoma
• Malignant granular cell tumor	
• Fibrosarcoma	

Source: Modified from Costa J, et al. *Cancer* 53:530–541, 1994.

respectively. Grade I tumors consistently had an excellent prognosis (20–24). Kulander et al. (27) presented results confirming necrosis as a predictor of survival.

Trojani et al. (24) used degree of differentiation, mitosis, and necrosis in their grading system, which also provided clinically significant prognostic information. Again, grade appears to be the most important prognostic factor of soft-tissue sarcomas. Coindre et al. (25), affiliated with the French Federation of Cancer Centres (FNCLCC), later tested the reproducibility of this grading system; overall agreement of tumor grade was 75%. This grading system is presented in Tables 18 and 19. A comparative study was done in 1997, using the grading systems of Costa (NCI) and Coindre, based on necrosis and mitotic counts, respectively, resulting in a slightly increased predictive utility in terms of distant metastasis and tumor mortality of the FNCLCC system (28).

The WHO does not necessarily advocate any one of the above grading systems but rather encourages the use of a regionally accepted system "in a stringent and consistent fashion" (10).

It is perhaps the ultimate goal in the grading of soft-tissue tumors to define a group of patients (such as those with grade II tumors) who may benefit from surgery alone or in combination with adjuvant therapy (29). It has been hypothesized

Table 18 French Federation of Cancer Centres

Histologic parameters
• Tumor differentiation
• Mitosis count
• Tumor necrosis

Grade
• I—Score 0–3
• II—Score 4–5
• III—Score 6–8

Source: Modified from Coindre JM, et al. *Cancer* 58:306–309, 1996.

Table 19 French Federation of Cancer Centres Scoring of Soft-Tissue Sarcomas

Score	Differentiation	Mitosis count	Necrosis
0			No necrosis
1	Well differentiated	0–9/field[a]	<50% necrosis
2	Uncertain histology	10–19/field	>50% necrosis
3	Poorly differentiated	>20/field	

[a] A field is 0.1734 mm^2.
Source: Modified from Coindre JM, et al. *Cancer* 58:306–309, 1996.

that proliferation markers and DNA analysis may play a role in this setting and in overall grading of soft-tissue tumors (29–31). Ki-67, a monoclonal antibody, identifies the nuclear antigen in proliferating cells in all phases of the cell cycle except G_o. Recently replacing Ki-67 is MIB-1, which can be utilized with paraffin-embedded tissue. Although several studies have examined the relationship of proliferative activity using Ki-67 and the prognosis of benign and malignant soft-tissue tumors (30), its exact relevance remains undetermined. AgNor counts (silver staining of nucleolar organizer regions) as well as mast cell counts in soft-tissue sarcomas have also been studied as additional factors in grade assessment (32). Tomita et al. (32) have shown both AgNor and mast cell counts to be prognostically significant by univariate analysis and the former significant as an independent prognostic factor by multivariate analysis. Further studies, however, are necessary to evaluate the role of proliferating markers, DNA analysis, and other molecular diagnostic techniques in the grading of soft-tissue tumors. As with histologic parameters, many of the above techniques also show intraobserver variation and inconsistent reproducibility.

It appears that overall the grade of soft-tissue tumors is prognostically significant (21–25,27). Despite the fact that numerous studies have been and continue to be done on this subject, grading remains somewhat of an enigma to many pathologists. Appropriate and adequate sampling, fixation and staining is necessary for accurate diagnosis and the subsequent grading of soft-tissue tumors.

III. CYTOGENETICS

As with many other tumor types, cytogenetic aberrations of soft-tissue tumors have been identified and continue to be studied. However, the role of molecular and cytogenetic abnormalities in soft-tissue tumors is yet to be clarified in terms of classification, diagnosis, and possible prognostication. Molecular studies of a variety of soft-tissue sarcomas have revealed several chromosomal defects, including amplified genes, mutated genes, novel gene products, and isolated deletions (33,34). Although in many cases these are nonspecific rearrangements, many specific chromosomal translocations have been identified (Table 20).

Many nonspecific chromosomal aberrations have been associated with soft-tissue tumors, including gene amplification and tumor suppressor gene mutations. Briefly, gene amplification is identifiable in the form of homogeneously staining regions (hsr) and double minutes (dmin) (33,34). Amplification, important in tumorogenesis, results in selective advantage of the tumor cell line (33). In many circumstances, the amplified gene interacts with a tumor suppressor gene, with the former inhibiting the function of the latter (33,34). Tumor suppressor genes relevant in soft-tissue tumors are the *TP53* gene and retinoblastoma gene (*RB1*). Altered expression of *RB1* has been reported in approximately half of soft-tissue sarcomas (35).

Table 20 Cytogenetic Abnormalities of Soft-Tissue Tumors

Tumor type	Chromosomal aberration	Involved genes
Clear cell sarcoma	t(12;22)(ql3;ql2),+8	*ATF1/EWS*
Chondrosarcoma		
(Extraskeletal myxoid)	t(9;22)(q22-q31;q12)	*TEC/EWS*
Desmoplastic small round	t(11;22)(p13;q12)	*WT1/EWS*
cell tumor		
Dermatofibrosarcoma protuberans	t(17;22)(q22;q15)	*COL1A1/PDGFB*
Ewing's sarcoma/PNET	t(11;22)(q24;q12)	*FLI1/EWS*
	t(21;22)(q22;q12)	ERG/EWS
	t(7;22)(p22;p12)	ETV1/EWS
Fibrosarcoma (infantile)	+8, +11, +17, +20	
Hemangiopericytoma	12q13-15	
Lipoma (ordinary)	t(3;12)(q27;q15)	*HMGI-C/LPP*
Liposarcoma (myxoid/round cell)	t(12;16)(q13;p11)	*CHOP/FUS*
	t(12;22)(q13;q12)	*CHOP/EWS*
Liposarcoma (well differentiated)	+r(12)	
Malignant fibrous histiocytoma	12q14-15 amplification	
(myxoid)		
Malignant fibrous histiocytoma	1q21-22 amplification	
(storiform)		
Malignant peripheral nerve	17p, 17q loss	
sheath tumor		
Rhabdomyosarcoma (alveolar)	t(2;13)(q35;q14)	*PAX3/FKHR*
	t(1;13)(p36;q14)	*PAX7/FKHR*
Rhabdomyosarcoma (embryonal)	+2, +8, +12, +20	
Synovial sarcoma	t(X;18)(p11;q11)	*SYT/SSX1 or SSX2*

Specific translocations, as previously mentioned, are known for a variety of soft-tissue tumors. Similarities are noted among several specific translocations for Ewing's sarcoma/primitive neuroectodermal tumor (PNET), t(11;22); clear cell sarcoma, t(12;22); and myxoid liposarcoma, t(12;16). There is gene fusion resulting in an RNA binding domain with a transcription factor gene (38). Other translocations of diagnostic relevance are t(X;18), present in synovial sarcomas, and t(2;13), characteristic of alveolar rhabdomyosarcoma (37–39). For example, poorly differentiated synovial sarcoma can be a diagnostic challenge by morphologic means alone. In a study by Sreekanhariah et al. (34), the t(X;18) was present in 90% of cases. It appears to be a diagnostic feature. Embryonal rhabdomyosarcoma and alveolar rhabdomyosarcoma each have distinct chromosomal abnormalities, numerical aberrations, and loss of p15 and the t(2;13) or t(1;13), respectively. Though often distinguishable clinically and morphologically, molecular genetics may aid in problematic cases. Other specific aberrant phenotypes may be useful in identifying small round blue cell tumors, including Ewing's sarcoma, PNET, neuroblastoma, and desmoplastic small round blue cell tumor (34). In addition, the detection of molecular abnormalities in primary tumors may provide the diagnostic link in the setting of metastatic disease.

IV. STAGING

Staging of any cancer describes its anatomical location and the extent of disease at the time of initial diagnosis. As one can imagine, the staging of soft-tissue sarcomas presents a set of unique problems given the rarity of these tumors, the wide variety of histologic types and anatomical locations, and, in some circumstances, the unpredictable biological behavior (37). Furthermore, the controversies surrounding histologic grade directly influence the stage of disease, as grade is prognostically the most important variable (21–25,27,38). The goals of any staging system should incorporate relevant prognostic factors and provide useful clinical information for the purposes of appropriate surgical management and adjuvant therapy. In addition, data accumulated over time should aid in predicting outcomes and allow for statistical comparisons worldwide (37–40).

The staging of cancers began in 1959 with the organization of the American Joint Committee for Cancer Staging and End-Results Reporting (AJC). The AJC used the TNM system for staging of cancers and published its first clinical and pathologic staging system for soft-tissue sarcomas in 1977 (41). Over time, the AJC became the American Joint Committee on Cancer (AJCC) and, together with the International Union Against Cancer, devised a four-stage system applicable to soft-tissue tumors in a variety of anatomical locations (40). In 1980, Enneking et al. (39) formatted an alternative three-stage system highlighting clinical perspectives and surgical management of soft-tissue sarcomas in the extremities. There are pros and cons of each of the above staging systems. Both, however, apply the basic principles of staging by incorporating the relevant prognostic variables. The emphasis placed on grade, tumor size, local extent, and metastasis varies for each staging system.

The AJCC staging system excludes sarcomas arising within the confines of the dura mater, including the brain, and sarcomas arising in parenchymatous organs and from hollow viscera (44). The same system included in its analysis the sarcomas listed in Table 21 (44). The AJCC four-tier staging system (Table 22) separates each stage on the basis of histologic grade: well differentiated, moderately differentiated, poorly differentiated, and undifferentiated. Letter designations A and B categorize tumors by size. Tumors 5 cm or less are labeled A and those greater than 5 cm are B. Both regional metastasis to lymph nodes and distant metastasis are considered in this system. No specific grading system is advocated. As mentioned, this system can be applied to sarcomas at any anatomical

Table 21 Tumors of the TNM Staging Analysis

Alveolar soft part sarcoma
- Angiosarcoma
- Epithelioid sarcoma
- Extraskeletal chondrosarcoma
- Extraskeletal osteosarcoma
- Fibrosarcoma
- Leiomyosarcoma
- Liposarcoma
- Malignant fibrous histiocytoma
- Malignant hemangiopericytoma
- Malignant schwannoma
- Rhabdomyosarcoma
- Synovial sarcoma
- Sarcoma (NOS)

Source: Modified from Beahrs OH, et al. Manual for staging of cancer, 1992.

Table 22 TNM Staging Classification and Grouping

TNM staging classification		Stage grouping
Primary tumor		Stage I
TX	Primary tumor cannot be assessed	A G1, T1, N0, M0
T0	No evidence of primary tumor	B G1, T2, N0, M0
T1	Tumor 5 cm or less	
T2	Tumor >5 cm	Stage II
		A G2, T1, N0, M0
Regional lymph nodes		B G2, T2, N0, M0
NX	Lymph nodes cannot be assessed	
N0	No regional lymph node metastasis	Stage III
N1	Regional lymph node metastasis	A G3–4, T1, N0, M0
		B G3–4, T2, N0, M0
Distant metastasis		
MX	Metastatic disease cannot be assessed	Stage IV
M0	No distant metastasis	A Any G, any T, N1, M0
M1	Distant metastasis	A Any G, any T, any N, M1
Histopathologic grade		
GX	Grade cannot be assessed	
G1	Well differentiated	
G2	Moderately differentiated	
G3	Poorly differentiated	

Source: Modified from Beahrs OH, et al. Manual for staging of cancer, 1992.

Table 23 Enneking Staging System and Grouping

Enneking staging system	Stage grouping
Surgical Sites (T)	Stage I
T1 Intracompartmental	A G1, T1, M0
T2 Extracompartmental	B G1, T2, M0
Extent of Disease (M)	Stage II
M0 No regional or distant metastasis	A G2, T1, M0
M1 Regional or distant metastasis	B G2, T2, M0
Surgical Grade (G)	Stage III
G1 Low grade	G1 or G2, T1 or T2, M1
G2 High grade	

Source: Modified from Enneking WF, et al. *Clin. Orthop* 153:106–120, 1980.

site; however, it does not address issues of compartmentalization for sarcomas arising in the extremities, which may have practical surgical utility.

Enneking describes a staging system based also on grade, emphasizes compartmentalization, and considers both regional and distant metastasis together (Table 23) (39). Grade, determined by histology as well as clinical and radiographic features, is designated high or low. Tumor site is regarded as either intra- or extracompartmental, limiting this system to sarcomas arising in the extremities. Size, per se, is not directly considered. Common to both systems is the accentuation on histologic grade and presence of metastasis.

Staging of soft-tissue sarcomas requires accurate histologic details as well as pertinent clinical and radiographic information. Input from the pathologist, surgeon, radiologist, and oncologist is necessary for management of the patient with a soft-tissue sarcoma. In the future, molecular and cytogenetic studies, as they affect the histologic grade, may also indirectly impact surgical staging. Incorporation of new and relevant prognostic factors will be essential.

V. PROGNOSTICATION

To reiterate many of the issues previously discussed in this chapter, prognostic factors that are predictive of overall survival include histologic grade (20–24,42,43), tumor size (42,44), local control and adequate margins (21,25,42,44), and necrosis (23,42,44). Depth and tumor site have also shown predictive value for overall survival by some authors (43).

In addition to predicting overall survival, many past and recent studies have focused on predicting local recurrence, metastasis, and survival after metastatic diagnosis and therapy. The most important factor in predicting local recurrence is the adequacy of the surgical procedure (42,45). Patients with local recurrence tend to have a worse prognosis than those without; however, if no detectable metastases are present, a favorable outcome may be postulated (45). Studies have shown that size and histologic grade may be predictive of metastatic risk (45,46). Survival rates after pulmonary metastatectomy may be of value, as surgical therapy for metastatic disease is increasingly common. Prognostic factors include the number of metastases and time from therapy of the primary tumor until diagnosis of metastatic disease (45).

It is certainly of clinical and academic interest to decipher useful prognostic factors for soft-tissue sarcomas. In the future, prospective studies, as well as the continued advances in knowledge of molecular biology, might allow for the development of more effective surgical and appropriate adjuvant therapeutic regimens.

REFERENCES

1. Enzinger FM, Weiss SW. Soft tissue tumors, 3rd ed. St. Louis: Mosby–Year Book, 1995:1–16.
2. Ackerman LV, Spjut HJ. Atlas of tumor pathology, Fascicle 4. Washington, DC: Armed Forces Institute of Pathology, 1962.
3. Stout AP, Lattes R. Atlas of tumor pathology, Fascicle 1. Washington, DC: Armed Forces Institute of Pathology, 1967.
4. Fisher, C. Soft tissue sarcomas: diagnosis, classification and prognostic factors. Br J Plast Surg 49:27–33, 1996.
5. Fletcher, CDM. Soft tissue tumors. In: CDM Fletcher, ed. Diagnostic histopathology of tumors. New York: Churchill Livingstone, 1995:1043–1096.
6. Evans, HL. Classification and grading of soft tissue sarcomas. A comment. Hematol/Oncol Clin North Amer 9(3):653–656, 1995.
7. Meister, P. Classification, grading and staging of soft tissue sarcomas. Recent Results Cancer Res 138:13–15, 1995.
8. Lattes R. Tumors of the soft tissue. In: Atlas of tumor pathology, 2nd Series, Fascicle 1, Revised. Armed Forces Institute of Pathology, 1983.
9. Enzinger FW, Lattes R, Torloni H. Histological typing of soft tissue tumors. World Health Organization, Geneva (International Histological Classification of Tumors, No. 3), 1969.
10. Weiss SW. Histological typing of soft tissue tumours. World Health Organiation, Berlin: Springer-Verlag, 1994.
11. Meis JM, Enzinger FM. Chondroid lipoma. A unique tumor simulating liposarcoma and myxoid chondrosarcoma. Am J Surg Pathol 17(11):1103–1112, 1993.
12. Meis JM, Enzinger FM. Myolipoma of soft tissue. Am J Surg Pathol 15(2):121–125, 1991.
13. Dei Tos AP, Mentzel T, Newman PL, Fletcher CDM. Spindle cell liposarcoma. A hitherto unrecognized variant of liposarcoma. Am J Surg Pathol 18(9):913–921, 1994.

14. Kilpatrick SE, Mentzel T, Fletcher CDM. Leiomyoma of deep soft tissue. Am J Surg Pathol 18(6):576–582, 1994.
15. Hachisgua T, Hashimoto H, Enjoji M. Angioleiomyoma Cancer 54:126–130, 1984.
16. Newton WA, Gehan EA, Webber BL, Marsden HB, van Unik AJM, Hamoudi AB, Tsokos MG, Simada H, Harms D, Schmidt D, Ninfo V, Cavazzaria AO, Gonzalez-Crussi F, Parham DM, Reiman HM, Asmar L, Beltangady MS, Sachs NE, Triche TJ, Maurer HM. Classification of rhabdomyosarcoma and related sarcomas. Cancer 76(6):1073–1085, 1995.
17. Fisher C. Synovial Sarcoma. Ann Diagn Pathol 1998; 2:401-421.
18. Suster S, Nascimento AG, Meittinen M, Sickel JZ, Moran CA. Solitary fibrous tumors of soft tissue. Am J Surg Pathol 19(11):1257–1266, 1995.
19. Nielsen GP, O'Connell JX, Dickersin GR, Rosenberg AE. Solitary fibrous tumor of soft tissue: a report of 15 cases, including 5 malignant examples with light microscopic, immunohistochemical and ultrastructural data. Mod Pathol 10(10):1028–1037, 1997.
20. Stout AP. Mesenchymoma, the mixed tumor of mesenchyme derivatives. Ann Surg 127:278–290, 1948.
21. Markhede G, Angervall L, Stener B. A multivariate analysis of the prognosis after surgical treatment of malignant soft tissue tumors. Cancer 49:1721–1733, 1982.
22. Myhre-Jensen O, Kaae S, Madsen EH, Sneppen U. Histopathological grading in soft tissue tomors. Acta Pathol Microbiol Immunol Scand A, 91:145–150, 1983.
23. Costa J, Wesley RA, Glatstein E, Rosenberg SA. The grading of soft tissue sarcomas. Cancer 53:530–541, 1984.
24. Trojani M, Contesso G, Coindre JM, Rouesse J, Bui NB, De Mascarel A, Goussot JF, David M, Bonichon J, Lagarde C. Soft tissue sarcomas of adults; study of pathological prognostic variables and definitions of a histopathological grading system. Int J Cancer 33:37–42, 1984.
25. Coindre JM, Trojani M, Contesso G, David M, Rouesse J, Bui NB, Bodaert A, De Mascarel I, De Mascarel A, Groussot JF. Reproducibility of a histopathological grading system for adult soft tissue sarcoma. Cancer 58:306–309, 1986.
26. Mhyre-Jensen O, Hogh J, Ostgaard SE, Nordentoft AM, Sneppen O. Histopathological grading of soft tissue tumors. Prognostic significance in a prospective study of 278 consecutive cases. J Pathol 163:19–24, 1991.
27. Kulander BJ, Polissar L, Yang CY, Woods JS. Grading of soft tissue sarcomas; necrosis as a determinant of survival. Mod Pathol 2(3):205–208, 1989.
28. Guillou L, Coindre JM, Bonichon F, Bui NB, Terrier P, Collin J, Vilain MO, Mandar AM, Le Doussal V, Leroux A, Jacquemier J, Duplay H, Sastre-Garau X, Costa J. Comparative study of the National Cancer Institute and the French Federation of Cancer Centers sarcoma group grading systems in a population of 410 adult patients with soft tissue sarcomas. J Clin Oncol 15(1):350–362, 1997.
29. Meister P. Grading of soft tissue sarcomas: a proposal for a reproducible, albeit limited scheme. Curr Top Pathol 89:153–173, 1995.
30. Kroese MCS, Rutgers DH, Wils IS, van Unik JAM, Roholl PJM. The relevance of the DNA index and proliferation rate in the grading of benign and malignant soft tissue tumors. Cancer 65:1782–1788, 1990.

31. Calonje E, Fletcher CDM. Immunohistochemistry and DNA flow cytometry in soft tissue sarcomas. Hematol/Oncol Clin North Am 9(3):657–675, 1995.

32. Tomita Y, Aozasa K, Myoui A, Kuratsn S, Uchida A, Ono K, Matsumota K. Histopathologic grading in soft tissue sarcomas. An analysis of 194 cases including AgNor count and mast cell count. In J Cancer 54:194–199, 1993.

33. Nilbert M. Molecular and cytogenetics of soft tissue sarcomas. Acta Orthop Scand (Supp 273) 68:60–67, 1997.

34. Sreekantaiah C, Ladanyi M, Rodriguez E, Chaganti RSK. Chromosomal aberrations in soft tissue tumors. Relevance to diagnosis, classification and molecular mechanisms. Am J Pathol 144:1121–1134, 1994.

35. Cance WG, Brennan MF, Dudas ME. Altered expression of the retinoblastoma gene product in human sarcomas. N Engl J Med 323:1457–1462, 1990.

36. Donnor LR. Cytogenetics of tumors of soft tissue and bone. Implication for pathology. Cancer Genet Cytogenet 78:115–126, 1994.

37. Peabody TD, Simon MA. Principles of staging of soft tissue sarcomas. Clin Orthop Rel Res 289:19–31, 1993.

38. Hashimoto H, Daimani Y, Takesluta S, Tsuneyoshi M, Enjoji M. Prognostic significance of histologic parameters of soft tissue sarcomas. Cancer 70:2816–2822, 1992.

39. Enneking WF, Spamer SS, Goodman MA. A system for the surgical staging of musculoskeletal sarcoma. Clin Orthop 153:106–120, 1980.

40. Beahrs OH, Henson DE, Hutter RVP. Manual for staging of cancer, 3rd ed. Philadelphia: JB Lippincott, 1992:131–133.

41. Russell WO, Cohen J, Enzinger F, Hajdu SI, Heise H, Martin RG, Meissner W, Miller WT, Schmitz RL, Suit HD. A clinical and pathological staging system for soft tissue sarcomas. Cancer 40:1562–1570, 1977.

42. Mandard AM, Petiot JP, Marnay J, Mandard JC, Chasle J, De Ranieri E, Dupin P, Herlin P, De Ranierei J, Tanguy A, Boulier N, Abbatucci JS. Prognostic factors in soft tissue sarcomas. A multivariate analysis of 109 cases. Cancer 63:1437–1451, 1989.

43. Ravaud A, Bui NB, Coindre JM, Lagarde P, Tramoud P, Bonichon F, Stockle E, Kantor G, Trojani M, Chauvergne J, Maree D. Prognostic variables for the selection of patients with operable soft tissue sarcomas to be considered in adjuvant chemotherapy trials. Br J Cancer 66(5):961–969, 1992.

44. El-Jabbour JN, Akhtar SS, Kerr GR, McLaren KM, Smyth JF, Rodger A, Leonard RCF. Prognostic factors for survival in soft tissue sarcomas. Br J Cancer 62(5):857–861, 1990.

45. Rydolm A. Prognostic factors in soft tissue sarcoma. Acta Orthop Scand (Suppl 273) 68:148–154, 1997.

46. Coindre JM, Terrier P, Bui NB, Bonichon F, Collin F, Le Donssal V, Mandard AM, Vilain MO, Jacquemier J, Duplay H, Sastre X, Barlier C, Henry-Amar M, Mace-Lesech J, Contesso F. Prognostic factors in adult patients with locally controlled soft tissue sarcomas. A study of 546 patients from the French Federation of Cancer Centers sarcoma group. J Clin Oncol 14:869–877, 1996.

5
Immunohistochemistry of Soft-Tissue Tumors

Kalisha A. Hill and William B. Laskin
Northwestern University Medical School and
Northwestern Memorial Hospital
Chicago, Illinois

I. INTRODUCTION

Although the diagnosis of a soft-tissue process is based principally on histomorphologic characteristics of the lesional tissue with support from surgical findings and clinical history, pathologists have become increasingly reliant on immunohistochemistry as a diagnostic adjunct, especially in helping to separate tumors with morphologic overlap and in determining cytodifferentiation.

The immunohistochemical procedure is based on the ability of an antibody (immunoreagent) to recognize and complex with an antigen site (epitope) on a molecule of interest located in tissue. Identification is then made by attaching a visually detectable second antibody onto the primary antigen–antibody complex.

The success of immunohistochemical detection of a target molecule is dependent on a variety of factors, including the concentration of the molecule in tissue, type of antibody used, mode of tissue fixation, type of technique used to expose or "unmask" the antigen site on the molecule (so-called antigen retrieval), and sensitivity of the immunohistochemical procedure.

There are two basic types of antibodies available for immunohistochemical procedures. Polyclonal antiserum consist of a mixture of antibodies that react with different epitopes on the molecule of interest. The monoclonal antibody, which is more widely used in general practice, reacts with only a single epitope. From a diagnostic standpoint, polyclonal antibodies suffer from a higher incidence of spurious immunoreactivity with similar antigens on other molecules (a phenomenon known as cross-reactivity), whereas the utility of monoclonal antibodies is more greatly affected by fixative-induced epitope alterations.

The method of fixation and techniques to expose antigens altered by fixation impact on immunohistochemical results. Presently, there is no universal fixative for immunohistochemistry. Formaldehyde (formalin), which forms covalent bonds with aminoacids and cross-links protein, is the most popular fixative because of its ability to preserve tissue morphology. However, it is less than adequate for the preservation of surface immunoglobulin molecules and the so-called intermediate filaments. Alcohol-based agents coagulate protein and are excellent fixatives for preservation of intermediate filaments and surface immunoglobulin molecules, but they tend to solubilize small peptide antigens. Bouin's and B5 fixative are superior to formaldehyde, but not to ethanol, for the preservation of some antigens, especially those present on lymphocytes. However, prolonged fixation often renders the tissue brittle and difficult to cut.

As antigen preservation is adversely affected by prolonged exposure to fixatives, especially formalin, methods of enhancing the exposure of antigen to the immunoreagent have been developed. Traditionally, pretreatment of tissue with proteolytic enzymes, such as Pronase and trypsin, was used. Recently, nonenzymatic heat-induced epitope retrieval using a microwave oven, a water bath, steam, autoclave, or a pressure cooker has gained acceptance as an effective method for improving immunohistochemical results with alcohol-fixed and, especially, formalin-fixed tissue.

The sensitivity of an immunohistochemical procedure is dependent on the concentration of the antibody and antigen, duration of incubation of the complex, overall stability of the antigen–antibody reaction, quality of antigen preservation, degree of antigen "unmasking" (see above), and sensitivity of the detection system. The detection system in immunohistochemistry involves linking a second antibody complexed with peroxidase to the primary antibody (bound to the antigen). The peroxidase enzyme reacts with a chromogen introduced later in the procedure, which yields a characteristic color indicating reactivity. The avidin-biotin conjugate and the peroxidase-antiperoxidase techniques are the two most widely used detection systems. Studies indicate that the former is a more sensitive detection method (1).

Lastly, it is important to understand the specificity of an antibody. In general, immunoreagents that have a restricted tissue distribution (greater degree of specificity) are more useful in diagnosis. However, when immunohistochemistry is used as a diagnostic tool, the investigator should order a panel of immunoreagents, including less specific antibodies capable of identifying each of the three major lines of cellular differentiation (epithelial, hematopoietic, or mesenchymal), particularly if the differential diagnosis is broad, and not rely solely on the results of one antibody test.

II. IMMUNOMARKERS USED IN THE DIAGNOSIS OF SOFT-TISSUE TUMORS

A. Vimentin

Vimentin is one of the five intermediate (8–12 nm in diameter) filament proteins (keratin, desmin, glial fibrillary acidic protein, and neurofilament protein), which are major structural proteins in the cell. Vimentin is a ubiquitous mesenchymal marker found in virtually all mesenchymal cells and in most mesenchymal neoplasms. It is the only intermediate filament present in mesenchymal cells during early embryologic development, and it is usually replaced by a type-specific intermediate filament as the cell undergoes differentiation (2). Although once thought to be a specific marker of mesenchymal differentiation, this protein has been found in a variety of nonmesenchymal tumors, including ovarian, thyroid, endometrial, renal, breast, adrenal, and lung adenocarcinomas (3,4), as well as melanoma (5), mesothelioma (6), and lymphoma (7). Moreover, spindle cell (metaplastic) or "sarcomatoid" carcinoma frequently exhibits vimentin expression within nonepithelial-appearing cells of the neoplasm. Along with its diagnostic potential, vimentin has been used as an internal control to determine the immunocompetence of the lesional cells. That is, immunocompetent tissue reacts with antibodies directed against vimentin, whereas tissue that is necrotic, autolyzed, or poorly fixed shows weak or no reactivity. Consequently, other immunoreagents do not demonstrate reliable staining.

B. Epithelial Markers

Cytokeratin is the principal cytoskeletal component of epithelial cells (8), and antibodies directed against cytokeratin are the most commonly used immunoreagents to detect epithelial differentiation. Cytokeratins are intermediate filaments composed of about 20 subtypes according to molecular weight and isoelectric point (9). Moll et al. (9) categorized the cytokeratins numerically, providing a convenient method of identification. Cytokeratins can also by subdivided into two major families: acidic (type I, cytokeratins 9–19) and basic (type II, cytokeratin 1–8) (10). All epithelial cells (and some mesenchymal cells) express pairs of keratins composed of one basic and one acidic molecule. For example, Moll number 7 and 8 (CK7/8) (type I) and 8 and 18 (CK8/18) (type II) keratins are expressed in pairs within simple epithelia, such as that lining mucosal surfaces. Mesenchymal neoplasms have the potential to express keratin, most commonly CK 8 and 18 (11). The soft-tissue neoplasms that most frequently express cytokeratin include synovial sarcoma (12), epithelioid sarcoma (13), mesothelioma (14), desmoplastic small round cell tumor (15), chordoma (16), parachordoma (17), melanotic neuroectodermal tumor (of infancy) (18), and extrarenal rhabdoid tumor (19).

Other sarcomas that variably express keratin include Ewing's sarcoma/primitive neuroectodermal tumor (20), leiomyosarcoma (21), epithelioid variant of angiosarcoma (22), malignant peripheral nerve sheath tumor (23), and, rarely, rhabdomyosarcoma (24) and malignant fibrous histiocytoma (8).

Analysis of cytokeratin subsets has been useful in the diagnosis of several types of sarcoma with histologic overlap. Some examples of poorly differentiated, monophasic synovial sarcoma can histologically resemble malignant peripheral nerve sheath tumor. Moreover, both neoplasms are known to express cytokeratin, epithelial membrane antigen (EMA), and S-100 protein. However, antibodies to cytokeratins 7 and 19 react with the spindle element of monophasic synovial sarcoma, whereas in malignant peripheral nerve sheath tumor, the lesional cells typically are nonreactive (25). Extraskeletal myxoid chondrosarcoma, chordoma, and parachordoma can display histomorphologic overlap. Parachordoma has been reported to express cytokeratins 8 and 18 (detected by immunoreagent CAM5.2), but not 7, 19, or the high molecular weight cytokeratins, 1/10, as does chordoma (17,26). On the other hand, extraskeletal myxoid chondrosarcoma is negative for virtually all cytokeratins (26).

EMA is a glycoprotein located in the apical plasma membrane of mammary epithelial cells (27). EMA, like cytokeratin, is expressed in a wide variety of epithelia and their tumors, and is typically located on the cell surface or delimiting intracytoplasmic lumina. The antigen has also been detected in plasma cells and in the malignant element of some large cell lymphomas, particularly the anaplastic large cell lymphoma (28,29) with translocation 2;5.

EMA expression generally parallels that of cytokeratin in soft-tissue neoplasms with the exception of a few notable differences. Antibodies against EMA may be more sensitive than cytokeratin for eliciting epithelial differentiation in poorly differentiated examples of monophasic synovial sarcoma (30). In contrast to cytokeratin, EMA is not helpful in differentiating extraskeletal myxoid chondrosarcoma from chordoma and parachordoma as all three neoplasms have the potential to express EMA (26). Extranodal examples of follicular dendritic cell tumor/sarcoma can mimic a mesenchymal or even an epithelial tumor. Neoplastic cells of this entity express EMA (along with compliment markers anti-CD21 and CD35) but not cytokeratin (31). EMA is also expressed by normal meningeal cells and perineurial fibroblast-like cells. Accordingly, EMA immunoreactivity has been documented in meningioma (32), malignant peripheral nerve sheath tumor (33), and perineurioma (34). While expression is generally diffuse in perineurioma, only limited expression of EMA is typically observed in malignant peripheral nerve sheath tumor. Nonneoplastic EMA-positive perineurial cells frequently surround tumor deposits in the nerve sheath myxoma, neurofibroma, and neurilemmoma (benign schwannoma).

C. Muscle Markers

Actins are contractile proteins that measure 6–7 nm in diameter and are a major component of the microfilamentous cytoskeleton. Six major isoforms of actin have been identified (35). However, from a diagnostic standpoint, antibodies have been generated that react with only four of them. Muscle-specific actin detects α-smooth, cardiac, and skeletal actins and γ-smooth muscle actin. α-Smooth muscle actin detects the α isoform of smooth muscle, whereas α-sarcomeric actin marks both α-cardiac and α-skeletal actin.

Antibodies to muscle-specific actin can assist in the evaluation of rhabdomyosarcoma. According to some investigators, muscle-specific actin stains virtually all rhabdomyosarcomas (36) and therefore helps distinguish the latter from other primitive, round cell neoplasms. Anti-α-smooth muscle actin is an excellent immunostain for tumors of smooth muscle differentiation. In addition, both muscle-specific actin and smooth muscle actin highlight cells with partial smooth muscle differentiation, such as pericytes, myoepithelial cells, and myofibroblasts (37). The identification of pericytes around vascular structures is a feature favoring a benign vascular process as most malignant vascular neoplasms lack pericytic cells. Moreover, the modified smooth muscle cells composing glomus tumor react with antibodies to both muscle-specific and smooth muscle actin (38,39). The presence of spindle cells with myofibroblastic features account for the reported expression of actin in a wide variety of reactive and neoplastic lesions, including nodular fasciitis and fibromatosis. Anti-α-sarcomeric actin is primarily used to identify skeletal muscle differentiation. It has been used to distinguish the pleomorphic rhabdomyosarcoma in the adult from poorly differentiated leiomyosarcoma and malignant fibrous histiocytoma (40), although its specificity has been questioned (41).

Desmin is an intermediate filament found in cardiac, skeletal, and smooth muscle fibers. In skeletal muscle cells, the desmin filaments are associated with the Z-disc material, whereas in smooth muscle cells, desmin filaments interconnect fusiform dense bodies that run parallel to actin filaments with the plasmalemmal dense plaques (8). Antidesmin is an excellent marker for smooth or skeletal muscle differentiation, although it is more frequently expressed in rhabdomyosarcoma than in leiomyosarcoma (36). Desmin expression characterizes angiomyofibroblastoma (42) of the vulva whose chief neoplastic element is believed to be a modified myofibroblast-like cell and the strictly nonmyogenic neoplasm, the desmoplastic small round cell tumor (15), in which the reaction with antibodies to desmin is best considered aberrant. Variable desmin expression has also been reported in alveolar soft-part sarcoma (43), epithelioid sarcoma (in particular, the "proximal" or large cell variant) (44), mesothelioma (45), myofibroblastoma (of the breast) (46), "angiomatoid" fibrous histiocytoma (47), and in a select cell population of tenosynovial giant cell tumor (48).

Myosins act as enzymes and structural proteins within muscle cells. They have the ability to bind the actin microfilament present in muscle and initiate muscle contraction. Muscle myosins can be divided into smooth and striated muscle types. The striated muscle types (skeletal and cardiac muscle myosins) are referred to as sarcomeric myosin. Antibodies to sarcomeric actin have found utility in the diagnosis of rhabdomyosarcoma (49).

The *MyoD* family of transcription factors play a pivotal role in the differentiation and development of the skeletal muscle cell by encoding a series of DNA-binding proteins that direct muscle differentiation in uncommitted mesenchymal stem cells (50). These myogenic regulatory proteins include MyoD1 (myf-3 is the human analog), myogenin (myf-4), myf-5, and myf-6. MyoD1 (Myf-3) and myogenin (myf-4) are up-regulated early in myogenesis, and antibodies to these factors have shown promise as very sensitive and specific immunohistochemical markers for diagnosing pediatric and adult rhabdomyosarcoma (51,52). The potential roles of Myf-5 and Myf-6 in the diagnosis of soft-tissue neoplasms have yet to be established.

Calponin and h-caldesmon are cytoskeleton-associated, actin-binding proteins found in smooth muscle that regulate muscle contraction. Antibodies to calponin and h-caldesmon react with parenchymal and vascular smooth muscle cells in a variety of organs and are a sensitive marker of myoepithelial cells (along with cytokeratin and S-100 protein). In an initial study evaluating calponin and h-caldesmon expression in mesenchymal tumors (53), all benign smooth muscle tumors, including angiomyolipoma, and most leiomyosarcomas expressed both antigens. Calponin expression was demonstrated in tumors with cells exhibiting myofibroblastic differentiation, whereas h-caldesmon expression was more prevalent in gastrointestinal stromal tumors.

D. Endothelial Markers

Factor VIII–related antigen (FVIII:RAg), also known as von Willebrand factor, is a large multimeric component of the factor VIII complex of the clotting system and is synthesized by endothelial cells, megakaryocytes, and platelets (8). The protein is produced in the Weibel-Palade body of the endothelial cell (36). Although anti-FVIII:RAg is considered a specific marker for endothelial differentiation, it is not very sensitive as it is not identified in endothelium-lining capillaries in a variety of organs (54) and stains lymphatic endothelium weakly (55). FVIII:RAg is convincingly expressed in most benign vascular tumors (54,56) and variably expressed in benign lesions of presumed lymphatic origin (57). In hemangiopericytoma, endothelial cells lining vascular channels express the protein, whereas the surrounding spindle cell element is negative (58). Cytoplasmic immunoreactivity with accentuation around intracytoplasmic vacuoles is a somewhat characteristic staining pattern observed in most examples of epithelioid hemangioendothelioma (59). However, angiosarcomas demonstrate inconsistent immunoreactivity, particularly in poorly differentiated, solid areas and foci composed of epithelioid cells (60,61), and in the spindle cell foci of Kaposi's sarcoma (56,60). These limitations indicate the need to test for additional endothelial cell–associated antigens (see below).

CD31 is a glycoprotein that belongs to the cell adhesion molecules of the immunoglobulin gene family. The protein is identical to adhesion molecule, PECAM-1 (platelet-endothelial cell adhesion molecule), present on platelets, granulocytes, and endothelial cells (8). It is considered slightly less specific for endothelial cell differentiation than is FVIII:RAg. However, CD31 is a more sensitive marker of malignant vascular tumors by virtue of its ability to immunolabel poorly differentiated foci in angiosarcomas (61) and spindle cell areas of Kaposi's sarcoma (56,61). Mesothelioma and some adenocarcinomas may show weak cytoplasmic staining with anti-CD31, but not the specific membranous pattern of staining observed in endothelial cells (56).

CD34 is a glycosylated transmembrane cell adhesion molecule present on human hematopoietic progenitor cells, vascular endothelial cells, and a subset of dendritic fibroblast-like cells within connective tissue (62,63). Evidence suggests that cells tend to lose their ability to express the protein as they mature or undergo further differentiation. As an endothelial marker, the CD34 immunoreagent shows sensitivity greater than FcVIII:RAg, but comparable to CD31, particularly in identifying poorly differentiated angiosarcoma (62), spindled foci of Kaposi's sarcoma (54,56,62), and marking the intracytoplasmic lumina of the neoplastic cells composing epithelioid hemangioendothelioma (62).

CD34 has utility in the diagnosis of a variety of nonvascular mesenchymal tumors. CD34 immunoexpression characterizes the solitary fibrous tumor (64,65), dermatofibrosarcoma protuberans (66), and the closely related giant cell fibroblastoma (67), and CD34 positivity is also found in epithelioid sarcoma (68), gastrointestinal stromal tumors (69), the spindle component of spindle cell lipoma (70), hemangiopericytoma (56), and "dedifferentiated" liposarcoma (71), as well as in two rare tumors—the giant cell angiofibroma (72) and pleomorphic hyalinizing angiectatic tumor (of soft parts) (73). A variable number of CD34-positive dendritic cells have been described in conventional neurofibroma and in the Antoni B areas of neurilemmoma (67).

CD34 has been used in the differential diagnosis of spindle cell lesions with histologic overlap. It can help distinguish dermatofibrosarcoma protuberans from benign fibrous histiocytoma, which only rarely contains CD34-positive cells (74), and examples of solitary fibrous tumor occurring in soft tissue from deep, monomorphic variants of fibrous histiocytoma. Monophasic synovial sarcoma occasionally features hemangiopericytomatous areas. The former neoplasm exhibits a keratin-positive/CD34-negative immunoprofile, whereas true hemangiopericytoma is usually CD34-positive/keratin-negative. Epithelioid sarcoma may be misinterpreted as a carcinoma both histologically and by the presence of EMA and keratin immunopositivity. However, 50% of the former express CD34 (68), whereas carcinomas are almost always negative (62). Gastrointestinal stromal tumors can share histologic features with smooth muscle tumors occurring in this region. However, 70–80% of the former express CD34 and virtually all express c-kit (see below) (75), in contrast to leiomyoma and leiomyosarcoma, in which these markers are typically negative.

Ulex europeus agglutinin I (UEAI) is a plant protein (lectin) that binds non-immunologically to the H antigen of the ABO system. It is an extremely sensitive marker for endothelial cells (regardless of blood group). Although UEAI, like CD34 and CD31, is more sensitive than FVIII:RAg in detecting neoplastic cells of angiosarcoma, it shares with CD34 a lack of specificity by virtue of its reactivity with tumor cells from a wide variety of carcinomas (58,60), thus necessitating its use with other endothelial markers.

Vascular endothelial growth factors (VEGFs) help regulate endothelial cell proliferation, angiogenesis, and vascular permeability through high-affinity tyrosinase receptors VEGF-R1, VEGF-R2, and VEGF-R3 (76). The VEGF-C receptor, VEGFR-3, plays a key role in lymphangiogenesis (77). Presence of this protein receptor has been reported in a select group of vascular tumors, including examples of lymphangioma and hemangioma, the spindle cell element of Kaposi's sarcoma, examples of angiosarcoma, Dakska tumor, and kaposiform hemangioendothelioma (77,78).

E. Neuroendocrine and Neuroectodermal Markers

Enolase is an enzyme found in the glycolytic pathway. The various enolase isoenzymes consist primarily of homodimers of α, β, and γ subunits and have a wide distribution throughout the body. The γ- or neuron-specific enolase is found in high concentrations in cells of the nervous system and in neuroendocrine cells. Although initially touted as a specific marker for endocrine or neuronal differentiation by virtue of its expression in neuroendocrine carcinoma, neuroblastoma, paraganglioma, and pheochromocytoma (79,80), later studies showed that NSE immunoreactivity was rather nonspecific as it was identified in normal nonneural tissue, in a variety of nonendocrine carcinomas, and in several types of sarcoma, including rhabdomyosarcoma, leiomyosarcoma, angiosarcoma, synovial sarcoma, melanoma and clear cell sarcoma, alveolar soft-part sarcoma (81–84), and lymphoma (85). Other mesenchymal tumors that express NSE include Ewing's sarcoma/primitive neuroectodermal tumor (79), desmoplastic small round cell tumor (15), gastrointestinal stromal tumor (86), and mesenchymal chondrosarcoma (87). Fortunately, more specific neural markers are now available commercially (see below).

Chromogranins are a group of calcium-binding proteins present in the secretory granules of endocrine cells. Chromogranin A, which has a wider distribution in hormone-producing cells than chromogranins B and C, has been employed as a marker of endocrine differentiation. It is found in pheochromocytoma, paraganglioma, a variety of endocrine tumors, carcinoid tumor, and pituitary adenomas (88–90). Some neuroendocrine and neuroectodermal tumors, such as Merkel cell carcinoma, neuroblastoma, and undifferentiated small cell carcinoma of the lung, stain weakly or not at all, as staining intensity is proportional to the number of neuroendocrine granules present in the cytoplasm (8). The prevalence of chromogranin expression is low in desmoplastic small round cell tumor and gastrointestinal stromal tumor. In the Ewing's sarcoma/primitive neuroectodermal family of tumors, it is more frequently found in tumors not harboring the *EWS/FLI-1* translocation (91).

Synaptophysin is a membrane glycoprotein found in presynaptic vesicles of neurons, vesicles of cells of the adrenal medulla, and neurosecretory granules of neuroendocrine cells (92). Synaptophysin is a sensitive and very specific marker of neuroendocrine and neuronal differentiation, and its reactivity often shows overlap with chromogranin. However, synaptophysin should be included in an immunopanel with chromogranin as its expression is present irrespective of other neuroendocrine markers (8).

Glial fibrillary acidic protein (*GFAP*) is an intermediate filament protein found chiefly in astrocytes and ependymal cells of the central nervous system. In soft tissue, GFAP is used to identify neurosustentacular (peripheral nerve sheath) differentiation in cells. Accordingly, it is expressed in some neurilemmomas (particularly the centrally located, cellular variant) (93,94), rarely in neurofibrom a (93), in most examples of nerve sheath myxoma (95), in ganglioneuromatous areas of neuroblastoma (96), and in glial hamartoma (of soft tissue) (36). GFAP also labels sustentacular (supportive) cells surrounding nests of tumor in paraganglioma and pheochromocytoma (97). As in the salivary gland, the ability of GFAP to identify neoplastic myoepithelial cells explains its expression in myoepitheliomas occurring in soft tissue (98).

Leu-7 or HNK-1 is a member of the CD57 group of antibodies. Although the antibody was first reported to react with lymphocytes exhibiting "natural killer" activity, it was later found to detect an epitope of a myelin-associated glycoprotein on Schwann cells (99). As a marker of schwannian differentiation, variable Leu-7 expression is detected in the majority of benign schwannomas (100), in over 50% of malignant peripheral nerve sheath tumors (101) and neurofibromas (102), in about one third of granular cell tumors (103), and in nerve sheath myxomas (95). It is also identified in the Ewing's sarcoma/primitive neuroectodermal family of tumors where its expression is more commonly observed in tumors without the EWS/FLI-1 translocation (91). However, Leu-7 is not very specific for neurosustentacular (peripheral nerve sheath) differentiation as it is also found in monophasic synovial sarcoma, leiomyosarcoma, and rhabdomyosarcoma (104,105), as well as a variety of endocrine and some nonendocrine carcinomas.

Neurofilament protein (*NFP*) is an intermediate filament protein composed of high, medium, and low molecular weight subunits. NFP is present in the axons of mature neurons in both the peripheral and central nervous systems (8). NFP, particularly the low molecular weight component, is chiefly expressed in soft-tissue tumors exhibiting neuronal differentiation, such as neuroblastoma, ganglioneuroma, ganglioneuroblastoma, and paraganglioma (106). In the Ewing's/primitive neuroectodermal family of tumors, NFP expression is more prevalent in tumors not bearing the type 1 EWS/FLI-1 translocation (91). Nonneural mesenchymal tumors known to express NFP include rhabdomyosarcoma (107) and epithelioid sarcoma (108). Neuroendocrine carcinomas can also express NFP. In particular, coexpression of CK20 and NFP in a paranuclear "dot" pattern is characteristic of neuroendocrine carcinoma of the skin (Merkel cell carcinoma) (109).

F. Macrophage and "Fibrohistiocytic" Markers

CD68 represents a group of antibodies that react to a glycoprotein antigen found in the lysosomal membrane of macrophages. KP1 is the CD68 antibody most commonly used in general practice and reacts with histiocytes, mast cells and their related tumors (110), and normal and neoplastic hematopoietic cells showing myelomonocytic differentiation (111). Early studies reported that the immunoreactivity of KP1 in cells of malignant fibrous histiocytoma is useful in its diagnosis (112). However, with the exception of tumors classified as "angiomatoid" fibrous histiocytoma, most examples of conventional malignant fibrous histiocytoma demonstrate little tumor cell reactivity (113). KP1 immunoexpression is not specific for histiocytic differentiation as it is been documented in carcinoma, melanoma, lymphoma (particularly small, diffuse B-cell and CD30-positive large cell lymphomas) (114), and a variety of soft-tissue neoplasms, including tenosynovial giant cell tumor (115) and the granular cell tumor (116).

Factor XIIIa, the "fibrin-stabilizing factor" of the coagulation cascade, identifies a monocyte-derived, dendritic macrophage that resides in most connective tissues throughout the body (117,118). Subsequently, a number of mesenchymal lesions contain a population of reactive factor XIIIa–positive dendritic cells. The presence of factor XIIIa–positive cells is useful in differentiating fibrous histiocytoma, a tumor known to have a large number of factor XIIIa–positive cells, from dermatofibrosarcoma protuberans, which typically has only a few (74). Some investigators have reported factor XIIIa–positive cells in juvenile xanthogranuloma (119), a finding that helps distinguish this lesion from Langerhans' histiocytosis and melanocytic lesions that lack factor XIIIa expression. The calcifying fibrous pseudotumor, a benign tumefaction that shares histologic features with inflammatory myofibroblastic tumor, differs immunohistochemically by its composition of factor XIIIa–positive cells (120).

G. Miscellaneous Immunomarkers

S-100 protein is a group of small calcium-binding proteins that are involved in cell cycle progression, cell differentiation, and cytoskeletal membrane interactions (8). Cell types relevant to the study of soft-tissue pathology that express S-100 protein include Schwann cells of the peripheral nervous system, histiocytes with antigen-processing function such as Langerhans' cells, adipocytes, chondrocytes, melanocytes, myoepithelial cells, sustentacular cells of the adrenal medulla, and the cellular remnants of the primitive notochord (121–123). From a diagnostic standpoint, S-100 protein is considered a sensitive but not a specific marker of peripheral nerve sheath and melanocytic differentiation, and thus should be used with a panel of other immunoreagents. Nuclear or cytoplasmic S-100 protein expression is typically strong and diffuse in neurilemmona (benign and cellular schwannoma) but is more variable in neurofibroma (36). Focal immunoexpression of S-100 protein is reported in 30–67% of malignant peripheral sheath tumors tested (124) and in almost all examples of clear cell sarcoma (125), granular cell tumor (125), and nerve sheath myxoma (95). As a marker of melanocytic neoplasms, anti-S-100 protein stains almost all benign melanocytic processes with the exception of some blue nevi, and melanomas (126), including the desmoplastic variant (127). S-100 protein expression (along with cytokeratin) is useful in the diagnosis of chordoma (125). S-100 protein immunoreactivity is found in most well-differentiated chondroid tumors, but it is generally weak or negative in extraskeletal myxoid chondrosarcoma (128). Its restricted expression in certain subsets of histiocytes facilitates its use in confirming the diagnosis of Langerhans' cell histiocytosis (125) and Rosai-Dorfman disease occurring in the soft tissues (129). S-100 protein immunoreactivity is also reported in myoepithelioma (of soft tissue) (98), parachordoma (17), and in about 30% of synovial sarcomas (130).

The immunoreagent *HMB-45* recognizes an antigen associated with the early stages of melanosome development. Although HMB-45 stains fetal melanocytes and junctional nevi, including the junctional component of compound nevi, it does not react with adult melanocytes or intradermal nevi (131). However, it is considered a specific and sensitive marker for malignant melanoma and complements S-100 protein and the antimelanoma markers Melan-A (MART-1) and tyrosinase (see below). In general, over 90% of examples of primary and metastatic melanoma (132) and most clear cell sarcomas (84) react with HMB-45, whereas less than 50% of spindle cell and desmoplastic melanomas are positive (133). The large pigmented cells of melanotic neuroectodermal tumor of infancy and the pigmented dendritic cells of the melanotic (pigmented) variant of neurofibroma also demonstrate reactivity with HMB-45 (18,134). The family of tumors purportedly derived from a distinctive perivascular epithelioid cell that expresses melanocytic and smooth muscle antigens all share HMB-45 positivity (135). These lesions include angiomyolipoma, lymphangioleiomyoma, and pulmonary and extrapulmonary clear cell (sugar) tumors (135).

Two recently described antimelanoma markers, *Melan-A* (*MART-1*) and *tyrosinase*, have proven to be highly sensitive and specific markers for melanocytic nevi and malignant melanoma (136,137). In one study, Melan-A appeared more sensitive than HMB-45 (but less sensitive than S-100 protein) for recognizing melanocytic differentiation in desmoplastic melanoma (136). Anti-Melan-A, which detects a melanosome-associated glycoprotein, also reacts with cells of angiomyolipoma (138) and the A103 antibody clone reacts with an antigen present on benign and neoplastic steroid hormone–producing cells (139). Both Melan-A and tyrosinase are expressed in pigmented dendritic cells of the melanotic variant of neurofibroma (134).

The *MIC2* gene located on the X and Y chromosomes encodes a cell surface glycoprotein, the p32/30 ^{MIC2} antigen (*CD99*), which is recognized by three commercially available antibodies: HBA-71, 12E7, and O13. CD99 is expressed chiefly in a membranous pattern in nearly 90% of Ewing's sarcoma and primitive neuroectodermal tumors (140,141) and therefore is most useful in distinguishing this family of tumors from neuroblastoma, which is negative. However, CD99 expression is not specific for Ewing's sarcoma/primitive neuroectodermal tumor as it has been reported in other small blue cell tumors including T-cell acute lymphoblastic leukemia/lymphoma, rhabdomyosarcoma (particularly the embryonal variant), Wilms' tumor, small cell osteosarcoma, mesenchymal chondrosarcoma, granulocytic sarcoma, and desmoplastic small round cell tumor (140–142). Other mesenchymal tumors, including hemangiopericytoma, solitary fibrous tumor, mesothelioma (with the exception of the sarcomatoid variant), synovial sarcoma, sex cord stromal tumors, and malignant peripheral nerve sheath tumor have all been reported to react with anti-CD99 (30,140,143).

C-kit encodes a transmembrane tyrosine kinase growth factor receptor (*KIT*, *CD117*), which is found on hematopoietic "stem" cells, mast cells, germ cells, melanocytes, interstitial cells of Cajal of the gastrointestinal tract, and certain epithelial cells (144–146). KIT and CD34 are typically expressed in gastrointestinal stromal tumors, but not in leiomyomas, which occasionally occur in this region (75). KIT along with tryptase is also expressed in most mast cell tumors and is also found in some examples of granulocytic sarcoma (147). CD68 and CD43 expression complement KIT in both disorders. In one study, more than 50% of angiosarcomas and 15% of Kaposi's sarcoma expressed KIT (148). In contrast to the "gain in function" c-kit mutations that predominate in gastrointestinal stromal tumors, seminomas, and mast cell tumors, the latter neoplasms overexpress KIT without mutagenesis (148).

The *basement membrane* is an extracellular structure composed of collagenous and noncollagenous proteins that separates epithelial cells from the adjacent stroma and also surrounds certain mesenchymal cells. Ultrastructural and immunohistochemical observations that mesenchymal cells such as smooth and striated muscle cells, adipocytes, Schwann cells, perineurial cells in the peripheral nervous system and endothelial cells, possess basement membrane, (149) are the rationale for evaluating its presence in mesenchymal tumors. Antibodies against collagen IV and laminin, two proteins ubiquitous to basement membranes, are generally employed for this task. Benign mesenchymal neoplasms that express collagen type IV or laminin include neurilemmoma (benign schwannoma), neurofibroma, perineurioma, nerve sheath myxoma, rhabdomyoma, leiomyoma, hemangioma, and lipoma (95,149,150). Malignant peripheral nerve sheath tumors, synovial sarcomas, leiomyosarcomas, and rhabdomyosarcomas demonstrate more variability in expression of these markers, whereas fibrosarcomas are typically negative (149). Collagen type IV surrounds nests of tumor cells in parachordoma, in contrast to its focal or absent expression in chordoma and myxoid chondrosarcoma (26) and it enclosed groups of cells undergoing early epithelial differentiation in synovial sarcoma (30). However, in everyday practice, immunohistochemical detection of basement membrane components has little value in the diagnostic workup of soft-tissue tumors.

REFERENCES

1. Shi Z-R, Itzkowitz SH, Kim YS. A comparison of three immunoperoxidase techniques for antigen detection in colorectal carcinoma tissues. J Histochem Cytochem 36:317–322, 1988.
2. Damjanov I. Antibodies to intermediate filaments and histogenesis. Lab Invest 47:215–217, 1982.
3. Azumi N, Battifora H. The distribution of vimentin and keratin in epithelial and nonepithelial neoplasms: a comprehensive immunohistochemical study on formalin and alcohol-fixed tumors. Am J Clin Pathol 88:286–296, 1987.
4. Wick MR, Cherwitz DL, McGlennen RC, Dehner LP. Adrenocortical carcinoma. An immunohistochemical comparison with renal cell carcinoma. Am J Pathol 122:343–352, 1986.
5. Ramaekers FC, Puts JJ, Moesker O, Kant A, Vooijs GP, Jap PH. Intermediate filaments in malignant melanomas. Identification and use as marker in surgical pathology. J Clin Invest 71:635–643, 1983.
6. Jasani B, Edwards RE, Thomas ND, Gibbs AR. The use of vimentin antibodies in the diagnosis of malignant mesothelioma. Virchow Arch A 406:441–448, 1985.
7. Giorno R, Sciotto CG. Use of monoclonal antibodies for analyzing the distribution of the intermediate filament protein vimentin in human non-Hodgkin's lymphomas. Am J Pathol 120:351–355, 1985.

8. Ordonez NG. Application of imunocytochemistry in the diagnosis of soft tissue sarcomas: a review and update. Adv Anat Pathol 5:67–85, 1998.
9. Moll R, France WW, Schiller DL, Geiger B, Krepler R. The catalog of human cytokeratins: patterns of expression in normal epithelia, tumors and cultured cells. Cell 31:11–24, 1982.
10. Cooper D, Schermer A, Sun TT. Classification of human epithelium and their neoplasms using monoclonal antibodies to keratin: strategies, applications and limitations. Lab Invest 52:243–256, 1985.
11. Van Muijen GNP, Ruiter DJ, Warnaar SO. Coexpression of intermediate filament polypeptides in human fetal and adult tissues. Lab Invest 57:134–141, 1987.
12. Corson JM, Weiss LM, Banks-Schlegel SP, Pinkus GS. Keratin proteins in synovial sarcoma, Am J Surg Pathol 7:107–109, 1983.
13. Chase DR, Enzinger FM, Weiss SW, Langloss JM. Keratin in epithelioid sarcoma: an immunohistochemical study. Am J Surg Pathol 8:435–441, 1984.
14. Corson JM, Pinkus GS. Mesothelioma: profile of keratin proteins and carcinoembryonic antigen: an immunoperoxidase study of 20 cases and comparison with pulmonary adenocarcinoma. Am J Pathol 108:80–87, 1982.
15. Gerald WL, Miller HK, Battifora H, Miettinen M, Silva EG, Rosai J. Intra-abdominal desmoplastic small round-cell tumor: report of 19 cases of a distinctive type of high-grade polyphenotypic malignancy affecting young individuals. Am J Surg Pathol 15:499–513, 1991.
16. Miettinen M, Lehto V, Dahl D, Virtanen I. Differential diagnosis of chordoma, chondroid, and ependymal tumours as aided by anti-intermediate filament antibodies. Am J Pathol 112:160–169, 1983.
17. Fisher C, Miettinen M. Parachordoma: a clinicopathologic and immunohistochemical study of four cases of an unusual soft tissue neoplasm. Ann Diagn Pathol 1:3–10, 1997.
18. Kapadia SB, Frisman DM, Hitchcock CL, Ellis GL, Popek EJ. Melanotic neuroectodermal tumor of infancy. Clinicopathological, immunohistochemical, and flow cytometric study. Am J Surg Pathol 17:566–573, 1993.
19. Kodet R, Newton WA, Sachs N, Hamoudi AB, Raney RB, Asmar L, Gehan EA. Rhabdoid tumors of soft tissues: a clinicopathologic study of 26 cases enrolled on the Intergroup Rhabdomyosarcoma Study. Hum Pathol 22:674–684, 1991.
20. Gu M, Antonescu CR, Guiter G, Huvos AG, Ladanyi M, Zakowski MF. Cytokeratin imunoreactivity in Ewing's sarcoma. Prevalence in 50 cases confirmed by molecular diagnostic studies. Am J Surg Pathol 24:410–416, 2000.
21. Norton AJ, Thomas JA, Isaacson PG. Cytokeratin-specific monoclonal antibodies are reactive with tumours of smooth muscle derivation: an immunocytochemical and biochemical study using antibodies to intermediate filament cytoskeletal proteins. Histopathology 11:487–499, 1987.
22. Gray MH, Rosenberg AE, Dickersin GR, Bhan AK. Cytokeratin expression in epithelioid vascular neoplasms. Hum Pathol 21:212–217, 1990.
23. Gray MH, Rosenberg AE, Dickersin GR, Bhan AK. Glial fibrillary acidic protein and keratin expression by benign and malignant nerve sheath tumors. Hum Pathol 20:1089–1096, 1989.

24. Coindre JM, de Mascarel A, Trojani M, de Mascarel I, Pages A. Immunohistochemical study of rhabdomyosarcoma. Unexpected staining with S100 protein and cytokeratin. J Pathol 155:127–132, 1988.

25. Smith TA, Machen SK, Fisher C, Goldblum JR. Usefulness of cytokeratin subsets for distinguishing monophasic synovial sarcoma from malignant peripheral nerve sheath tumor. Am J Clin Pathol 112:641–648, 1999.

26. Folpe AL, Agoff SN, Willis J, Weiss SW. Parachordoma is immunohistochemically and cytogenetically distinct from axial chordoma and extraskeletal myxoid chondrosarcoma. Am J Surg Pathol 23:1059–1067, 1999.

27. Imam A, Tokes ZA. Immunoperoxidase localization of a glycoprotein on plasma membrane of secretory epithelium from human breast. J Histochem Cytochem 29:581–584, 1981.

28. Pinkus GS, Kurtin PJ. Epithelial membrane antigen—a diagnostic discriminant in surgical pathology: immunohistochemical profile in epithelial, mesenchymal, and hematopoietic neoplasms using paraffin sections and monoclonal antibodies. Hum Pathol 16:929–940, 1985.

29. Delson G, Al Saati T, Gatter KC, Gerdes J, Schwarting R, Caveriviere P, Rigal-Huguet F, Robert A, Stein H, Mason DY. Coexpression of epithelial membrane antigen (EMA), Ki-1, and interleukin-2 receptor by anaplastic large cell lymphomas. Diagnostic value in so-called malignant histiocytosis. Am J Pathol 130:59–70, 1988.

30. Folpe AL, Schmidt RA, Chapman D, Gown AM. Poorly differentiated synovial sarcoma. Immunohistochemical distinction from primitive neuroectodermal tumors and high-grade malignant peripheral nerve sheath tumors. Am J Surg Pathol 22:673–682, 1998.

31. Chan JKC, Fletcher CDM, Nayler SJ, Cooper K. Follicular dendritic cell sarcoma. Clinicopathologic analysis of 17 cases suggesting a malignant potential higher than currently recognized. Cancer 79:294–313, 1997.

32. Schmitt SJ, Vogel H. Meningiomas. Diagnostic value of immunoperoxidase staining for epithelial membrane antigen. Am J Surg Pathol 10:640–649, 1986.

33. Wick MR, Swanson PE, Scheithauer BW, Manivel JC. Malignant peripheral nerve sheath tumor. An immunohistochemical study of 62 cases. Am J Clin Pathol 87:425–433, 1987.

34. Tsang WYW, Chan JKC, Chow LTC, Tse CCH. Perineurioma: an uncommon soft tissue neoplasm distinct from localized hypertrophic neuropathy and neurofibroma. Am J Surg Pathol 16:756–763, 1992.

35. Vandekerckhove J, Weber K. At least six different actins are expressed in a higher mammal: an analysis based on the amino acid sequence of the amino-terminal tryptic peptide. J Mol Biol 126:783–802, 1978.

36. Enzinger FM, Weiss SW. Immunohistochemistry of soft tissue lesions. In: FM Enzinger, SW Weiss, eds. Soft tissue tumors. 3rd ed. St. Louis: Mosby, 1995:139–163.

37. Skalli O, Schurch W, Seemayer T, Lagace R, Montandon D, Pittet B, Gabbiani G. Myofibroblasts from diverse pathologic settings are heterogeneous in their content of actin isoforms and intermediate filament proteins. Lab Invest 60:275–285, 1989.

38. Schurch W, Skalli O, Lagace R, Seemayer TA, Gabbiani G. Intermediate filament proteins and actin isoforms as markers for soft tissue differentiation and origin. III. Hemangiopericytomas and glomus tumors. Am J Pathol 136:771–786, 1990.

39. Porter PG, Bigler SA, McNutt M, Gown AM. The immunophenotype of heman-giopericytoma and glomus tumors with special reference to muscle protein expression: an immunohistochemical study and review of the literature. Mod Pathol 4:46–52, 1991.

40. Gaffney EF, Dervan PA, Fletcher CDM. Pleomorphic rhabdomyosarcoma in adulthood. Analysis of 11 cases with definition of diagnostic criteria. Am J Surg Pathol 17:601–609, 1993.

41. Hollowood K, Fletcher CDM. Rhabdomyosarcoma in adults. Semin Diagn Pathol 11:47–57, 1994

42. Fletcher CD, Tsang WY, Fisher C, Lee KC, Chan JK. Angiomyofibroblastoma of the vulva: a benign neoplasm distinct from aggressive angiomyxoma. Am J Surg Pathol 16:373–382, 1992.

43. Hirose T, Kudo E, Hasegawa T, Abe J, Hizawa K. Cytoskeletal properties of alveolar soft part sarcoma. Hum Pathol 21:204–211, 1990.

44. Guillou L, Wadden C, Coindre J-M, Krausz T, Fletcher CD. "Proximal-type" epithelioid sarcoma, a distinctive aggressive neoplasm showing rhabdoid features: clinicopathologic, immunohistochemical, and ultrastructural study of a series. Am J Surg Pathol 21:130–146, 1997.

45. Truong LD, Rangdaeng S, Cagle P, Ro JY, Hawkins H, Font RL. The diagnostic utility of desmin: a study of 5854 cases and review of the literature. Am J Clin Pathol: 93:305–314, 1990.

46. Wargotz ES, Weiss SW, Norris HJ. Myofibroblastoma of the breast. Sixteen cases of a distinctive benign mesenchymal tumor. Am J Surg Pathol 11:493–502, 1987.

47. Fletcher CDM. Angiomatoid "malignant" fibrous histiocytoma: an immunohistochemical study indicative of myoid differentiation. Hum Pathol 22:563–568, 1991.

48. Folpe AL, Weiss SW, Fletcher CD, Gown AM. Tenosynovial giant cell tumors: evidence for a desmin-positive dendritic cell subpopulation. Mod Pathol 11:939–944, 1998.

49. Skalli O, Gabbiani G, Babai F, Seemayer TA, Pizzolato G, Schurch W. Intermediate filament proteins and actin isoforms as markers for soft tissue tumor differentiation and origin. II. Rhabdomyosarcomas. Am J Pathol 130:515–531, 1988.

50. Dias P, Dilling M, Houghton P. The molecular basis of skeletal muscle differentiation. Semin Diagn Pathol 11:3–14, 1994.

51. Tallini G, Parham DM, Dias P, Cordon-Cardo C, Houghton PJ, Rosai J. Myogenic regulatory protein expression in adult soft tissue sarcomas. A sensitive and specific marker of skeletal muscle differentiation. Am J Pathol 144:693–701, 1994.

52. Cui S, Hano H, Harada T, Takai S, Masui F, Ushigome S. Evaluation of new monoclonal anti-MyoD1 and anti-myogenin antibodies for the diagnosis of rhabdomyosarcoma. Pathol Int 49:62–68, 1999.

53. Miettinen MM, Sarlomo-Rikala M, Kovatich AJ, Lasota J. Calponin and h-caldesmon in soft tissue tumors: consistent h-caldesmon immunoreactivity in gastrointestinal stromal tumors indicates traits of smooth muscle differentiation. Mod Pathol 12:756–762, 1999.

54. Kuru I, Bicknell R, Harris A, Jones M, Gatter K, Mason D. Heterogeneity of vascular endothelial cells with relevance to diagnosis of vascular tumors. J Clin Pathol 45:143–148, 1992.

55. Nagle RB, Witte MH, Maritnez AP, Witte CL, Hendrix MJ, Way D, Reed K. Factor VIII-associated antigen in human lymphatic endothelium. Lymphology 20:20–24, 1987.
56. Miettinen M, Lindenmayer AE, Chaubal A. Endothelial cell markers CD31, CD34, and BNH9 antibody to H- and Y-antigens–evaluation of their specificity and sensitivity in the diagnosis of vascular tumors and comparison with von Willebrand factor. Mod Pathol 7:82–90, 1994.
57. Burgdorf WH, Mukai K, Rosai J. Immunohistochemical identification of factor VIII–related antigen in endothelial cells of cutaneous lesions of alleged vascular nature. Am J Clin Pathol 75:167–171, 1981.
58. Leader M, Collins M, Patel J, Henry K. Staining for factor VIII-related antigen and Ulex europaeus agglutinin I (UEA-I) in 230 tumours. An assessment of their specificity for angiosarcoma and Kaposi's sarcoma. Histopathology 10:1153–1162, 1986.
59. Weiss SW, Ishak KG, Dail DH, Sweet DE, Enzinger FM. Epithelioid hemangioendothelioma and related lesions. Semin Diagn Pathol 3:259–287, 1986.
60. Ordonez NG, Batsakis JB. Comparison of Ulex europaeus I lectin and factor VIII–related antigen in vascular lesions. Arch Pathol Lab Med 108:129–132, 1984.
61. Ohsawa M, Naka N, Tomita Y, Kawamori D, Kanno H, Aozasa K. Use of immunohistochemical procedures in diagnosing angiosarcoma. Evaluation of 98 cases. Cancer 75:2867–2874, 1995.
62. Ramani P, Bradley N, Fletcher C. Qbend/10. A new monoclonal antibody to endothelium: assessment of its diagnostic utility in paraffin sections. Histopathology 17:237–242, 1990.
63. van de Rijn M, Rouse RV. CD34: a review. Appl Immunohistochem 2:71–80, 1994.
64. Renshaw AA, Pinkus GS, Corson JM. CD34 and AE1/AE3: diagnostic discriminants in the distinction of solitary fibrous tumor of the pleura from sarcomatoid mesothelioma. Appl Immunohistochem 2:94–102, 1994.
65. Westra WH, Gerald WL, Rosai J. Solitary fibrous tumor: consistent CD34 immunoreactivity and occurrence in the orbit. Am J Surg Pathol 18:992–998, 1994.
66. Aiba S, Tabata N, Ishii H, Ootani H, Tagami H. Dermatofibrosarcoma protuberans is a unique fibrohistiocytic tumor expressing CD34. Br J Cancer 127:79–84, 1992.
67. Weiss SW, Nickoloff BJ. CD34 is expressed by a distinctive cell population in peripheral nerve, nerve sheath tumors, and related lesions. Am J Surg Pathol 17:1039–1045, 1993.
68. Traweek ST, Kandalaft PL, Mehta P, Battifora H. The human hematopoietic progenitor cell antigen (CD34) in vascular neoplasia. Am J Clin Pathol 96:25–31, 1991.
69. Mikhael AI, Bacchi CE, Zarbo RJ, Ma CK, Gown AM. CD34 expression in stromal tumors of the gastrointestinal tract. Appl Immunohistochem 2:89–93, 1994.
70. Templeton SF, Solomon AR. Spindle cell lipoma is strongly CD34 positive. An immunohistochemical study. J Cutan Pathol 23:546–550, 1996.
71. Suster S, Fisher C, Moran CA. Expression of bcl-2 oncoprotein in benign and malignant spindle cell tumors of soft tissue, skin, serosal surfaces, and gastrointestinal tract. Am J Surg Pathol 22:863–872, 1998.
72. Dei Tos AP, Seregard S, Calonje E, Chan JK, Fletcher CD. Giant cell angiofibroma. A distinctive orbital tumor in adults. Am J Surg Pathol 19:1286–1293, 1995.

73. Smith MEF, Fisher C, Weiss SW. Pleomorphic hyalinizing angiectatic tumor of soft parts. A low-grade neoplasm resembling neurilemmoma. Am J Surg Pathol 20:21–29, 1996.

74. Altman DA, Nickoloff BJ, Fivenson DP. Differential expression of factor XIIIa and CD34 in cutaneous mesenchymal tumors. J Cutan Pathol 20:154–158, 1993.

75. Miettinen M, Sarlomo-Rikala M, Lasota J. Gastrointestinal stromal tumors: recent advances in understanding of their biology. Hum Pathol 30:1213–1220, 1999.

76. Klagsbrun M, D'Amore PA. Vascular endothelial growth factor and its receptors. Cytokine Growth Factor Rev 7:259–270, 1996.

77. Folpe AL, Veikkola T, Valtola R, Weiss SW. Vascular endothelial growth factor receptor-3 (VEGFR-3): a marker of vascular tumors with presumed lymphatic differentiation, including Kaposi's sarcoma, kaposiform and dabska-type hemangioendotheliomas, and a subset of angiosarcomas. Mod Pathol 13:180–185, 2000.

78. Fanburg-Smith JC, Michal M, Partanen TA, Alitalo K, Miettinen M. Papillary intralymphatic angioendothelioma (PILA). A report of twelve cases of a distinctive vascular tumor with phenotypic features of lymphatic vessels. Am J Surg Pathol 23:1004–1010, 1999.

79. Tsokos M, Linnoila RI, Chandra RS, Triche TJ. Neuron-specific enolase in the diagnosis of neuroblastoma and other small, round-cell tumors in children. Hum Pathol 15:575–584, 1984.

80. Thomas P, Battifora H, Manderino GL, Patrick J. A monoclonal antibody against neuron-specific enolase. Immunohistochemical comparison with a polyclonal antiserum. Am J Clin Pathol 88:146–152, 1987.

81. Haimoto H, Takahashi Y, Koshikawa T, Nagura H, Kato K. Immunohistochemical localization of gamma-enolase in normal human tissues other than nervous and neuroendocrine tissues. Lab Invest 52:257–263, 1985.

82. Leader M, Collins M, Patel J, Henry K. Antineuron specific enolase staining reactions in sarcomas and carcinomas: its lack of neuroendocrine specificity. J Clin Pathol 39:1186–1192, 1986.

83. Ordonez NG, Ro JY, Mackay B. Alveolar soft part sarcoma: an ultrastructural and immunocytochemical investigation of its histogenesis. Cancer 63:1721–1736, 1989.

84. Swanson PE, Wick MR. Clear cell sarcoma: an immunohistochemical analysis of six cases and comparison with other epithelioid neoplasms of soft tissue. Arch Pathol Lab Med 113:55–60, 1989.

85. Nemeth J, Galian A, Mikol J, Cochand-Priollet B, Wassef M, Lavergne A. Neuron-specific enolase and malignant lymphomas (23 cases). Virchows Arch A 412:89–93, 1987.

86. Newman PL, Wadden C, Fletcher CDM. Gastrointestinal stromal tumors: correlation of immunophenotype with clinicopathological features. J Pathol 164:107–117, 1991.

87. Devaney K, Vinh TN, Sweet DE. Small cell osteosarcoma of bone: an immunohistochemical study with differential diagnostic considerations. Hum Pathol 24:1211–1225, 1993.

88. DeStephano DB, Lloyd RV, Pike AM, Wilson BS. Pituitary adenomas. An immunohistochemical study of hormone production and chromogranin localization. Am J Pathol 116:464–472, 1984.

89. Lloyd RV, Mervak T, Schmidt K, Warner TF, Wilson BS. Immunohistochemical detection of chromogranin and neuron-specific enolase in pancreatic endocrine neoplasms. Am J Surg Pathol 8:607–614, 1984.

90. Said JW, Vimadalal S, Nash G, Shintaku IP, Heusser RC, Sassoon AF, Lloyd RV. Immunoreactive neuron-specific enolase, bombesin, and chromogranin as markers for neuroendocrine lung tumors. Hum Pathol 16:236–240, 1985.

91. Amann G, Zoubek A, Salzer-Kuntschik M, Windhager R, Kovar H. Relation of neurological marker expression and EWS gene fusion types in MIC2/CD99-positive tumors of the Ewing family. Hum Pathol 30:1059–1064, 1999.

92. Wiedenmann B, Franke WW, Kuhn C, Moll R, Gould VE. Synaptophysin: a marker protein for neuroendocrine cells and neoplasms. Proc Natl Acad Sci USA 83:3500–3504, 1986.

93. Memoli VA, Brown EF, Gould VE. Glial fibrillary acidic protein (GFAP) immunoreactivity in peripheral nerve sheath tumors. Ultrastruct Pathol 7:269–275, 1984.

94. Lodding P, Kindblom L-G, Angervall L, Stenman G. Cellular schwannoma. A clinicopathologic study of 29 cases. Virchow Arch A 416:237–248, 1990.

95. Laskin WB, Fetsch JF, Miettinen M. The "neurothekeoma": immunohistochemical analysis distinguishes the true nerve sheath myxoma from its mimics. Hum Pathol (in press).

96. Molenaar WM, Baker DL, Pleasure D, Lee VM, Trojanowski JQ. The neuroendocrine and neural profiles of neuroblastomas, ganglioneuroblastomas, and ganglioneuromas. Am J Pathol 136:375–382, 1990.

97. Achilles E, Padberg BC, Holl K, Kloppel G, Schroder S. Immunocytochemistry of paragangliomas—value of staining for S-100 protein and glial fibrillary acid protein in diagnosis and prognosis. Histopathology 18:453–458, 1991.

98. Kilpatrick SE, Hitchcock MG, Kraus MD, Calonje E, Fletcher CD. Mixed tumors and myoepitheliomas of soft tissue: a clinicopathologic study of 19 cases with a unifying concept. Am J Surg Pathol 21:13–22, 1997.

99. McGarry RC, Helfand SL, Quarles RH, Roder JC. Recognition of myelin-associated glycoprotein by the monoclonal antibody HNK-1. Nature 306:376–378, 1983.

100. Johnson MD, Glick AD, Davis BW. Immunohistochemical evaluation of Leu-7, myelin basic-protein, S100-protein, glial-fibrillary acidic-protein, and LN3 immunoreactivity in nerve sheath tumors and sarcomas. Arch Pathol Lab Med 112:155–160, 1988.

101. Wick MR, Swanson PE, Scheithauer BW, Manivel JC. Malignant peripheral nerve sheath tumor. An immunohistochemical study of 62 cases. Am J Clin Pathol 87:425–433, 1987.

102. Perentes E, Rubinstein LJ. Immunohistochemical recognition of human nerve sheath tumors by anti-Leu 7 (HNK-1) monoclonal antibody. Acta Neuropathol 69:227–233, 1986.

103. Mazur MT, Shultz JJ, Myers JL. Granular cell tumor. Immunohistochemical analysis of 21 benign tumors and one malignant tumor. Arch Pathol Lab Med 114:692–696, 1990.

104. Swanson PE, Manivel JC, Wick MR. Immunoreactivity for Leu-7 in neurofibrosarcoma and other spindle cell sarcomas of soft tissue. Am J Pathol 126:546–560, 1987.

105. Pettinato G, Swanson PE, Insabato L, DeChiara A, Wick MR. Undifferentiated small round-cell tumors of childhood: the immunocytochemical demonstration of myogenic differentiation in fine-needle aspirates. Diagn Cytopathol 5:194–199, 1989.

106. Mukai M, Torikata C, Iri H, Morikawa Y, Shimizu K, Shimoda T, Nukina N, Ihara Y, Kageyama K. Expression of neurofilament triplet proteins in human neural tumors. An immunohistochemical study of paraganglioma, ganglioneuroma, ganglio-neuroblastoma, and neuroblastoma. Am J Pathol 122:28–35, 1986.

107. Molenaar WM, Muntinghe FL. Expression of neural cell adhesion molecules and neurofilament protein isoforms in Ewing's sarcoma of bone and soft tissue sarcomas other than rhabdomyosarcoma. Hum Pathol 30:1207–1212, 1999.

108. Gerharz CD, Moll R, Meister P, Knuth A, Gabbert H. Cytoskeletal heterogeneity of an epithelioid sarcoma with expression of vimentin, cytokeratins, and neurofilaments. Am J Surg Pathol 14:274–283, 1990.

109. Schmidt U, Muller U, Metz KA, Leder LD. Cytokeratin and neurofilament protein staining in Merkel cell carcinoma of the small cell type and small cell carcinoma of the lung. Am J Dermatopathol 20:346–351, 1998.

110. Horny H-P, Schaumburg-Lever G, Bolz S, Geerts ML, Kaiserling E. Use of monoclonal antibody KP1 for identifying normal and neoplastic human mast cells. J Clin Pathol 43:719–722, 1990.

111. Warnke RA, Pulford KA, Pallesen G, Ralkiaer E, Brown DC, Gatter KC, Mason DY. Diagnosis of myelomonocytic and macrophage neoplasms in routinely processed tissue biopsies with monoclonal antibody KP1. Am J Pathol 135:1089–1095, 1989.

112. Binder SW, Said JW, Shintaku IP, Pinkus GS. A histiocyte-specific marker in the diagnosis of malignant fibrous histiocytoma. Use of monoclonal antibody KP-1 (CD68). Am J Clin Pathol 97:759–763, 1992.

113. Smith ME, Costa MJ, Weiss SW. Evaluation of CD68 and other histiocytic antigens in angiomatoid malignant fibrous histiocytoma. Am J Surg Pathol 15:757–763, 1991.

114. Gloghini A, Rizzo A, Zanette I, Canal B, Rupolo G, Bassi P, Carone A. KP1/CD68 expression in malignant neoplasms including lymphomas, sarcomas, and carcinomas. Am J Clin Pathol 103:425–431, 1995.

115. Maluf HM, DeYoung BR, Swanson PE, Wick MR. Fibroma and giant cell tumor of tendon sheath: a comparative histological and immunohistological study. Mod Pathol 8:155–159, 1995.

116. Kurtin PJ, Bonin DM. Immunohistochemical demonstration of the lysosome associated glycoprotein CD68 (KP-1) in granular cell tumors and schwannomas. Hum Pathol 25:1172–1178, 1994.

117. Grassi F, Dezutter-Dambuyant C, McIlroy D, Jacquet C, Yoneda K, Imamura S, Boumsell L, Schmitt D, Autran B, Debre P, Hosmalin A. Monocyte-derived dendritic cells have a phenotype comparable to that of dermal dendritic cells and display ultrastructural granules distinct from Birbeck granules. J Leukocyte Biol 64:484–493, 1998.

118. Derrick EK, Barker JN, Khan A, Price ML, Macdonald DM. The tissue distribution of factor XIIIa positive cells. Histopathology 22:157–162, 1993.

119. Misery L, Boucheron S, Clandy AL. Factor XIIIa expression in juvenile xanthogranuloma. Acta Derm Venereol 74:43–44, 1994.

120. Hill KA, Gonzalez-Crussi F, Crawford S, Chou P. Calcifying fibrous pseudotumor versus inflammatory myofibroblastic tumor: A histological and immunohistochemical comparison. Pathol Res Prac (in press)

121. Nakajima T, Watanabe S, Sato Y, Kemeya T, Hirota T, Shimosato Y. An immunoperoxidase study of S-100 protein distribution in normal and neoplastic tissues. Am J Surg Pathol 6:715–727, 1982.

122. Kahn HJ, Marks A, Thom H, Baumal R. Role of antibody to S100 protein in diagnostic pathology. Am J Clin Pathol 79:341–347, 1983.

123. Nakamura Y, Becker LE, Marks A. S100 protein in human chordoma and human and rabbit notochord. Arch Pathol Lab Med 107:118–120, 1983.

124. Scheithauer BW, Woodruff JM, Erlandson RA. Primary malignant tumors of peripheral nerve. In: BW Scheithauer, JM Woodruff, RA Erlandson, eds. Tumors of the peripheral nervous system, 3rd series. Washington, DC: Armed Forces Institute of Pathology, 1997:303–372.

125. Weiss SW, Langloss JM, Enzinger FM. Value of S-100 protein in the diagnosis of soft tissue tumors with particular reference to benign and malignant Schwann cell tumors. Lab Invest 49:299–308, 1983.

126. Nakajima T, Watanabe S, Sato Y, Kameya T, Shimosato Y, Ishihara K. Immunohistochemical demonstration of S100 protein in malignant melanoma and pigmented nevus, and its diagnostic application. Cancer 50:912–918, 1982.

127. Warner TF, Lloyd RV, Hafez GR, Angevine JM. Immunocytochemistry of neurotropic melanoma. Cancer 53:254–257, 1984.

128. Dei Tos AP, Wadden C, Fletcher CDM. Extraskeletal myxoid chondrosarcoma: an immunohistochemical reappraisal of 39 cases. Appl Immunohistochem 5:73–77, 1997.

129. Montgomery EA, Meis JM, Frizzera G. Rosai-Dorfman disease of soft tissue. Am J Surg Pathol 16:122–129, 1992.

130. Guillou L, Wadden C, Krausz T, Dei Tos AP, Fletcher CDM. S-100 protein reactivity in synovial sarcomas—a potentially frequent diagnostic pitfall. Appl Immunohistochem 4:167–175, 1996.

131. Gown AM, Vogel AM, Hoak D, Gough F, McNutt MA. Monoclonal antibodies specific for melanocytic tumors distinguish subpopulations of melanocytes. Am J Pathol 123:195–203, 1986.

132. Bacchi CE, Bonetti F, Pea M, Martignoni G, Gown AM. HMB-45. A review. Appl Immunohistochem 4:73–85, 1996.

133. Skelton HG, Maceira J, Smith KJ, McCarthy WF, Lupton GP, Graham JH. HMB45 negative spindle cell malignant melanoma. Am J Dermatopathol 19:580–584, 1997.

134. Fetsch JF, Michal M, Miettinen M. Pigmented (melanotic) neurofibroma. A clinicopathologic and immunohistochemical analysis of 19 lesions from 17 patients. Am J Surg Pathol 24:331–343, 2000.

135. Pea M, Martignoni G, Zamboni G, Bonetti F. Perivascular epithelioid cell [letter]. Am J Surg Pathol 20:1149–1155, 1996.

136. Busam KJ, Chen YT, Old LJ, Stockert E, Iversen K, Coplan KA, Rosai J, Barnhill RL, Jungbluth AA. Expression of Melan-A (MART1) in benign melanocytic nevi and primary cutaneous malignant melanoma. Am J Surg Pathol 22:976–982, 1998.

137. Hofbauer GF, Kamarshev J, Geertsen R, Boni R, Dummer R. Tyrosinase expression in formalin-fixed paraffin-embedded primary and metastatic melanoma: frequency and distribution. J Cutan Pathol 25:204–209, 1998.

138. Jungbluth AA, Iversen K, Coplan K, Williamson B, Chen YT, Stockert E, Old LJ, Busam KJ. Expression of melanocyte-associated markers gp-100 and Melan-A/MART-1 in angiomyolipomas. Virchows Archiv. 434:429–435, 1999.

139. Busam KJ, Iversen K, Coplan KA, Old LJ, Stockert E, Chen YT, McGregor D, Jungbluth A. Immunoreactivity for A103, an antibody to Melan-A (MART-1), in adrenocortical and other steroid tumors. Am J Surg Pathol 22:57–63, 1998.

140. Stevenson AJ, Chatten J, Bertoni F, Miettinen M. CD99 (p30/32 ^{MIC2}) neuroectodermal/Ewing's sarcoma antigen as an immunohistochemical marker. Review of more than 600 tumors and the literature experience. Appl Immunohistochem 2:231–240, 1994.

141. Scotlandi K, Serra M, Manara MC, Benini S, Sarti M, Maurici D, Lollini P-L, Picci P, Bertoni F, Baldini N. Immunostaining of the p30/32 ^{MIC2} antigen and molecular detection of EWS rearrangements for the diagnosis of Ewing's sarcoma and peripheral neuroectodermal tumor. Hum Pathol 27:408–416, 1996.

142. Cooper K, Haffajee Z. Immunohistochemical assessment of MIC2 gene product in granulocytic sarcoma using six epitope retrieval system. Appl Immunohistochem 3:198–201, 1995.

143. Renshaw AA. O13 (CD99) in spindle cell tumors, reactivities with hemangiopericytoma, solitary fibrous tumor, synovial sarcoma, and meningioma but rarely with sarcomatoid mesothelioma. Appl Immunohistochem 3:250–256, 1995.

144. Ashman LK, Cambareri AC, To LB, Levinsky RJ, Juttner CA. Expression of the YB5.B8 antigen (c-kit proto-oncogene product) in normal human bone marrow. Blood 78:30–37, 1991.

145. Tsuura Y, Hiraki H, Watanabe K, Igarashi S, Shimamura K, Fukuda T. Preferential localization of c-kit product in tissue mast cells, basal cells of skin, epithelial cells of breast, small cell lung carcinoma, and seminoma/dysgerminoma in humans: immunohistochemical study of formalin-fixed, paraffin-embedded tissues. Virchows Archiv. 424:135–141, 1994.

146. Maeda H, Yamagata A, Nishikawa S, Yoshinaga K, Kobayshy S, Nishi K, Nishikawa S. Requirement of c-kit for development of intestinal pacemaker system. Development 116:369–375, 1992.

147. Yang F, Tien-Anh T, Carlson JA, Hsi ED, Ross CW, Arber DA. Paraffin section immunophenotype of cutaneous and extracutaneous mast cell disease. Comparison to other hematopoietic neoplasms. Am J Surg Pathol 24:703–709, 2000.

148. Miettinen M, Sarlomo-Rikala M, Lasota J. KIT expression in angiosarcomas and fetal endothelial cells: lack of mutations of exon 11 and exon 17 of c-kit. Mod Pathol 13:536–541, 2000.

149. Nerlich AG, Haraida S, Wiest I. Basement membrane components as differential markers for mesenchymal tumors of various origin. Anticancer Res 14:683–692, 1994.

150. Scheithauer BW, Woodruff JM, Erlandson RA. Miscellaneous benign neurogenic tumors. In: BW Scheithauer, JM Woodruff, RA Erlandson, eds. Tumors of the peripheral nervous system, 3rd series. Washington, DC: Armed Forces Institute of Pathology, 1997:219–282.

6
Fibroblastic Lesions

Salwa S. Sheikh
Dhahran Health Center
Dhahran, Saudi Arabia

Elizabeth Montgomery
The Johns Hopkins University
Baltimore, Maryland

Fibrous lesions, including tumors and nontumorous lesions, form a large group of entities with diverse clinical behavior ranging from entirely benign to locally aggressive to frankly malignant with metastases (1,2). Therefore, these lesions may be divided into four categories:

1. Benign fibrous tissue proliferations.
2. Fibromatoses.
3. Malignant tumors, including fibrosarcoma and myofibrosarcoma.
4. Fibrous proliferations of infancy and childhood. As this group of lesions primarily occurs during the first year of life and has a distinct histologic picture, it will be discussed separately.

Fibrous connective tissue consists primarily of fibroblasts and extracellular matrix. Fibroblasts most commonly appear as spindle-shaped cells with pale-staining nuclei with one or two small nucleoli. The cytoplasmic borders are indistinct because of long slender processes, and the cytoplasm is eosinophilic to slightly basophilic depending on the state of activity. Myofibroblasts are modified fibroblasts with features of both fibroblasts and smooth muscle cells. These cells are involved in a variety of reactive and neoplastic proliferations. Both fibroblasts and myofibroblasts produce procollagen and collagen.

I. BENIGN FIBROUS TISSUE PROLIFERATIONS

Benign fibroblastic proliferations constitute a diverse group of disorders that are mostly considered as reactive rather than neoplastic. Pseudosarcomatous proliferative lesions of soft tissue are fascia-based fibroblastic and myofibroblastic lesions that have the potential to be overdiagnosed as sarcoma. They are usually subtyped according to the location, depth of involvement, age at presentation, and histologic features. They are presumed to be reactive, and recurrences are only rarely encountered after surgical excision (3). For example, a flow cytometric study of several of these benign proliferations, including 13 examples of nodular fasciitis, 3 of proliferative myositis, 1 of proliferative fasciitis, and 12 other benign fibrous lesions, showed uniform diploidy. Cell cycle analysis did not correlate with mitotic counts (4).

A. Nodular Fasciitis

Nodular fasciitis is the most frequently encountered pseudosarcomatous lesion. It is sometimes mistaken for a sarcoma because of its rapid growth, increased cellularity, and high mitotic index (1,2,5). Nodular fasciitis occurs mostly in the third to fourth decades as a rapidly growing solitary mass of the upper extremities (6,7). The second most common site is the head and the neck region, which is the most frequently reported site in infants and children. No gender predilection has been observed.

Grossly the lesion is a well-circumscribed, nonencapsulated nodule usually less than 2 cm in diameter. The cut surface varies from fibrous to gelatinous or mucoid. Histologically, nodular fasciitis usually involves subcutaneous tissue, but intramuscular and fascial forms also occur. The nodule consists primarily of plump fibroblasts that appear similar to those seen in tissue culture or granulation tissue. The fibroblasts are arranged in a whorled/storiform pattern (Fig. 1), or haphazardly. The cells are bland in appearance, with pale nuclei and small nucleoli. The mitotic rate is fairly high but atypical mitoses are absent. Intermixed with the fibroblasts are lymphocytes and extravasated erythrocytes, with variable numbers of macrophages and giant cells (Fig. 2) in the central portion of the lesion. The intervening matrix is myxoid, imparting a feathery appearance, whereas cellular forms exhibit dense cellularity and have less matrix (8). Microcysts and/or macrocysts as well as areas of microhemorrhages can be seen, but hemosiderin is absent. Lesions of short duration usually are myxoid, whereas those of longer duration are more fibrotic or hyalinized with cyst formation. These fibroblasts stain positive with vimentin, smooth muscle actin, and muscle-specific actin.

Other variants of nodular fasciitis merit a brief description (8). *Ossifying fasciitis* is a nodular fasciitis-like fibroblastic proliferation with osseous metapla-

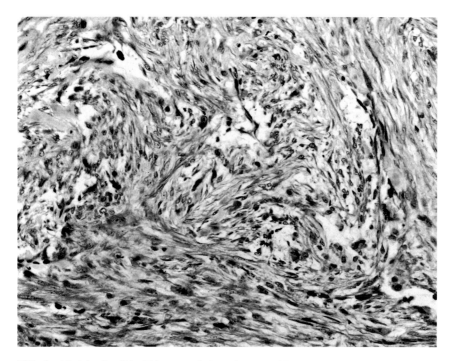

FIG. 1 Nodular fasciitis. This example has a loose storiform pattern, small cystic spaces, and cells with scattered mitoses and uniform small nucleoli.

sia (7). Most of these lesions show features of both nodular fasciitis and myositis ossificans. *Intravascular fasciitis* is a rare variant of nodular fasciitis arising from small or medium-size vessels (9,10). The lesion presents as a soft-tissue mass with focal intravascular extension or as a multinodular predominantly intravascular mass. Despite the intravascular location, the lesion behaves in a benign fashion with no tendency to recur or metastasize. *Cranial fasciitis* involves soft tissues of the scalp and underlying skull of infants. It usually erodes the bone but may penetrate through the bone to involve the meninges. Fragments of bone may be seen at the periphery of this lesion. Birth trauma is presumed to be the inciting stimulus of this benign reactive process (11).

The differential diagnosis of nodular fasciitis includes a number of entities, including malignant ones. *Myxoma*, although it may appear similar to the myxoid form of nodular fasciitis, is paucicellular and poorly vascularized. *Fibrous histiocytoma* is usually less well circumscribed with cells arranged in a storiform pattern, hyalinized collagen, and abundant chronic inflammatory cells, siderophages,

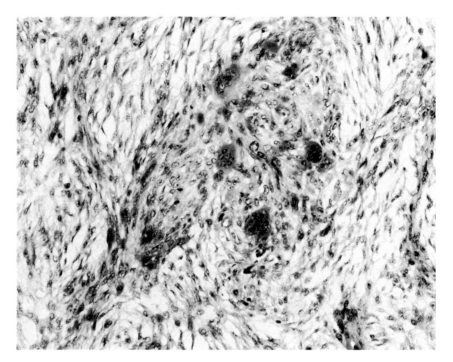

FIG. 2   Osteoclast-like giant cells are frequently found in nodular fasciitis.

and Touton-type giant cells. *Fibromatosis* is usually a larger lesion that is less well circumscribed with infiltration into the muscle. The fibroblasts are arranged in long sweeping fascicles separated by bundles of collagen with infrequent mitotic figures. *Fibrosarcomas* are large, deeply located masses that are almost always more cellular. The cells are arranged in a herringbone pattern. The nuclei are hyperchromatic with increased numbers of mitoses as well as atypical ones.

   Myxoid malignant fibrous histiocytoma/myxofibrosarcoma (MFH) occurs principally in older patients (>50 years). There is close association between the myxoid and the cellular areas and cellular pleomorphism (12,13).

B.   Proliferative Fasciitis

Proliferative fasciitis is another pseudosarcomatous lesion that poses diagnostic problems. It is less common than nodular fasciitis (7,14,15). It occurs mainly in adults with no sex predilection. The lesion often presents as a palpable, mobile, rapidly growing, subcutaneous nodule in the extremities, especially the forearm and the thigh.

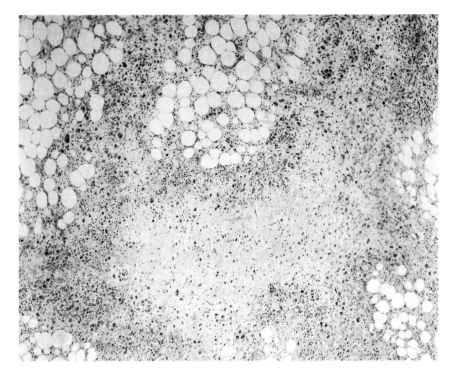

FIG. 3 Proliferative fasciitis. The lesion tracks along connective tissue septa.

Grossly it appears as a poorly circumscribed elongated mass mainly involving the interlobular fibrous tissue septa of the subcutis.

Histologically, in addition to stellate cells, there are large characteristic ganglion-like cells (Figs. 3 and 4) with basophilic cytoplasm, one or two nucleoli, and occasional cytoplasmic inclusions. There is variable myxoid stroma that becomes more collagenized as lesions persist.

The differential diagnosis includes *malignant fibrous histiocytoma*, which has more atypia and pleomorphic-looking giant cells as opposed to ganglion-like cells. *Ganglioneuroblastoma* contains, in addition to small round cells, aberrantly formed ganglion cells and may resemble proliferative myositis. However, ganglion cells express neuroendocrine markers, whereas the ganglion-like cells in proliferative fasciitis are modified fibroblasts, thus retaining the same staining characteristics. *Rhabdomyosarcoma* also enters into the differential diagnosis as the ganglion-like cells may bear resemblance to the rhabdomyoblasts, a consideration apt to arise in pediatric examples (14). Immunohistochemistry can assist in any doubtful case as rhabdomyoblasts are desmin-positive whereas ganglion-like cells of proliferative fasciitis are typically desmin-negative.

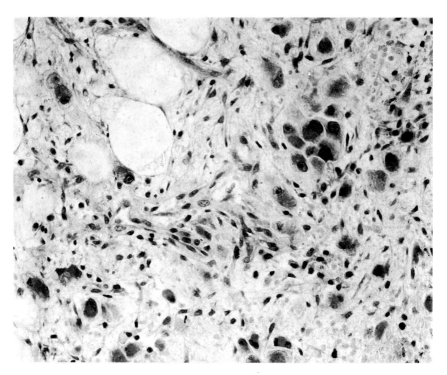

FIG. 4 In proliferative fasciitis, the enlarged cells with macronucleoli are referred to as "ganglion-like." Note that, despite the impressive appearance of the ganglion-like cells, the background myofibroblasts resemble those seen in nodular fasciitis.

C. Proliferative Myositis

Proliferative myositis is the deep or intramuscular counterpart of proliferative fasciitis (14). It typically presents as a rapidly growing mass affecting the muscles of the trunk and the limb girdles. Grossly the tumor/nodule is poorly circumscribed, appearing as a pale, scar-like induration of the muscle and overlying fascia. Histologically, it is a poorly demarcated process with fibroblastic proliferation involving the epimysium, perimysium, and endomysium, with scattered large basophilic ganglion-like giant cells. At low magnification, alternating areas of proliferated fibroblasts and remnants of infiltrated muscle tissue produce a "checker board" pattern. Variable amounts of myxoid to collagenized stroma are usually present. Focal areas of ossification can be seen, although this finding is less conspicuous in proliferative myositis than in myositis ossificans.

The differential diagnosis is that of proliferative fasciitis.

D. Atypical Decubital Fibroplasia/Ischemic Fasciitis

Atypical decubital fibroplasia, also known as ischemic fasciitis, has some resemblance to proliferative fasciitis and is considered a degenerative and reparative process (16,16a). It occurs as a mass lesion over bony prominences (e.g., sacrum or ischial tuberosities) and has been attributed to prolonged pressure and impaired circulation, mainly in elderly debilitated, immobilized, or wheelchair-bound patients. Microscopically there is a lobular or zonal pattern with central fibrinous and myxoid areas rimmed by ingrowing thin-walled ectatic vascular channels. There is proliferation of fibroblasts with scattered ganglion-like giant cells with basophilic cytoplasm, large hyperchromatic nuclei with smudged nuclear chromatin and prominent nucleoli. These cells are intermixed with inflammatory cells, areas of hemorrhage, granulation tissue, focal fibrinoid necrosis with fibrosis, and cystic changes (seen more often in older patients).

From a practical standpoint, recognition of atypical decubital fibroplasia and its distinction from sarcoma is critical. The differential diagnosis includes *myxoid liposarcoma*, which is characterized by organized arborizing delicate vasculature and the presence of lipoblasts in majority of the cases. Although distinction from *myxoid MFH* can be problematic, the cells in atypical decubital fibroplasia are usually less bizzare and there are accompanying secondary/reactive features, including hemorrhage, fat necrosis, and fibrin deposition. Cells of *extraskeletal myxoid chondrosarcoma* are, ironically, more uniform and bland than those of atypical decubital fibroplasia. Myxoid chondrosarcoma has a distinct multilobular architecture with fibrous bands and an inconspicuous vascular pattern. Other considerations include nonneoplastic fibroblastic proliferations, such as *proliferative fasciitis* and *decubitus ulcer*/bed sore. The former lacks fibrinoid necrosis and the latter features skin ulceration without a mass lesion; the skin overlying atypical decubital fibroplasia is intact.

E. Fibroma

Fibroma is a generic term denoting any polypoid or localized tumorous lesion with abundant collagen associated with sparse fibroblasts. Various subtypes have been recognized depending on their characteristic location or clinical presentation. Examples include fibroma of tendon sheath that involves the tendon sheaths on the digits of the hands and feet, and nuchal fibroma, typically occurring in a midline location at the nape of the neck (17).

1. Fibroma of Tendon Sheath

Fibroma of tendon sheath is a slow-growing, painless, reactive, fibrous proliferation with characteristic location and histologic appearance. It is firmly attached to the tendons of the hands and feet. It is seen most commonly in adults between the ages of 20 and 50 years. Its lobular architecture resembles that of giant cell tumor of tendon sheath, which is a fibrohistiocytic lesion. Some authors believe that both entities are different stages of the same pathologic process as some studies show that both lesions demonstrate some degree of monocyte-macrophage and (myo)-fibroblastic differentiation, although fibromas of tendon sheath show more fibroblastic differentiation whereas giant cell tumors of tendon sheaths have more monocyte-macrophage differentiation (18). Fibromas of tendon sheath are usually less cellular than giant cell tumor of tendon sheath and are devoid of giant cells or xanthoma cells. About 25% of these lesions recur locally.

Grossly the tumor/nodule appears as a well-circumscribed, lobulated, rubbery, pearly, white mass resembling cartilage. Histologically, at low magnification, the distinct lobular configuration can be appreciated (Fig. 5). Although most nodules are densely collagenized or hyalinized, a cellular phase may be seen early in some cases, which resembles nodular fasciitis (Fig. 6). The lobules have cleft-

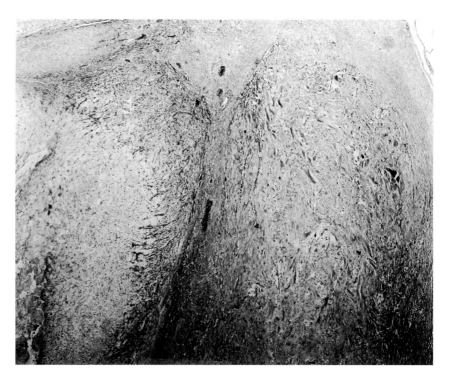

FIG. 5 At scanning magnification, fibroma of tendon sheath is a lobulated lesion with central dense collagen within individual lobules.

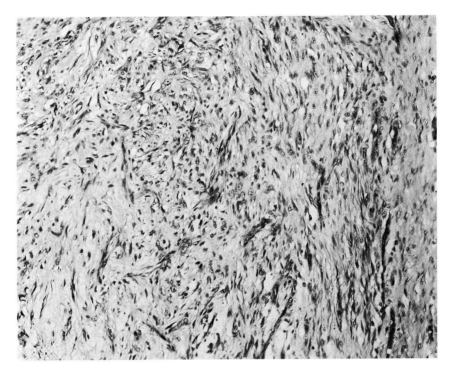

FIG. 6 The more cellular tissue at the periphery of the lobules of fibroma of tendon sheath resembles nodular fasciitis.

like spaces with scattered chondro-osseous foci seen occasionally. Myxoid change with interspersed stellate-shaped fibroblasts may be a prominent feature.

Confusion with other lesions is less likely due to the distinct microscopic appearance of these densely hyalinized fibromas. More cellular cases can be confused with *fibrous histiocytoma*, *nodular fasciitis*, *fibromatosis*, and *fibrosarcoma*, but close attention to the lobular configuration, circumscription, attachment to tendon sheaths, and gradual transition from cellular to hyalinized areas allows recognition of this lesion.

2. Nuchal Fibroma

Benign soft-tissue tumors with a predilection for the head and neck region include spindle cell lipomas, pleomorphic lipomas, and nuchal fibromas. Nuchal fibroma is a rare fibrous proliferation of subcutis that mainly involves the interscapular and paraspinal regions of adult patients. If incompletely excised, the lesion may recur.

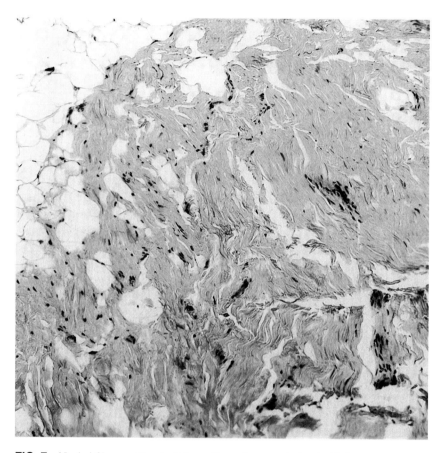

FIG. 7   Nuchal fibroma. Paucicellular collagen is seen admixed with fat.

The tumor lacks a capsule and shows paucicellular dense collagen with inter-spersed mature fat and entrapment of nerve fibers (Fig. 7). A variable amount of calcification and, rarely, ossification may be present.

Distinction from *fibrolipoma* can be difficult; however, fibrolipoma usu-ally has a fibrous capsule with more adipose tissue and also nuchal fibromas have a characteristic location. Nuchal fibroma can be distinguished from *extra-abdominal fibromatosis* by its superficial location and low cellularity (19). *Nuchal fibrocartilaginous pseudotumor* is a distinctive soft-tissue lesion that occurs in the posterior aspect of the base of the neck (Figs. 8–10), at the junction of the nuchal ligament and the deep cervical fascia. It was first believed to be a variant of nuchal fibroma, although several differences were noted. Nuchal fibroma is not confined to the midline, lacks an association with ligaments, and occurs superficial to the

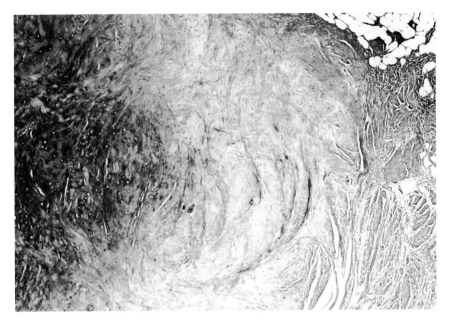

FIG. 8 Nuchal fibrocartilaginous tumor. Hypocellular fibrocartilaginous nodule adjacent to the nuchal ligament.

fascia. Nuchal fibrocartilaginous pseudotumor is associated with prior neck injury and histologically shows fibrocartilaginous metaplasia (20).

3. Elastofibroma

Elastofibroma is a slowly growing fibroelastic proliferation resulting from mechanical friction between the scapula and the chest wall, and is hence considered reactive. Lesions typically occur on the backs of elderly patients, usually female, with a history of mechanical labor (21). Grossly the mass is usually firm, ill defined, with glistening surface showing foci of cystic degeneration and interspersed fatty areas. Microscopically, the mass consists of interwining eosinophilic hyalinized collagen and thickened, serrated, deeply eosinophilic elastic fibers that have a degenerated beaded appearance or are fragmented into globules (*chenille*, or "caterpillar" bodies) or flower-like arrangements. Elastin stain characteristically highlights the degenerated appearance of these elastic fibers (Fig. 11). The differential diagnosis would include other elastic tissue disorders, such as *pseudoxanthoma elasticum*, which is an autosomal recessive disorder and presents as multiple xanthoma-like papules. *Fibrolipoma* and *fibromatosis* both lack the characteristic degenerated elastic fibers.

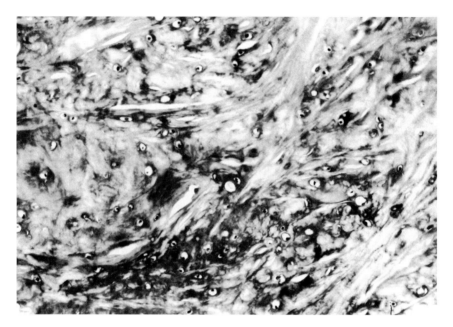

FIG. 9   Nuchal fibrocartilaginous tumor. Irregular fibrillated cartilage matrix.

4.   Nasopharyngeal Angiofibromas

Nasopharyngeal angiofibroma is a richly vascular fibrous proliferation that typically presents in the second decade in males as a lobulated polypoid mass of the
nasopharynx or paranasal sinuses leading to nasal obstruction and epistaxis. It may
erode the bone or extend from the antrum into cheek and orbit, causing visual disturbance, protrusion of the eye, and swelling (22).

    Grossly the tumor is polypoid, smooth, firm-rubbery in consistency, with a
spongy appearance of the cut surface due to the rich vascularity. Microscopically,
the lesion consists of fibrous tissue proliferation with variable cellularity and interspersed slit-like or gaping vascular channels. The vessels are thin-walled and
are usually devoid of smooth muscle lining and elastic membrane, a feature that
probably is responsible for the profuse hemorrhage.

5.   Keloid

A keloid is a benign overgrowth of scar tissue with a predilection for individuals
with darkly pigmented skin; it may also show a familial tendency. It usually occurs
in adolescents and young adults after trauma or surgery. In addition, there are idiopathic forms that are considered secondary to occult minor infections or injuries.

    Grossly, the lesion appears as a well-circumscribed, polypoid, fleshy mass
often, extending with multiple processes into the surrounding tissue. Although it

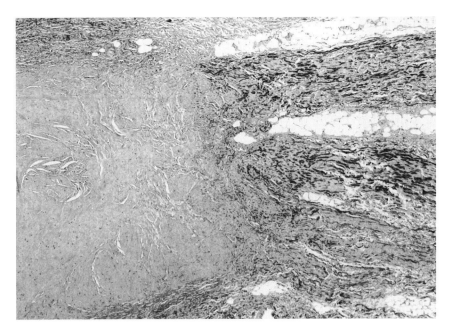

FIG. 10 Nuchal fibrocartilaginous tumor. Fibrocartilage nodule juxtaposed to the nuchal ligament demonstrating degenerative fragmentation of elastic fibers (elastic stain).

may be asymptomatic, most keloids cause itching, pain, and tenderness. Histologically, there is haphazard arrangement of collagen fibers with a glassy hyalinized appearance and myxoid matrix. Early lesions tend to be more vascular, especially at the periphery. Longstanding cases may show variable amounts of calcification and ossification.

The differential diagnosis includes *hypertrophic scar*, which in the early stage may resemble keloid microscopically but in later stage usually flattens out and has less mucoid matrix and scant or no glassy collagen. *Collagenoma* is a connective tissue nevus that presents clinically as multiple discrete nodules with no history of trauma or scar but microscopically may resemble keloid and hypertrophic scar. *Scleroderma* may enter into the histologic differential diagnosis as it leads to thickening and altered staining of existing collagen, but it usually lacks glassy fibers and differs clinically by being flat and retracted rather than protuberant.

6.   Collagenous Fibroma (Desmoplastic Fibroblastoma)

Collagenous fibroma/desmoplastic fibroblastoma is a distinctive soft-tissue tumor that is poorly recognized and may be mistaken for other benign or even malignant spindle cell tumors because of the small number of reported cases. The tumors

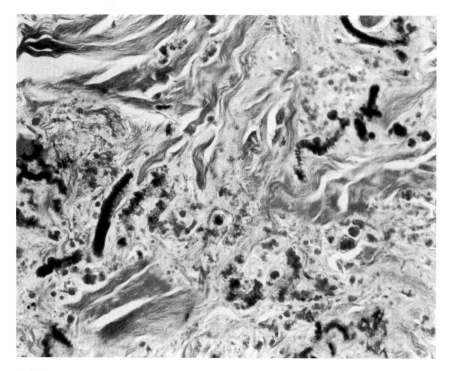

FIG. 11   Chenille bodies in elastofibroma, so named for their resemblance to caterpillars (elastic stain).

usually present as well-circumscribed, firm masses that are hypocellular with spindle- and stellate-shaped fibroblasts embedded in a hypovascular, densely fibrous stroma. Mitotic figures and necrosis are not identified. The lesions reported to date have not recurred (23,24). The most significant differential diagnostic consideration is probably *desmoid tumor (fibromatosis)*. Desmoid tumors are more cellular, more vascular, and more infiltrative at their periphery.

II. FIBROMATOSES

The fibromatoses are a distinctive and broad group of benign fibrous proliferations that are intermediate in their biological behavior between benign fibrous proliferations and fibrosarcoma in that they tend to invade locally and recur after surgical excision but do not metastasize (25,26). Fibromatoses/desmoids are considered a truly neoplastic process as clonality has been demonstrated by several studies, including traditional cytogenetics and polymerase chain reaction (PCR) amplification of *HUMARA* for analysis of patterns of X-chromosome inactivation (27,28). Reported cytogenetic abnormalities have included trisomy 8, trisomy 20, and abnormalities of the Y chromosome (29). A specific history of trauma at the precise point of growth is often elicited. Hormonal effects and pregnancy are believed to influence the growth of this tumor. A generalized (inherited or mutant) defect in growth regulation of connective tissue has also been suggested as an underlying cause. Patients have also been shown to have radiographic evidence of minor skeletal anomalies (30,31). Some tumors express hormone receptors (estrogen and progestrone receptors); therefore tamoxifen and other hormonal manipulations are among the adjuvant therapies that have been used for this tumor (31–35).

Fibromatoses are categorized as superficial or deep based on their distinctive features:

1. Superficial fibromatoses (fascial)
   a. Palmar fibromatosis
   b. Plantar fibromatosis
   c. Penile fibromatosis
   d. Knuckle pads
2. Deep fibromatoses (musculoaponeurotic)
   a. Extra-abdominal fibromatosis/desmoid
   b. Abdominal fibromatosis/desmoid
   c. Intra-abdominal fibromatosis/desmoid

A. Superficial Fibromatoses

1. Palmar Fibromatosis (Dupuytren's Disease)

Palmar fibromatosis is probably the commonest of all fibromatoses. Its incidence is 1–2%, and lesions present as a slowly growing small subcutaneous nodules or plaques involving the dermis or underlying fascia of the palm. These nodules may lead to contractures (36). They may be bilateral, familial, and multiple. There is an association between Dupuytren's contractures and alcoholism, epilepsy, diabetes, chronic lung disease, and painful shoulders. Coexistence with other superficial fibromatoses (plantar and penile) has been described but not with deep fibromatoses. There is a tendency to local recurrence after surgical excision.

Grossly the lesion usually consists of a single nodule or a multinodular mass closely associated with thickened palmar aponeurosis. Microscopically, the palpable nodule or plaque consists of multiple tiny fibrovascular nodules with narrow blood vessels surrounded by a thin cuff of collagen situated near the center of these nodules. Lesions of short duration are more cellular, with plump immature-appearing fibroblasts that are uniform in appearance and contain variable numbers of mitotic figures. Lesions of longer duration are less cellular and contain an increased amount of dense collagen. Variable myxoid matrix is present and, rarely, longstanding lesions may develop cartilaginous or osseous metaplasia.

2. Plantar Fibromatosis (Ledderhose's Disease)

Plantar fibromatosis, like palmar fibromatosis, is a nodular fibrous proliferation. It involves plantar aponeuroses but is less likely to develop contractures and has a higher rate of recurrence than palmar fibromatosis. Its incidence is increased in patients with palmar or penile fibromatosis. Although the lesions may be entirely asymptomatic, they may cause mild pain or paresthesia if there is superficial plantar nerve entrapment.

Grossly and histologically the lesion is essentially indistinguishable from palmar fibromatosis, although the presence of striking cellularity and numerous mitoses can raise the possibility of malignancy—an interpretation avoided by attention to the clinical history.

3. Penile Fibromatosis (Peyronie's Disease/Plastic Induration of the Penis)

Peyronie's disease is a localized fibromatosis that affects the tunica albuginea of the penis. It begins as an inflammatory disorder, subsequently leading to fibrous plaques on the dorsum of the penis causing it to curve toward the affected side. Often there is difficulty in passing urine and pain on erection and intercourse. It is much less common than palmar and plantar fibromatosis but is seen more frequently in patients with these other superficial fibromatoses. Multiple clonal chromosomal abnormalities have been described in Peyronie's disease (37).

Histologically there is relatively little fibrosis with inflammatory cells in earlier lesions, as opposed to older lesions which are more fibrotic with only scant inflammatory cells. Patchy deposition of elastic fibers, thickened fibrous plaques, destruction of smooth muscle, and/or ossification (Fig. 12) may all be encountered in older lesions.

4. Knuckle Pads

Knuckle pads are uncommon flat or dome-shaped fibrous thickenings of the dorsal aspect of proximal interphalangeal or metacarpophalangeal joints. They are seen more frequently in patients with palmar or plantar fibromatosis. Microscopically they resemble palmar fibromatosis but there are no contractures. Knuckle pads should be distinguished from Heberdon's nodes of osteoartheritis and hyperkeratosis secondary to chronic irritation or trauma.

B. Deep Fibromatoses

1. Extra-Abdominal Fibromatosis (Desmoid)

Extra-abdominal desmoid has a deceptively bland histomorphology but a tendency to recur locally and infiltrate the surrounding tissue; hence the name "ag-

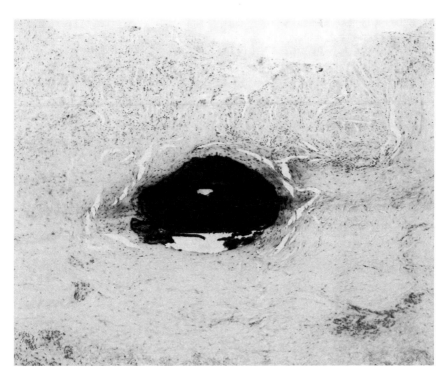

FIG. 12 Peyronie's disease (penile fibromatosis). Ossification is not uncommon in these lesions.

gressive fibromatosis" (38). It arises primarily in the connective tissue of muscle and the overlying fascia or aponeurosis (musculoaponeurotic fibromatosis). Although many organs can be involved, such as breast, vulva, and spermatic cord, the most common location is the shoulder girdle followed by chest wall and back, thigh, and neck (39–45). The tumor has rarely been associated with breast implants (46). Fibromatosis of the head and neck is seen more commonly in children, in which case the lesions tend to be more cellular and may grow more aggressively, even encroaching on the trachea with destruction of adjacent bone and a fatal outcome. Although these tumors do not metastasize, multicentricity has been described (47,48).

Clinically the lesions present as deep-seated, firm, nonencapsulated, slowly growing, locally invasive, painless masses. They are seen most commonly in young women, although, as above, children and even infants may be affected.

Grossly the tumor is firm with coarse white trabeculation resembling a scar and cuts with a gritty sensation. Microscopically, the lesion is poorly defined with

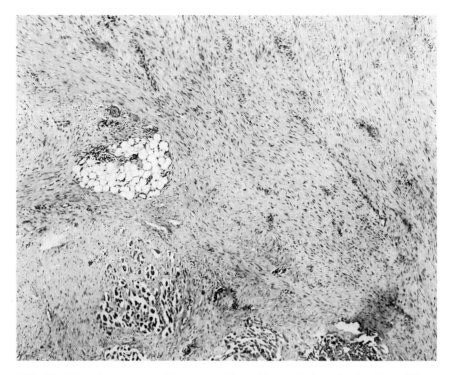

FIG. 13 Musculoaponeurotic fibromatosis (desmoid tumor). Sweeping fascicles of fibro-blasts, punctuated by small, prominent vessels, infiltrate between skeletal muscle bundles.

infiltrative margins consisting of spindled fibroblasts separated by abundant col-lagen (Figs. 13 and 14). Cells and collagen are organized in a sweeping fashion. Keloid-like collagen and hyalinization may be so extensive as to obscure the orig-inal pattern of the tumor. Scattered thin-walled, elongated, and compressed vessels are usually seen with focal areas of hemorrhage, lymphoid aggregates, and, rarely, calcification or chondro-osseous metaplasia. Mitotic figures are uncommon.

The differential diagnosis includes fibrosarcoma and benign fibroblastic proliferative lesions. Classic high-grade *fibrosarcomas* are, in general, more cellu-lar with a herringbone pattern, have increased mitotic figures (i.e., one mitosis per high-power field), and atypical mitoses. The challenge is to separate fibromatoses from low-grade fibrosarcomas. Both lesions have infiltrative margins, although well-differentiated fibrosarcoma may appear less invasive to the adjacent struc-tures and has a tendency to form a pseudocapsule. Well-differentiated fibrosar-coma tumor cells and collagen are arranged in bundles and bands in a manner re-sembling fibromatoses. Mitoses are rare, and the classic herringbone pattern may

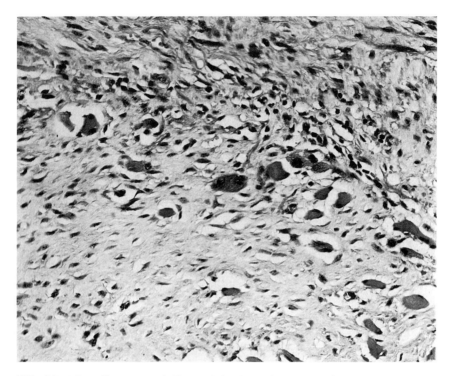

FIG. 14 When fibromatoses infiltrate skeletal muscle, degenerating myocytes may appear atypical and even have large nucleoli.

not be a prominent feature in better differentiated tumors. The distinction between these two entities, which revolves around identification of subtle nuclear atypia in fibrosarcomas, may be extremely difficult, if not impossible, on small biopsy specimens (49). A *scar* may also resemble a fibromatosis, especially in a small biopsy where the relationship with adjacent tissue cannot be assessed. Fibromatosis may focally exhibit a whorled/storiform pattern mimicking *nodular fasciitis*, but never with the prominence or uniformity as that seen in nodular fasciitis. *Myxomas* may enter the differential diagnosis as fibromatoses may have areas of myxoid degeneration. However, fibromatoses are typically more cellular and have more collagen than myxomas. *Desmoplastic fibromas* of bone are histologically indistinguishable from fibromatoses.

2. Abdominal Fibromatosis (Desmoid)

Abdominal fibromatosis has identical morphology to the extra-abdominal desmoids but is given separate consideration as it has a characteristic location and presentation. It usually occurs in the abdominal wall of women of childbearing age during or after pregnancy (50). It typically manifests as a slow-growing progressive mass, which becomes more prominent on abdominal muscle contraction.

The gross and microscopic features are identical to those of extra-abdominal fibromatosis. In this location, recurrences are less frequent than in extra-abdominal presentations.

3.   Intra-abdominal Fibromatosis (Desmoid)

Intra-abdominal fibromatosis includes several entities that have similar morphologic findings but distinct clinical presentations (51). *Pelvic fibromatosis* typically involves the lower portion of the pelvis where it presents as a slowly growing mass in young females but has no relationship to gestation. *Mesentric fibromatosis* is probably the commonest among the intra-abdominal fibromatoses. It usually presents as a slowly growing mass that involves small-bowel mesentery or retroperitoneum where distinction may become extremely difficult due to retropritoneal fibrosis. There are cases associated with pregnancy and Crohn's disease, although the majority are considered to be secondary to trauma (52). Mesentric fibromatosis in patients with *Gardner's syndrome* appears to have a substantially higher recurrence rate than in patients without this syndrome (51,53,54). Gardner's syndrome is an autosomal dominant familial disease with a female predilection. It consists of numerous colorectal adenomatous polyps, osteomas, cutaneous cysts, soft-tissue masses, and other manifestations (55), and is related to *familial adenomatous poyposis*, a disorder caused by germ line adenomatous polyposis coli (APC) gene mutations associated with an 8–12% incidence of fibromatosis (56,57). Fibromatosis in familial adenomatous polyposis is one of the manifestations of Gardner's syndrome (58). As above, unresectability and recurrence of fibromatoses seem more common in this group of patients (59).

III.   MALIGNANT TUMORS

A.   Fibrosarcoma

Fibrosarcoma is a deep-seated, slowly growing, painless mass occurring primarily in lower extremities of patients in their fourth through sixth decades (60). It usually involves the intramuscular fibrous tissue, aponeuroses, or tendons. Involvement of the subcutis is unusual and occurs mostly in cases where the tumor is seen in association with dermatofibrosacoma protuberans, cicatrix, burn, or history of exposure to radiation (2,61). In fact, the tumor may arise anywhere in the body where fibrous tissue is present. The skin overlying superficial tumors is generally intact, but focal ulceration may be seen in the case of rapid growth or trauma. Deep-seated tumors, on the other hand, may encircle bone and cause periosteal and cortical thickening, making distinction from parosteal osteosarcoma difficult at best. The overall survival rate seems to be closely related to the degree of tumor differentiation (grade). The recurrence rate is mainly related to adequacy of surgical excision. As for most sarcomas, metastasis occurs almost exclusively hematogenously, with lung the most common site. Only rare examples of lymph node metastasis have been reported (62). Spontaneous development of fibrosarcoma from a benign lesion, e.g., desmoid, is a vanishingly rare complication, with few such cases reported (63,64). Review of the illustrations in one of these reportedly occurring 28 years after resection of a fibromatosis (63) casts some doubt on the accuracy of the original diagnosis.

Grossly the tumor consists of a gray–white, fleshy-to-firm, lobulated, well-circumscribed mass with focal or complete pseudoencapsulation that is especially prominent in small lesions. Microscopically, in high-grade examples, there is a rather uniform growth pattern with fibroblasts separated by intervening collagen arranged in the classic "herringbone" pattern. The number of mitotic figures is variable. Rarely, chondroid or osseous metaplasia can be seen. The prognosis in regard to recurrence and metastasis is least favorable in cases with rich cellularity, decreased amount of collagen, necrosis, and more than two mitotic figures per high-power field (61).

Well-differentiated fibrosarcomas have a uniform growth pattern markedly resembling fibromatoses with bland-appearing fibroblasts, subtle nuclear atypia, and only rare mitotic figures (Figs. 15–17). *Sclerosing epithelioid fibrosarcoma* is another variant of fibrosarcoma that consists of nests and strands of epithelioid fibroblasts with clear cytoplasm, round cells, and small nuclei simulating infiltrating carcinoma. These tumor nests and cords are surrounded by collagen. Focal areas of myxoid degeneration and more cellular areas resembling desmoids can be seen. The majority of cases do exhibit at least focal areas of conventional fibrosarcoma (65). *Poorly differentiated fibrosarcomas* are more cellular with less intervening collagen. Although there is some cellular atypia, marked pleomorphism is not a typical feature. Mitotic figures are numerous, with a less prominent herringbone pattern and areas of hemorrhage and necrosis. Although the most common postirradiation sarcoma is probably malignant fibrous histiocytoma, there is a higher incidence of fibrosarcoma in patients exposed to radiation. In such cases, the surrounding tissue typically shows signs of radiation injury, such as fibrosis, intimal proliferation, and fat necrosis. The lag time between exposure to radiation and development of *postirradiation fibrosarcoma* is 4–15 years (61,66). These tumors typically have a low-grade fibrosarcoma appearance and are peculiar in that they often cause death of the patient by local infiltration rather than by distant metastasis (67). Occasionally, fibrosarcomas may arise as a result of *thermal injury* in patients with extensive burns. As carcinoma is a more common late consequence of thermal injury, the possibility of spindle cell carcinoma should be excluded before making the diagnosis of fibrosarcoma. *Inflammatory fibrosarcoma* occurs primarily but not exclusively in children and young adults, typically pre-

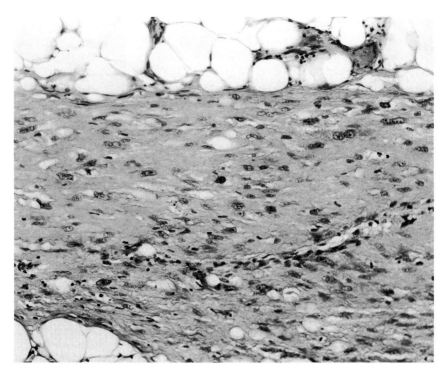

FIG. 15 Low-grade fibrosarcoma. Compare the cytologic features to those in Fig. 14, taken at the same magnification. Despite similar cellularity, the low-grade fibrosarcoma features larger nuclei than the fibromatosis.

senting as multiple nodules within the abdominal cavity involving the mesentery and the retroperitoneum. There are associated systemic symptoms, such as anemia, fever, weight loss, and high erythrocyte sedimentation rate. These tumors are locally aggressive, potentially metastasizing lesions that may lead to the patient's death (68). Immunohistochemistry and ultrastructural studies show fibroblastic/myofibroblastic differentiation. Inflammatory fibrosarcoma has a low proliferative activity, which is in keeping with the impression that this is a low-grade sarcoma, and no association has been demonstrated thus far with viral agents such as cytomegalovirus and Epstein-Barr virus (69). *Inflammatory fibrosarcoma* is essentially the same lesion as the so-called *inflammatory myofibroblastic tumor*; the latter term is generally applied to lesions lacking cytologic atypia, but a clinicopathologic continuum exists between these entities (69). A key subtype of low-grade fibrosarcoma is the *low-grade fibromyxoid sarcoma*. These lesions appear similar to fibromatoses and, in fact, one of the initially reported cases was first di-

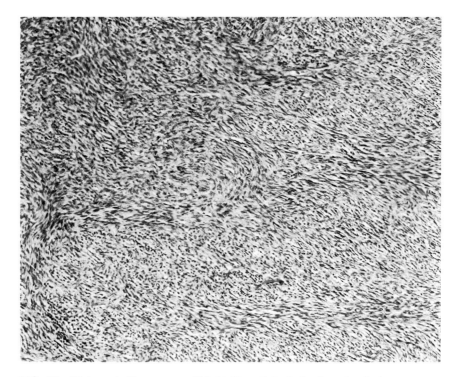

FIG. 16 High-grade fibrosarcoma. This highly cellular lesion has a herringbone pattern.

agnosed as fibromatosis, but they differ by having swirled architecture, myxoid zones, and subtle cytologic atypia (70). These tumors are capable of metastasis and de-differentiation to high-grade lesions. It is now clear that the *hyalinizing spindle cell tumor with giant rosettes* is a variant, the latter characterized by unusual giant collagen rosettes (71).

Fibrosarcoma is sometimes difficult to distinguish from a variety of benign as well as malignant conditions. *Nodular fasciitis* is a rapidly growing lesion with smaller size than fibrosarcoma, cells arranged in short bundles rather than long sweeping fascicles or in a herringbone pattern, more myxoid stroma and scattered chronic inflammatory cells, and no tendency for invasion of the adjacent structures. *Dermatofibroma/fibrous histiocytoma* exhibits cells in storifom configuration, absence of atypical mitotic figures, and presence of secondary characteristics such as xanthoma cells, giant cells, and siderophages. *Fibromatosis* may closely resemble fibrosarcoma, especially the well-differentiated type, but is usually less cellular and has more collagen. The distinction between these two entities can be

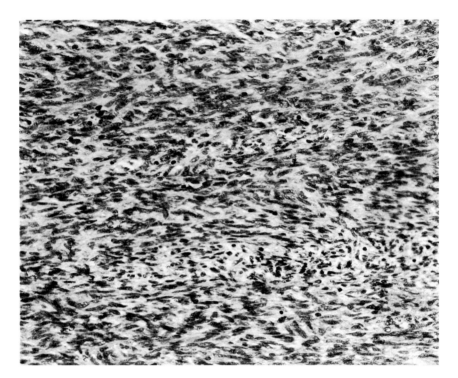

FIG. 17   High-grade fibrosarcoma. Note the nuclear hyperchromasia.

extremely difficult as both have bland-appearing fibroblasts, rare mitotic figures, and a uniform growth pattern. *Malignant fibrous histiocytoma* is commonly seen in the elderly population and histologically has a more storiform pattern with bizarre giant cells and often abundant eosinophilic collagen. Although *malignant peripheral nerve sheath tumor* may have areas indistinguishable from fibrosarcoma, it typically does show features suggestive of its neural origin. The nuclei are often buckled and bullet-shaped. The cells are long and slender, arranged in fascicular pattern, and show perivascular cuffing and nuclear palisading. Myxoid matrix is also more prominent, and often neurofibroma-like areas are seen focally. Malignant peripheral nerve sheath tumor may also be attached to a nerve and may be associated with neurofibromatosis. Monophasic *synovial sarcoma* can generally be separated by application of an appropriate immunohistochemical panel since synovial sarcomas generally exhibit at least focal expression of cytokeratin or epithelial membrane antigen. As immunohistochemical and molecular genetic techniques have improved and allowed more precise separation of other types of sarcomas, the incidence of fibrosarcoma, once the most commonly diagnosed sarcoma subtype, has become rare.

B. Myofibrosarcoma

Several malignant soft-tissue tumors may show myofibroblastic differentiation, including some fibrosarcomas, malignant fibrous histiocytomas, and well-differentiated sclerosing liposarcomas. Recently, attention has been drawn to a group of sarcomas showing a predominance of myofibroblastic differentiation (72–76). Cases often occur in the head and neck region, but involvement of other sites, such as breast, soft tissue of cheek, and trunk, has been reported (77–79). Clinically, although few cases have been reported so far, the behavior tends to be more indolent than that of fibrosarcoma and leiomyosarcoma (80). High-grade examples of this tumor type may comprise a significant percentage of tumors presently classified as *malignant fibrous histiocytomas*.

Microscopically, the myofibroblasts are arranged in a storiform pattern mimicking nodular fasciitis and areas of herringbone pattern simulating *fibrosarcoma*. The cells are usually plump, elongated, and have lightly eosinophilic cytoplasm. Cytologically, the tumor cells vary from having a low-grade appearance with a few mitotic figures and tissue culture–like spindle cells, to a high-grade appearance with pleomorphic features, necrosis, and abundant mitotic figures. By immunohistochemistry, these cells stain for smooth muscle actin and may be positive for desmin.

The major differential of low-grade examples is *nodular fasciitis* and its other pseudosarcomatous congeners. The pseudosarcomatous processes are generally less infiltrative and lack nuclear atypia and, with the exception of atypical decubital fibroplasia, lack necrosis. *Sarcomas*, such as fibrosarcoma, rhabdomyosarcoma, malignant fibrous histiocytoma, malignant peripheral nerve sheath tumor, and *carcinosarcoma*, may also come into differential diagnosis, in which case a panel of immunohistochemical tests along with careful search for diagnostic or classic patterns by light microscopy may lead to the final diagnosis.

IV. FIBROUS TUMORS OF INFANCY AND CHILDHOOD

Fibrous tumors of infancy and childhood can be divided into two groups: lesions similar to those occurring in adults, and fibroblastic soft-tissue lesions peculiar to infants and children. The latter will be discussed in this section (22,81).

A. Fibrous Hamartoma of Infancy

Fibrous hamartoma of infancy is an uncommon benign fibroblastic and myofibroblastic proliferation that typically occurs in the axillary or shoulder region of boys in their first 2 years of life (82–84), usually presenting as a solitary, small, rapidly growing, soft-to-firm mass. About 20% of cases are congenital. The lesion only rarely occurs on the hands and feet (2,22,84).

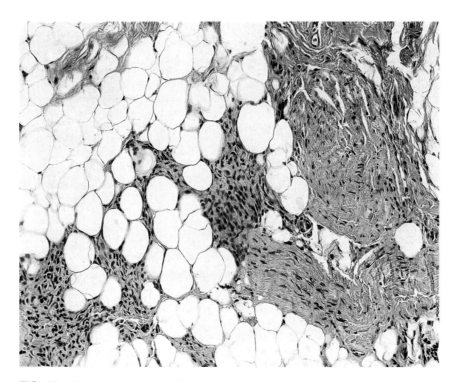

FIG. 18   Fibrous hamartoma of infancy displays three elements: fat, fibrous tissue, and whorls of primitive-appearing cells with low mitotic activity.

Grossly the lesion is poorly circumscribed with firm gray–white tissue ad-mixed with fat. Histologically the lesion consists of three cell types: (a) fibroblasts and myofibroblasts, (b) primitive mesenchymal cells, and (c) haphazardly distrib-uted fat. The three tissue components are seen in varying proportions appearing as follows: (a) fibrous trabeculae or septae composed of spindle cells separated by collagen; (b) myxoid foci containing primitive round or stellate mesenchymal cells; and (c) interspersed mature fat. The lesion has an organoid pattern (Fig. 18).

Generally, this entity is recognized by most pathologists as a benign process; however, examples with predominant myofibroblastic differentiation and sparse numbers of primitive cells may be confused with *infantile fibromatosis*. The latter is a locally aggressive tumor whereas fibrous hamartoma of infancy is cured by local excision and is not locally destructive. Areas of fibrous hamartoma with ser-pentine nuclei and wiry collagen may mimic *neural tumors*, especially neurofi-bromas, but these cells lack expression of neural markers, such as S-100 protein. Occasionally, fibrous hamartoma of infancy can occur in the genital region (83), where it may mimic *embryonal rhabdomyosarcoma* clinically, although the pathologic features are quite distinct if the pathologist is aware of this presentation. The characteristic organoid pattern helps distinguishing fibrous hamartoma of infancy from rhabdomyosarcoma and other sarcomas such as *infantile fibrosarcoma*. *Calcifying aponeurotic fibroma* may have histologic resemblance, especially in earlier lesions when the tumor may grow in a trabecular manner and lack calcifications. However, these lesions occur in the palms of older children.

B. Infantile Digital Fibromatosis

Infantile digital fibromatosis is a distinct tumor of the dermis and subcutis of the fingers and toes of infants. Approximately 30% of cases are congenital. The salient feature of this tumor is the presence of cytoplasmic inclusion bodies. The lesion may be single or multiple and has a tendency to recur. The ultimate prognosis is excellent, and most tumors eventually regress spontaneously after the initial growth period. These tumors are capable of causing contracture deformities.

Grossly the tumor is poorly circumscribed and is attached to the overlying skin. Microscopically, there are fascicles of bland-appearing fibroblasts that look similar to those of other superficial fibromatoses. The characteristic globular, eosinophilic cytoplasmic inclusion bodies can be seen on routine staining (Fig. 19) but appear bright red with the Masson trichrome stain and stain with actin antibodies on immunohistochemical investigation. The inclusions are variable in number and are seen less frequently in cases involving more fibrosis (85).

C. Myofibroma and Myofibromatosis

Myofibroma and myofibromatosis are hamartomatous myofibroblastic proliferations, typically presenting during the first few weeks of life, which can be congenital (2,81). Adult counterparts are also well known. The lesion presents as a single mass or, less commonly, with multicentric involvement (myofibromatosis). Lesions usually involve the dermis or subcutis. The solitary examples most commonly occur in the head and neck region, whereas multicentric cases can involve the skeleton and internal organs in addition to the skin. Involvement of the internal organs may lead to the patient's demise through secondary complications.

Grossly, the nodules are firm, gray–white or pink, and have a scar-like consistency. Microscopically, the nodules show a biphasic pattern with multiple lobules separated by richly vascular or spindle cell areas. There is a myoid appearance at the periphery of the lobules, with leiomyoma-like short fascicles of plump, eosinophilic myofibroblasts and fibroblasts. The central portions are richly vascular, with round polygonal cells arranged around blood vessels mimicking hemangiopericytoma (Fig. 20). Variable amount of necrosis, calcification, and intravascular growth can be present.

Several benign as well as malignant neoplasms can be confused with myofibroma/myofibromatosis. *Nodular fasciitis* arises from the fascia and has more

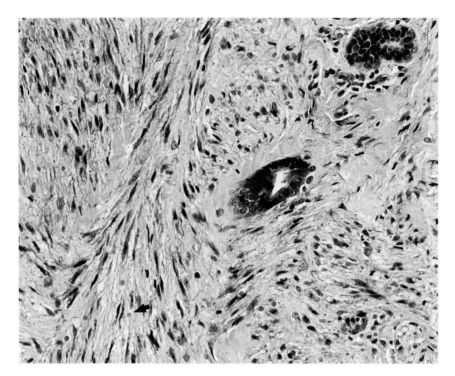

FIG. 19 Infantile digital fibromatosis. This lesion infiltrates between skin appendages and contains the characteristic cytoplasmic inclusions (*arrow*).

prominent myxoid matrix and inflammatory cells, whereas myofibroma has a biphasic pattern with plump eosinophilic myofibroblasts and hemangiopericytoma-like areas. Although prominent mitotic figures, intravascular growth, and necrosis may bring malignant neoplasms such as *fibrosarcoma* and *hemangiopericytoma* into the differential, the presence of alternating nodular and spindle cell patterns should call the correct diagnosis to mind. The multifocal form/myofibromatosis is unlikely to be confused with other entities. *Neurofibromatosis* in general affects older children and shows other stigmata of the disease. *Juvenile hyaline fibromatosis* usually affects children older than 2 years, does not involve internal organs, and is associated with joint deformities.

D. Juvenile Hyaline Fibromatosis

Juvenile hyaline fibromatosis is a rare autosomal recessive disorder related to abnormal collagen metabolism. The disease usually manifests between the age of 2

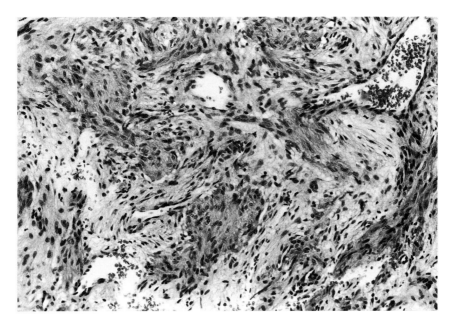

FIG. 20   Myofibroma/myofibromatosis. The biphasic histology is the same in both solitary (myofibroma) and multiple (myofibromatosis) lesions.

and 5 years with multiple slowly growing skin nodules on the head, neck, and extremities. In addition, patients may have flexion contractures of large joints, gingival thickening, muscle weakness, and multiple osteolytic bone lesions (86).

Grossly, the tumors are poorly circumscribed with small scattered spindle cells in an abundant amorphous extracellular eosinophilic collagen-poor matrix. Older lesions tend to be less cellular with more abundant extracellular matrix. Variable amounts of calcification may be seen.

In contrast, *neurofibromatosis* usually presents in older children with other stigmata of the disease. *Myofibromatosis* occurs during infancy, is well circumscribed, affects skin as well as bones and internal organs, and microscopically shows a biphasic pattern. *Gingival fibromatosis*, which is also a hereditary lesion, is limited to gingival areas and consists of scar-like dense connective tissue. *Lipoid proteinosis* is another rare disorder characterized by multiple plaques, papules, or nodules associated with dysphonia and hoarseness. The lesions consist of amorphous eosinophilic infiltrates that tend to surround the sweat glands and small blood vessels, and lack the spindle cell component seen in juvenile hyaline fibromatosis. *Winchester syndrome* is another rare hereditary disorder with poorly circumscribed cellular fibrous proliferations that lack the extracellular matrix component. There are associated corneal opacities and severe skeletal deformities.

E.   Gingival Fibromatosis

Gingival fibromatosis is a rare and distinct disease that mainly affects young individuals and has a tendency for local recurrence. Most cases are transmitted as an autosomal dominant trait, although sporadic cases do occur. The lesion usually presents as a slowly enlarging, poorly defined mass of the gingiva, usually at the time of tooth eruption. The disease may be *localized* with limitation to a small area of the gum or *generalized* with bilateral and extensive involvement. Occasional cases are associated with hypertrichosis, and mental or physical growth retardation (22).

Grossly, the tumor consists of scar-like tissue with a glistening gray–white surface. Histologically, the nodules are paucicellular with dense collagenization, and there may be overlying acanthosis.

There is a striking resemblance between gingival fibromatosis and gingival hypertrophy secondary to *phenytoin*, and gingival lesions seen during *pregnancy*. Clinical and family history are critical to reach a correct diagnosis. *Juvenile hyaline fibromatosis* has multiple nodules, skeletal deformities, and characteristic abundant eosinophilic, amorphous matrix.

F.   Fibromatosis Colli

Fibromatosis colli is fibrous growth involving the distal portion of the sternocleidomastoid muscle. In about half of cases, a history of a complicated delivery is elicited. The lesion typically presents between the second to fourth week of life, is more common in males, and, for obscure reasons, affects the right side more frequently than the left side. It is characterized by a rapid growth phase leading to a stationary phase and eventually to regression such that, in a matter of 1 or 2 years, the lesion is no longer palpable (22).

If the lesion is excised it shows partial replacement of the sternocleidomastoid muscle by a bland-appearing fibrous proliferation without inflammatory cells.

Fibrosing myositis characteristically has an inflammatory infiltrate. *Fibromatosis* has an infiltrative margin and a more monotonous growth pattern rather than admixture of fibroblasts and skeletal muscle cells as seen in fibromatosis colli.

G.   Calcifying Aponeurotic Fibroma

Calcifying aponeurotic fibroma primarily affects the hands and feet of children between birth and 16 years. Only rare cases are reported outside the acral location (87). It has a tendency for local recurrence. The lesion usually presents as a slowly growing, poorly circumscribed mass. On radiologic examination, calcific stippling is often appreciated (22).

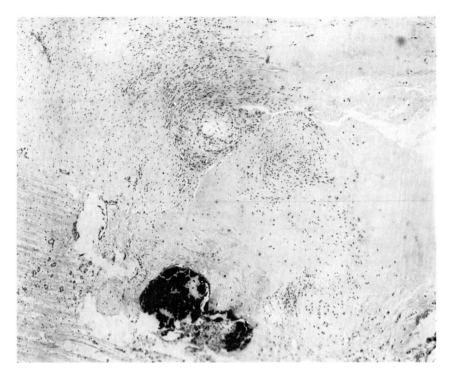

FIG. 21 Calcifying aponeurotic fibroma. These tumors are lobulated with hypercellular zones and foci of calcification/ossification.

Grossly, the tumor consists of an ill-defined gritty mass with punctate calcification. Microscopically, the nodules are characterized by infiltrative fibrous growth of plump oval fibroblasts arranged in cords. There is rich cellularity and dense collagen. Not infrequently, the nodule may be attached to the aponeurosis or tendon. Focal calcification is present (Fig. 21), except in early cases occurring in infants or small children. There is band-like or serpinginous central calcification often associated with chondroid matrix. The number of giant cells seen in association with the calcification may vary.

Cases with no calcification may cause a diagnostic dilemma in differentiation from *infantile fibromatosis*. However, calcifying aponeurotic fibroma has plumper spindle cells, is associated with dense collagen, and occurs in the hands and feet. *Palmar and plantar fibromatoses*, which are rare in children, have a nodular growth pattern and lack calcification and chondroid matrix. *Soft-part chondroma* may cause significant diagnostic problem because both entities commonly involve the hands; however, soft-part chondroma usually occurs in older patients and microscopically displays a lobulated fibrous proliferation that undergoes cal-cification in a diffuse rather than linear manner.

H. Infantile Fibromatosis

Infantile fibromatosis is the childhood counterpart of the adult-type fibromatosis (abdominal or extra-abdominal) (88). It usually presents as a deep, poorly defined, rapidly growing, solitary mass involving the skeletal muscle or fascia. It occurs in children between birth and the age of 5 years, most commonly in the head and neck, followed by the proximal extremities and limb girdles. It is slightly more common in males. Although the tumor does not metastasize, it tends to recur if in-completely excised; it may behave in a locally aggressive fashion, or involve adja-cent bones and entrap neighboring nerves and vessels. Complete excision, which is the treatment of choice, is sometimes very difficult and may not be feasible with-out disfiguring surgery (22).

Grossly, the tumor consists of an ill-defined, scar-like, gray–white mass with infiltrative margins. Histologically, the morphologic appearance ranges from primitive myxoid mesenchymal lesions (immature diffuse form), typically seen in infants, to that resembling an adult desmoid tumor (mature adult form), which is more commonly seen in older children. Admixtures of these types can also be seen. The *immature diffuse form* is characterized by small, round to oval, fibro-blast-like cells arranged in haphazard fashion in a myxoid background. There is often a rich reticulin network with tumor diffusely infiltrating the muscle. There is often intimate association with the residual atrophic-appearing skeletal muscle and adipose tissue representing fatty replacement of the muscle. Scattered lym-phoid aggregates are often seen. The *mature adult-like form* is more cellular, with plump spindle-shaped fibroblasts arranged in short fascicles. Variable collagen is present and rare cases may even show ossification. The tumor has a scar-like ap-pearance and features scattered thin-walled ectatic blood vessels.

The immature diffuse form is frequently confused with myxoid or lipoma-tous tumors. *Myxoid liposarcoma* is only rarely seen in children under the age of 5 years and typically has plexiform vasulature and lipoblasts. *Botryoid rhabdo-myosarcoma* involves the same age group as infantile fibromatosis but almost al-ways occurs in the walls of mucosa-lined cavities and does not involve the deep musculature. *Lipoblastomatosis* has a distinctly lobular pattern and uniform ap-pearance of the constituent lipoblasts. Confusion may also occur with early stages of *calcifying aponeurotic fibroma*, which characteristically occurs in the hands and feet, and *fibrodysplasia ossificans progressiva*, a lesion associated with bilat-eral malformations of fingers and toes. The mature adult-like form may pose the most difficult problem, differentiating this lesion from *infantile fibrosarcoma* (89). Fibromatosis usually has a more infiltrating pattern with alternating areas of cellularity and more collagenous areas with intimate association with residual muscle and fat. In some cases, the distinction may be impossible. Rapidly growing, destructive tumors with high cellularity and increased mitotic activity should probably be classified as infantile fibrosarcoma (81).

I. Calcifying Fibrous Pseudotumor (with Psammomatous Calcifications)

Calcifying fibrous pseudotumor a recently described rare, distinctive, benign, fibrous pseudotumor that occurs in children and young adults and closely mimics fibromatosis clinically (90,91). It usually presents as a slowly growing, deep-seated, firm, highly collagenized mass that commonly situates in the extremities. The tumor recurs only rarely following even incomplete excision.

The tumor has well-defined margins with hypocellular tissue exhibiting scattered fibroblasts in densely hyalinized collagenous matrix. Variable number of plasma cells, Russell bodies, lymphoid aggregates, and histiocytes are seen. Characteristically there is concentric psammomatous or dystrophic calcification of this unique lesion (Fig. 22).

Certain paucicellular lesions may enter the differential diagnosis. *Amyloidoma* has demonstrable amyloid and typically contains giant cells. *Fibroma of tendon sheath* usually involves tendons of hands and feet and has a multilobular architecture with cleft-like spaces in between.

J. Congenital and Infantile Fibrosarcoma

Infantile fibrosarcoma primarily presents during infancy, and about 20% of cases are congenital (2,92). Although the tumor closely resembles adult fibrosarcoma, it must be considered as a separate entity due to the marked difference in the clinical behavior. Infantile fibrosarcoma has a much better prognosis than its adult counterpart despite its ominous histologic features. Rarely, the tumor has the potential to recur and even metastasize. It is slightly more common in boys (93). A comparative study of apoptosis and cell proliferation in infantile and adult fibrosarcomas showed a significantly lower proliferative index and a higher apoptotic index in infantile cases when compared with adult lesions (94).

Grossly, the tumor usually consists of a large, rapidly growing, poorly circumscribed, painless mass commonly involving the distal extremities that may even entirely replace the distal portion of the limb. Microscopically, the lesion consists of spindled to round, small, primitive fibroblasts arranged in vague fascicles or bundles and separated by variable amounts of collagen. Mitotic figures are common. Scattered lymphocytes are often seen. Necrosis and hemorrhage are

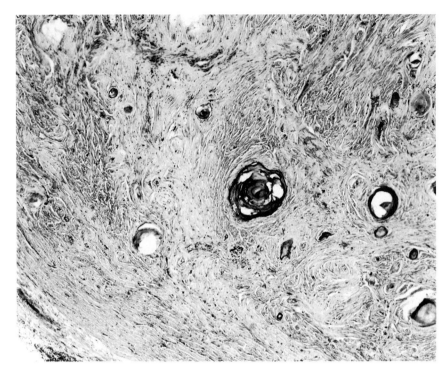

FIG. 22   Calcifying fibrous tumor. Note the psammomatous (in concentric whorls) calcification.

commonly present, which often leads to marked distortion of larger tumors. Areas of rich vascularity are often seen. Larger number of undifferentiated mesenchymal cells and slit-like blood vessels have been correlated with a tendency of the tumor to local recurrence (95).

Other mesenchymal lesions can often be confused with infantile fibrosarcoma, although the solid growth pattern with spindle cells in fascicles with lack of cell differentiation are fairly characteristic. Application of a panel on immunohistochemical stains can be helpful in excluding other pediatric sarcomas. *Rhabdomyosarcoma* is seen in a similar age group, but it lacks the solid growth and often contains rhabdomyoblasts and intracellular glycogen. Rhabdomyosarcomas also express skeletal muscle markers. Areas of rich vascularity may mimic *infantile hemangiopericytoma*, a tumor characterized by distinct lobulation and staghorn-like dilated vessels. *Infantile fibromatosis*, especially the mature-adult form, may be difficult to distinguish from fibrosarcoma. Infantile fibromatoses in general have a more infiltrating border with alternating areas of cellularity with collagenized areas rather than the more uniform solid growth of fibrosarcoma. However, in some cases the distinction is almost impossible to make. However, since the treatments of the two entities are essentially identical, divergences of diagnostic opinion on such cases do not alter therapy.

ACKNOWLEDGMENT

The authors thank Drs. Cyril Fisher and John X. O'Connell for generously providing examples from their slide collections for illustrative purposes.

REFERENCES

1. Enzinger F, Weiss S. Benign fibrous tissue tumors. In: Enzinger F, Weiss S, eds., Soft tissue tumors. St. Louis: Mosby, 1995.
2. Meis-Kindblom J, Enzinger F, eds. Color atlas of soft tissue tumors. St. Louis: Mosby-Wolfe, 1996.
3. Batsakis J, El-Naggar A. pseudosarcomatous proliferative lesions of soft tissues. Ann Otol Rhinol Laryngol 103:578–582, 1994.
4. El-Jabbour J, Wilson G, Bennett M, Burke M, Davey A, Eames K. Flow cytometric study of nodular fasciitis, proliferative fasciitis, and proliferative myositis. Hum Pathol 22:1146–1149, 1991.
5. Montgomery E, Meis J. Nodular fasciitis. Its morphologic spectrum and immunohistochemical profile. Am J Surg Pathol 15(10):942–948, 1991.
6. Shimizu S, Hashimoto H, Enjoji M. Nodular fasciitis: an analysis of 250 patients. Pathology 16:161–166, 1984.
7. Samaratunga H, Searle J, O'Loughlin B. nodular fasciitis and related pseudosarcomatous lesions of soft tissues. Aust N Z J Surg 66(1):22–25, 1996.
8. Allen P. Nodular fasciitis. Pathology 4:9–26, 1972.
9. Sheikh SS, Henderson F, Gomes M, Montgomery E. Intravascular fasciitis clinically mimicking an axillary peripheral nerve sheath tumor. Case report with discussion. Vascular surgery 33:439–446, 1999.
10. Patchefsky AS, Enzinger, FM. Intravascular fasciitis. A report of 17 cases. Am J Surg Pathol 5:29–36, 1981.
11. Clapp C, Dodson E, Pickett B, Lambert P. Cranial fasciitis presenting as an external auditory canal mass. Arch Otolaryngol Head Neck Surg 123(2):223–225, 1997.
12. Mentzel T, Calonje E, Wadden C, Camplejohn R, Beham A, Smith M, Fletcher C. Myxofibrosarcoma. Clinicopathologic analysis of 75 cases with emphasis on the lower-grade variant. Am J Surg Pathol 20(4):391–405, 1996.
13. Meck C, Angervall L, Kindblom L, Oden A. Myxofibrosarcoma. A malignant soft tissue tumor of fibroblastic-histiocytic origin. A clinicopathologic and prognostic study of 110 cases using multivariate analysis. Acta Pathol 282(91):9–39, 1983.

14. Meis J, Enzinger F. Proliferative fasciitis and myositis of childhood. Am J Surg Pathol 16(4):364–372, 1992.

15. Chung E, Enzinger F. Proliferative fasciitis. Cancer 36(4):1450–1458, 1975.

16. Montgomery E, Meis J, Mitchell M, Enzinger F. Atypical decubital fibroplasia. A distinctive fibroblastic pseudotumor occuring in debilitated patients. Am J Surg Pathol 16(7):708–715, 1992.

16a. Perosio PM, Weiss SW. Ischemic fasciitis: a juxta-skeletal proliferation with a predilection for elderly patients. Mod Pathol 6:69–72, 1993.

17. Weiss S, Sobin L, eds. Histologic classification of soft tissue tumors. Berlin: Springer-Verlag, 1994.

18. Maluf H, DeYoung B, Swanson P, Wick M. Fibroma and giant cell tumor of tendon sheath: a comparative histological and immunohistological study. Mod Pathol 8(2):155–159, 1995.

19. Balachandran K, Allen P, MacCormac L. Nuchal fibroma. A clinicopathological study of nine cases. Am J Surg Pathol 19(3):313–317, 1995.

20. O'Connell J, Janzen D, Hughes T. Nuchal fibrocartilagenous pseudotumor: a distinctive soft-tissue lesion associated with prior neck injury. Am J Surg Pathol 2(7):836–840, 1997.

21. Kransdorf M, Meis J, Montgomery E. Elastofibroma: MR and CT appearance with radiologic-pathologic correlation. AJR Am J Roentpensl 159:575–579, 1992.

22. Allen P. The fibromatoses: a clinicopathologic classification based on 140 cases. Part 2. Am J Surg Pathol 1:305–321, Dec 1977.

23. Hasegawa T, Hirohashi S, Hizawa K, Sano T. Collagenous fibroma (desmoplastic fibroblastoma): report of four cases and review of the literature. Arch Pathol Lab Med 122(5):455–460, 1998.

24. Evans H. Desmoplastic fibroblastoma. A report of seven cases. Am J Surg Pathol 19(9):1077–1081, 1995.

25. Posner M, Shiu M, Newsome J, Hajdu S, Gaynor J, Brennan M. The desmoid tumor. Not a benign disease. Arch Surg 124:191–196, 1989.

26. Reitamo J, Hayry P, Nykyri E, Saxen E. The desmoid tumor. I. Incidence, sex-, age-, and anatomical distribution in the Finnish population. Am J Clin Pathol 77(6):665–673, 1981.

27. Lucas D, Shroyer K, McCarthy P, Markham N, Fujita M, Enomoto T. Desmoid tumor is a clonal cellular proliferation: PCR amplification of HUMARA for analysis of patterns of X-chromosome inactivation. Am J Surg Pathol 21(3):306–311, 1997.

28. Bridge J, Sreekantaiah C, Mouron B, Neff J, Sandberg A, Wolman S. Clonal chromosomal abnormalities in desmoid tumors. Cancer 69:430–436, 1992.

29. Fletcher J, Naeem R, Xiao S, et al. Chromosomal aberrations in desmoid tumors: trisomy 8 may be a predictor of recurrence. Cancer Genet Cytogenet 79:139, 1995.

30. Hayry P, Reitamo J, Totterman S, Hopfner-Hallikainen D, Sivula A. The desmoid tumor. II. Analysis of factors possibly contributing to the etiology and growth behavior. Am J Clin Pathol 77(6):674–680, June 1982.

31. Hayry P, Reitammo J, Vihko R, Janne O, Schein T, Totterman S, Ahonen J, Norio R, Alan A. The desmoid tumor. III. A biochemical and genetic analysis. Am J Clin Pathol 77(6):681–685, 1982.

32. Gelmann E. Tamoxifen for the treatment of malignancies other than breast and endometrial carcinoma. Semin Oncol 24(1):S1-65–S1-70, 1997.

33. Lanari C, Molinolo A, Kordon E, Pasualini C, Charreau E. Progesterone receptors in estrogen-induced fibromatosis of guinea pigs. Cancer 51:235–245, 1990.

34. Waddell W, Gerner R, Reich M. Nonsteroid antiinflammatory drugs and tamoxifen for desmoid tumors and carcinoma of the stomach. J Surg Oncol 22:197–211, 1983.

35. Reitamo J. The desmoid tumor. IV. Choice of treatment, results, and complications. Arch Surg 118:1318–1322, 1983.

36. Allen P. The fibromatoses: a clinicopathologic classification based on 140 cases. Part 1. Am J Surg Pathol 1:255–270, Sept 1977.

37. Guerneri S, Stioui S, Mantovani F, Austoni E, Simoni G. Multiple clonal chromosome abnormalities in Peyronie's disease. Cancer Genet Cytogenet 52:181–185, 1991.

38. Pereyo N, Heimer W. Extraabdominal desmoid tumor. J Am Acad Dermatol 34(2):352–6, 1996.

39. Das Gupta T, Brasfield R, O'Hara J. Extra-abdominal desmoids: a clinicopathological study. Ann Surg 109–121, July 1969.

40. Mac-Moune F, Allen P, Chan P, Cooper J, Mackenzie T. Aggressive fibromatosis of the spermatic cord. A typical lesion in a "new" location. Am J Clin Pathol 104:403–407, 1995.

41. Wargotz E, Norris H, Austin R, Enzinger F. Fibromatosis of the breast. A clinicopathological study of 28 cases. Am J Surg Pathol 11(1):38–45, 1987.

42. Allen M, Novotny D. Desmoid tumor of the vulva associated with pregnancy. Arch Lab Med 121:512–514, 1997.

43. Masson J, Soule E. Desmoid tumors of the head and neck. Am J Surg Pathol 112:615–622, 1966.

44. Conley J, Healey W, Purdy Stout A. Fibromatosis of the head and neck. Am J Surg 112:609–614, 1966.

45. Enzinger F, Shiraki M. Musculo-aponeurotic fibromatosis of the shoulder girdle (extraabdominal desmoid). Cancer 20:1131–1140, 1967.

46. Aaron A, O'Mara J, Legendre K, Evans S, Attinger C, Montgomery E. Chest wall fibromatosis associated with silicone breast implants. Surg Oncol 5:93–99, 1996.

47. Enzinger F, Weiss S. Fibromatoses. In: Enzinger F, Weiss S, eds. Soft tissue tumors. St. Louis: Mosby, 1995.

48. Zayid I, Dihmis C. Familial multicentric fibromatosis-desmoids. A report of three cases in a Jordanian family. Cancer 24:786–795, 1969.

49. Stiller D, Katenkamp D. Cellular features in desmoid fibromatosis and well-differentiated fibrosarcomas. An electron microscopic study. Virchows Arch A 369:155–164, 1975.

50. Brasfield R, Das Gupta T. Desmoid tumors of the anterior abdominal wall. Surg 65(2):241–246, 1969.

51. Burke A, Sobin L, Helwig E. Intra-abdominal fibromatosis. A pathologic analysis of 130 tumors with comparison of clinical subgroups. Am J Surg Pathol 14(4):335–341, 1990.

52. DiGaiacomo J, Lazenby A, Salloum L. Mesentric fibromatosis associated with Crohn's disease. Am J Gastroentrol 89(7):1103–1105, 1994.

53. Burke A, SobinL, Shekitka K. Mesentric fibromatosis. A follow-up study. Arch Pathol Lab Med 114:832–835, 1990.

54. Harvey J, Quan S, Fortner J. Gardner's syndrome complicated by mesentric desmoid tumors. Surgery 85:475–477, April 1979.

55. Gardner E. Follow-up study of a family group exhibiting dominant inheritance for a syndrome including intestinal polyps, osteomas, fibromas, and epidermal cysts. Am J Hum Genet 14:376–390, 1962.

56. Garbuz A, Giardiello F, Petersen G, Krush, A, Offerhaus G, Booker S, Kerr M, Hamilton S. Desmoid tumors in familial adenomatous polyposis. Gut 35:377–381, 1994.

57. Miyaki M, Konishi M, Kikuchi-Yanoshita R, Enomoto M, Tanaka K, Takahashi H, Muraoka M, Mori T, Konishi F, Iwama T. Coexistence of somatic and germline mutations of APC gene in desmoid tumors from patients with familial adenomatous polyposis. Cancer Res 53:5079–5082, 1993.

58. Simpson R, Harrison E, Mayo C. Mesentric fibromatosis in familial polyposis. A variant of Gardner's syndrome. Cancer 17:526–534, April 1964.

59. Rogriguez-Bigas M, Mahoney M, Karakousis C, Petrelli N. Desmoid tumors in patients with familial adenomatous polyposis. Cancer 74:1270–1274, 1994.

60. Purdy Stout A. Fibrosarcoma: the malignant tumor of fibroblasts. Cancer 1:30–63, 1948.

61. Enzinger F, Weiss S. Fibrosarcoma. In: Enzinger F, Weiss S, eds. Soft tissue tumors. St. Louis: Mosby, 1995.

62. Scott S, Reiman H, Pritchard D, Ilstrup D. Soft tissue fibrosarcoma. A clinicopathologic study of 132 cases. Cancer 64:925–931, 1989.

63. Mooney E, Meagher P, Edwards G, Cahalane S, Gaffney E. Fibrosarcoma of the thigh 28 years after excision of fibromatosis. Histopathology 23:498–500, 1993.

64. Soule E, Scanlon P. Fibrosarcoma arising in an extra-abdominal desmoid tumor: report of case. Staff Meet Mayo Clin 37(17):443–451, 1962.

65. Meis-Kindblom J, Kindblom L, Enzinger F. Sclerosing epithelioid fibrosarcoma. A variant of fibrosarcoma simulating carcinoma. Am J Surg Pathol 19(9):979–993, 1995.

66. Borman H, Safak T, Ertoy D. Fibrosarcoma following radiotherapy for breast carcinoma: a case report and review of the literature. Ann Plast Surg 41(2):201–4, 1998.

67. Pettit V, Chamness J, Ackerman L. Fibromatosis and fibrosarcoma following irradiation therapy. Cancer 7:149–158, 1954.

68. Meis J, Enzinger F. Inflammatory fibrosarcoma of the mesentry and retroperitoneum. A tumor closely simulating inflammatory pseudotumor. Am J Surg Pathol 15(12):1146–1156, 1991.

69. Meis-Kindblom J, Kjellstrom C, Kindblom L. Inflammatory fibrosarcoma: update, reappraisal, and perspective on its place in the spectrum of inflammatory myofibroblastic tumors. Semin Diagn Pathol 15(2):133–143, 1998.

70. Evans, HL. Low-grade fibromyxoid sarcoma. A report of two metastasizing neoplasms having a deceptively bland appearance. Am J Clin Pathol 88:615–619, 1987.

71. Folpe AL, Lane KL, Paull G, Weiss SW. Low-grade fibromyxoid sarcoma and hyalinizing spindle cell tumor with giant rosettes. A clinicopathologic study of 73 cases sup-

porting their identity and assessing the impact of high-grade areas. Am J Surg Pathol 24:1353–1360, 2000.

72. Lagace R, Schürch W, Seemayer T. Myofibroblasts in soft tissue sarcomas. Virchows Arch A 389:1–11, 1980.

73. Coffin C, Dehner L, Meis-Kindblom J. Inflammatory myofibroblastic tumor, inflammatory fibrosarcoma, and related lesions: an historical review with differential diagnostic considerations. Semin Diagn Pathol 15(2):102–110, 1998.

74. Eyden B. Brief review of the fibronexus and its significance for myofibroblastic differentiation and tumor diagnosis. Ultrastruct Pathol 17:611–622, 1993.

75. Schürch W, Seemayer T, Gabbiani G. The myofibroblast. A quarter century after its discovery. Am J Surg Pathol 22(2):141–147, 1998.

76. Mentzel T, Dry S, Katenkamp D, Fletcher C. Low-grade myofibroblastic sarcoma. Analysis of 18 cases in the spectrum of myofibroblastic tumors. Am J Surg Pathol 22(10):1228–1238, 1998.

77. Smith D, Mahmoud H, Jenkins J, Rao B, Hopkins K, Parham D. Myofibrosarcoma of the head and neck in children. Pediatr Pathol Lab Med 15:403–418, 1995.

78. Taccagni G, Rovere E, Masullo M, Christensen L, Eyden B. Myofibrosarcoma of the breast. Review of the literature on myofibroblastic tumors and criteria for defining myofibroblastic differentiation. Am J Surg Pathol 21(4):489–496, 1997.

79. Eyden B, Christensen L, Tagore V, Harris M. Myofibrosarcoma of subcutaneous soft tissue of the cheek. Submicros Cytol Pathol 24:307–313, 1992.

80. Montgomery E, Goldblum JR, Fisher C. Myofibrosarcoma: A clinicopathologic study. Am J Surg Pathol (in press).

81. Enzinger F, Weiss S. Fibrous tumors of infancy and childhood. In: Enzinger F, Weiss S, eds. Soft tissue tumors. St. Louis: Mosby, 1995.

82. Groisman G, Lichtig C. Fibrous hamartoma of infancy: an immunohistochemical and ultrastructural study. Hum Pathol 22:914–918, 1991.

83. Popek E, Montgomery E, Fourcroy J. Fibrous hamartoma of infancy in the genital region: findings in 15 cases. J Urol 152:990–993, 1994.

84. Jebson P, Louis D. Fibrous hamartoma of infancy in the hand: a case report. J Hand Surg 22(4):740–742, 1997.

85. Hayashi T, Tsuda N, Chowdhury P, Anami M, Kishikawa M, Iseki M, Kobayashi K. Infantile digital fibromatosis: a study of the development and regression of cytoplasmic inclusion bodies. Mod Pathol 8(5):548–552, 1995.

86. Senzaki H, Kiyozuka Y, Uemura Y, Shikata N, Ueda S, Tsubura A. Juvenile hyaline fibromatosis: a report of two unrelated adult sibling cases and a literature review. Pathol Int 48(3):230–236, 1998.

87. Murphy B, Kilpatrick S, Panella M, White W. Extra-acral calcifying aponeurotic fibroma: a distinctive case with 23 year follow-up. J Cutan Pathol 23(4):369–372, 1996.

88. Karakousis C, Mayordomo J, Zografos G, Driscoll D. Desmoid tumors of the trunk and extremity. Cancer 72:1637–1641, 1993.

89. Fisher C. Fibromatosis and fibrosarcoma in infancy and childhood. Eur J Cancer 32A(12):2094–2100, 1996.

90. Chen K. Intraabdominal calcifying fibrous pseudotumor. Int J Surg Pathol 4(1):9–12, 1996.

91. Fetsch J, Montgomery E, Meis J. Calcifying fibrous pseudotumor. Am J Surg Pathol 17(5):502–508, 1993.
92. Kodet R, Stejskal J, Pilat D, Kocourkova M, Smelhaus V, Eckschlager T. Congenital infantile fibrosarcoma: a clinicopathological study of five patients entered on the Prague Children's Tumor Registry. Pathol Res Praect 192(8):845–853, 1996.
93. Chung E, Enzinger F. Infantile fibrosarcoma. Cancer 38:729–739, 1976.
94. Kihara S, Nehlsen-Cannarella S, Kirsch W, Chase D, Garvin J. A comparative study of apoptosis and cell proliferation in infantile and adult fibrosarcomas. Am J Clin Pathol 106:493–497, 1996.
95. Schmidt D, Klinge P, Leuschner I, Harms D. Infantile desmoid-type fibromatosis. Morphological features correlate with biological behavior. J Pathol 164:315–319, 1991.

7
Fibrohistiocytic Tumors

Cyril Fisher
The Royal Marsden NHS Trust
London, England

I. INTRODUCTION

Fibrohistiocytic tumors are a large and varied group of benign, intermediate-grade, and malignant soft-tissue neoplasms that involve skin or deeper tissues. The category includes numerous common and rare entities that are composed of different proportions of spindled fibroblast-like cells that often display a storiform pattern, rounded histiocyte-like cells, and admixtures of giant, foamy, and inflammatory cells. The 1994 World Health Organization (WHO) classification of fibrohistiocytic tumors (Table 1) is based on a combination of clinical and morphologic features (1). Tumors in the intermediate or "borderline" group have appreciable potential for recurrence but only a small likelihood of metastasis.

The concept of a fibrohistiocytic cell, with features of both fibroblasts and histiocytes, is based on erroneous interpretations of early tissue culture and electron microscopic studies and is now considered to be incorrect (2,3). In fact, the principal cells of fibrohistiocytic lesions are, ultrastructurally, fibroblasts and myofibroblasts in various morphologic manifestations, including increased cytoplasm with lysosomes (as well as rough endoplasmic reticulum, intermediate filaments, and Golgi apparatus), which renders them histiocyte-like. In addition, there is often a nonneoplastic infiltrate of true histiocytes with their variants (multinucleated osteoclast-like cells, and those containing lipid or hemosiderin).

It is also clear from immunohistochemical studies that the lesional cells are mesenchymal and not truly histiocytic (4). So-called histiocytic markers previously considered of value, including α_1-antitrypsin and antichymotrypsin and CD68, relate to nonspecific antigens that reflect lysosomal content, and their diagnostic use in this context is limited because they are also detectable in many other

163

TABLE 1   WHO Classification of Fibrohistiocytic Tumors (1994) and Newer Variants of BFH

Benign	*Intermediate*
Benign fibrous histiocytoma	Atypical fibroxanthoma
Cutaneous[a]	Dermatofibrosarcoma protuberans
Atypical	Pigmented dermatofibrosarcoma protuberans
Cellular	Giant cell fibroblastoma
Epithelioid	Plexiform fibrohistiocytic tumor
Aneurysmal or angiomatoid	Angiomatoid fibrous histiocytoma
Myxoid	
Clear cell	*Malignant*
Granular cell	Malignant fibrous histiocytoma
Deep	Storiform-pleomorphic
Juvenile xanthogranuloma	Myxoid
Reticulohistiocytoma	Giant cell
Xanthoma	Xanthomatous (inflammatory)

[a] Additional variants in italics.

types of tumor (5). Infiltrating macrophages, perhaps chemoattracted by tumor cells, must not be confused with neoplastic cells.

There are no specific immunohistochemical markers for fibrohistiocytic lesions. However, smooth muscle action (SMA) is often (and desmin and cytokeratin occasionally) positive when there is myofibroblastic differentiation.

In many tumors in this group, the lesional cells are rounded or short spindly cells, often with an irregularly ovoid vesicular nucleus, and for these the term *fibrohistiocytic cell* (although histogenetically meaningless) is useful as it has a reasonably consistent and recognizable morphology that allows distinction from similar cell types. Benign and malignant fibrous histiocytomas appear to have a similar mixture of cell types, and the terminology has remained acceptable for benign lesions and some intermediate ones. However, the so-called malignant fibrous histiocytomas compose a heterogeneous group of malignancies that continue to undergo revision, and this term, though still descriptively convenient, is in decline at the present time (6).

II. BENIGN LESIONS

A. Benign Cutaneous Fibrous Histiocytoma

Benign cutaneous fibrous histiocytoma includes the common dermatofibroma and a number of variants of both clinical and pathologic interest (7–14). However, it is of concern to surgical pathologists principally for its atypical and cellular forms, which can present diagnostic difficulties with dermatofibrosarcoma protuberans

(DFSP) and malignant fibrous histiocytoma. The regular dermatofibroma presents as a firm dermal thickening or elevation. It comprises an ill-defined dermal infiltrate of spindly fibroblasts, with foamy cells, siderophages, multinucleated giant cells of Touton type (i.e., with a peripheral rim of nuclei), and blood vessels, in variable proportions related to the age of the lesion. In the more fibrous stages the lesion is also known as dermatofibroma or sclerosing hemangioma. Mitotic figures are occasionally seen, usually in small numbers, but without abnormal forms. The presence of the latter raises the possibility of atypical fibroxanthoma or of another type of mesenchymal tumor.

These lesions lack CD34, but many have immunoreactivity for factor XIIIa (FXIIIa), and rarely a case displays desmin and cytokeratin (15). Scattered atypical cells and the epithelioid variant are clinically insignificant, but the very cellular forms, which may infiltrate into subcutis, have an appreciable recurrence rate; some of these, when monomorphic and storiform, may resemble dermatofibrosarcoma protuberans. Also, at the periphery they may develop plexiform features. Similar tumors occurring in deeper soft tissue are more circumscribed and have a variety of patterns, including hemangiopericytomatous, myxoid, and giant cell morphology (16).

1. Atypical BFH

Some lesions have atypical large cells, with abundant cytoplasm, without mitoses (Fig. 1). These have been termed atypical benign fibrous histiocytoma (7) but are of no clinical significance as the reported cases did not recur. The presence of frequent or atypical mitoses raises the question of atypical fibroxanthoma. It is also important in such cases to exclude other tumors, such as melanoma or carcinoma, by immunohistochemistry for S-100 protein and cytokeratin, respectively.

2. Cellular Cutaneous Fibrous Histiocytoma

a. General and Clinical Features Cellular cutaneous fibrous histiocytoma is a variant of dermatofibroma that is often mistaken for sarcoma (17). It occurs more commonly in men, in young or middle-aged adults, as a flat or polypoid lesion in the upper or lower limbs, trunk, or head and neck region, including face. The history can be short, in weeks, or up to 2 years or more. Cellular cutaneous fibrous histiocytomas recur in about 25% of cases, generally within 3 years, although usually no more than once. Two metastasizing examples have, however, been reported, with spread to lymph node and lung (18). The metastases histologically resembled the primary lesions, which lacked abnormal mitoses, necrosis, or vascular invasion. In fact, neither patient died at the time of the report: one was disease-free 4 years after pulmonary resections, and the other was alive with stable bilateral lung metastases 8 years after the first diagnosis.

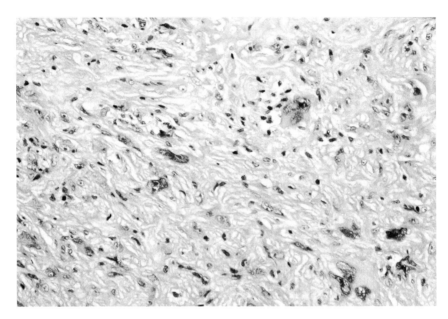

FIG. 1 Atypical cutaneous fibrous histiocytoma. Scattered cells have large atypical nuclei, but there are no mitotic figures.

b. Microscopic Features Cellular benign fibrous histiocytomas can arise at various anatomical levels. Most lesions are located in the dermis, and the overlying epidermis is often hyperplastic, as with other cutaneous benign fibrous histiocytomas (Fig. 2). Some lesions arise in deeper dermis (Fig. 3), at the dermal–subcutaneous junction, or adjacent to interlobular septa in the superficial subcutis. The lesions are markedly cellular, with fascicles of somewhat uniform, thin, tapered, spindle cells, which involve superficial and deep dermis and can extend into subcutaneous fat. In parts the cells are sometimes more plump, with discernible cytoplasm imparting a "myoid" appearance (17). Although necrosis with or without ulceration occurs, cytologic atypia and abnormal mitoses are not seen. Normal mitoses can number up to 10 per high-power field (hpf). There are occasionally small aggregates of lymphocytes or, more rarely, of foamy cells, but giant cells are scarce. The patterns of infiltration of adjacent tissues are characteristic. Laterally, where the lesion infiltrates the dermis, it is associated with thickened dermal collagen bundles (Fig. 4). At the deep aspect, in deeper or cellular examples of benign fibrous histiocytoma (BFH), the infiltrating edge may be rounded (Fig. 2), but more often forms a wedge-shaped point radial to the lesion (Fig. 3). Immunostains are positive for SMA at least focally but not for desmin, CD34, or S-100 protein.

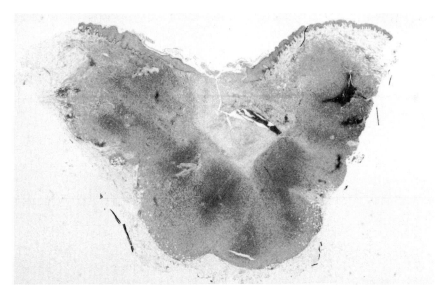

FIG. 2 Cellular cutaneous fibrous histiocytoma. The epidermis is hyperplastic over a cellular lesion with central necrosis and ulceration, and a rounded lower border showing some infiltration into fat.

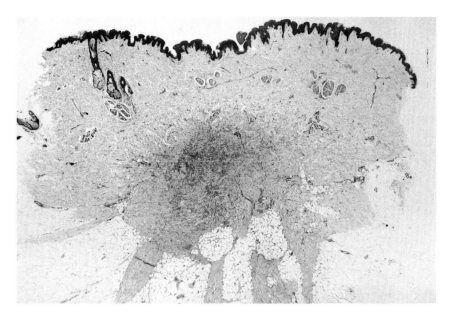

FIG. 3 Cellular fibrous histiocytoma in deep dermis, showing characteristic radial extensions into fat.

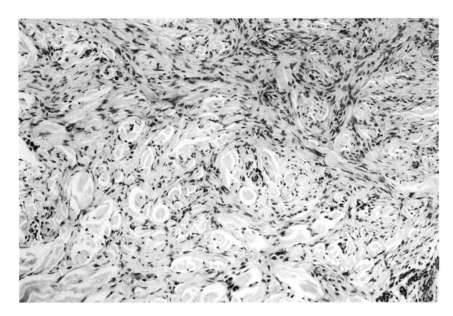

FIG. 4   Cellular cutaneous fibrous histiocytoma. There are thickened collagen bundles at the lateral edges of the lesion.

c. Differential Diagnosis   The cellularity and fascicular architecture resemble those of smooth muscle tumors, and in the presence of mitotic figures an erroneous diagnosis of leiomyosarcoma can be made. However, the cells of cellular fibrous histiocytoma are more tapered and the nuclei more pointed, whereas those of smooth muscle cells have square-ended nuclei, with more abundant, eosinophilic, and parallel-sided cytoplasm and distinct cell boundaries. Muscle tumors do not infiltrate adjacent tissues in the same way that cellular benign fibrous histiocytoma does, and they are not accompanied by epidermal hyperplasia. Finally, most superficial leiomyosarcomas are desmin-positive, and the absence of this marker argues against such a diagnosis.

In DFSP, the epidermis is thinned, the cells are uniform and more elongated, and the histiocytic epiphenomena seen in BFH are sparse or absent. At the deep edge, layers of cells infiltrate along interlobular septa parallel to the skin surface, with honeycomb involvement of the intervening fat. These morphologic features nearly always facilitate distinction between BFH and DFSP, but the use of CD34 can be extremely helpful as the majority of DFSP are strongly positive, especially at the infiltrating edge, whereas BFH is usually negative. The variants of DFSP (myxoid, Bednar or pigmented, and myoid; and giant cell fibroblastoma) are unlikely to be confused with cellular BFH.

3.   Aneurysmal BFH

Aneurysmal BFH is a variant with hemorrhage [angiomatoid, aneurysmal (10,19)] and heavy iron pigmentation that is sometimes misdiagnosed as angiosarcoma but lacks angiogenesis, atypia, and endothelial markers. It is a benign lesion that must be distinguished from the intermediate lesion angiomatoid fibrous histiocytoma, which has recurrent and low metastatic potential. Angiomatoid fibrous histiocytoma is located more deeply, is circumscribed with a fibrous and chronic inflammatory cuff, and in many cases is desmin-positive.

B.   Deep Benign Fibrous Histiocytoma

BFHs can arise in the subcutis and, occasionally in deep soft tissues (16), especially in lower limb or head and neck. They are usually circumscribed rather than infiltrative (Fig. 5) and can be encapsulated. There are sheets of bland cells, sometimes with a storiform pattern (Fig. 6), and with hemangiopericytic areas. Foamy macrophages, osteoclast-like giant cells, and even bone formation (20) are occasionally seen. These lesions are generally CD34-negative, which distinguishes them from solitary fibrous tumors. In one series, 4 of 12 tumors recurred locally, at intervals of 4 months to 17 years, but none metastasized (21).

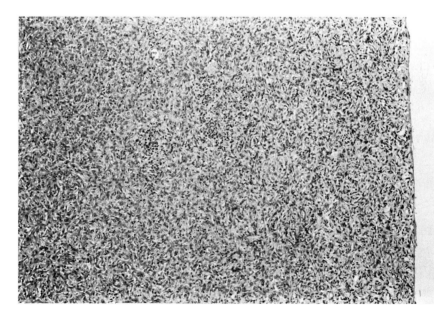

FIG. 5   Deep fibrous histiocytoma. The lesion is sharply circumscribed and uniformly cellular.

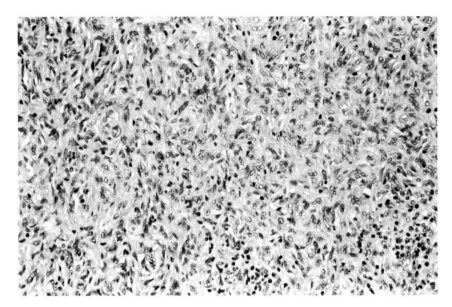

FIG. 6 Deep fibrous histiocytoma. Bland ovoid "fibrohistiocytic" cells with a storiform pattern.

C. Juvenile Xanthogranuloma (Nevoxanthoendothelioma)

1. General and Clinical Features

Juvenile xanthogranuloma (nevoxanthoendothelioma) is a lesion predominantly of infancy that occasionally occurs in adolescents or adults. It is characterized by one or more cutaneous lesions that appear at or shortly after birth and are sometimes associated with similar lesions in deep soft tissue or viscera, including especially the eye, but also epicardium, lung, oral cavity, and testis. The cutaneous lesions are typically found in the head and neck region. The prognosis is excellent as the lesions ultimately regress. Intramuscular juvenile xanthogranuloma has been described (22) as a rare, benign solitary lesion involving the skeletal muscles of the trunk in young children.

2. Microscopic Features

In cutaneous lesions, the epidermis is thinned over a dermal infiltrate of histiocyte-like cells with rounded vesicular nuclei, pale eosinophilic cytoplasm, and indistinct margins without atypia and with rare mitoses (Fig. 7). Variable numbers of lipid-laden xanthomatous cells with foamy cytoplasm and multinucleated giant

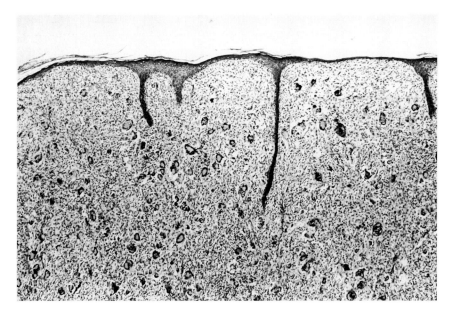

FIG. 7   Juvenile xanthogranuloma. The epidermis is thinned, with fine prolongations into a cellular lesion with frequent Touton giant cells.

cells, including those of Touton type, are also seen, with mixed inflammatory cells, notably lymphocytes and eosinophils, and fibroblasts (Fig. 8). The deeply located lesions are composed of a more homogeneous population of histiocytic cells. Skin lesions entrap adnexa and extend into subcutaneous tissues, and intramuscular lesions infiltrate adjacent muscle. The lesional cells display immunoreactivity for CD68 (more so for the PG-M1 clone than for KP-1) and for FXIIIa. Interestingly, about half of the lesions so studied have shown focal membranous staining in the histiocyte-like cells for the endothelial marker CD31 (22).

3.   Differential Diagnosis

Older lesions resemble regular BFH, but the predominantly histiocytic aspect and the clinical features are distinctive. The principal differential diagnosis is from Langerhans cell histiocytosis (LCH), which also has eosinophils. The nuclei of the histiocytes in LCH are typically grooved, and immunohistochemically they are S-100 protein–positive. Electron microscopy shows Birbeck granules, which are absent from the histiocytes of juvenile xanthogranuloma. Intramuscular lesions must be distinguished from childhood sarcomas and lymphoproliferative disorders by morphologic examination and appropriate immunohistochemical panels.

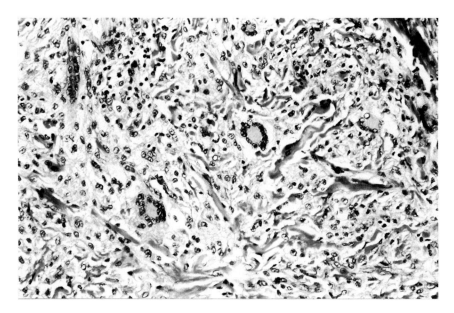

FIG. 8 Juvenile xanthogranuloma. This is composed of a mixture of inflammatory cells including macrophages, Touton giant cells, and fibroblasts.

D. Reticulohistiocytoma

1. General and Clinical Features

Reticulohistiocytoma is a lesion of adult life composed of nodules of eosinophilic histiocytes, often showing multinucleation. It occurs either as red or brown papular skin nodules, or as part of a systemic disease (multicentric reticulohistiocytosis), which includes mucocutaneous lesions and arthritis, as well as systemic symptoms.

The skin nodule is usually solitary, in the upper part of the body, and forms a small, raised red or brown nodule. The lesion is benign and can regress, although an occasional one recurs after excision. However, multicentric reticulohistiocytosis is characterized by a fluctuating but progressive arthritis, affecting especially the distal interphalangeal joint.

2. Microscopic Features

The appearances are similar in the cutaneous and systemic forms. In the dermis, and occasionally involving subcutis or even epidermis, there are circumscribed, nonencapsulated aggregates of characteristic, large multinucleated histiocyte-like cells with abundant eosinophilic or pale cytoplasm. The cells vary in size and number of nuclei, and occasionally are spindled. Nuclear pleomorphism can be seen, but there are rarely mitotic figures. A variable but usually light infiltrate of inflammatory cells, including eosinophils, is usually present. The cytoplasm of the lesional cells is periodic acid–Schiff (PAS)–positive (diastase-resistant) but does not have any specific immunohistochemical markers.

3. Differential Diagnosis

The differential includes Langerhans cell histiocytosis (which is S-100 protein positive), Erdheim-Chester disease, juvenile xanthogranuloma, and even melanoma (which displays cytologic atypia, as well as positivity for S-100 protein and, often, HMB-45).

III. INTERMEDIATE FIBROHISTIOCYTIC TUMORS

A. Atypical Fibroxanthoma

1. General and Clinical Features

Atypical fibroxanthoma is a dermal tumor that is sometimes considered to be the most superficial counterpart of malignant fibrous histiocytoma, since it has a similar cellular composition. Atypical fibroxanthoma typically arises in sun-damaged (or therapeutically irradiated) skin of elderly persons, and is therefore common in the head and neck and especially the scalp. However, there is another peak in young adults, with lesions arising on the trunk (23). The overall excellent prognosis is attributed to the superficial location, but rarely metastases do occur (24).

2. Microscopic Features

The epidermis is thinned or ulcerated over a dome-shaped or flat lesion (Fig. 9). In the superficial dermis there are atypical spindle and polygonal cells with mitoses, including atypical forms (Fig. 10). The lesion can reach the subcutis but does not usually extend more deeply. Those that do, or have necrosis, are prone to recurrence and even metastasis, and might best be regarded as superficial forms of pleomorphic sarcoma (malignant fibrous histiocytoma). A spindle cell nonpleomorphic variant (25) and one with osteoclast-like giant cells (26) have been described. Immunohistochemically, atypical fibroxanthoma occasionally has actin positivity, but desmin, S-100 protein, cytokeratin (27), and CD34 are lacking.

3. Differential Diagnosis

The differential includes melanoma (which has junctional activity and S-100 protein positivity), spindle cell carcinoma (adjacent epidermal dysplasia, positivity for cytokeratin, especially of high molecular weight), leiomyosarcoma (fascicular

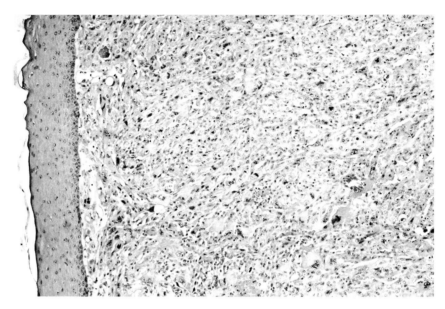

FIG. 9 Atypical fibroxanthoma. The epidermis has lost its rete pegs, and the lesion is variably cellular.

architecture, paranuclear vacuoles, desmin), and angiosarcoma (vasoformation and endothelial marker positivity, including FVIIIRAg, CD34, and CD31).

B. Dermatofibrosarcoma Protuberans

1. General and Clinical Features

DFSP is a relatively common lesion, with a peak age incidence at 20–40 years, which is more common in males, and occurs especially on the trunk and upper limbs. It begins as a dermal plaque or nodule and grows slowly, sometimes becoming multinodular and attaining a large size. DFSP recurs, especially if incompletely excised; surgical clearance can require a wider excision than the clinical appearance might suggest (28). Metastasis occurs in fewer than 5% of cases and follows multiple recurrences; exceptionally, there is fibrosarcomatous or malignant fibrous histiocytoma–like transformation (29), usually in recurrent tumors, which is associated with a more aggressive course (30).

2. Microscopic Features

The epidermis overlying DFSP is generally thinned. The lesion is composed of uniform elongated thin spindle cells with minimal cytoplasm and indistinct mar-

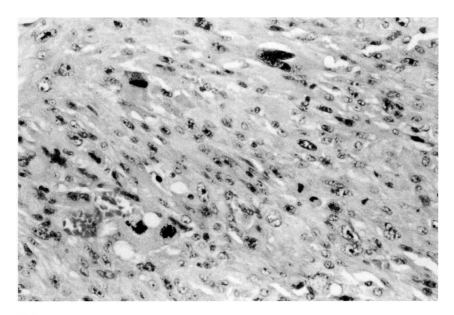

FIG. 10 Atypical fibroxanthoma. Atypical spindle and polygonal cells and abnormal mitotic figures are present.

gins, usually arranged in a striking and monotonous "tight" storiform pattern (Fig. 11). The tumor forms a nodule or ill-defined plaque in the dermis that extends into subcutaneous fat with a characteristic honeycomb pattern, including trabeculae or layers of infiltrating tumor parallel to the skin surface (Fig. 12). The advancing edge is often hypocellular, imparting a deceptively bland appearance. Immunostaining shows strong diffuse positivity for CD34 (31) and focal reactivity for smooth muscle actin, but usually no significant staining for S-100 protein.

3. Differential Diagnosis

DFSP, especially in the early stages, needs distinction from deeper or cellular examples of BFH, and sometimes from neural or smooth muscle tumors. Cellular BFH is generally smaller and associated with epidermal hyperplasia, and its infiltrating edge often forms a wedge-shaped point, radial to the lesion, and associated with thickened dermal collagen bundles. In DFSP, the epidermis is usually thinned, the infiltration is more extensive and parallel to the skin surface, and the histiocytic epiphenomena seen in BFH are sparse or absent. Sometimes there are fascicular or fibrosarcoma-like areas, unlike in BFH. These morphologic features nearly always facilitate distinction between BFH and DFSP, but the use of CD34 can be extremely helpful as BFH is usually negative (but positive for FXIIIa).

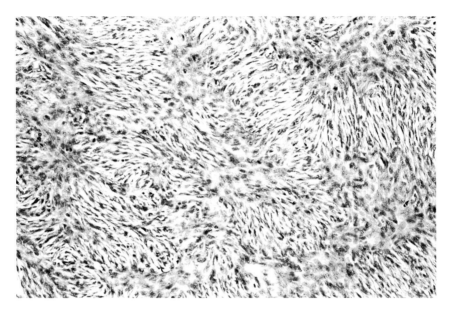

FIG. 11 Dermatofibrosarcoma protuberans. Long spindle cells with tapering nuclei arranged in a repetitive and uniform storiform ("cartwheel") pattern are present.

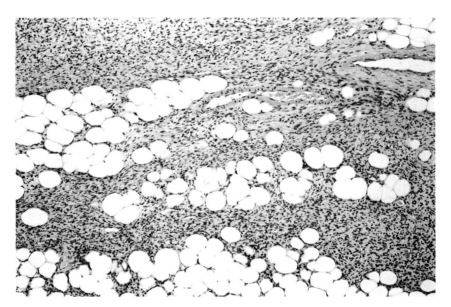

FIG. 12 Dermatofibrosarcoma protuberans. Subcutaneous fat is infiltrated by parallel layers of tumor cells, with intervening "honeycombing."

Occasional cells are S-100 protein–positive but widespread staining is absent, helping to exclude neurofibroma, particularly the diffuse type. Smooth muscle and muscle-specific actins are sometimes found focally in DFSP, but desmin is absent, unlike in cutaneous smooth muscle tumors.

4. Nature

The cell type of DFSP is not clearly characterized ultrastructurally: a histiocytic origin had been suggested, but most now agree that there are variably developed features of fibroblasts (rough endoplasmic reticulum) with focal presence of myofilament bundles indicating myofibroblastic differentiation in some instances (32). In keeping with this, many DFSP are actin-positive. FXIIIa (which stains dermal "dendrocytes") is generally not detectable in DFSP, but immunostaining for CD34 is generally positive (especially at the growing edges, but less so in myxoid areas or centrally). This allows the further hypothesis that the tumor might be derived from any of the local populations of normal CD34-positive fibroblasts: intradermal, periadnexal, or endoneurial. However, DFSP is at present still included in the fibrohistiocytic canon.

Variants of dermatofibrosarcoma protuberans include the following:

1. *Myxoid DFSP* (33,34) (Fig. 13), which can be diagnosed by the characteristic cytology as well as the (variable) CD34 positivity but which requires distinction from myxoid malignant fibrous histiocytoma (by absence of nuclear pleomorphism and the different vascular pattern) as well as a range of benign myxoid lesions.
2. *Pigmented DFSP* (*Bednar's tumor*) (35), which has melanin-containing S-100-positive cells singly or in small clusters (Fig. 14). This variant is incidentally more common in individuals with pigmented skin.
3. *Myoid foci* are infrequently seen in DFSP, and are more common in fibrosarcoma-DFSP (36). In these, the cells have short, blunt-ended nuclei with discernible eosinophilic cytoplasm that is SMA-positive but desmin- and CD34-negative, and electron microscopy has shown myofibroblastic differentiation (37). This feature has no clinical significance.
4. *Fibrosarcoma* occasionally arises in DFSP, more commonly de novo but also in recurrent lesions (29,30). This is characterized by a cellular, fascicular architecture and increased mitotic activity. CD34 can be positive or negative in the fibrosarcomatous area (38). The fibrosarcomatous component behaves relatively aggressively, with local recurrence in over 50% and metastasis in 15% of cases in a recent report that included 34 cases with follow-up (30).

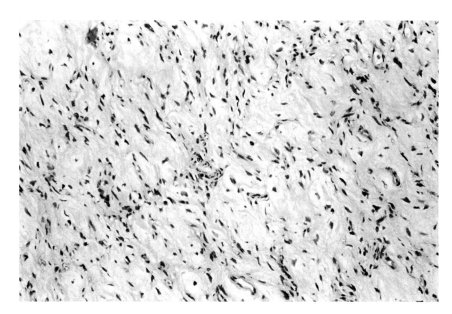

FIG. 13 Dermatofibrosarcoma protuberans, myxoid variant. Though separated by myxoid stroma, the cytologically uniform and bland spindle cells retain an ill-defined storiform pattern.

C. Giant Cell Fibroblastoma

1. General and Clinical Features

This is a rare childhood (and occasionally adult) lesion of dermis/subcutis, which has spindle and bland multinucleate cells in a fibrous and myxoid stroma (Fig. 15), and focally forms cystic spaces lined by tumor (not endothelial) cells (Fig. 16) (39,40). The lesional cells are CD34-positive. Giant cell fibroblastoma has been recorded as either associated with (41) or recurring (partially or completely) as DFSP, of either classical (42–44) or pigmented (45) types, and examples have displayed the same cytogenetic abnormality, t(17;22)(q22;q13), as in DFSP (46), of which it is therefore currently considered to represent a juvenile variant (47).

D. Plexiform Fibrohistiocytic Tumor

1. General and Clinical Features

Plexiform fibrohistiocytic tumor is a relatively recently described entity, with 65 cases in the original 1988 report by Enzinger and Zhang (48) and about 30 additional cases in the subsequent literature (49–52). One case arose in an irradia-

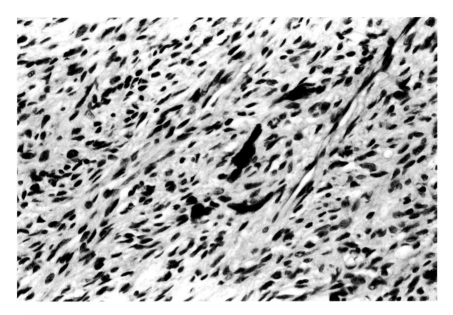

FIG. 14   Dermatofibrosarcoma protuberans, pigmented variant (Bednar tumor). Scattered cells contain melanin pigment.

tion field 7 years after treatment for malignant hemangiopericytoma. It is a slowly growing tumor that occurs mainly in adolescents and young adults, favoring the shoulder and arm region. The tumor is multinodular (hence the term plexiform) and arises at the dermal–subcutaneous junction (Fig. 17), but sometimes extends into deeper tissue, and discrete dermal and subcutaneous variants have been reported (53). Over one third (37%) of plexiform fibrohistiocytic tumors in the original series recurred, usually within 2 years, and two cases (3%) involved metastasis to regional lymph nodes. Thus, the tumor is categorized as of borderline malignancy. In aggregate, the recurrence rate in the subsequent literature has been about 23%, and adequate local excision (with a margin sufficient to ensure removal of peripheral tongues of tumor) is required. One case has recently been reported with systemic (pulmonary) as well as nodal metastases (54). There seems to be no correlation between histologic features and behavior.

2. Microscopic Features

Two principal histologic patterns are described. In the original report (48), 43% displayed a fibrohistiocytic picture with nodules of round or spindle cells with scattered osteoclast-like multinucleate giant cells, chronic inflammation, and hemosiderin pigment (Fig. 18). A predominantly fibroblastic pattern with plexiform

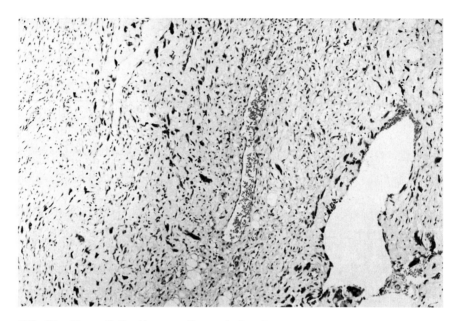

FIG. 15 Giant cell fibroblastoma. Short spindle cells, some with hyperchromatic nuclei, and small multinucleated cells are dispersed in a fibromyxoid stroma with distinct cystic spaces.

bundles of spindle cells was seen in 17% of cases (Fig. 19), and 40% had a mixed pattern. Mitotic figures up to 7–10 per hpf are described. Occasionally pleomorphic cells are seen, and even atypical mitoses, but this feature appears not to worsen the prognosis (55).

Immunohistochemically, as well as with vimentin, some of the spindle cells have smooth muscle actin positivity, and CD68 is found in rounded cells and in the multinucleate giant cells, which are probably histiocytic and nonneoplastic. The spindle cells display focal reactivity for smooth muscle actin, but not for desmin or muscle-specific actin. S-100 protein is nearly always negative, though detected in one case in the original series. FXIIIa is also reportedly negative in lesional cells, but there is no published information on CD34 positivity. The few reports of ultrastructure indicate fibroblastic or myofibroblastic differentiation, or undifferentiated mesenchymal cells. One patient displayed histiocyte-like cells with smooth muscle–type cytoplasmic filaments. These findings are similar to those in other fibrohistiocytic tumors.

3. Differential Diagnosis

Plexiform fibrohistiocytic tumor with nodular pattern and a prominent giant cell component may have to be distinguished from other giant cell tumors, including

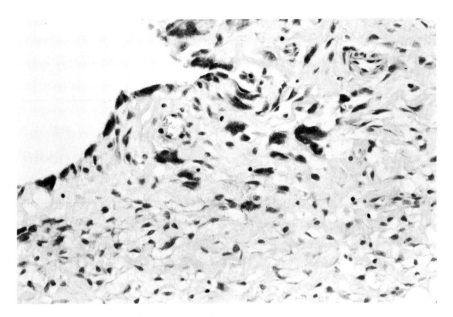

FIG. 16 Giant cell fibroblastoma. Multinucleated cells, as well as cystic space lined by lesional cells, are present.

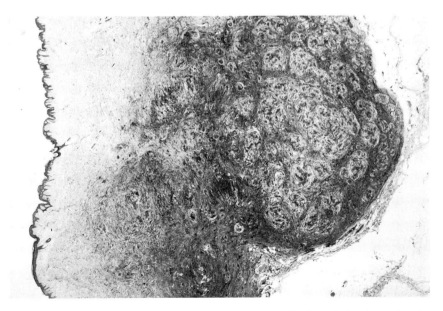

FIG. 17 Plexiform fibrohistiocytic tumor. This is a multinodular lesion located at the dermal–subcutaneous junction and extends into subcutis.

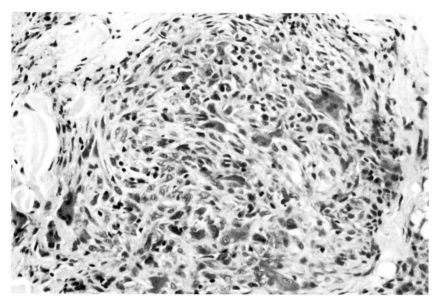

FIG. 18   Plexiform fibrohistiocytic tumor. The nodules are composed of fibroblastic spindle cells, ovoid histiocyte-like cells, and multinucleated cells.

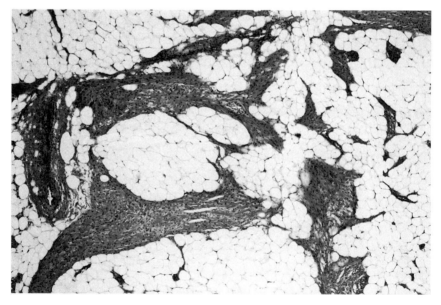

FIG. 19   Plexiform fibrohistiocytic tumor. A minority of cases have plexiform bundles of fibroblastic cells.

TABLE 2 Tumors with Osteoclast-like Giant Cells

Benign and intermediate	Malignant
Fibrohistiocytic	Giant cell MFH
Benign fibrous histiocytoma	Leiomyosarcoma
Cutaneous	Osteosarcoma
Deep	Carcinoma (breast, pancreas)
Plexiform fibrohistiocytic tumor	
Atypical fibroxanthoma	
Giant cell tumor	
of soft tissues	
of tendon sheath	
Nodular fasciitis	

those of tendon sheath, and malignant fibrous histiocytoma, giant cell type (Table 2). In the fibroblastic variant, the differential diagnosis includes fasciitis, fibromatosis, other neoplasms with a plexiform pattern, other types of fibrohistiocytic tumor, and perhaps epithelioid sarcoma. Nodular fasciitis has a very short history, sometimes of only a few days, and a loose myxoid stroma with myofibroblasts. Fibromatosis is infiltrative but displays evenly spaced, parallel-aligned cells in a collagenous stroma, with mast cells and a characteristic vasculature. Plexiform variants of several other soft-tissue tumors have been described (Table 3). Among nerve sheath tumors, these include neurofibroma, schwannoma, malignant peripheral nerve sheath tumor of infancy and childhood, perineurial cell tumor, and granular cell tumor. The first two have characteristic morphology and S-100 protein immunostaining, and perineurial cell tumors display epithelial membrane antigen (EMA) and the typical ultrastructure, with long processes, pinocytosic behavior, and external lamina. Plexiform types of xanthomatous tumor and spindle cell nevus should not cause difficulties.

TABLE 3 Tumors with Plexiform Pattern

Plexiform fibrohistiocytic tumor
Cellular neurothekeoma
Xanthoma
Spindle cell nevus
Nerve sheath tumors
Neurofibroma
Schwannoma
MPNST, childhood
Granular cell schwannoma
Ossifying fibromyxoid tumor

The combination of patterns, morphology, and location bring several other fibrohistiocytic tumors into consideration. Cellular cutaneous fibrous histiocytomas occasionally develop peripheral plexiform features, particularly when extending into subcutis. However, they tend to be more superficial; they have spindle fascicular or storiform morphology, with little collagen, and normal mitoses, but no atypical forms or significant pleomorphism. Atypical cutaneous BFH is more superficial, and has scattered pleomorphic cells, but usually without mitoses. Deep BFH is better circumscribed, with epiphenomena, haemangiopericytomatous pattern, and no significant atypia. BFHs may be immunoreactive for α-smooth muscle actin, but not usually for CD34. DFSP has infiltrative margins, but with honeycombing or in parallel layers rather than in a plexiform fashion. Also, it is characterized by a more marked and uniform storiform pattern, with few epiphenomena, and cytologic pleomorphism is not a feature. DFSP is usually CD34-positive. Atypical fibroxanthoma is intradermal and more markedly pleomorphic. The fibroma-like variant of epithelioid sarcoma may need consideration, but such cases display cytokeratin and EMA positivity.

F. Angiomatoid Fibrous Histiocytoma

1. General and Clinical Features

The term angiomatoid fibrous histiocytoma is applied both to "aneurysmal" cutaneous fibrous histiocytoma and to the more deeply located tumor formerly known as angiomatoid malignant fibrous histiocytoma (56–58); it is used in the latter sense here. In the 1994 WHO classification, angiomatoid malignant fibrous histiocytoma has been removed from the malignant fibrous histiocytoma group in recognition of its generally good prognosis and placed in the intermediate category as angiomatoid fibrous histiocytoma. It is a distinct entity that affects children and adolescents, usually in the upper limb girdle and trunk, and is mostly located in the mid- or deep subcutis with occasional cases in the muscle. A small number of patients have associated systemic symptoms. Ten percent of tumors recur locally, but fewer than 5% metastasize (58); in the original report, a patient with inguinal lymph node metastasis was disease-free 5 years after excision. The studied cases have been diploid (59).

2. Microscopic Features

This tumor is characterized by featureless (or occasionally storiform) sheets of generally uniform histiocyte-like cells with hemorrhagic cyst formation, and a distinct fibrous cuff with chronic inflammatory cells and lymphoid tissue formation (Figs. 20–22). The latter feature often gives the erroneous impression of metastasis within a lymph node, especially in the epitrochlear region. Myxoid change is occasionally seen, and, rarely, focal nuclear pleomorphism and signifi-

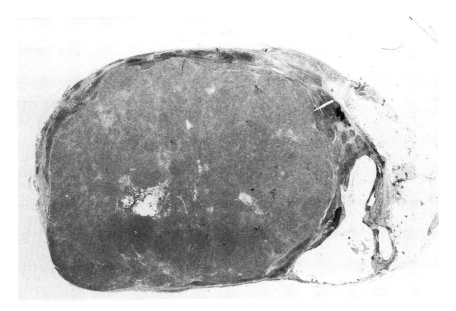

FIG. 20 Angiomatoid fibrous histiocytoma. The tumor is well circumscribed with a fibrous capsule containing lymphoid tissue. The lesion is cellular with minimal hemorrhage in this example.

cant mitotic activity. Some examples display CD68, but desmin and SMA have also been demonstrated (57), whereas endothelial markers are lacking. The few examined by electron microscopy have shown a mixture of vascular, fibroblastic, and histiocyte-like differentiation, but there is no thorough correlative immuno/ electron microscopy study, and the nature of the tumor cells remains uncertain.

3. Differential Diagnosis

The differential diagnosis is principally from cutaneous fibrous histiocytoma, the various hemangiomas and angiosarcoma, as well as from other tumors that can occasionally have hemorrhagic cysts, notably synovial sarcoma and melanoma. Cutaneous fibrous histiocytoma, which can be angiomatoid or aneurysmal, is more superficially located, with typical changes in the overlying epidermis. It displays a mixed cellular composition and an irregular infiltrative margin with stromal collagenous reaction, and usually lacks desmin immunoreactivity. Angiosarcomas are more vasoformative and variably atypical, and the lesional cells are immunoreactive for some or all endothelial markers, including CD34, CD31, and FVIIIRAg. Synovial sarcoma and melanoma can be distinguished by detection of epithelial antigens or S-100 protein and HMB-45, respectively.

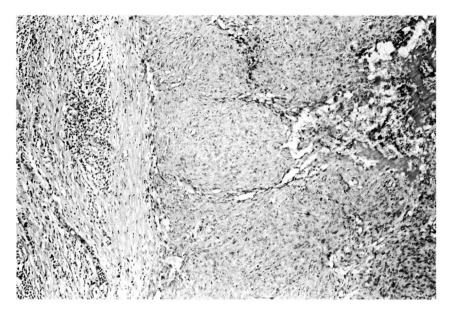

FIG. 21 Angiomatoid fibrous histiocytoma. Nodules and sheets of uniform cells within an inflamed fibrous capsule are present. There is a central area of hemorrhage.

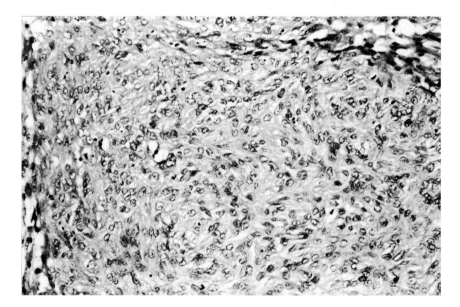

FIG. 22 Angiomatoid fibrous histiocytoma. The lesional cells are bland and histiocyte-like and display a vague storiform architecture.

IV. MALIGNANT FIBROUS HISTIOCYTOMA

A. Introduction

Malignant fibrous histiocytoma (MFH) is classified into storiform-pleomorphic (S-PMFH), myxoid, giant cell, and xanthomatous subtypes; angiomatoid MFH has currently been reclassified as an intermediate fibrohistiocytic tumor. S-PMFH is a category that includes many tumors previously considered as fibrosarcoma, pleomorphic rhabdomyosarcoma, or undifferentiated pleomorphic sarcoma. It was the most frequently diagnosed adult soft-tissue sarcoma from the late 1970s to the early 1990s, but with current techniques and thorough investigation, the number of cases assigned as MFH has been reduced in recent years. Since a number of other types of sarcoma and even some carcinomas and melanomas can have a similar pattern, it has been suggested that pleomorphic MFH is not an entity but merely a collection of poorly differentiated neoplasms, many of which can be categorized by thorough examination (6). While this group might not be homogeneous, its natural history and management, as well as its relationship to other soft-tissue tumor types, have been well documented. The findings in the hundreds of cases studied are, within a range, remarkably similar; for cases with these features, the term malignant fibrous histiocytoma remains descriptively reasonable within awareness of its limitations and while attempts continue to define and characterize further subgroups. It is pertinent that the terms *fibrous histiocytoma* and *fibrohistiocytic* remain accepted and useful for benign and borderline tumors with similar features.

B. Storiform-Pleomorphic MFH

1. General and Clinical Features

S-PMFH is a tumor of older adults that presents as a soft-tissue mass usually deeply located in the limbs, limb girdles, retroperitoneum, trunk, or head and neck. Similar tumors in visceral organs are usually sarcomatoid carcinomas, a diagnosis that can be confirmed by demonstration of cytokeratins (especially high molecular weight subtypes) or epithelial features on electron microscopy. MFH commonly reaches a large size and shows areas of hemorrhage and necrosis, within a pale cream or tan tumor surface. Deeper tumors are circumscribed and have a pseudocapsule formed by compression of adjacent tissue by expansile growth of the tumor, whereas some superficial (subcutaneous) tumors have infiltrative growth margins, so that wide local excision is necessary to ensure complete removal (60).

2. Microscopic Features

There is at least focally a storiform pattern, which sometimes predominates, imparting a resemblance to DFSP (Fig. 23). Characteristically, S-PMFH is composed

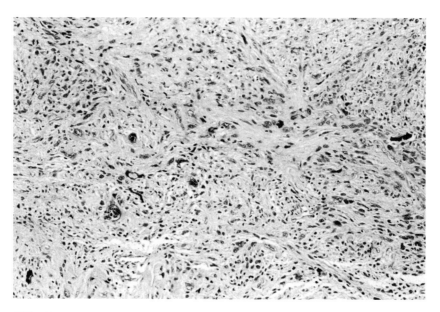

FIG. 23   Malignant fibrous histiocytoma, storiform-pleomorphic subtype. The spindle cells form a storiform pattern with scattered polygonal cells.

of a variable proportion of atypical pleomorphic spindle cells and polygonal cells, often multinucleated and with abundant eosinophilic cytoplasm, and with atypical and typical mitoses (Fig. 24). The stroma has variable amounts of collagen, myxoid change, and inflammatory cells, as well as hemorrhage and necrosis.

There is still no diagnostically specific antibody to fibroblasts or "MFH cells." Antibodies reactive with subsets of dermal dendrocytic or fibroblast-like cells (FXIIIa, CD34) have not proved useful in MFH. By definition, the tumor should display no specific line of differentiation (61,62), but multiple intermediate filament (IF) subtypes have been found singly and coexpressed in examples of MFH. All display vimentin, and some desmin. Neurofilament and cytokeratin have also been detected in a series of ultrastructurally confirmed MFHs (63). Those tumors that are desmin- or keratin-positive might conceivably represent pleomorphic leiomyosarcoma, or undifferentiated carcinoma or synovial sarcoma, respectively, but both of these antigens are on occasion detectable in myofibroblasts. Furthermore, IF subtypes have been shown in MFH without ultrastructural or light microscopic evidence of specific differentiation (63–65). In diagnosing pleomorphic sarcomas, a panel of antibodies should be employed, and a specific diagnosis should not be made in the absence of relevant histomorphologic features. These may be detected only after extensive sampling.

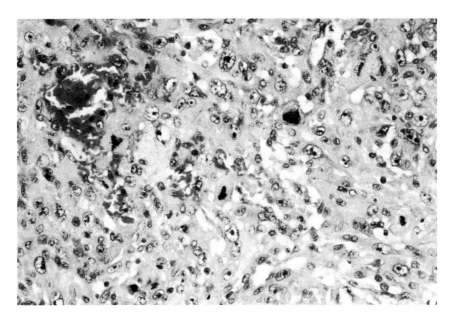

FIG. 24 Malignant fibrous histiocytoma, storiform-pleomorphic subtype. This area has polygonal histiocyte-like cells with nuclear pleomorphism and atypical mitoses.

There is no diagnostic cytogenetic or molecular genetic abnormality specific for MFH. Many have structural and numerical rearrangements (66), some relating to behavior, but generally the changes relate nonspecifically to tumorigenesis.

3. Differential Diagnosis

Pleomorphic MFH-like areas are found in many other types of soft-tissue tumor, including those that represent dedifferentiated examples of specific sarcoma subtypes. Pleomorphic liposarcoma is identified by the presence of lipoblasts, and pleomorphic rhabdomyosarcoma, which occasionally occurs in adults, by the presence of cross-striations or ultrastructural evidence of sarcomeric differentiation. Immunohistochemically, desmin and sarcomeric actin are positive in pleomorphic rhabdomyosarcoma, but neither is specific for this tumor type and a panel of antibodies, including those to myogenin and myogenic regulatory protein (MyoD1), should be employed. Similar considerations apply to the diagnosis of pleomorphic leiomyosarcoma, since smooth muscle actin is detectable in numerous tumor types; fascicles of spindle cells with typical smooth muscle morphology should preferably be identified.

MFH-like patterns are also seen in some carcinomas, melanomas, and lymphomas. A detailed clinical history, adequate sampling, and judicious use of appropriate antibody panels will help to prevent diagnostic errors.

C. Myxoid MFH

Myxoid MFH (20% of MFH) was originally defined as having myxoid stromal change in more than 50% of the lesion (67). It occurs mostly in the limbs of older subjects and has a tendency to superficial location, as a multinodular subcutaneous unencapsulated mass (Fig. 25), which is usually slow growing. Prognostic factors include size (for metastasis, but not recurrence—60% recur locally), and depth: tumors in subcutis may recur but do not metastasize, whereas those involving deep fascia or muscle are more likely to recur and metastasize. The likelihood of metastasis is inversely proportional to the amount of myxoid change.

There is overlap or identity with higher grades of myxofibrosarcoma. This lesion was originally defined as having four grades (68), of which the lower ones are relatively bland angiomyxoid lesions, while higher ones have features of pleomorphic sarcomas. More recently, three grades of malignancy have been defined

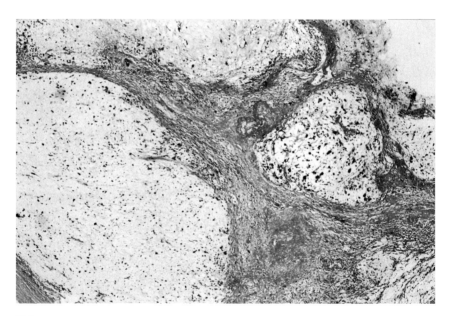

FIG. 25 Malignant fibrous histiocytoma, myxoid subtype, low grade (myxofibrosarcoma). Variably sized myxoid nodules are separated by more cellular and fibrous areas.

in myxofibrosarcoma, and a smaller percentage of myxoid change (10%) has been suggested as definitional (69).

1. Microscopic Features

There are typical cytologic and vascular features. Within the myxoid nodules, spindle-shaped cells with hyperchromatic nuclei are irregularly dispersed (Fig. 26). Nuclear pleomorphism is always present at least focally, but this is highly variable, and in some areas the cells may look remarkably bland. Mitotic figures are usually found relatively easily, especially in the pleomorphic areas, and abnormal forms are seen. In the higher grade lesions, there is an increasing proportion of nonmyxoid tumor, with pleomorphic cells as in storiform-pleomorphic MFH. These initially form solid cellular areas between the myxoid nodules and can be fibrous, hemorrhagic or necrotic.

The vascular pattern in myxoid areas is characteristic. Vessels are typically fairly numerous, short, separate, curved, and relatively thick-walled rather than delicate; a plexiform vascular pattern is lacking, and the tumor cells are not closely related to the blood vessels.

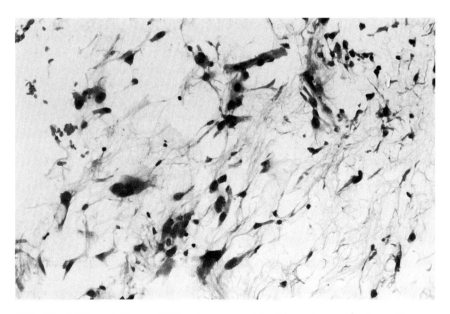

FIG. 26 Malignant fibrous histiocytoma, myxoid subtype, low grade (myxofibrosarcoma). Spindle cells with pleomorphic hyperchromatic nuclei in a myxoid stroma with scanty, short curved blood vessels are present.

Immunohistochemical markers are usually negative, although a few scattered cells are sometimes actin-positive, implying possible myofibroblastic differentiation, and there is sometimes focal immunoreactivity for the fibroblastic marker CD34. Ultrastructurally, there are fibroblasts, myofibroblasts, and histiocyte-like cells, as with typical MFH. In some, dilated vesicles contain granular secretion identical to the stromal ground substance, with which the vesicles can be seen to communicate. Myofibroblastic differentiation is, however, rarely seen in myxoid MFH or myxofibrosarcoma.

2. Differential Diagnosis

The differential diagnosis for superficial tumors includes nodular fasciitis (which lacks pleomorphism and atypia); myxoma (same, and lacks vessels and mitoses); neurothekeoma (S-100 protein–positive, with a rim of EMA-positive perineurial cells around the nodules); myxoid DFSP (less pleomorphic, with straight rather than curved vessels, and usually CD34-positive). Deeply located myxoid MFH is often misdiagnosed as myxoid liposarcoma, but the latter (Fig. 11) has more uniform and more uniformly distributed cells, a more delicate vasculature, and definite lipoblasts. These can be distinguished by their rounded, empty vacuoles, which lack stainable acid mucopolysaccharide in the cytoplasm and which indent the cell's nucleus. The recently described inflammatory myxohyaline tumor with virocyte or Reed-Sternberg-like cells (70) [acral myxoinflammatory fibroblastic sarcoma (71)], which predominantly involves extremities (especially hand and wrist) and sometimes infiltrates tendon sheaths, might represent a subset of myxoid MFH. These tumors have myxoid nodules with markedly vacuolated fibroblasts, separated by cellular fibrous tissue containing mixed inflammatory cells and polygonal cells with nuclei (sometimes binucleate) containing prominent eosinophilic nucleoli. These atypical cells are immunoreactive only for vimentin and are thought to represent modified fibroblasts. These tumors recur locally but rarely metastasize.

D. Giant Cell MFH

Giant cell MFH (8%) (72) is multinodular and, in addition to atypical spindle and polygonal cells, has numerous osteoclast-like giant cells (Fig. 27), sometimes with peripheral bone formation. This tumor requires distinction from leiomyosarcoma with osteoclast-like giant cells (73), and from other types of tumor in which giant cells are an occasional or regular feature, such as plexiform fibrohistiocytic tumor and giant cell tumor of tendon sheath (Table 2). The bone, which is also seen on occasion in storiform-pleomorphic MFH, is sometimes metaplastic and sometimes neoplastic (this distinction is not always obvious). The latter occurrence might indicate a diagnosis of extraskeletal osteosarcoma, but some (72,74) distin-

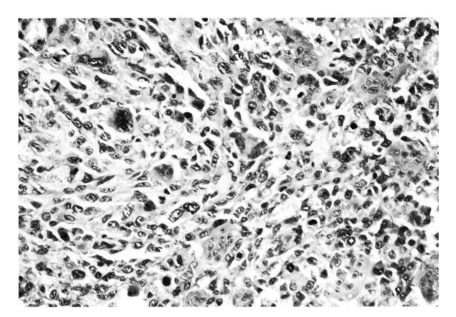

FIG. 27 Malignant fibrous histiocytoma, giant cell subtype. Scattered osteoclast-like giant cells in a pleomorphic cellular background are present.

guish the two entities by the differing patterns and distribution of the osteoid or osteochondroid component. As with myxoid MFH, the behavior of the giant cell variant relates to tumor size and depth.

E. Xanthomatous (Inflammatory) MFH

Xanthomatous (inflammatory) MFH (4%), which is often located in the retroperitoneum, forms a large mass and also behaves in an aggressively malignant fashion (75,76). This tumor is composed of sheets of large histiocyte-like cells, often deceptively bland looking with abundant clear or granular cytoplasm, but focally with atypical nuclei (Fig. 28). There is often an intense, predominantly neutrophilic inflammatory infiltration, but little collagen is seen, and sometimes there are transitions to more typical pleomorphic MFH. These tumors are rare and not well studied. However, some reportedly produce cytokines (77), including neutrophil chemotactic factors and granulocyte-macrophage colony-stimulating factor (GM-CSF), as do histiocytes. This type of MFH requires distinction not only from inflammatory processes, including pseudotumors, but also from lymphomas (especially those of T-cell type), true histiocytic tumors, and other mesenchymal tumors

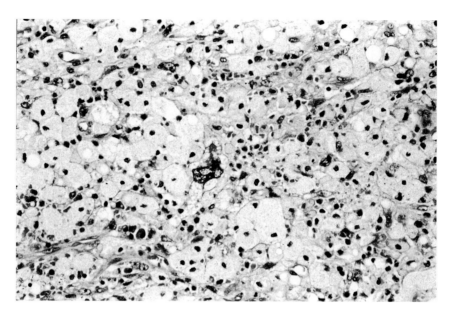

FIG. 28 Malignant fibrous histiocytoma, xanthomatous (inflammatory) subtype. Foamy cells, some with atypical nuclei, and mixed acute and chronic inflammatory cells are present.

that can have a marked inflammatory infiltrate, such as liposarcoma, leiomyosarcoma, and fibrosarcoma (78).

REFERENCES

1. Weiss SW. Histological Typing of Soft Tissue Tumours, 2nd ed. Berlin: Springer-Verlag, 1994.
2. Fletcher CDM. Commentary. Malignant fibrous histiocytoma? Histopathology 11: 433–437, 1987.
3. Fisher C. Fibrohistiocytic tumors. Monogr Pathol 38:162–180, 1996.
4. Wood GS, Beckstead JH, Turner RR, Hendrickson MR, Kempson RL, Warnke RA. Malignant fibrous histiocytoma tumor cells resemble fibroblasts. Am J Surg Pathol 10:323–335, 1986.
5. Weiss LM, Arber DA, Chang KL. CD68—a review. Appl Immunohistochem 2:2–8, 1994.
6. Fletcher CDM. Pleomorphic malignant fibrous histiocytoma: fact or fiction? A critical reappraisal based on 159 tumors diagnosed as pleomorphic sarcoma. Am J Surg Pathol 16:213–228, 1992.

7. Leyva WH, Santa Cruz DJ. Atypical cutaneous fibrous histiocytoma. Am J Dermatopathol 8:467–471, 1986.
8. Zelger BG, Calonje E, Zelger B. Myxoid dermatofibroma. Histopathology 34:357–364, 1999.
9. Zelger BW, Öfner D, Zelger BG. Atrophic variants of dermatofibroma and dermatofibrosarcoma protuberans. Histopathology 26:519–527, 1995.
10. Santa Cruz DJ, Kyriakos M. Aneurysmal ("angiomatoid") fibrous histiocytoma of the skin. Cancer 47:2053–2061, 1981.
11. Wambacher-Gasser B, Zelger B, Zelger BG, Steiner H. Clear cell dermatofibroma. Histopathology 30:64–69, 1997.
12. Zelger BG, Steiner H, Kutzner H, Rutten A, Zelger B. Granular cell dermatofibroma. Histopathology 31:258–262, 1997.
13. Glusac EJ, McNiff JM. Epithelioid cell histiocytoma: a simulant of vascular and melanocytic neoplasms. Am J Dermatopathol 21:1–7, 1999.
14. Glusac EJ, Barr RJ, Everett MA, Pitha J, Santa Cruz DJ. Epithelioid cell histiocytoma. A report of 10 cases including a new cellular variant. Am J Surg Pathol 18:583–590, 1994.
15. Soini Y. Cell differentiation in benign cutaneous fibrous histiocytomas. An immunohistochemical study with antibodies to histiomonocytic cells and intermediate filament proteins. Am J Dermatopathol 12:134–140, 1990.
16. Enzinger FM, Weiss SW. Soft Tissue Tumors, 3rd ed. St Louis: Mosby, 1995, pp. 215–296.
17. Calonje E, Mentzel T, Fletcher CDM. Cellular benign fibrous histiocytoma. Clinicopathologic analysis of 74 cases of a distinctive variant of cutaneous fibrous histiocytoma with frequent recurrence. Am J Surg Pathol 18:668–676, 1994.
18. Colome-Grimmer MI, Evans HL. Metastasizing cellular dermatofibroma: a report of two cases. Am J Surg Pathol 20:1361–1367, 1996.
19. Calonje E, Fletcher CDM. Aneurysmal benign fibrous histiocytoma: clinicopathological analysis of 40 cases of a tumour frequently misdiagnosed as a vascular neoplasm. Histopathology 26:323–331, 1995.
20. Smith NM, Davies JB, Shrimankar JS, Malcolm AJ. Deep fibrous histiocytoma with giant cells and bone metaplasia. Histopathology 17:365–381, 1990.
21. Fletcher CDM. Benign fibrous histiocytoma of subcutaneous and deep soft tissue: a clinicopathologic analysis of 21 cases. Am J Surg Pathol 14:801–809, 1990.
22. Nascimento AG. A clinicopathologic and immunohistochemical comparative study of cutaneous and intramuscular forms of juvenile xanthogranuloma. Am J Surg Pathol 21:645–652, 1997.
23. Kempson RL, McGavran MH. Atypical fibroxanthomas of the skin. Cancer 17:1463–1471, 1964.
24. Helwig EB, May D. Atypical fibroxanthoma of the skin with metastasis. Cancer 57:368–376, 1986.
25. Calonje E, Wadden C, Wilson-Jones E, Fletcher CDM. Spindle-cell non-pleomorphic atypical fibroxanthoma: analysis of a series and delineation of a distinctive variant. Histopathology 22:247–254, 1993.
26. Khan ZM, Cockerell CJ. Atypical fibroxanthoma with osteoclast-like multinucleated giant cells. Am J Dermatopathol 19:174–179, 1997.

27. Longacre TA, Smoller BR, Rouse RV. Atypical fibroxanthoma. Multiple immunohistologic profiles. Am J Surg Pathol 17:1199–1206, 1993.

28. Arnaud EJ, Perrault M, Revol M, Servant JM, Banzet P. Surgical treatment of dermatofibrosarcoma protuberans. Plast Reconstr Surg 100:884–895, 1997.

29. Connelly JH, Evans HL. Dermatofibrosarcoma protuberans. A clinicopathologic review with emphasis on fibrosarcomatous areas. Am J Surg Pathol 16:921–925, 1992.

30. Mentzel T, Beham A, Katenkamp D, Dei Tos AP, Fletcher CD. Fibrosarcomatous ("high-grade") dermatofibrosarcoma protuberans: clinicopathologic and immunohistochemical study of a series of 41 cases with emphasis on prognostic significance. Am J Surg Pathol 22:576–587, 1998.

31. Brathwaite C, Suster S. Dermatofibrosarcoma protuberans. A critical reappraisal of the role of imunohistochemical stains for diagnosis. Appl Immunohistochem 2:36–41, 1994.

32. Dominguez-Malagón HR, Ordoñez NG, Mackay B. Dermatofibrosarcoma protuberans: ultrastructural and immunocytochemical observations. Ultrastructural Pathol 19:281–289, 1995.

33. Frierson HF, Cooper PH. Myxoid variant of dermatofibrosarcoma protuberans. Am J Surg Pathol 7:445–450, 1983.

34. Orlandi A, Bianchi L, Spagnoli LG. Myxoid dermatofibrosarcoma protuberans: morphological, ultrastructural and immunohistochemical features. J Cutan Pathol 25:386–393, 1998.

35. Dupree WB, Langloss JM, Weiss SW. Pigmented dermatofibrosarcoma protuberans (Bednar tumor): a pathologic, ultrastructural, and immunohistochemical study. Am J Surg Pathol 9:630–639, 1985.

36. Calonje E, Fletcher CDM. Myoid differentiation in dermatofibrosarcoma protuberans and its fibro-sarcomatous variant: clinicopathologic analysis of 5 cases. J Cutan Pathol 23:30–36, 1996.

37. Morimitsu Y, Hisaooka M, Okamoto S, Hashimoto H, Ushijima M. Dermatofibrosarcoma protuberans and its fibrosarcomatous variant with areas of myoid differentiation: a report of three cases. Histopathology 32:547–551, 1998.

38. Goldblum JR. CD34 positivity in fibrosarcomas which arise in dermatofibrosarcoma protuberans. Arch Pathol Lab Med 119:238–241, 1995.

39. Abdul-Karim FW, Evans HL, Silva EG. Giant cell fibroblastoma: a report of three cases. Am J Clin Pathol 83:165–170, 1985.

40. Dymock RB, Allen PW, Stirling JW, Gilbert EF, Thornbery JM. Giant cell fibroblastoma. A distinctive, recurrent tumor of childhood. Am J Surg Pathol 11:263–272, 1987.

41. Michal M, Zamecnik M. Giant cell fibroblastoma with a dermatofibrosarcoma protuberans component. Am J Dermatopathol 14:549–552, 1992.

42. Alguacil-Garcia A. Giant cell fibroblastoma recurring as dermatofibrosarcoma protuberans. Am J Surg Pathol 15:798–801, 1991.

43. Goldblum JR. Giant cell fibroblastoma—a report of three cases with histologic and immunohistochemical evidence of a relationship to dermatofibrosarcoma protuberans. Arch Pathol Lab Med 120:1052–1055, 1996.

44. Harvell JD, Kilpatrick SE, White WL. Histogenetic relations between giant cell fibroblastoma and dermatofibrosarcoma protuberans. CD34 staining showing the spectrum and a simulator. Am J Dermatopathol 20:339–345, 1998.

45. Chadarévian J-P, Coppola D, Billmire DF. Bednar tumor pattern in recurring giant cell fibroblastoma. Am J Clin Pathol 100:164–166, 1993.

46. Simon MP, Pedeutour F, Sirvent N, Grosgeorge J, Minoletti F, Coindre JM, Terrier-Lacombe MJ, Mandahl N, Craver RD, Blin N, Sozzi G, Turc-Carel C, O'Brien KP, Kedra D, Fransson I, Guilbaud C, Dumanski JP. Deregulation of the platelet-derived growth factor B-chain gene via fusion with collagen gene COL1A1 in dermatofibrosarcoma protuberans and giant cell fibroblastoma. Nat Genet 15:95–98, 1997.

47. Shmookler BM, Enzinger FM, Weiss SW. Giant cell fibroblastoma. A juvenile form of dermatofibrosarcoma protuberans. Cancer 64:2154–2161, 1989.

48. Enzinger FM, Zhang R. Plexiform fibrohistiocytic tumor presenting in children and young adults. An analysis of 65 cases. Am J Surg Pathol 12:818–826, 1988.

49. Hollowood K, Holley MP, Fletcher CDM. Plexiform fibrohistiocytic tumour: clinicopathological, immunohistochemical, and ultrastructural analysis in favour of a myofibroblastic lesion. Histopathology 19:503–513, 1991.

50. Hibon E, Verzeaux E. Plexiform fibrohistiocytic tumor: a case report. Am J Dermatopathol 13:206–207, 1991.

51. Angervall L, Kindblom LG, Lindholm K, Eriksson S. Plexiform fibrohistiocytic tumor. Report of a case involving preoperative aspiration cytology and immunohistochemical and ultrastructural analysis of surgical specimens. Pathol Res Pract 188:350–356, 1992.

52. Herring SM. Plexiform fibrohistiocytic tumor of skin. Ann Plast Surg 30:459–461, 1993.

53. Zelger B, Weinlich G, Steiner H, Zelger BG, Egarter-Vigl E. Dermal and subcutaneous variants of plexiform fibrohistiocytic tumor. Am J Surg Pathol 21:235–241, 1997.

54. Salomao DR, Nascimento AG. Plexiform fibrohistiocytic tumor with systemic metastases. A case report. Am J Surg Pathol 21:469–476, 1997.

55. Fisher C. Atypical plexiform fibrohistiocytic tumour. Histopathology 30:271–273, 1997.

56. Enzinger FM. Angiomatoid malignant fibrous histiocytoma. A distinct fibrohistiocytic tumor of children and young adults simulating a vascular neoplasm. Cancer 44:2147–2157, 1979.

57. Smith MEF, Costa MJ, Weiss SW. Evaluation of CD68 and other histiocytic antigens in angiomatoid malignant fibrous histiocytoma. Am J Surg Pathol 15:757–763, 1991.

58. Costa MJ, Weiss SW. Angiomatoid malignant fibrous histiocytoma. A follow up study of 108 cases with evaluation of possible histologic predictors of outcome. Am J Surg Pathol 14:1126–1132, 1990.

59. Pettinato G, Manivel JC, De Rosa G, Petrella G, Jaszcz W. Angiomatoid malignant fibrous histiocytoma: cytologic, immunohistochemical, ultrastructural, and flow cytometric study of 20 cases. Mod Pathol 3:479–487, 1990.

60. Fanburg-Smith JC, Spiro IJ, Katapuram SV, Mankin HJ, Rosenberg AE. Infiltrative subcutaneous malignant fibrous histiocytoma: a comparative study with deep malignant fibrous histiocytoma and an observation of biologic behavior. Ann Diagn Pathol 3:1–10, 1999.

61. Weiss SW. Malignant fibrous histiocytoma: a reaffirmation. Am J Surg Pathol 6:773–784, 1982.

62. Meister P. Malignant fibrous histiocytoma; history, histology, histogenesis. Pathol Res Pract 183:1–7, 1988.

63. Lawson CW, Fisher C, Gatter K. An immunohistochemical study of differentiation in malignant fibrous histiocytoma. Histopathology 11:375–383, 1987.

64. Miettinen M, Soini Y. Malignant fibrous histiocytoma, Heterogeneous patterns of intermediate filament proteins by immunohistochemistry. Arch Pathol Lab Med 113:1363–1366, 1989.

65. Rosenberg AE, O'Connell JX, Dickersin GR, Bhan AK. Expression of epithelial markers in malignant fibrous histiocytoma of the musculoskeletal system. An immunohistochemical and electron microscopic study. Hum Pathol 24:284–293, 1993.

66. Mertens F, Fletcher CD, Dal Cin P, De Wever I, Mandahl N, Mitelman F, Rosai J, Rydholm A, Sciot R, Tallini G, Van den Berghe H, Vanni R, Willen H. Cytogenetic analysis of 46 pleomorphic soft tissue sarcomas and correlation with morphologic and clinical features: a report of the CHAMP Study Group. Chromosomes and Morphology. Genes Chromosomes Cancer 22:16–25, 1998.

67. Weiss SW, Enzinger FM. Myxoid variant of malignant fibrous histiocytoma. Cancer 39:1672–1685, 1977.

68. Angervall L, Kindblom L-G, Merck C. Myxofibrosarcoma. A study of 30 cases. Acta Pathol Microbiol Scand. 85:127–140, 1977.

69. Mentzel T, Calonje E, Wadden C, Camplejohn RS, Beham A, Smith MA, Fletcher CDM. Myxofibrosarcoma: clinicopathologic analysis of 75 cases with emphasis on the low-grade variant. Am J Surg Pathol 20:391–405, 1996.

70. Montgomery EA, Devaney K, Weiss SW. Inflammatory myxohyaline tumor of distal extremities with virocyte or Reed-Sternberg-like cells: a distinctive lesion with features simulating inflammatory conditions, Hodgkin disease, and various sarcomas. Mod Pathol 11:384–391, 1998.

71. Meis-Kindblom JM, Kindblom L-G. Acral myxoinflammatory fibroblastic sarcoma. A low-grade tumor of the hands and feet. Am J Surg Pathol 22:911–924, 1998.

72. Guccion JG, Enzinger FM. Malignant giant cell tumor of soft parts. An analysis of 32 cases. Cancer 29:1518–1528, 1972.

73. Mentzel T, Calonje E, Fletcher CDM. Leiomyosarcoma with prominent osteoclast-like giant cells. Analysis of eight cases closely mimicking the so-called giant cell variant of malignant fibrous histiocytoma. Am J Surg Pathol 18:258–265, 1994.

74. Bhagavan B, Dorfman H. The significance of bone and cartilage formation in malignant fibrous histiocytoma of soft tissue. Cancer 49:480–488, 1982.

75. Kyriakos M, Kempson RL. Inflammatory fibrous histiocytoma. An aggressive and lethal lesion. Cancer 37:1584–1606, 1976.

76. Merino MJ, Livolsi VA. Inflammatory malignant fibrous histiocytoma. Am J Clin Pathol 73:276–281, 1980.

77. Melehm MF, Meisler AI, Saito R, Finley GG, Hockman HR, Koski RA. Cytokines in inflammatory malignant fibrous histiocytoma presenting with leukaemoid reaction. Blood 82:2038–2044, 1993.

78. Meis JM, Enzinger FM. Inflammatory fibrosarcoma of the mesentery and retroperitoneum. A tumor closely simulating inflammatory pseudotumor. Am J Surg Pathol 15:1146–1156, 1991.

8
Tumors Demonstrating Adipocytic Differentiation

John X. O'Connell
Surrey Memorial Hospital
Surrey, British Columbia, Canada

G. Petur Nielsen
Massachusetts General Hospital
Boston, Massachusetts

I. INTRODUCTION

Lipomas and liposarcomas are the commonest mesenchymal neoplasms of the somatic soft tissue that exhibit specific lineage differentiation (1). Although neoplasms classified as variants of fibrous histiocytoma (benign and malignant) outnumber adipose tissue tumors, the former group includes a mixture of entities, often exhibiting different lines of differentiation. Like virtually all other soft-tissue neoplasms, the benign variants of adipose tumors (lipomas) greatly outnumber their malignant counterparts (liposarcomas). The vast majority of both of these neoplasms occur in adulthood and only rare specific subtypes occur in children. As with virtually all other soft-tissue tumors, the cell of origin of adipose neoplasms is unknown. In this regard, these neoplasms, like most other soft-tissue tumors, are classified based on the resemblance of the lesional neoplastic cells to normal cells (in this case the adipocyte and its various precursor cells) and not the cell of origin. Mature adipocytes are spherical cells whose cytoplasm is distended by a single lipid vacuole. The vacuole compresses the nucleus, which is seen microscopically at the periphery of the cell as a thin dark crescent. Immunohistochemically mature fat cells label for vimentin and S-100 protein and typically are negative for most other markers used in the standard immunohistochemial investigation of soft-tissue tumors. In embryologic development mature fat cells are

199

derived from fibroblastic or pericytic cells that undergo progressive accumulation of multiple cytoplasmic lipid droplets, which eventually coalesce into a single vacuole (2,3). Immature fat cells thus contain multiple lipid vacuoles and exhibit a higher nuclear-to-cytoplasmic ratio by virtue of their smaller size. A variety of adipose neoplasms contain cells resembling these precursor cells. Such multivacuolated cells are termed *lipoblasts* when they occur in the setting of liposarcoma and *lipoblast-like cells* when present in benign neoplasms or reactive conditions. The diagnostic significance of these multivacuolated cells, particularly regarding their specificity for liposarcoma, has been overemphasized in the past, and it is apparent that lipoblast-like cells are present as a typical finding in several variants of lipoma (see below) and even in nonneoplastic conditions (1).

II. CYTOGENETIC EVALUATION OF ADIPOSE TISSUE NEOPLASMS

Although the diagnosis and classification of adipose tissue neoplasms is based on their microscopic morphology, in recent years cytogenetic evaluation of cultured cells from many different types of benign and malignant adipose tissue tumors has revealed that many demonstrate specific, reproducible karyotypic abnormalities (4,5). These chromosomal abnormalities include numerical deletions, translocations, and acquisition of marker chromosomes (4,5). Since these have a high frequency and in many instances appear to be specific to tumor types, it is likely that these structural and numerical chromosomal abnormalities play an important role in the development of the neoplasms (4,5). However, the exact molecular mechanism whereby these result in the benign or malignant phenotype is unclear. While the specific karytoypic abnormalities that characterize the individual tumors were discovered using classical cytogenetic techniques, these aberations may now be detected using the alternative technologies of fluorescent in situ hybridization, reverse transcriptase polymerase chain reaction, and other chromosmal labeling methodologies. The specific chromosomal abnormalities that characterize individual neoplasms will be reported in each of the relevent sections.

III. BENIGN TUMORS

A. Lipoma

1. General and Clinical Features

Lipomas, benign tumors composed of cells resembling mature adipocytes, are the most common soft-tissue tumors of adulthood. Most lipomas occur in adults between the ages of 40 and 60 years, and they are more common in obese individuals. The tumors may arise in the subcutaneous tissue (*superficial lipoma*) or within deep soft tissues (*deep lipoma*) or even from the surfaces of bone (*parosteal lipoma*) (6,7). Occasionally, lipomas can have areas of bone formation (*osteolipoma*) (8), nodules of cartilage (*chondrolipoma*), abundant fibrous tissue (*fibrolipoma*), extensive myxoid change (*myxolipoma*), or a smooth muscle component (*myolipoma*) (9). These microscopic subtypes do not have clinical significance with regard to the behavior of the tumors. Superficial lipomas present as painless, soft, mobile masses that are generally small at the time of diagnosis (<5.0 cm). They are treated by simple excision. Recurrences are extremely uncommon. Deep lipomas are generally larger at the time of diagnosis (>5.0 cm). They are typically painless but occasionally cause symptoms when they compress peripheral nerves. Deep-seated lipomas that arise within or between skeletal muscles are called intramuscular and intermuscular lipomas, respectively (10). *Intramuscular lipomas* affect patients in middle to late adult life. They occur in various locations, including the trunk and the upper and lower extremities (10). Intramuscular lipomas may be infiltrative or well circumscribed. This clinicopathologic distinction is important, as the infiltrative type has a tendency to recur locally following incomplete excision. Total removal of the involved muscle or a compartmental resection has been suggested for these infiltrating tumors in order to minimize the risk of recurrence (11). The *intermuscular lipoma*, as the name implies, arises between muscles. It also affects adults and arises most often in the anterior abdominal wall. These are usually cured by local excision alone.

2. Pathologic Findings

Grossly, lipoma is well circumscribed and encapsulated and has a yellow, greasy cut surface (Fig. 1). The superficial lipomas are generally small (<5.0 cm), whereas the deep ones often exceed 5.0 cm. Basically, they all have a similar gross appearance; however, areas of bone formation can be seen in osteolipomas and gray glistening nodules of cartilage may be seen in chondrolipoma. Intermuscular lipomas do not demonstrate any specific gross features, except that a portion of skeletal muscle is often attached to the periphery of the tumor. Intramuscular lipomas may appear as ill-defined regions of pallor within skeletal muscles and typically these lack a capsule (Fig. 2). Microscopically, conventional lipoma is composed of lobules of mature adipocytes (Fig. 3). In the infiltrative type of intramuscular lipoma the mature adipocytes are arranged between skeletal muscle fibers and therefore appear to infiltrate these (Fig. 4). The majority of lipomas demonstrate karyotypic abnormalities involving 12 q (4,12–14).

3. Differential Diagnosis

The most important pathologic differential diagnosis, especially for deep-seated lipomas, is low-grade liposarcoma. *Well-differentiated liposarcoma* (see below)

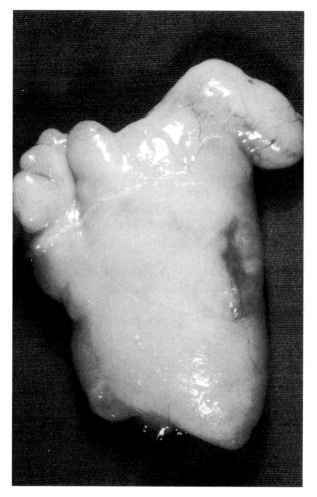

FIG. 1 Typical circumscribed encapsulated appearance of a superficial lipoma.

generally shows areas of fibrosis that contains cells with bizarre, hyperchromatic nuclei and occasional lipoblasts, whereas deep lipomas are composed only of mature univacuolated adipocytes that do not demonstrate hyperchromasia or atypia. Intramuscular *arteriovenous hemangioma* can have a prominent fatty component that can simulate intramuscular lipoma. Microscopically, however, medium and large vessels are present in addition to mature adipose tissue and atrophic skeletal muscle—features that are not present in conventional deep-seated lipoma.

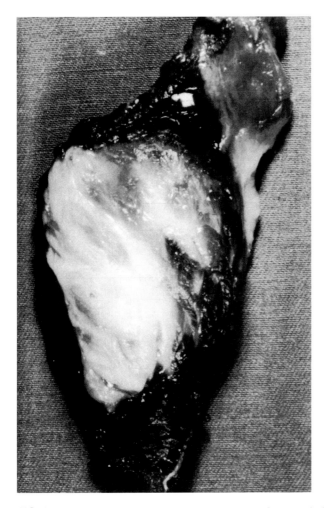

FIG. 2 Deep intramuscular lipoma. Note the lack of encapsulation and the pale gray tissue within the tumor that represents entrapped skeletal muscle.

B. Multiple Lipomas/Lipomatosis

1. General and Clinical Features

Approximately 5% of patients with lipomas have multiple tumors, each of which is clinically, grossly, and microscopically identical to conventional lipoma. Up to several hundred of these lipomas can be present in lipomatosis. The back, shoul-

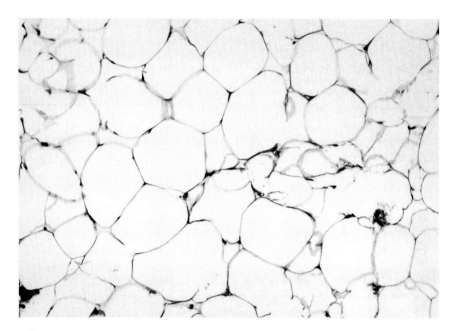

FIG. 3 Uniform mature adipocytes that lack cytologic atypia.

der, and upper arms are the most common location, and men are affected more frequently than women. Familial cases of multiple lipomas have been described that seem to have a dominant inheritance pattern (15,16). In lipomatosis, there is diffuse, nonlobular proliferation of fat in the affected tissues. The subcutaneous fat of the back of the neck and shoulder are involved in nearly every individual (17). Lipomatosis is thought to be secondary to a defect in lipid metabolism (17). Patients with diffuse lipomatosis have the clinical appearance of obesity; mediastinal involvement can cause venous obstruction with stasis and airway obstruction (17).

2. Pathologic Findings

The lipomas in multiple lipomas have the same gross and histologic features as conventional lipomas. The adipocytes have the appearance of normal adipocytes, except for slightly smaller size. In lipomatosis the proliferation is nonencapsulated (17).

C. Spindle Cell Lipoma

1. General and Clinical Features

Spindle cell lipoma is a histologically distinct type of lipoma that was first recognized as a benign variant of lipoma in 1975 (18). Although spindle cell lipoma can occur in various locations, the classic presentation is that of a painless subcutaneous mass involving the shoulder, back, or posterior neck in a middle-aged to elderly man (18,19). Most tumors are solitary, but occasionally they can be multiple. In rare cases, there may be a familial tendency to multiple lesions (20). The treatment of choice is simple excision. Recurrences are extremely rare.

2. Pathologic Findings

Grossly, the tumors are well circumscribed and typically measure between 3 and 5 cm although occasionally larger examples occur. On sectioning they have yellow areas, representing the mature fat, and gray-gelatinous areas representing the spindle cell component. Microscopically, spindle cell lipoma is usually well circumscribed; however, focal infiltration into surrounding tissue can be seen, espe-

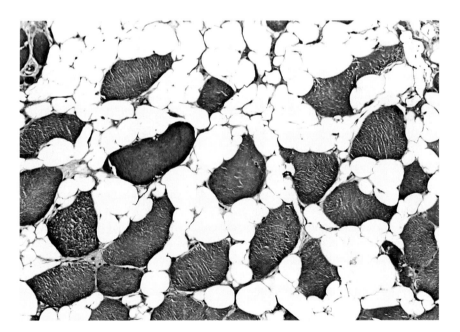

FIG. 4 Intramuscular lipoma demonstrating mature adipocytes separating individual skeletal myocytes.

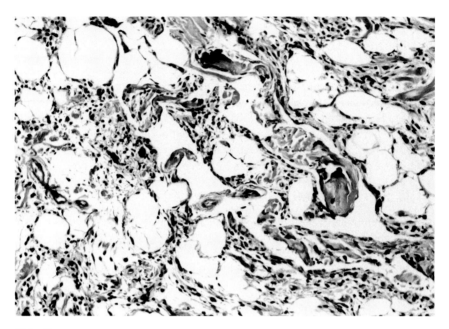

FIG. 5 Spindle cell lipoma exhibiting mature adipocytes, numerous uniform spindle cells, and bands of dense collagen.

cially in those spindle cell lipomas that involve the deeper structures. Spindle cell lipoma is, as its name implies, composed of an admixture of mature adipocytes and spindle cells embedded in myxoid matrix that contains birefringent collagen fibers (Fig. 5). The spindle cell component can occupy only a portion of the tumor or can involve almost the entire lesion, obscuring its lipomatous nature (18). The mature adipocytes have identical features to those seen in conventional lipoma. The spindle cells have oval to elongated uniform dark-staining nuclei and bipolar eosinophilic cytoplasm (21). Mitotic figures are rare. The matrix is variably myxoid and characteristically contains bright eosinophilic collagen fibers. Scattered mast cells are present. The vascular pattern is usually inconspicuous but occasionally can have a "pseudoangiomatous" appearance secondary to myxoid degenerative changes (22,23). Immunohistochemically, the mature adipocytes, but not the spindle cells, stain for S-100 protein (24). In contrast, the spindle cells, and not the adipocytes, stain for CD34. Cytogenetic studies have shown abnormalities involving 13q and 16q (4,25,26).

3. Differential Diagnosis

The differential diagnosis includes a variety of benign and malignant tumors. When spindle cell lipoma is extensively myxoid it can mimic a myxoma. *Myxomas*, however, generally arise in skeletal muscle, although they can sometimes show areas of hypercellularity they do not contain the birefringent collagen fibers or fat that is present in spindle cell lipomas (27). In addition, although intramuscular myxomas are grossly well circumscribed, they are not encapsulated. Microscopically myxoid material can be seen infiltrating and encasing adjacent skeletal muscle fibers (27), *Neurofibroma* is also composed of spindle cells, myxoid stroma that contains collagen fibers, and mast cells. Unlike spindle cell lipoma, in neurofibroma the spindle cells have "wavy" nuclei, are more haphazardly arranged, and the extracellular collagen fibers are more delicate. In addition, many of the spindle cells in neurofibroma stain for S-100 protein. Spindle cell lipoma with a myxoid stroma is distinguishable from *myxoid liposarcoma* by the lack of lipoblasts and the presence of the characteristic plexiform vascular pattern (see below).

D. Pleomorphic Lipoma

1. General and Clinical Features

Pleomorphic lipoma is clinically, morphologically, and cytogenetically related to spindle cell lipoma and can be considered a pleomorphic variant of spindle cell lipoma (4,25,26,28). Like spindle cell lipoma, pleomorphic lipoma generally occurs in males and involves the posterior neck, shoulder, and back (29,30). Patients typically present with a solitary subcutaneous mass often of many years' duration. As is the case with spindle cell lipoma, treatment is by simple excision. Recurrence is rare.

2. Pathologic Findings

Grossly, pleomorphic lipomas are well circumscribed and have a yellow or grayish tan cut surface. Microscopically, they closely resemble spindle cell lipoma. However, unlike spindle cell lipoma, pleomorphic lipoma contains variable numbers of hyperchromatic multinucleated giant cells that frequently demonstrate a concentric or floret-like arrangement of the nuclei (Fig. 6). These cells have eosinophilic cytoplasm with the nuclei arranged peripherally and circumferentially. The nuclei overlap and have finely dispersed or, less frequently, smudgy chromatin and small eosinophilic nucleoli. These pleomorphic cells may be few and widely scattered or they may occupy a large portion of the tumor. Like spindle cell lipoma, the extracellular matrix is myxoid and contains thick eosinophilic colla-

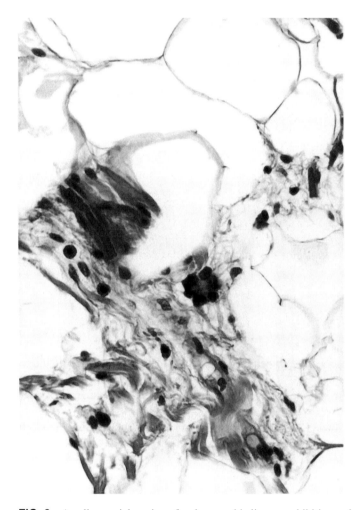

FIG. 6 A collagen-rich region of a pleomorphic lipoma exhibiting a characteristic multinucleated "florette" cell.

gen fibers. Lipoblast-like cells may be present. Cytogenetic studies have shown
chromosomal abnormalities similar to those of spindle cell lipoma (4,25,26).

3. Differential Diagnosis

Distinguishing pleomorphic lipoma from *well-differentiated sclerosing liposarcoma* (see below) can be problematic, especially as lipoblast-like cells (see
above) can be seen in pleomorphic lipoma. However, the clinical setting of a slow-

growing tumor arising in the subcutaneous tissue of the posterior neck, shoulder, or back is very characteristic for pleomorphic lipoma, whereas sclerosing liposarcoma arises in the deep soft tissues or the retroperitoneum. Also, sclerosing liposarcoma has large areas of collagen deposition (sclerosis), more easily identified multivacuolated lipoblasts, and fewer floret-like giant cells. In practical terms, the diagnosis of pleomorphic lipoma should not be considered outside of the appropriate clinical setting of a superficial shoulder/neck adipose tissue tumor.

E. Chondroid Lipoma

1. General and Clinical Features

Chondroid lipoma is a recently described distinctive subtype of lipoma (31). Prior to its recognition as a variant of lipoma, an example of this tumor had been reported as an "extraskeletal chondroma with lipoblast-like cells" because of the unusual cartilage-like appearance that is characteristic of this unusual neoplasm (32). These tumors occur more frequently in females than males. They usually arise in the extremities but can also involve other sites, such as the trunk and the head and neck region (31,33,34). Radiographic studies show mixed-signal characteristics (35). All reported examples of chondroid lipoma have behaved in a benign fashion. The treatment is simple excision.

2. Pathologic Findings

Grossly, chondroid lipoma is well circumscribed and has a yellow cut surface. Microscopically, it is lobulated, with the neoplastic cells growing in sheets, cords, or as single cells, separated by extracellular eosinophilic ("chondroid") matrix (Fig. 7). The cells have well-defined cell membranes and small, dark-staining nuclei surrounded by granular eosinophilic cytoplasm. Many cells contain clear intracytoplasmic fat vacuoles indenting the nucleus, making them indistinguishable from lipoblasts (lipoblast-like cells) (Fig. 8). However, mature adipocytes are present in all of the tumors. Immunohistochemically, the chondroid-like cells stain for vimentin and S-100 protein in a manner similar to that of normal adipocytes. Ultrastructural studies have shown a spectrum of differentiation, with the cells showing features of prelipoblasts and chondroblasts (34,36). Cytogenetic studies have shown t(12,16); however, the break points are different from those present in the t(12;16) of myxoid liposarcoma (see below) (37,38).

3. Differential Diagnosis

Because of the myxoid ground substance and multivacuolated lipoblast-like cells, chondroid lipoma may simulate myxoid liposarcoma. *Myxoid liposarcoma*, however, contains a prominent plexiform vascular pattern and a myxoid stroma

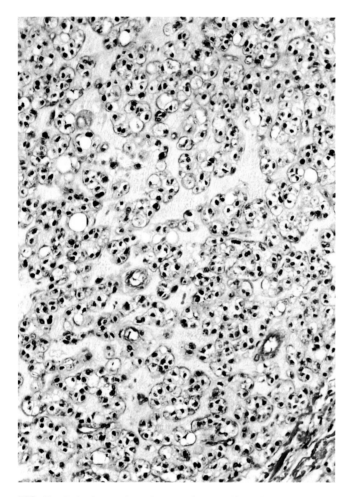

FIG. 7 Cohesive cords and nests of oval cells embedded within a uniform granular extracellular ground substance. The clustering of the cells highlights their resemblance to chondrocytes.

instead of the eosinophilic, "chondroid" stroma seen in chondroid lipoma (see below).

F. Angiolipoma

1. General and Clinical Features

Angiolipoma characteristically arises in the subcutaneous tissue of young adults, most frequently the forearm, trunk, and upper arm. These tumors are often mul-

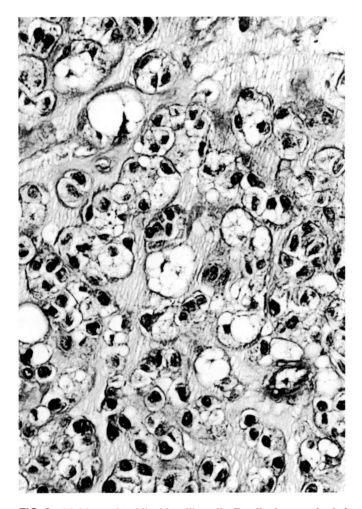

FIG. 8 Multivacuolated lipoblast-like cells. Focally the vacuoles indent the nuclei.

tiple and painful. The pain is more severe during the initial tumor growth phase but decreases in severity with time. Rare cases of familial angiolipomatosis have been described (39).

2. Pathologic Findings

Grossly, angiolipoma is well circumscribed and has a yellow or often slightly pink or reddish cut surface. It is rarely larger than 2 cm. Microscopically, it is composed of an admixture of mature adipocytes and tangles of capillaries. These tend to be most numerous at the periphery (subcapsular area) of the tumor. A characteristic feature is the presence of fibrin thrombi within vascular lumina (Fig. 9). Eventually the stroma around the vessels may become fibrotic. Sometimes the vascular component can occupy almost the entire tumor, with only few scattered mature adipocytes present. The term "cellular angiolipoma" has been used for this variant (40). Cytogenetic studies have shown a normal karyotype, which is in striking contrast with other lipomas (41). This and the fact that angiolipomas differ from other lipomas by virtue of their high vascular content has resulted in the proposal that angiolipomas may represent vascular tumors with a prominent fatty component (41).

3. Differential Diagnosis

Conventional angiolipoma should not cause diagnostic difficulties. Cellular angiolipoma can be confused with vascular tumors such as Kaposi's sarcoma or angiosarcoma. Both *Kaposi's sarcoma* and *angiosarcoma* are poorly circumscribed, demonstrate more cytologic atypia, usually do not demonstrate prominent intravascular fibrin thrombi, and in addition do not contain an adipocytic component. The clinical setting of multiple painful small subcutaneous lesions in the upper extremities in a young individual should help clarify the diagnosis.

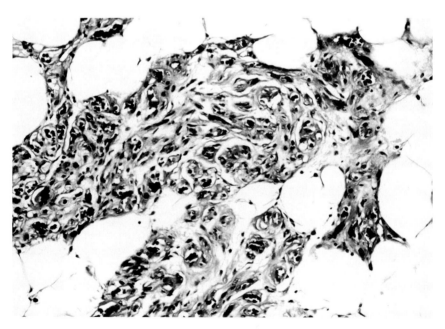

FIG. 9 A tangle of capillaries that focally exhibit intraluminal fibrin thrombi. A typical feature of angiolipoma.

G. Hibernoma

1. General and Clinical Features

Hibernoma is an uncommon benign tumor in which the lesional cells demonstrate morphologic features of brown fat cells (42). Other names that have been used for this tumor include lipoma of immature adipose tissue, lipoma of embryonic fat, and fetal lipoma. Hibernomas generally arise in locations where brown fat is found in fetuses and infants, such as the interscapular region, neck, mediastinum, axilla, posterior abdominal wall, and retroperitoneum adjacent to the kidney and adrenal gland (43). They can also arise in areas that normally do not harbor brown fat, such as the thigh. Like other fatty tumors, hibernoma presents as a painless, slow-growing mass. Hibernomas always pursue a benign course. The treatment of choice is local excision.

2. Pathologic Findings

Grossly, hibernomas are tan or red–brown, usually measuring between 5 and 10 cm; larger tumors measuring more than 20 cm occasionally occur (42). Microscopically, hibernoma demonstrates a lobular architecture and is composed of large polygonal cells supported by small branching capillaries. Three cell types can be identified, with their morphologic variations depending on the relative cytoplasmic amounts of mitochondria and fat (44). Cells with abundant mitochondria have a granular eosinophilic cytoplasm. Other cells have granular eosinophilic cytoplasm and numerous lipid vacuoles that typically indent the centrally located nucleus. The third type resembles a mature univacuolar adipocyte (Fig. 10). Cytogenetically, hibernomas demonstrate aberrations of chromosome 11q13 (45).

3. Differential Diagnosis

Other benign soft-tissue tumors that can have abundant eosinophilic cytoplasm and enter into the differential diagnosis of hibernoma are granular cell tumor and rhabdomyoma. *Granular cell tumor* is generally superficial in location. Unlike hibernoma, granular cell tumor is poorly circumscribed and infiltrates surrounding tissue. The cytoplasm in cells of granular cell tumor is eosinophilic, but it lacks the lipid vacuoles that are seen in hibernoma. Ultrastructurally, granular cell tumor contains abundant secondary lysosomes that give the tumor its eosinophilic granularity. *Rhabdomyoma* is a very rare benign tumor showing skeletal muscle differentiation. Histologically and ultrastructurally the cells in rhabdomyoma contain cross-striations due to the presence of organized sarcomeres. Immunohistochemically, rhabdomyomas stain for muscle markers.

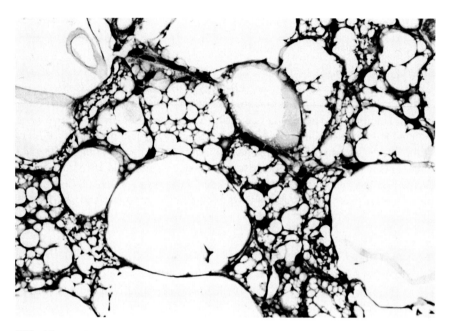

FIG. 10 A mixture of mature adipocytes and multivacuolated brown fat cells, typical of hibernoma.

H. Lipoblastoma/lipoblastomatosis

1. General and Clinical Features

Lipoblastoma is a benign tumor that arises exclusively in infants, typically during the first 3 years of life (46). The term *lipoblastomatosis* is used to describe poorly circumscribed masses of similar immature-appearing adipose tissue. Patients with lipoblastoma tend to be slightly older than patients with lipoblastomatosis (47). Lipoblastoma is more common in boys. It most frequently involves the extremities and presents as a slow-growing painless mass (48). Other locations include the neck, trunk, retroperitoneum, groin, axilla, back, labia, flank, and mediastinum (47,48). Lipoblastoma generally involves the subcutaneous tissue but can also involve deeper tissue, especially the diffuse (lipoblastomatosis) form (46). Lipoblastoma and lipoblastomatosis are treated by local resection. Local recurrence has been reported in 9–22% of patients; recurrences are more common in patients with the diffuse (lipoblastomatosis) form (47). Metastases do not occur.

2. Pathologic Findings

Grossly, lipoblastomas have a lobulated, myxoid, or pale cut surface. Occasionally, they can have cystic areas filled with mucoid material. They are typically well circumscribed. However, lipoblastomatosis is poorly circumscribed, infiltrating the subcutaneous tissue and, occasionally, the underlying skeletal muscle. Most tumors are smaller than 5.0 cm in diameter, but tumors measuring more than 20 cm rarely occur (47). Microscopically, lipoblastoma is lobular, with the individual lobules separated by fibrous connective tissue septa (Fig. 11). The former are composed of lipoblasts in varying stages of development. A wide array of cell types are present, including morphologically primitive stellate and spindle-shaped cells, multivacuolated adipocytes, and univacuolated "signet ring" cell adipocytes (48,49). Mitotic figures are rare and always normal in appearance. The supporting extracellular stroma is myxoid and commonly demonstrates a plexiform vascular pattern. Maturation to conventional lipoma rarely supervenes (47). Rearrangements of chromosome 8q have been identified in lipoblastomas (4,50–53).

3. Differential Diagnosis

The main differential diagnosis of lipoblastoma/lipoblastomatosis is myxoid liposarcoma. However, *myxoid liposarcoma* is extremely rare in children and lacks the well-formed lobular growth pattern seen in lipoblastoma (see below).[a]

IV. MALIGNANT TUMORS

A. Liposarcoma

The World Health Organization (WHO) recognizes the following subtypes of liposarcoma (54).

1. Well-differentiated liposarcoma
2. Myxoid liposarcoma
3. Round cell liposarcoma
4. Pleomorphic liposarcoma
5. Dedifferentiated liposarcoma

Well-differentiated liposarcoma and dedifferentiated liposarcoma are histogenetically related because the latter arises from the former. These two tumors, though linked, will be discussed separately because their treatment and clinical outcome are different. Myxoid and round cell liposarcoma represent two biological and clinical ends of a spectrum. Both tumors are characterized by a single cytogenetic abnormality. Therefore, although these lesions have been historically considered separate entities, it is clear that they represent low- and high-grade variants of the same neoplasm. For this reason, myxoid and round cell liposarcoma will be discussed as a single entity.

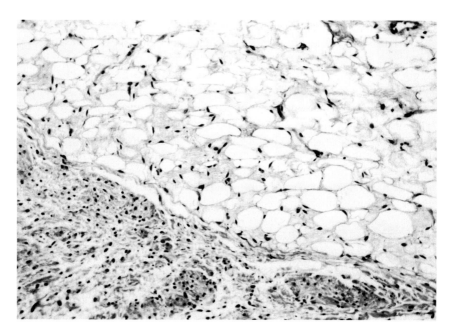

FIG. 11 A low-power view of the edge of a lobule within a lipoblastoma. The adipose component of the tumor exhibits varying sized adipocytes embedded in a myxoid extracellular ground substance.

B. Well-Differentiated Liposarcoma

1. General and Clinical Features

Well-differentiated liposarcoma represents the commonest histologic subtype of liposarcoma (1). These tumors virtually always occur in adults (55–59). Males and females are equally affected, and the patients are usually in the fifth through eight decades of life (55–59). Well-differentiated liposarcomas may arise in any site; however, the most common location for these tumors is the deep soft tissues of the proximal extremities and the retroperitoneum (55–59). By convention, when well-differentiated liposarcomas occur in the subcutaneous tissues they are classified as *atypical lipomas* (59). Although these tumors are histologically and cytogenetically identical to their deeply located counterparts, the natural history of the superficial tumors is sufficiently different for them to be considered as a separate group (see "Differential Diagnosis," below) (59). Most patients with well-differentiated liposarcomas present with painless, slow-growing, soft-tissue masses (55–59). Intra-abdominal tumors typically are larger than extremity tumors, and patients with abdominal tumors may present with altered abdominal girth or symptoms related to altered gastrointestinal tract function (55–59). Groin tumors commonly simulate inguinal or femoral herniae. The extremity tumors are typically soft; however, tumors that arise within muscle groups may become hard upon action of the affected muscles. Plain radiographs may demonstrate fat density masses distorting tissue planes. Mineralization within these tumors occurs only rarely. Computed tomography (CT) and magnetic resonance imaging (MRI) effectively demonstrate these neoplasms, highlighting their relationship to muscle, bone, and neurovascular structures (60–64). Using both of these modalities, the vast majority of well-differentiated liposarcomas exhibit signal qualities similar to those of normal subcutaneous fat. Strands of soft tissue with signal characteristics similar to muscle are often present in these tumors. These may represent entrapped skeletal muscle fibers or collagen-rich regions of the neoplasm (see "Sclerosing Liposarcoma," below) (60–64) (Fig. 12). If large volumes of this intermediate signal material are present in a neoplasm that otherwise is composed predominantly of fat, then this suggests the possibility of a dedifferentiated liposarcoma (see below) (64). The treatment of well-differentiated liposarcoma is greatly influenced by the location of the tumor and the presence or absence of dedifferentiation (see below). The following comments pertain to non-dedifferentiated tumors only. The resectability of these neoplasms is principally determined by their location, size, proximity to neurovascular structures, and the functional status of the patient. Any treatment option must encompass the fact that distant metastases from this family of neoplasms virtually never occur and although local recurrence commonly supervenes, it is often many years after the original surgical procedure. Local recurrence in the extremities is typically not associated with destructive growth. For these reasons, extremity well-differentiated liposarcoma is managed by wide local excision, if technically possible. Local or marginal excision is preferable to ablative surgical procedures that result in major functional compromise. Retroperitoneal tumors, by virtue of their location, are not usually amenable to radical resection. Patients are typically treated by debulking that virtually always results in residual gross or microscopic tumor following excision. Treated in this way, well-differentiated liposarcoma of the extremity demonstrates a recurrence rate of approximately 40–50%, whereas groin and retroperitoneal tumors exhibit an even higher rate of local recurrence, i.e., 80–90% (55–59). The behavior of these neoplasms, regardless of locaton, is characterized by multiple recurrences that occur over many years (55–59). The extremity tumors do not result in patient deaths; however, the retroperitoneal and groin tumors have a poor long-term prognosis, with the majority of affected patients ultimately dying of disease due to uncontrolled local growth in the abdominal cavity (55–59).

Well-differentiated liposarcomas demonstrate consistent karyotypic abnormalities in greater than 90% of examined cases (4,65). These abnormalities include the presence of ring chromosomes and long marker chromosomes derived from the q13-15 region of chromosome 12 (4,5,65). These findings are present

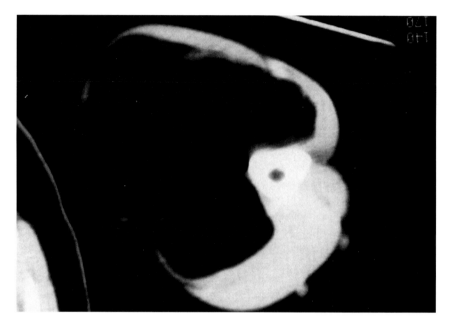

FIG. 12 A CT image of a large, well-differentiated (lipoma-like) liposarcoma of the upper arm. The faint strands within the tumor represent collagenous septae. A typical imaging finding in these types of tumors.

in tumors regardless of their anatomical location, including those that arise in the suprerficial soft tissue and which by convention are classified as atypical lipoma (4).

2. Pathologic Findings

Well-differentiated liposarcomas are usually large tumors with a mean size greater than 10 cm (1,55,58). Tumors in excess of 20 cm are not uncommon. They typically demonstrate a multinodular growth within and between skeletal muscles. Individual lobules of tumor are typically separated from adjacent structures by a "pseudocapsule" of compressed collagen. This layer results in a "plane" that facilitates the enucleation or shelling out of these neoplasms when they are located in regions that do not allow wide excision. The tumors are typically soft and pale yellow on cut section (Fig. 13). The cut surface often is a paler yellow than adjacent normal fat due to the presence of excessive interstitial collagen in the tumor in comparison to the normal fat. Three microscopic variants of well-differentiated liposarcoma occur.

The most common is the *lipoma-like variant*. As the name suggests, this tumor resembles lipoma morphologically. As such, this subtype is composed pre-

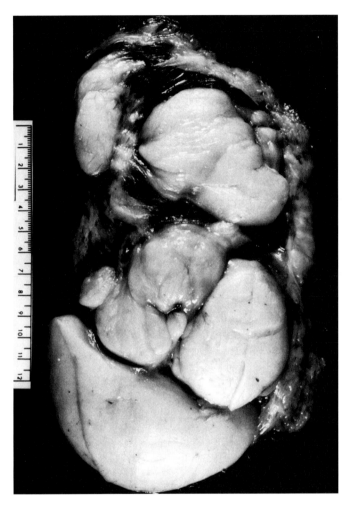

FIG. 13 Characteristic gross appearance of a large multinodular lipoma–like liposarcoma. The tumor exhibits intramuscular growth.

dominantly of cells that resemble mature adipocytes. In contrast to lipoma, there is a greater variability in adipocyte size. In addition, there is usually an increase in interstitial collagen within the tumor, within thickened fibrous bands that traverse the tumor as well as diffusely in the extracellular space (Fig. 14). It is this collagen that results in the gross pallor that is frequently a feature of well-differentiated liposarcoma. The diagnostic hallmark of lipoma-like liposarcoma is the presence of atypical hyperchromatic nuclei within the cells showing adipose differentiation in addition to nonspecific spindle cells embedded in the collagenous bands and

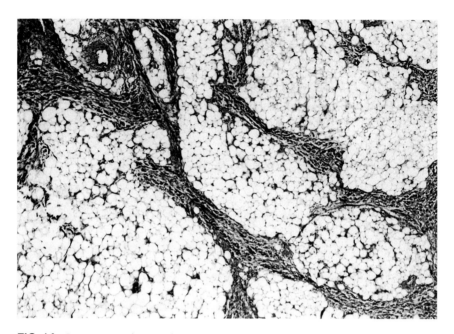

FIG. 14 Low-power microscopic appearance of the tumor from Fig. 13. Note the collagenous septae that traverse the lobules of tumor tissue.

interstitial matrix (Fig. 15). These latter nuclei are often markedly enlarged and characterized by the presence of intense hyperchromasia, coarsely clumped chromatin, and convoluted nuclear membranes. Subtle degrees of hyperchromatism and cytologic atypia are often present in the spindle cells that surround these markedly irregular nuclei. Lipoblasts are neoplastic cells resembling immature adipocyte precursors. These exhibit hyperchromatic atypical nuclei and one or more intracytoplasmic lipid vacuoles that indent the nuclear membrane. Lipoblasts are usually present in lipoma-like liposarcoma, particularly adjacent to the collagenous septae; however, their identification is not a requirement for the diagnosis of well-differentiated liposarcoma (1) (Fig. 16). Mitotic figures are typically few in number in pure well-differentiated liposarcoma. Focal regions of fat necrosis with cystic change and a histiocytic inflammatory reaction are commonly present. Other microscopic findings that may be present include the presence of the atypical stromal cells in the muscular walls of veins in the tumor (55,59) (Fig. 17), stromal myxoid change (66), and focal myoid differentiation (67). The latter finding, though rare, is more commonly present in dedifferentiated tumors (see below).

The second most common histologic variant of well-differentiated liposarcoma is the so-called *sclerosing type* (59). As its name suggests, these tumors are associated with intense collagen production. When exclusively sclerosing, the radiographic and gross appearance of the neoplasm suggests a nonfatty tumor because the adipocytic differentiation present may be extremely scant. Typically, however, there are transitions between lipoma-like and sclerosing regions in a single neoplasm. In sclerosing regions the tumor is dominated by the presence of abundant interstitial collagen that separates the widely spaced tumor cells. Only a minority of the embedded cells exhibit recognizable adipocytic differentiation. The majority appear as nonspecific spindle cells or markedly atypical stromal cells similar to the type present in the lipoma-like variant (Fig. 18). The extracellular collagen that separates the lesional cells will vary from fibrillary to hyalinized in appearance; however, the cellularity remains relatively low. Hypercellularity with fascicular growth suggests dedifferentiation (see below). As with the more common lipoma-like variant, mitotic figures are infrequently found.

The least common histologic subtype of well-differentiated liposarcoma is the *inflammatory type* (68,69). Both lipoma-like and sclerosing well-differentiated liposarcoma may rarely contain focal regions of tumor with extensive lymphoid infiltrates (Fig. 19). These regions may exhibit follicle formation with germinal centers, sheets and clusters of plasma cells, and even admixed neutrophils and eosinophils. The atypical stromal cells that characterize all types of well-differentiated

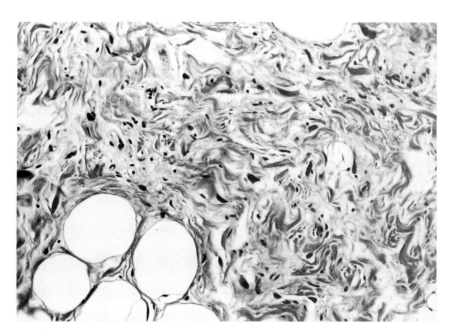

FIG. 15 Interstitial distribution of atypical spindled stromal cells within the collagenous septae. Note how the majority of these cells lack intracytoplasmic lipid.

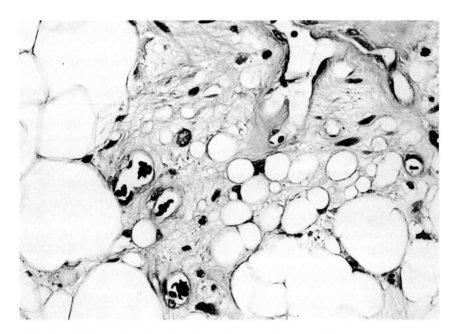

FIG. 16 Multivacuolated lipoblasts in a collagen-rich region of the tumor.

liposarcoma are found admixed with these inflammatory cells, which may cause confusion with malignant lymphoma. However, the lymphoid cells are reaction B and T cells.

None of the histologic variants of low-grade liposarcoma are clinically or prognostically relevant. The importance in their appropriate classification is that they not be confused with nonadipocytic neoplasms or more aggressive neoplasms, such as dedifferentiated liposarcoma.

3. Differential Diagnosis

The term *atypical lipoma* is applied to well-differentiated liposarcomas that occur in the subcutis (59). This is because tumors in this location have an excellent prognosis and an extremely low rate of dedifferentiation (see dedifferentiated liposarcoma below). Historically, the term atypical lipoma was applied to well-differentiated liposarcomas of the deep soft tissues of the extremities; however, the current favored terminology is as stated above (56). Finally, the term "atypical lipomatous tumor" has been suggested as an encompassing term for well-differentiated liposarcomas regardless of their location (57). However, we discourage the use of this term because of its nonspecificity and its application to tumors of different biological potential, including pleomorphic lipoma. *Pleomor-*

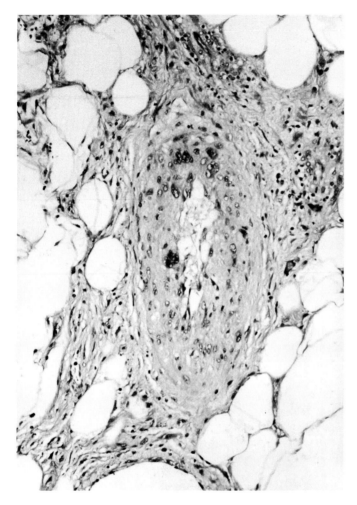

FIG. 17 Markedly atypical stromal cells in the muscular wall of a medium-size artery. This is a typical feature of lipoma-like liposarcoma.

phic lipoma is distinguished from well-differentiated liposarcoma principally by virtue of its location and the presence of spindle cell lipoma-like regions in these tumors (see above). Myxoid change in well-differentiated liposarcoma of the lipoma-like variant may occasionally simulate *myxoid liposarcoma*; however, the latter tumor may be distinguished morphologically and cytogenetically as described below. *Dedifferentiated liposarcoma* is histogenetically related to well-differentiated liposarcoma, as described below. It is distinguished from the well-differentiated tumors by virtue of its greater cellularity, atypia, and mitotic activ-

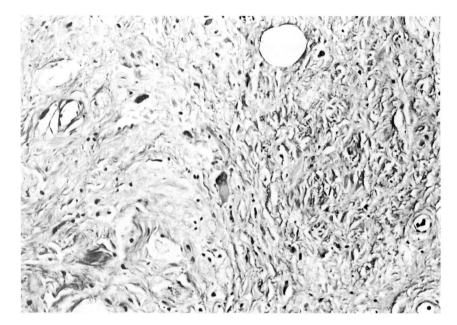

FIG. 18 A densely sclerotic sclerosing well-differentiated liposarcoma. Note the virtual absence of adipocytic differentiation in this field.

ity. Finally, well-differentiated liposarcoma must be distinguished from a number of nonneoplastic *inflammatory conditions* that are characterized by the infiltrates of so-called lipoblast-like histiocytes. This pattern of inflammation is often associated with the injection of lipid material or silicone implants of various types. The multivacuolated cells that form in reaction to the foreign material may closely resemble lipoblasts.

C. Myxoid and Round Cell Liposarcoma

1. General and Clinical Features

Up to half of all liposarcomas are of myxoid/round cell type (M/RC). Although these two lesions have historically been considered to be separate histologic entities, it is now apparent that these two diagnostic terms describe different histologic and clinical ends of a spectrum that is genetically homogeneous (56,57,70–74). Tumors with a pure myxoid liposarcoma morphology tend to demonstrate a better prognosis than those with a round cell appearance (56,57,70,71). In practical terms, pure round cell morphology is extremely uncommon, and most tumors classified as round cell liposarcoma are composed of mixtures of myxoid and

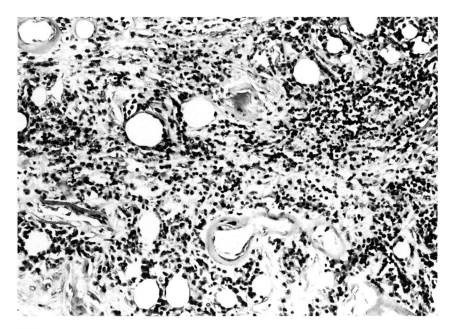

FIG. 19 A region of dense lymphocytic inflammation in a well-differentiated inflammatory liposarcoma. The degree of inflammation may obscure the correct diagnosis.

round cell components. The clinical presentation of patients with M/RC liposarcoma is independent of the proportion of each histologic variant represented. These tumors typically affect adults and are most common in the fifth decade of life (70,71). Rarely, MR/C occurs in children in the second decade of life; however, tumors in children younger than 10 years are exceptionally rare (75). Males are affected more commonly than females (56,57,70,71). The tumors most commonly arise in the extremities. The deep soft tissue of the thigh is the single most common location for these neoplasms (56,57,70,71). Primary tumors also arise in the soft tissue of the arms, trunk, and retroperitoneum. The majority of tumors occur deep to the fascia; however, occasionally tumors present as subcutaneous masses. Patients typically complain of a painless soft-tissue mass. Plain radiographs demonstrate only nonspecific soft-tissue swelling. Mineralization or obvious fat densities are typically not evident. MRI and CT effectively demonstrate these tumors and illustrate their typically lobulated outline and sharp demarcation from adjacent muscles and neurovascular structures (60–64) (Fig. 20). Recognizable fat is often difficult to identify and usually occupies less than 25% of the volume of the tumor (60–64). Up to 50% of tumors will not contain radiographically detectable fat (60–64). These tumors characteristically demonstrate inhomogene-

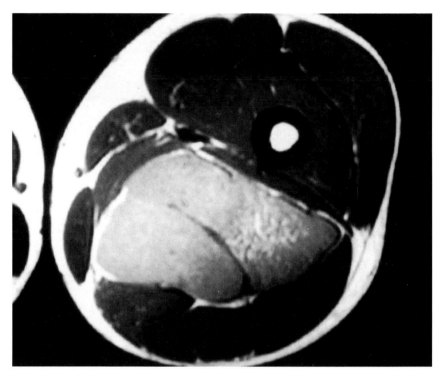

FIG. 20 A magnetic resonance image of a posterior thigh myxoid liposarcoma. Note the well-circumscribed outline of the tumor and the intermediate signal in comparison to the subcutaneous fat. Recognizable fat typically comprises only a minority of these tumors.

ous signal by CT and with T1- and T2-weighted MRI sequences (60–64). M/RC liposarcoma is treated by wide surgical excision with or without radiation therapy. If the pathologic margins are widely free of tumor, then local control is typically achieved. Approximately 30% of patients treated in this manner develop distant metastases (56,57,70,71). Like most other sarcomas, these often involve the lungs; however, M/RC liposarcoma often metastasizes to nonpulmonary sites, including retroperitoneum, soft tissue, and skeleton (76,77). Histologic grading appears to be of value in predicting those patients at risk for metastases. Specifically, as the cellularity of the tumor increases (see below) and the degree of tumor composed of round cell liposarcoma or so-called cellular myxoid liposarcoma increases, then there is an increased risk of metastasis (57,70,71).

Greater than 90% of MR/C liposarcomas demonstrate the chromosomal translocation t(12;16)(q13;p11) that results in the rearrangement of the *CHOP* and *FUS* genes (4,5,72). This translocation appears to be specific for these tumors. A

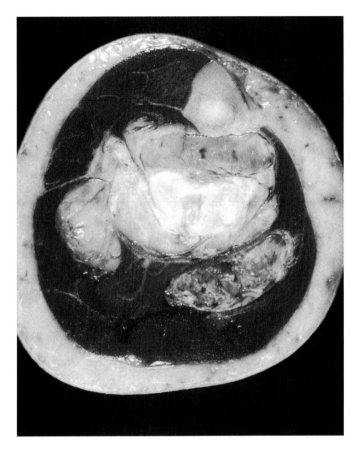

FIG. 21   A large lobulated gelatinous myxoid liposarcoma of the posterior calf. The tumor is relatively well defined; however, the neurovascular structures are extensively involved in this case, explaining the amputation.

minority of MR/C tumors may demonstrate variants of this translocation that typically also involve 12q13 break point (73).

2.   Pathologic Findings

Grossly, M/RC liposarcomas have a wide range in size; however, most measure greater than 10.0 cm (56,57,70,71). They typically demonstrate a lobulated smooth outline and may appear encapsulated. The cut surface of the tumor varies from gelatinous and tan to opaque and yellow (Fig. 21). The latter regions represent the parts of the tumor with the most adipose differentiation. Focal hemorrhage is common; however, necrosis or gross cystic change is unusual. It is usu-

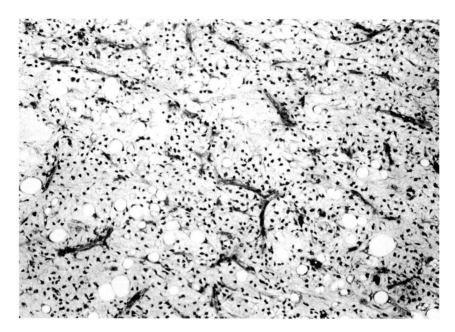

FIG. 22 A moderately cellular myxoid liposarcoma exhibiting the characteristic acute angle branching (plexiform) capillary pattern.

ally not possible to grossly distinguish those parts of the tumor that harbor round cell foci. As stated above, virtually all tumors in the M/RC spectrum contain myxoid regions. Round cell foci are present only in a minority. These two components of the tumor will be described separately. Myxoid liposarcoma is composed of aggregated lobules of low to moderately cellular uniform small spindle and oval tumor cells embedded in a richly myxoid ground substance. The tumor cells are arranged as cords and clusters, although individual cells are usually readily separable from adjacent ones by ground substance. Characteristically, an acute angle (plexiform) branching capillary vasculature is present in the ground substance (Fig. 22). The majority of the tumor cells have scant cytoplasm and uniform dark-staining nuclei. Nucleoli or mitotic figures are typically not prominent. Tumor cells tend to aggregate closer to each other at the periphery of individual tumor lobules and adjacent to blood vessels. Univacuolar and multivacuolar lipoblasts are scattered throughout the tumor (Fig. 23). The number and distribution of these cells varies considerably; however, they are often most prominent at the periphery of the tumor lobules. Histologic variations that may be present include acellular "mucin" pools separated by hypocellular strands of tumor producing a "sieve-like" appearance (56,71) (Fig. 24), a more hyalinized eosinophilic ground sub-

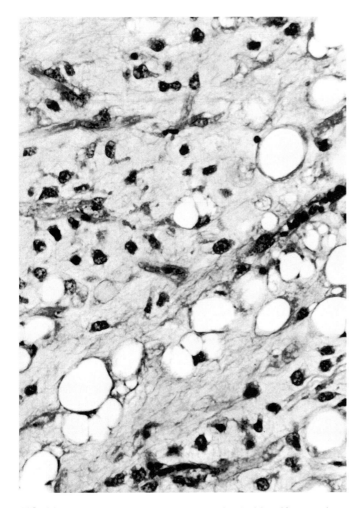

FIG. 23   Multivacuolated tumor cells admixed with uniform oval tumor cells lacking recognizable adipose differentiation.

stance that may resemble osteoid (56), and prominent adipose differentiation that results in larger tumor cell size and a corresponding relative paucity of myxoid matrix and inconspicuous capillary network (56). The latter finding may superficially resemble well-differentiated liposarcoma; however, it is readily distinguished from it by the absence of the atypical stromal cells that are present in the latter tumor, in addition to the presence of more conventional myxoid liposarcoma elsewhere. Round cell liposarcoma is characterized by a relative increase in cellu-

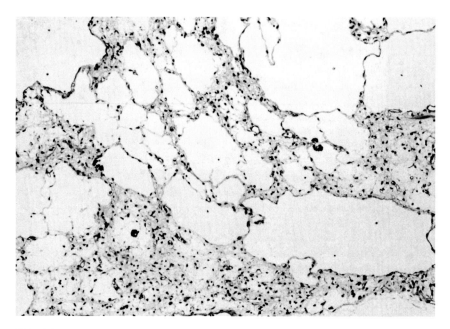

FIG. 24   In this myxoid liposarcoma, there are numerous "stroma empty spaces" produc-ing a sieve-like appearance.

larity of the tumor such that individual tumor cells lie in direct apposition to each other without intervening matrix (57,70,71). When this occurs the capillary vas-culature becomes less distinct and the tumor cell nuclei often are enlarged and ex-hibit pale-staining nuclear chromatin with prominent nucleoli (Fig. 25). Mitotic figures are typically more visible in these round cell regions. One of the difficul-ties in precise classification of M/RC liposarcoma is that there are no universally acceptable criteria for minimal levels of cellularity and nuclear atypia that define round cell foci within these tumors. Although virtually all authors agree with the definition as stated above, the cutoff as to when a cellular myxoid liposarcoma be-comes a round cell liposarcoma is imprecise (57,70,71). This has resulted in the introduction of terms such as "transitional regions" and "cellular mxyoid liposar-coma" to define tumors that demonstrate greater cellularity than the usual myxoid liposarcoma but in which ground substance continues to separate individual tumor cells (57,70,71).

3.   Differential Diagnosis

The differential diagnosis of M/RC liposarcoma is extremely wide because it en-compasses all *myxoid soft-tissue tumors*. This includes myxoid variants of nerve

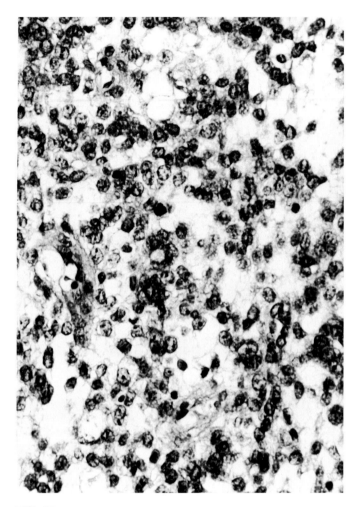

FIG. 25   In round cell liposarcoma, the ratio of cells to extracellular stroma increases dramatically and neighboring tumor cells are directly apposed. Typically, the supporting vasculature becomes indistinct, as in this example.

sheath tumors, smooth and skeletal muscle tumors, fibroblastic tumors, and fibrohistiocytic tumors. These are discussed in detail in the sections devoted to these neoplasms. M/RC liposarcoma is usually readily distinguished from *well-differentiated liposarcoma* by absence of the atypical stromal cells that characterize the latter tumor as well as the considerably lesser degrees of adipose differentiation in MR/C liposarcoma. *Dedifferentiated liposarcoma* (see below) contains histologically high-grade nonlipogenic spindle cell sarcoma as one of its components, a feature that is not present in M/RC liposarcoma. *Pleomorphic liposarcoma* contains numerous markedly atypical lipoblasts and exhibits a high mitotic rate. Neither feature is present in M/RC. Finally, pure round cell liposarcoma regions may simulate *undifferentiated malignant tumors* or even small blue cell tumors such as *Ewing's sarcoma/primitive neuroectodermal tumor.* Correct diagnosis is possible by searching for regions of conventional myxoid liposarcoma which are usually present even in predominantly round cell tumors, or by performing cytogenetic analysis. *Lipoblastoma,* which occurs exclusively in the first decade of life, demonstrates many overlapping histologic features with MR/C liposarcoma (see above); however, it can be distinguished from these tumors by appropriate clinical history, careful histologic evaluation, and the absence of t(12;16). *Spindle cell lipoma* commonly demonstrates myxoid change. The differential diagnosis is discussed above.

D. Dedifferentiated Liposarcoma

1. General and Clinical Features

Dedifferentiated liposarcoma is the term used to describe a spindle cell nonlipogenic sarcoma occurring in association with a well-differentiated low-grade liposarcoma (56). In the majority of cases, the spindle cell sarcoma and low-grade liposarcoma regions are represented in the same "tumor" at the time of diagnosis (56,78). This is termed a "primary dedifferentiated liposarcoma" (78). In a minority of cases, the spindle cell sarcoma is identified at the time of a local recurrence of a previously resected low-grade liposarcoma. This is termed a "secondary dedifferentiated liposarcoma" (78). In the latter situation, the dedifferentiated tumor may contain a mixture of well-differentiated liposarcoma and spindle cell sarcoma or be composed solely of the nonlipogenic component. Dedifferentiated liposarcoma affects the same patient population as differentiated liposarcomas (56,58,59,78–80). There is no sex predilection. In the past, it was suggested that dedifferentiation occurred only in the setting of retroperitoneal low-grade liposarcoma and that therefore this phenomenon was site-dependent; however, more recent experience has shown that well-differentiated liposarcomas in all locations may undergo dedifferentiation (55,56,58,78,79). Currently, the concept that dedifferentiation is time-dependent rather than site-dependent has been proposed (78). It is difficult to precisely determine the risk or incidence of dedifferentiation in well-differentiated liposarcoma. In a study of 92 low-grade liposarcomas of multiple sites with at least 2 years follow-up, the rate of dedifferentiation for tumors located in the retroperitoneum was 17%, the groin 29%, and the deep soft tissues of the extremities 7% (59). Incidence rates of dedifferentiation for retroperitoneal well-differentiated liposarcomas as high as 85% have been reported (80). It is clear that the risk of dedifferentiation is highest for retroperitoneal tumors and lowest for superficial (suprafacial) tumors (i.e., atypical lipomas) (58,59,78–81). The clinical significance of dedifferentiation is that, once it occurs in a well-differentiated liposarcoma, the tumor acquires the capacity for distant metastases and hence should be considered biologically high grade. The metastatic rate for dedifferentiated liposarcoma ranges between 15% and 30% (56,58,78,79). Dedifferentiation also typically portends more aggressive local growth, an increased risk of local recurrence, and higher tumor-related mortality (56,58,78,79).

As stated above, dedifferentiated liposarcoma is cytogenetically related to low-grade liposarcoma, and although these tumors may demonstrate complex karyotypes similar to those found in undifferentiated sarcomas, such as malignant fibrous histiocytoma, the majority of dedifferentiated liposarcomas exhibit the ring chromosomes characteristic of well-differentiated liposarcoma (4,5,65). Imaging of dedifferentiated liposarcomas tends to demonstrate findings similar to those of the well-differentiated tumors; however, as the volume of nonlipogenic sarcoma increases, the resemblance of the tumors to well-differentiated liposarcoma diminishes. As stated above, if a tumor exhibits large amounts of "nonfat" signal material on CT or MRI, the suspicion of dedifferentiation should increase. Dedifferentiated liposarcoma is treated by radical surgical excision, if feasible (57,78). Adjuvant radiation therapy and/or chemotherapy may also be considered as for other high-grade soft-tissue sarcomas (58,78).

2. Pathologic Findings

Like well-differentiated liposarcomas (see above), the dedifferentiated tumors are typically large (greater than 10 cm) and demonstrate multinodular growth (56,58, 78,79). There is no minimal amount of nonlipogenic spindle cell sarcoma that must be present for a tumor to be classified as dedifferentiated. Approximately 90% of these tumors are primary dedifferentiated liposarcomas, and these often show admixtures of pale soft yellow fat representing the well-differentiated liposarcoma component and firmer tan tissue representing the nonlipogenic spindle cell sarcoma (58,78,79) (Fig. 26). Secondary dedifferentiated tumors may consist of only nonlipogenic sarcoma at the time of recurrence or contain an admixture of adipose and nonadipose components (78,79). The adipose components of the dedifferentiated tumors are histologically identical to the usual well-differentiated liposarcoma (see above). In the majority of instances, the spindle cell sarcoma component is undifferentiated and histologically high grade, resembling malignant fibrous histiocytoma (56,58,78,79). These two components may show abrupt interfaces, gradual transitions, or a more diffuse admixture (58,78,79) (Fig. 27). The first of these is the most typical and the last the least common (78). The dedifferentiated component of the tumor characteristically demonstrates marked hypercellularity, nuclear pleomorphism, and a high mitotic rate (Fig. 28). All of the different patterns of malignant fibrous histiocytoma may be found in these re-

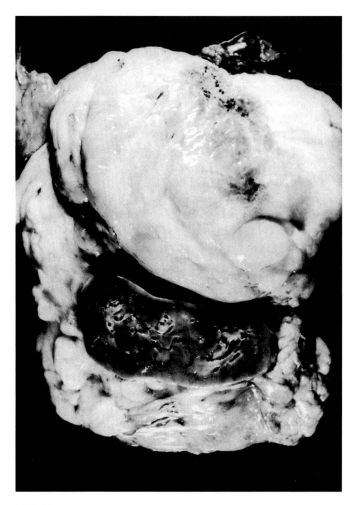

FIG. 26 An enormous retroperitoneal dedifferentiated liposarcoma that completely surrounds the kidney. Most of the tumor has the appearance of a well-differentiated lipoma-like liposarcoma; however, nodules of white tumor adjacent to the convex aspect of the kidney represent the high-grade dedifferentiated component.

gions. Recently, a number of morphologic variations of the dedifferentiated foci of the tumor have been described. It is now clear that in a minority of cases the dedifferentiated regions may appear histologically lower grade, resembling fibromatosis or low-grade fibrosarcoma (78,80). In addition, occasionally the dedifferentiated regions may exhibit a microscopic nodularity resembling meningioma (82,83). Finally, heterologous differentiation toward leiomyosarcoma, rhabdomy-

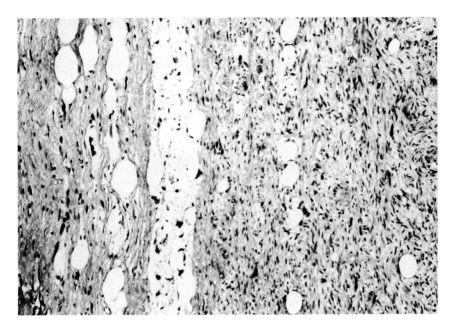

FIG. 27   The hypercellular dedifferentiated component of the tumor is present on the right side of the field. A sclerosing component of low-grade liposarcoma is present on the left of the field.

osarcoma, and/or osteosarcoma rarely occurs (84–86) (Fig. 29). These histologic variants of dedifferentiation do not appear to be prognostically relevant; in particular, the so-called low-grade dedifferentiated foci are associated with the same poor prognosis as the conventional high-grade tumors. Usually, when a dedifferentiated liposarcoma recurs the histologically higher grade component is present; however, on occasion a dedifferentiated tumor recurs as well-differentiated liposarcoma (78,79).

3.   Differential Diagnosis

The differential diagnosis of dedifferentiated liposarcoma *includes well-differentiated liposarcoma* and *spindle cell sarcomas* such as malignant fibrous histiocytoma. By definition, primary dedifferentiated tumors, which account for the majority, contain mixtures of low-grade liposarcoma and nonlipogenic spindle cell sarcoma. Although the latter may be confused with sclerosing regions of well-differentiated liposarcoma, the high-grade dedifferentiated foci demonstrate consistently greater cellularity and mitotic activity. The low-grade dedifferentiated foci characteristically exhibit greater cellularity and a fascicular growth pattern

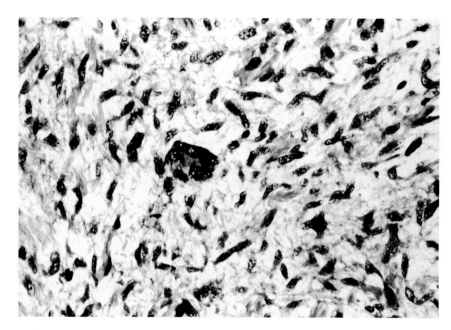

FIG. 28 The dedifferentiated component of the tumor typically resembles high-grade storiform pleomorphic malignant fibrous histiocytoma, as in the current example.

not seen in well-differentiated liposarcoma. Secondary dedifferentiated liposarcoma may be histologically indistinguishable from a variety of spindle cell sarcomas because the well-differentiated liposarcoma component is not consistently present in these tumors. Appropriate classification of these tumors in the absence of the adipose component requires history and clinical information. Dedifferentiated tumors with heterologous differentiation can be distinguished from the various sarcomas they resemble by the presence of the well-differentiated liposarcoma that accompanies the spindle cell components.

E. Pleomorphic Liposarcoma

1.   General and Clinical Features

Pleomorphic liposarcoma represents the rarest subtype of liposarcoma (1,56). Few series of this variant of liposarcoma have been reported, and most published examples have been as small numbers of tumors included within larger series of the more common types of liposarcoma (1,56,87). Despite the relative rarity of these neoplasms, certain consistent features are present (1,56,87,88). They typically occur in adults over the age of 50 years (1,56,88). Males and females are both affected. Pleomorphic liposarcoma in childhood is extremely uncommon (89). Most tumors arise in the deep soft tissues of the thigh, trunk, or retroperitoneum where they produce symptoms related to a painless mass. These tumors are often large and typically exceed 10 cm in maximum size (1,56,87,88). CT and MRI demonstrate a multinodular tumor with inhomogeneous signal characteristics (60–64). Recognizable fat within the tumor is often not present using these imaging modalities, imparting a somewhat nonspecific appearance (60–64). There are no consistent or specific cytogenetic abnormalities within this subgroup of liposarcoma. Pleomorphic liposarcomas are treated in a similar manner to other high-grade soft-tissue sarcomas by wide surgical excision with or without adjuvent radiation therapy. The role of chemotherapy in the management of patients with these tumors is not clear. Pleomorphic liposarcomas have a very high incidence of metastases and tumor-related mortality. In the largest reported series to date, five of eight patients with known follow-up information died of their disease (88). Metastatic and mortality rates of 100% have been described in earlier reports (57).

2. Pathologic Findings

Pleomorphic liposarcomas are large multinodular tumors that typically are yellow to tan on their cut surface. Grossly recognizable fat is usually not present; however,

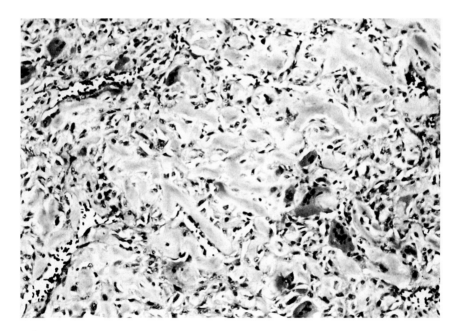

FIG. 29 In this tumor, the dedifferentiated component exhibits heterologous high-grade osteosarcoma. Note the bands of tumor osteoid and the multinucleated osteoclast-like giant cells.

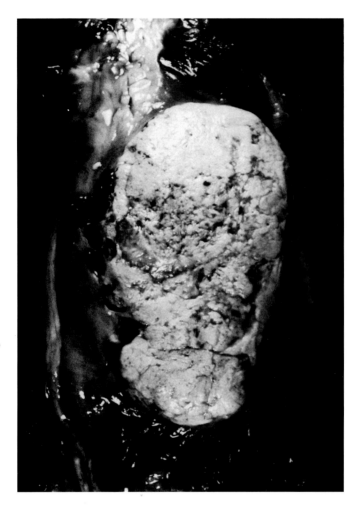

FIG. 30   A large thigh pleomorphic liposarcoma. These tumors are typically pale yellow and soft.

regions of hemorrhage and/or necrosis are common (Fig. 30). There are two microscopic subtypes of pleomorphic liposarcoma (1). In both, clusters of markedly atypical pleomorphic multivacuolated lipoblasts are present. In fact, pleomorphic liposarcoma is the variant of liposarcoma in which the most numerous and atypical lipoblasts are found. These are characterized by intensely hyperchromatic, variably sized nuclei, many with prominent nucleoli. Mitotic figures, including atypical forms, are readily found (88). Lipoblasts with in excess of 20 separate cytoplasmic vacuoles arranged around a central atypical nucleus are not uncommon.

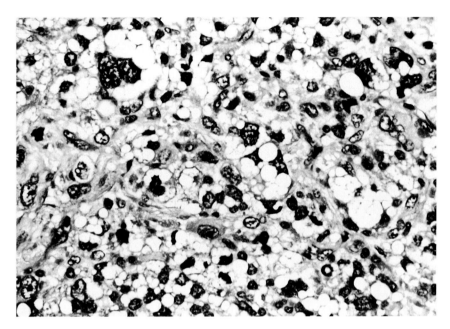

FIG. 31 Multiple bizzare pleomorphic lipoblasts typical of this variant of high-grade liposarcoma.

In the more common variant of pleomorphic liposarcoma these cells compose the majority of the tumor (Fig. 31). In the other histologic variant, clusters of these bizarre lipoblasts are embedded in a background of otherwise undifferentiated pleomorphic spindle cell sarcoma resembling malignant fibrous histiocytoma (1) (Fig. 32). There is usually an abrupt transition between these two microscopically distinct regions. Both variants of pleomorphic liposarcoma may exhibit a well-developed capillary vascular pattern that may appear somewhat "plexiform."

3. Differential Diagnosis

The differential diagnosis of pleomorphic liposarcoma includes *other variants of liposarcoma* and undifferentiated soft-tissue sarcoma, such as *malignant fibrous histiocytoma*. Well-differentiated and M/RC liposarcomas lack the large number of markedly atypical pleomorphic lipoblasts that characterize pleomorphic liposarcoma. Although bizarre enlarged hyperchromatic stromal cells are consistently seen in all of the histologic variants of well-differentiated liposarcoma, the majority of these cells lack fat vacuoles. In addition, these "atypical stromal cells" in well-differentiated liposarcomas are widely dispersed and lack mitotic activity. Myxoid and round cell liposarcoma never demonstrate the range of cytologic

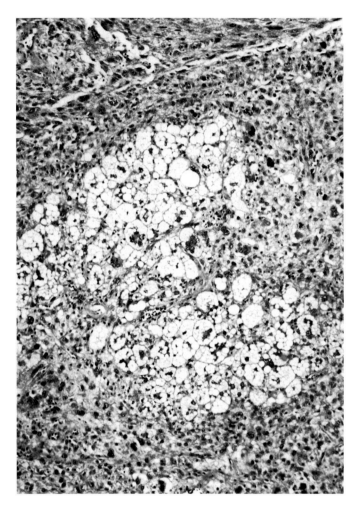

FIG. 32   In this histologic variant, islands of pleomorphic lipoblasts are surrounded by sheets of undifferentiated malignant fibrous histiocytoma–like sarcoma.

atypia that is a consistent hallmark and diagnostic feature of pleomorphic liposarcoma. Pleomorphic liposarcoma may be distinguished from undifferentiated sarcomas such as malignant fibrous histiocytoma by the presence of pleomorphic lipoblasts. Clearly, if the microscopically examined tissue lacks these cells, then appropriate diagnosis is not possible. A minority of myxoid malignant fibrous histiocytomas (high-grade myxofibrosarcomas) contain vacuolated oval pleomorphic tumor cells. These vacuoles, which correspond to markedly dilated rough endoplasmic reticulum, may simulate the lipid vacuoles of pleomorphic liposarcoma.

Careful microscopic examination usually reveals the presence of basophilic flocculent material within the vacuole in contrast to the completely "empty" appearance of a genuine lipid vacuole. The basophilic material is microscopically and ultrastructurally identical to the abundant extracellular matrix found in myxoid malignant fibrous histiocytoma.

REFERENCES

1. Weiss SW. Lipomatous tumors. In: Weiss SW, Brooks, JSJ, eds. Monographs in pathology, Soft tissue tumors. Baltimore: Williams & Wilkins, 1996, pp. 207–239.
2. Iyama K, Ohzono K, Usuku G. Electron microscopical studies on the genesis of white adipocytes: differentiation of immature pericytes into adipocytes in transplanted preadipose tissue. Virchows Arch B 1979; 31:143–155.
3. Cinti S, Cigolini M, Bosello O, Bjorntorp P. A morphological study of the adipocyte precursor. J Submicrosc Cytol 1984; 16:243–251.
4. Fletcher CDM, Akerman M, Dal Cin P, de Wever I, Mandahl N, Mertens F, Mitelman F, Rosai J, Rydholm A, Sciot R, Tallini G, van den Berghe H, van de Ven W, Vanni R, Willen H. Correlation between clinicopathological features and karyotype in lipomatous tumors. A reprot of 178 cases from the chromosomes and morphology (CHAMP) collaborative study group. Am J Pathol 1996; 148:623–630.
5. Rubin BP, Fletcher CDM. The cytogenetics of lipomatous tumours. Histopathology 1997; 30:507–511.
6. Kawashima A, Magid D, Fishman EK, Hruban RH, Ney DR. Parosteal ossifying lipoma: CT and MR findings. J. Comput Assist Tomogr 1993; 17:147–150.
7. Rodriguez-Peralto JL, Lopez-Barea F, Gonzalez-Lopez J, Lamas-Lorenzo M. Case report 821: Parosteal ossifying lipoma of femur. Skeletal Radiol 1994; 23:67–69.
8. Obermann EC, Bele S, Brawanski A, Knuechel R, Hofstaedter F. Ossifying lipoma. Virchows Arch 1999; 434:181–183.
9. Meis JM, Enzinger FM. Myolipoma of soft tissue. Am J Surg Pathol 1991; 15:121–125.
10. Kindblom LG, Angervall L, Stener B, Wickbom I. Intermuscular and intramuscular lipomas and hibernomas. A clinical, roentgenologic, histologic, and prognostic study of 46 cases. Cancer 1974; 33:754–762.
11. Bjerregaard P, Hagen K, Daugaard S, Kofoed H. Intramuscular lipoma of the lower limb. Long-term follow-up after local resection. J Bone Joint Surg Br 1989; 71:812–815.
12. Willen H, Akerman M, Dal Cin P, et al. Comparison of chromosomal patterns with clinical features in 165 lipomas: a report of the CHAMP study group. Cancer Genet Cytogenet 1998; 102:46–49.
13. Sreekantaiah C, Leong SP, Chu D, Sandberg AA. Translocation (X;12)(q27;q14) in a lipoma. Cancer Genet Cytogenet 1990; 49:235–239.
14. Heim S, Mandahl N, Rydholm A, Willen H, Mitelman F. Different karyotypic features characterize different clinico-pathologic subgroups of benign lipogenic tumors. Int J Cancer 1988; 42:863–867.

15. Shanks JA, Paranchych W, Tuba J. Famjilial multiple lipomatosis. Can M A J 1957; 77:881–884.
16. Kurzweg FT, Spender R. Familial multiple lipomatosis. Am J Surg 1951; 82: 762–765.
17. Enzi G. Multiple symmetric lipomatosis: an updated clinical report. Medicine (Baltimore) 1984; 63:56–64.
18. Enzinger FM, Harvey DA. Spindle cell lipoma. Cancer 1975; 36:1852–1859.
19. Angervall L, Dahl I, Kindblom LG, Save S. Spindle cell lipoma. Acta Pathol Microbiol Scand A 1976; 84:477–487.
20. Fanburg-Smith JC, Devaney KO, Miettinen M, Weiss SW. Multiple spindle cell lipomas: a report of 7 familial and 11 nonfamilial cases. Am J Surg Pathol 1998; 22: 40–48.
21. Bolen JW, Thorning D. Spindle-cell lipoma. A clinical, light- and electron-microscopical study. Am J Surg Pathol 1981; 5:435–441.
22. Hawley IC, Krausz T, Evans DJ, Fletcher CD. Spindle cell lipoma—a pseudoangiomatous variant. Histopathology 1994; 24:565–569.
23. Richmond I, Banerjee SS. Spindle cell lipoma—a pseudoangiomatous variant [letter]. Histopathology 1995; 27:201.
24. Templeton SF, Solomon AR Jr. Spindle cell lipoma is strongly CD34 positive. An immunohistochemical study. J Cutan Pathol 1996; 23:546–550.
25. Mandahl N, Mertens F, Willen H, Rydholm A, Brosjo O, Mitelman F. A new cytogenetic subgroup in lipomas: loss of chromosome 16 material in spindle cell and pleomorphic lipomas. J Cancer Res Clin Oncol 1994; 120:707–711.
26. Dal Cin P, Sciot R, Polito P, et al. Lesions of 13q may occur independently of deletion of 16q in spindle cell/pleomorphic lipomas. Histopathology 1997; 31: 222–225.
27. Nielsen GP, O'Connell JX, Rosenberg AE. Intramuscular myxoma: a clinicopathologic study of 51 cases with emphasis on hypercellular and hypervascular variants. Am J Surg Pathol 1998; 22:1222–1227.
28. Beham A, Schmid C, Hodl S, Fletcher CD. Spindle cell and pleomorphic lipoma: an immunohistochemical study and histogenetic analysis. J Pathol 1989; 158: 219–222.
29. Shmookler BM, Enzinger FM. Pleomorphic lipoma: a benign tumor simulating liposarcoma. A clinicopathologic analysis of 48 cases. Cancer 1981; 47:126–133.
30. Azzopardi JG, Iocco J, Salm R. Pleomorphic lipoma: a tumour simulating liposarcoma. Histopathology 1983; 7:511–523.
31. Meis JM, Enzinger FM. Chondroid lipoma. A unique tumor simulating liposarcoma and myxoid chondrosarcoma. Am J Surg Pathol 1993; 17:1103–1112.
32. Chan JK, Lee KC, Saw D. Extraskeletal chondroma with lipoblast-like cells. Hum Pathol 1986; 17:1285–1287.
33. Gomez-Ortega JM, Rodilla IG, Basco Lopez de Lerma JM. Chondroid lipoma. A newly described lesion that may be mistaken for malignancy. Oral Surg Oral Med Oral Pathol Oral Radio Endod 1996; 81:586–589.
34. Nielsen GP, O'Connell JX, Dickersin GR, Rosenberg AE. Chondroid lipoma, a tumor of white fat cells. A brief report of two cases with ultrastructural analysis. Am J Surg Pathol 1995; 19:1272–1276.

35. Logan PM, Janzen DL, O'Connell JX, Munk PL, Connell DG. Chondroid lipoma: MRI appearances with clinical and histologic correlation. Skeletal Radiol 1996; 25:592–595.

36. Kindblom LG, Meis-Kindblom JM. Chondroid lipoma: an ultrastructural and immunohistochemical analysis with further observations regarding its differentiation [see comments]. Hum Pathol 1995; 26:706–715.

37. Gisselsson D, Domanski HA, Hoglund M, et al. Unique cytological features and chromosome aberrations in chondroid lipoma: a case report based on fine-needle aspiration cytology, histopathology, electron microscopy, chromosome banding, and molecular cytogenetics. Am J Surg Pathol 1999; 23:1300–1304.

38. Thomson TA, Horsman D, Bainbridge TC. Cytogenetic and cytologic features of chondroid lipoma of soft tissue. Mod Pathol 1999; 12:88–91.

39. Cina SJ, Radentz SS, Smialek JE. A case of familial angiolipomatosis with Lisch nodules. Arch Pathol Lab Med 1999; 123:946–948.

40. Hunt SJ, Santa Cruz DJ, Barr RJ. Cellular angiolipoma. Am J Surg Pathol 1990; 14:75–81.

41. Sciot R, Akerman M, Dal Cin P, et al. Cytogenetic analysis of subcutaneous angiolipoma: further evidence supporting its difference from ordinary pure lipomas: a report of the CHAMP Study Group. Am J Surg Pathol 1997; 21:441–444.

42. Rigor VU, Goldstone SE, Jones J, Bernstein R, Gold MS, Weiner S. Hibernoma. A case report and discussion of a rare tumor. Cancer 1986; 57:2207–2211.

43. Levine GD. Hibernoma. An electron microscopic study. Hum Pathol 1972; 3:351–359.

44. Gaffney EF, Hargreaves HK, Semple E, Vellios F. Hibernoma: distinctive light and electron microscopic features and relationship to brown adipose tissue. Hum Pathol 1983; 14:677–687.

45. Gisselsson D, Hoglund M, Mertens F, Dal Cin P, Mandahl N. Hibernomas are characterized by homozygous deletions in the multiple endocrine neoplasia type I region. Metaphase fluorescence in situ hybridization reveals complex rearrangements not detected by conventional cytogenetics. Am J Pathol 1999; 155:61–66.

46. Mentzel T, Calonje E, Fletcher CD. Lipoblastoma and lipoblastomatosis: a clinicopathological study of 14 cases. Histopathology 1993; 23:527–533.

47. Collins MH, Chatten J. Lipoblastoma/lipoblastomatosis: a clinicopathologic study of 25 tumors. Am J Surg Pathol 1997; 21:1131–1137.

48. Chung EB, Enzinger FM. Benign lipoblastomatosis. An analysis of 35 cases. Cancer 1973; 32:482–492.

49. Bolen JW, Thorning D. Benign lipoblastoma and myxoid liposarcoma: a comparative light- and electron-microscopic study. Am J Surg Pathol 1980; 4:163–174.

50. Dal Cin P, Sciot R, De Wever I, Van Damme B, Van den Berghe H. New discriminative chromosomal marker in adipose tissue tumors. The chromosome 8q11-q13 region in lipoblastoma. Cancer Genet Cytogenet 1994; 78:232–235.

51. Miller GG, Yanchar NL, Magee JF, Blair GK. Tumor karyotype differentiates lipoblastoma from liposarcoma. J Pediatr Surg 1997; 32:1771–1772.

52. Miller GG, Yanchar NL, Magee JF, Blair GK. Lipoblastoma and liposarcoma in children: an analysis of 9 cases and a review of the literature. Can J Surg 1998; 41:455–458.

53. Fletcher JA, Kozakewich HP, Schoenberg ML, Morton CC. Cytogenetic findings in pediatric adipose tumors: consistent rearrangement of chromosome 8 in lipoblastoma. Genes Chromosomes Cancer 1993; 6:24–29.

54. Weiss SW. Lipomatous tumours. In: Weiss SW, ed. World Health Organization International Histological Classification of Tumors. Histological Typing of Soft Tissue Tumours, 2nd ed. Berlin: Springer-Verlag, 1994, pp. 23–25.

55. Evans HL, Soule EH, Winkleman RK. Atypical lipoma, atypical intramuscular lipoma and well differentiated retroperitoneal liposarcoma. A reappraisal of 30 cases formerly classified as well differentiated liposarcoma. Cancer 1979; 43:574–584.

56. Evans HL. Liposarcoma. A study of 55 cases with a reassesment of its classification. Am J Surg Pathol 1979; 3:507–523.

57. Evans HL. Liposarcomas and atypical lipomatous tumros: a study of 66 cases followed for a minimum of 10 years. Surg Pathol 1988; 1:41–54.

58. Lucas DR, Nascimento AG, Sanjay BKS, Rock MG. Well-differentiated liposarcoma. The Mayo Clinic experience with 58 cases. Am J Clin Pathol 1994; 102: 677–683.

59. Weiss SW, Rao VK. Well-differentiated liposarcoma (atypical lipoma) of deep soft tissue of the extremities, retroperitoneum and micellaneous sites. A follow-up study of 92 cases with analysis of the incidence of "dedifferentiation." Am J Surg Pathol 1992; 16:1051–1058.

60. Jelinek JS, Kransdorf MJ, Shmookler BM, Aboulafia AJ, Malawer MM. Liposarcoma of the extremities: MR and CT findings in the histological subtypes. Radiology 1993; 186:455–459.

61. Kransdorf MJ, Moser RP, Meis JM, Meyer CA. Fat containing soft-tissue masses of the extremities. Radiographics 1991; 11:81–106.

62. London J, Kim EE, Wallace S, Shirkhoda A, Coan J, Evans H. J Comput Assist Tomogr 1989; 13:832–835.

63. Arkun R, Memis A, Akalin T, Ustun EE, Sabah D, Kandiloglu G. Liposarcoma of the soft tissue: MRI findings with pathologic correlation. Skeletal Radiol 1997; 26:167–172.

64. Munk PL, Lee MJ, Janzen DL, Connell DG, Logan PM, Poon PY, Bainbridge TC. Lipoma and liposarcoma: evaluation using CT and MR imaging. AJR Am J Roentgenol 1997; 169:589–594.

65. Rosai J, Akerman M, Dal Cin P, DeWever I, Fletcher CDM, Mandahl N, Mertens F, Mitelman F, Rydholm A, Sciot R, Tallini G, van den Berghe H, van de Ven W, Vanni R, Willen H. Combined morphologic and karyotypic study of 59 atypical lipomatous tumors. Evaluation of their relationship and differential diagnosis with other adipose tissue tumors (a report of the CHAMP study group). Am J Surg Pathol 1996; 20: 1182–1189.

66. Hisaoka M, Morimitsu Y, Hashimoto H, Ishida T, Mukai H, Satoh H, Motoi T, Machinami R. Retroperitoneal liposarcoma with combined well-differentiated and myxoid malignant fibrous histiocytoma-like myxoid areas. Am J Surg Pathol 1999; 23:1480–1492.

67. Evans HL. Smooth muscle in aytpical lipomatous tumors. A report of three cases. Am J Surg Pathol 1990; 14:714–718.

68. Argani P, Facchetti F, Inghirami G, Rosai J. Lymphocyte-rich well-differentiated liposarcoma: report of nine cases. Am J Surg Pathol 1997; 21:884–895.

69. Kraus MD, Guillou L, Fletcher CDM. Well-differentiated inflammatory liposarcoma: An uncommon and easily overlooked variant of a common sarcoma. Am J Surg Pathol 1997; 21:518–527.

70. Smith TA, Easley KA, Goldblum JR. Myxoid/Round cell liposarcoma of the extremeties. A clinicopathologic study of 29 cases with particular attention to extent of round cell liposarcoma. Am J Surg Pathol 1996; 20:171–180.

71. Kilpatrick SE, Doyon J, Choong PFM, Sim FH, Nascimento AG. The clinicopathologic spectrum of myxoid and round cell liposarcoma. A study of 95 cases. Cancer 1996; 77:1450–1458.

72. Tallini G, Akerman M, Dal Cin P, DeWever I, Fletcher CDM, Mandahl N, Mertens F, Mitelman F, Rosai J, Rydholm A, Sciot R, Van Den Berghe H, Van Den Ven W, Vanni R, Willen H. Combined morphologic and karyotypic study of 28 myxoid liposarcomas. Implications for a revised morphologic typing (a report of the CHAMP group). Am J Surg Pathol 1996; 20:1047–1055.

73. Gibas Z, Miettinen M, Limon J, Nedoszytko B, Mrozek K, Roszkiewicz A, Rys J, Niezabitowski A, Debiec-Rychter M. Cytogenetic and immunohistochemical profile of myxoid liposarcoma. Am J Clin Pathol 1995; 103:20–26.

74. Mrozek K, Szumigala J, Brooks JSJ, Crossland DM, Karakousis CP, Bloomfield CD. Round cell liposarcoma with the insertion (12;16)(q13;p11.2p13). Am J Clin Pathol 1997; 108:35–39.

75. La Quaglia MP, Spiro SA, Ghavimi F, Hajdu SI, Meyers P, Exelby PR. Liposarcoma in patients younger than or equal to 22 years of age. Cancer 1997; 72:3114–3119.

76. Cheng EY, Springfield DS, Mankin HJ. Frequent incidence of extrapulmonary sites of intial metastasis in patients with liposarcoma. Cancer 1995; 75:1120–1127.

77. Pearlstone DB, Pisters PWT, Bold RJ, Feig BW, Hunt KK, Yasko AW, Patel S, Pollack A, Benjamin RS, Pollack RE. Patterns of recurrence in extremity liposarcoma. Implications for staging and follow-up. Cancer 1999; 85:85–92.

78. Henricks WH, Chu YC, Goldblum JR, Weiss SW. Dedifferentiated liposarcoma. A clinicopathological analysis of 155 cases with a proposal for an expanded definition of dedifferentiation. Am J Surg Pathol 1997; 21:271–281.

79. McCormick D, Mentzel T, Beham A, Fletcher CDM. Dedifferentiated liposarcoma. Clinicopathologic analysis of 32 cases suggesting a better prognosis subgroup among pleomorphic sarcomas. Am J Surg Pathol 1994; 18:1213–1223.

80. Elgar F, Goldblum JR. Well-differentiated liposarcoma of the retroperitoneum: a clinicopathologic analysis of 20 cases, with particular attention to the extent of low-grade dedifferentiation. Mod Pathol 1997; 10:113–120.

81. Yoshikawa H, Ueda T, Mori S, Araki N, Myoui A, Uchida A, Fukuda H. Dedifferentiated liposarcoma of the subcutis. Am J Surg Pathol 1996; 20:1525–1530.

82. Nascimento AG, Kurtin PJ, Guillou L, Fletcher CDM. Dedifferentiated liposarcoma. Report of nine cases with a peculiar neural-like whorling pattern associated with metaplastic bone formation. Am J Surg Pathol 1998; 22:945–955.

83. Fanburg-Smith JC, Miettinen M. Liposarcoma with meningothelial-like whorls: a study of 17 cases of a distinctive histological pattern associated with dedifferentiated liposarcoma. Histopathology 1998; 33:414–424.

84. Evans HL, Khurana KK, Kemp BL, Ayala AG. Heterologous elements in the dedifferentiated component of dedifferentiated liposarcoma. Am J Surg Pathol 1994; 18:1150–1157.

85. Tallini G, Erlandson RA, Brennan MF, Woodruff JM. Divergent myosarcomatous differentiation in retroperitoneal liposarcoma. Am J Surg Pathol 1993; 17:546–556.
86. Suster S, Wong TY, Moran CA, Sarcomas with combined features of liposarcoma and leiomyosarcoma. Study of two cases of an unusual soft-tissue tumor showing dual lineage differentiation. Am J Surg Pathol 1993; 17:905–911.
87. Golledge J, Fisher C, Rhys-Evans PH. Head and neck liposarcoma. Cancer 1995; 76:1051–1058.
88. Miettinen M, Enzinger FM. Epithelioid variant of pleomorphic liposarcoma: a study of 12 cases of a distinctive variant of high-grade liposarcoma. Mod Pathol 1999; 12:722–728.
89. Pawel BR, de Chadarevian JP, Inniss S, Kalwinski P, Paul SR, Weintraub WH. Mesenteric pleopmorphic liposarcoma in an adolescent. Arch Pathol Lab Med 1997; 121:173–176.

9

Tumors of Peripheral Nerves and the Nerve Sheath

James M. Woodruff
Memorial Sloan-Kettering Cancer Center and
Cornell University Medical College
New York, New York

I. INTRODUCTION

The peripheral nerve (Fig. 1) consists of nerve fibers (axons and encasing Schwann cells) and external to these three sheaths: the endoneurium, containing capillaries, fibroblasts, macrophages and mast cells; the perineurium, consisting of layered highly specialized and unique perineurial cells; and the epineurium, composed of ordinary fibroadipose tissue. Peripheral nerve tumor is here defined as any primary alteration causing a mass in the peripheral nerve, and therefore includes reactive and inflammatory lesions, hyperplasias, hamartomas, choristomas, and neoplasms. The present discussion will be confined to reactive lesions and neoplasms, the two groups of peripheral nerve tumors most often encountered by clinicians.

II. REACTIVE LESIONS

A. Amputation Neuroma (Traumatic Neuroma)

Amputation neuroma, the most common reactive lesion of peripheral nerves, and the prototypic true neuroma, is formed by the disorganized growth of peripheral nerve tissue after nerve disruption. Following partial or complete severance of a peripheral nerve, axons and myelin sheaths distal to the point of injury degenerate

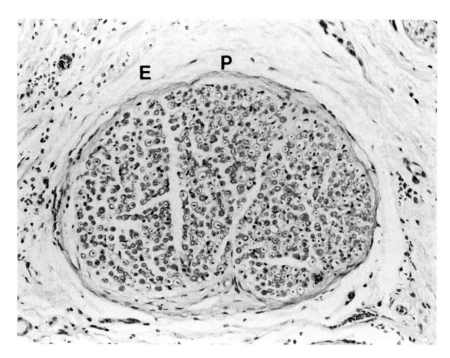

FIG. 1 Peripheral nerve, consisting of a single transected nerve fascicle enclosed by a perineurium (P). The perineurium surrounds a field of nerve fibers: axons are represented by dots, small circles are transected cylinders of Schwann cells encasing axons, and short hyperchromatic specks next to small circles are Schwann cell nuclei. Endoneurium is tissue between and around Schwann cell cylinders, and epineurium (E) is fibrous tissue encasing the perineurium.

(37). Residual Schwann cells lined by basement membrane form tubes that await the extension of regenerating axons emanating from the intact proximal portion of the nerve. If for some reason the proximal and distal portions of the nerve have been widely displaced or the path of regeneration has been blocked, the proliferating proximal nerve elements will not reach the distal nerve tubes and instead will grow in an aimless disorganized manner (47). The resulting disordered growth is referred to as an amputation neuroma. The development of an amputation neuroma takes several weeks, and the clinical finding is a painful nodule at the site of prior trauma or surgery.

Pathologic findings are distinctive. The gross appearance is a bulbous gray–white mass to which macroscopically is attached a segment of peripheral nerve (Fig. 2). Most amputation neuromas are incidental findings and identified only microscopically. Microscopically, the mass consists of a haphazard tangle of peripheral nerve tissue arranged in microfascicles (Fig. 3). Immunostaining for neuro-

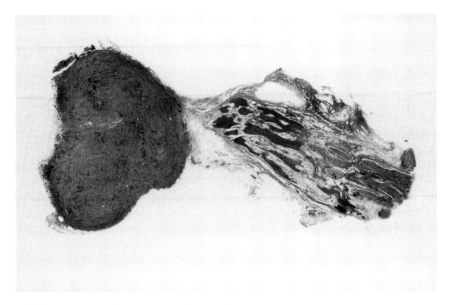

FIG. 2 Macroscopic appearance of amputation neuroma.

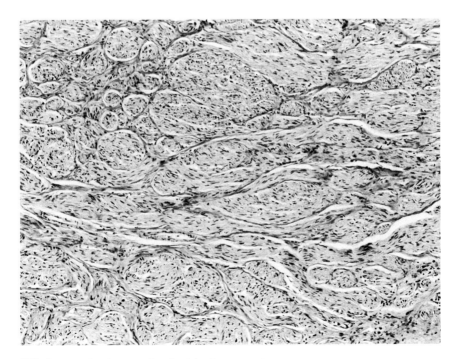

FIG. 3 Tangle of nerve microfascicles in amputation neuroma.

filament and S-100 protein demonstrates normal nerve fibers. Elongated nerve fascicles are closely packed but can be distinguished from one another by a stain for epithelial membrane antigen (EMA). This identifies perineurial tissue outlining each fascicle. Fibrosis is not a prominent component of the lesion.

The differential diagnosis of amputation neuroma includes localized interdigital neuritis (Morton's neuroma), various other true neuromas, schwannoma, and neurofibroma. Localized interdigital neuritis is a primarily fibrosing and degenerative change affecting the endoneurium, perineurium, and epineurium of a nerve. The palisaded encapsulated neuroma differs from amputation neuroma in that it is not subdivided by microfascicles of nerves. Instead, the entire lesion is encased by a perineurium. Schwannomas commonly have Antoni B or loose areas in addition to cellular areas (Antoni A) and, unlike amputation neuroma, usually are devoid of nerve fascicles and encapsulated. Rarely, amputation neuroma may be mistaken for neurofibroma. Neurofibromas, however, are not rich in axons, do not have closely packed layers of nerve microfascicles, and the uncommon plexi-

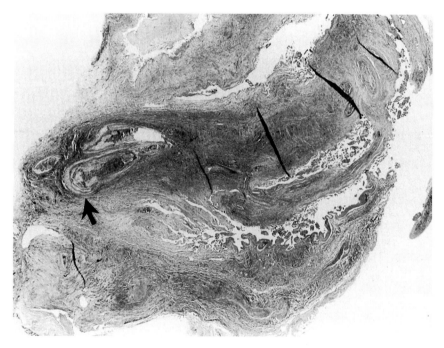

FIG. 4 Localized interdigital neuritis (LIN) with extensive fibrosis in nerve (*arrow*) and in surrounding fibrous tissue. Note papillary hyaline degenerative changes of adjacent intermetatarsal bursa, a finding easily mistaken for a ganglion cyst.

form neurofibroma simulating amputation neuroma will be less cellular and often focally myxoid.

B. Localized Interdigital Neuritis (Morton's Neuroma)

Localized interdigital neuritis (LIN) (47) is a degenerative change of a plantar digital nerve with associated fibrosis and enlargement of affected tissues. The lesion should not be referred to simply as a neuroma. LIN primarily affects women with tight, ill-fitting shoes. The typical clinical presentation is a woman with unilateral burning pain that is localized to the plantar aspect of a foot, sometimes radiates to a toe, and is relieved by resting the foot or removing the shoe. The nerves most often affected are digital nerves of the second and third metatarsophalangeal interspaces. Chronic compression with vascular compromise is thought to be the cause of the disorder.

Grossly, the process presents as a nodule or fusiform soft-tissue enlargement. Microscopically, all nerve sheaths—epineurium, perineurium, and endoneurium—are fibrosed to varying degrees (Fig. 4). Obvious thickening of the perineurium is a key finding (Fig. 5). In addition to endoneurial fibrosis, which

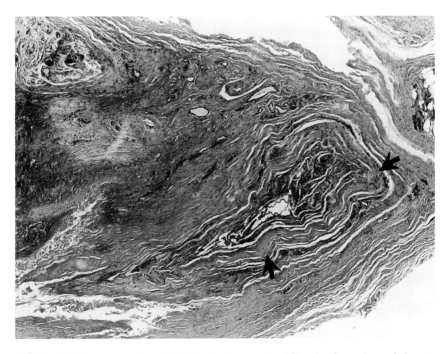

FIG. 5   LIN showing perineurial thickening (*arrows*) and fibrosis of encasing soft tissues.

leads to a decrease in axon number, myxoid changes in the endoneurium may be seen. There may also be evidence of thickened or occluded small digital arteries. In many cases the adjacent intermetatarsal bursa exhibits degenerative changes. Thus, myxoid changes may be seen in both altered nerve bundles and metatarsal-bursa.

As a clinicopathologic entity, LIN is highly specific. However, the lesion is sometimes mistaken for two other disorders. In surgical specimens in which degenerative bursal tissue is conspicuous (Fig. 4), an erroneous interpretation of ganglion cyst may be made. Ganglion cysts do not show degenerative changes of nearby neurovascular tissue, a histologic feature of LIN. The other lesion for which LIN is mistaken is amputation neuroma. Distinction from amputation neuroma is based on the fact that in LIN there is no proliferation of neural tissue. The interdigital neurovascular compartment is enlarged because of fibrosis; the affected nerve is not thickened due to an increase in the number of nerve fascicles. The problem of distinction from an amputation neuroma is compounded by the occasional development of an amputation neuroma at the site of a resected LIN.

III. NEOPLASMS

Primary neoplasms of the peripheral nerve arise from nerve sheaths and have a varied histology, attributed mainly to a remarkably diverse histologic differentiation exhibited by neoplastic Schwann cells. Neoplasia of Schwann cells is thought to be responsible for the vast majority of peripheral nerve sheath neoplasms, with most of the remainder accounted for by the perineurial cell. Peripheral nerve neoplasms are currently classified according to their combined immunohistochemical and ultrastructural features. Schwann cells and perineurial cells are readily distinguishable immunohistochemically: Schwann cells express S-100 protein (51) but not epithelial membrane antigen (3), while perineurial cells have the reverse staining profile (3). Ultrastructurally, neoplastic Schwann cells have convoluted cell processes almost devoid of pinocytotic vesicles and are lined by a continuous basal lamina, whereas the cell processes of neoplastic perineurial cells are very thin, contain numerous pinocytotic vesicles, and are lined by an interrupted basal lamina (14,22).

A. Schwannoma

Schwannomas are neoplasms consisting of differentiated Schwann cells as demonstrated ultrastructurally and immunohistochemically. Four subtypes of schwannoma are recognized (47,53): (a) conventional schwannoma, (b) cellular schwannoma, (c) plexiform schwannoma, and (d) melanotic schwannoma. The first three subtypes are benign, whereas slightly more than 10% of melanotic schwannomas follow a malignant clinical course (47).

1. Conventional Schwannoma

Also referred to as neurilemoma, this is a widely distributed, usually solitary tumor. The peak incidence is the third through sixth decades, and there is no sex prevalence. Multiple or numerous schwannomas are seen in patients with type 2 neurofibromatosis (NF-2) where cranial and spinal nerves, notably the vestibular branch of the eighth cranial nerve, are most often affected (Fig. 6). Multiple schwannomas unassociated with other stigmata of NF-2 characterize a newly de-

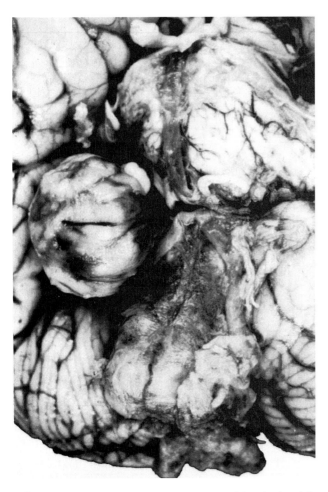

FIG. 6 Eighth cranial nerve schwannoma arising in the right cerebellopontine angle; pons (above), cerebellum (below).

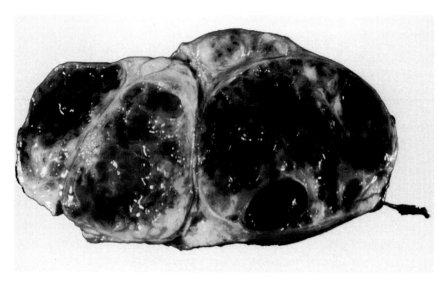

FIG. 7   Encapsulated, cystic, hemorrhagic conventional schwannoma.

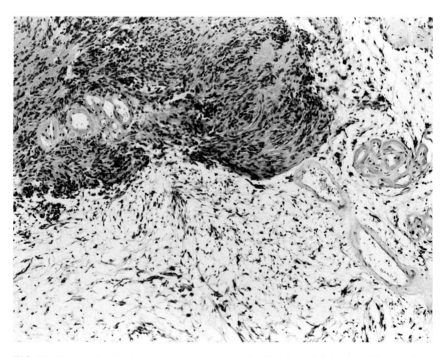

FIG. 8   Conventional schwannomas are characterized by Antoni A (*top*) and B areas (*bottom*). Note hyalinized thick-walled blood vessels.

scribed disorder, referred to as schwannomatosis, in which the schwannomas are usually cutaneous. Affected individuals are thought to have somatic alterations of the *NF2* gene (38).

Grossly, schwannomas are usually globoid, encapsulated tumors that may be attached to a nerve. Gross appearance of the cut surface is quite varied. Often there are cysts and obvious hemorrhage, but a constant finding is some firm, homogeneously tan tissue (Fig. 7). Yellow patches are common. When adjacent to bone, the tumor may cause bone erosion.

Microscopically, characteristic features are a thick fibrous encapsulation, a cellular component designated Antoni A area (Fig. 8) consisting of spindle cells with elongated nuclei, ample eosinophilic cytoplasm, and Verocay bodies [formed by two lines of palisaded nuclei separated by densely eosinophilic tissue (Fig. 9)], a loosely cellular component designated Antoni B area (Fig. 8), and thick-walled hyalinized blood vessels (Fig. 8). Collections of lipid-laden histiocytes may be present in either Antoni A or B areas. The tumor cells are routinely diffusely and strongly reactive for S-100 protein (47). Perivascular hemorrhage is common, and

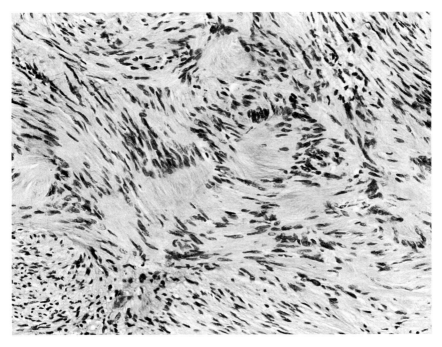

FIG. 9 Verocay bodies. Each Verocay body is outlined by palisaded Schwann cell nuclei and the center of the body is dense and eosinophilic. On ultrastructural study the body center consists of parallel, tightly packed, elongated individual Schwann cell cytoplasmic processes alternating with thick basal lamina (14).

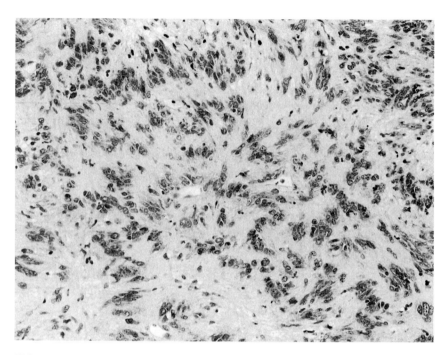

FIG. 10 This palisaded malignant gastrointestinal tumor (GIST) of the rectum masqueraded as a conventional schwannoma.

some cases show extensive fibrosis. Rare examples are predominantly myxoid (47) or have epithelioid tumor cells (47). Hyperchromasia, some pleomorphic nuclei, and mitotic figures may be seen but usually have no bearing on the clinical behavior of this benign tumor (47,53). Glandular metaplasia has been reported, but such schwannomas invariably are cutaneous in location and the "glandular" component is consistent with trapped sweat gland tissue (47,55).

The histology of most conventional schwannomas is highly specific, and confusion with other lesions rarely occurs unless the tumor is mainly myxoid or the cells are predominantly epithelioid (47). If cytologically malignant cells are identified in a schwannoma, the tumor may represent a rare example of a schwannoma with malignant transformation (61). The malignant component in such transformed schwannomas consists of either epithelioid or primitive neuroepithelial cells (47,61). Uncommonly, other soft-tissue tumors, such as smooth muscle and gastrointestinal stromal tumors (GIST), exhibit a striking nuclear palisading (Fig. 10), sometimes leading to misinterpretation for conventional schwannoma.

2. Cellular Schwannoma

Cellular schwannoma is highly cellular, consists mostly of Antoni A tissue, and is devoid of formed Verocay bodies (7,18,36,52,58). Identification of this subtype is important because the tumor is easily mistaken for sarcoma or malignant peripheral nerve sheath tumor (MPNST). Like conventional schwannoma, the tumor is usually solitary, but it has a propensity to involve paravertebral areas of the mediastinum, retroperitoneum, and pelvis where it may cause bone erosion. Cranial nerves are also affected (8) and many cutaneous schwannomas are this subtype. The tumor is more prone to occur in females, and the peak incidence is in the fourth and fifth decades.

Like conventional schwannomas, cellular schwannomas are usually globoid and encapsulated. An attached nerve may be found. Some cases are multinodular. However, they differ on cut section. The cut surface is commonly solid, tan, and firm (Fig. 11). Cysts and large areas of hemorrhage are uncommon, but patches of

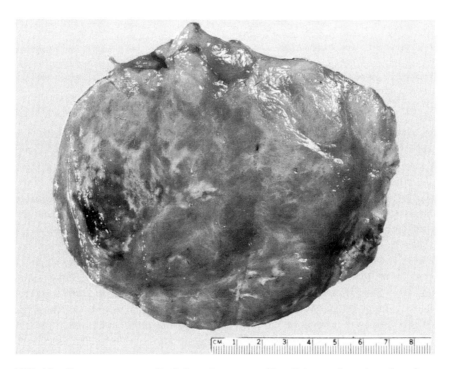

FIG. 11 Gross appearance of cellular schwannoma. Note light streaks and patches: these represent collections of lipid-laden histiocytes, a frequent gross finding common to both conventional and cellular schwannomas. (Reprinted from Ref. 47, p. 139.)

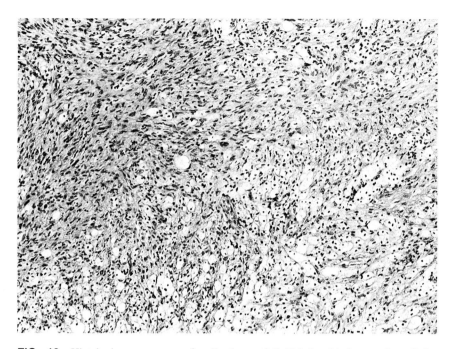

FIG. 12 Histologic appearance of collections of lipid-laden histiocytes in cellular schwannoma.

yellow may be present. Unless the clinician or pathologist are familiar with their appearance, gross distinction from a sarcoma may be difficult.

Microscopic features of the tumor are quite distinctive and include those shared with conventional schwannoma and those relatively specific for cellular schwannoma (53). Shared features are a true capsule, thick-walled hyalinized blood vessels, collections of lipid-laden histiocytes (Fig. 12), and a diffuse, strong immunoreactivity for S-100 protein. Relatively specific histologic features are sheets of quasi-fasciculated spindle cells with abundant eosinophilic cytoplasm (Fig. 13), cellular whorls (Fig. 14), and perivascular and capsular lymphoid cell deposits (Fig. 13). Palisaded nuclei may be present but well-formed Verocay bodies are absent. Worrisome features largely responsible for misinterpretation for a malignant tumor include bone erosion, the presence in large areas of hyperchromatic cells with scattered pleomorphic nuclei (54) (Fig. 15), occasional focal necrosis, and, in over half of cases, mitotic figures. The presence of mitotic figures, regardless the number, in this tumor has no prognostic import.

Histologic distinction from sarcoma and MPNST is important and may be difficult. The two sarcomas for which cellular schwannoma is most often mistaken

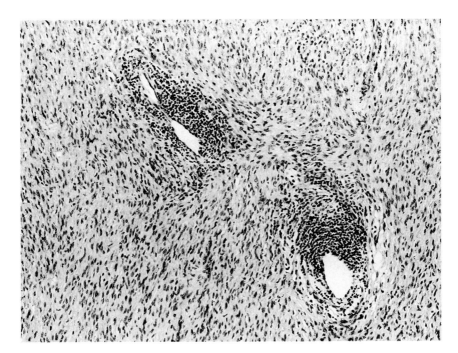

FIG. 13 Sheets of closely arranged spindle tumor cells in cellular schwannoma. Note typical perivascular lymphoid deposits.

are low-grade fibrosarcoma and differentiated leiomyosarcoma. Both sarcomas commonly have a fascicular growth pattern, so histologic distinction rests on identifying features typical of cellular schwannoma (see above). Perivascular and capsular lymphoid deposits are especially helpful in distinguishing a cellular schwannoma from leiomyosarcoma in sites least frequently involved by schwannoma (54). Neither fibrosarcoma nor leiomyosarcoma will be diffusely and strongly reactive for S-100 protein. Also, ultrastructural features of schwannoma cells are unlike those of fibrosarcoma or leiomyosarcoma. More difficult is distinguishing a cellular schwannoma from MPNST (54). Unlike cellular schwannoma, a majority of MPNSTs arise in individuals with NF-1 and are associated with a neurofibroma. MPNSTs have a pseudo-, not a true capsule. The cells of MPNST are more crowded, more diffusely hyperchromatic, and contain a coarser chromatin. Necrosis in MPNST is typically geographic in type. A diffuse strong reactivity for S-100 protein usually supports a diagnosis of schwannoma, but rare low-grade MPNSTs may have the same immunostaining characteristics. Ultrastructural evidence of differentiated Schwann cells favors schwannoma.

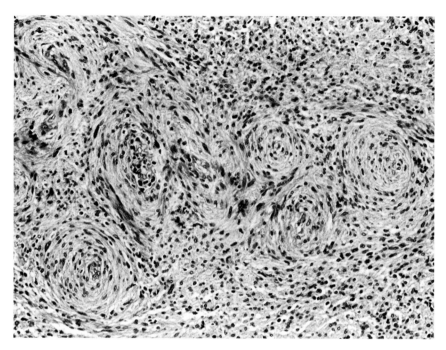

FIG. 14 Type of cellular whorls present in some cellular schwannomas.

3.   Plexiform Schwannoma

Either conventional or cellular schwannoma can present as a multinodular or plexiform tumor (17,24,59). Before 1983, such tumors were probably labeled plexiform neurofibroma, and some hypercellular and mitotically active examples may
have been classified as plexiform neurofibrosarcoma. This variety of schwannoma
is unassociated with neurofibromatosis and most commonly presents as a cutaneous lesion (17,27). Cellular examples arising in soft tissues in the pediatric age
group are controversial. Such tumors were designated by one group of investigators as "plexiform malignant peripheral nerve sheath tumor of infancy and childhood" (39,40). However, although the tumor may recur locally, no example has yet
metastasized, and it is difficult to see how the behavior of this variety of schwannoma differs from that of cellular schwannoma. For these reasons, this author (53)
and others (47) consider the tumor benign, irrespective of the number of mitoses
present.

Plexiform schwannomas are multinodular (Fig. 16). Their cut surface is
solid, infrequently focally cystic, tan, and firm. Microscopically, spindle tumor

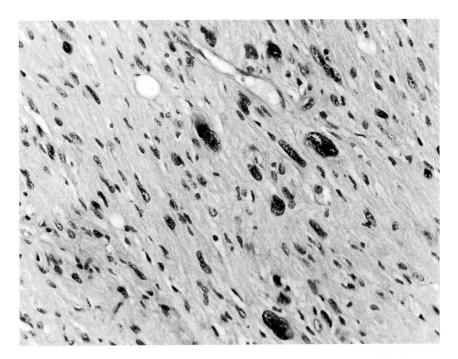

FIG. 15 Worrisome histologic features in some cellular schwannomas include pleomorphic hyperchromatic nuclei.

cells commonly grow in compact sheets or fascicles (Fig. 17). Encapsulation is not the rule. The overall appearance may be that of blunt finger-like processes in the dermis, subcutaneous tissue, or deeper soft tissues. Hyperchromasia may be evident, but there is no associated tumor necrosis. Recurrent tumor can erode adjacent bone (47).

Plexiform schwannomas can be mistaken for plexiform neurofibroma and plexiform palisaded neuroma (PEN), but also for neurotropic melanoma. Invariably, plexiform neurofibromas are far less cellular, the cells are smaller, mucinous matrix is a common finding, and lesional borders are outlined by a rim of eosinophilic fibrous tissue. S-100 protein staining is also less prominent. PEN is more difficult to distinguish but, unlike plexiform schwannoma, it contains numerous axonal processes demonstrable by a neurofilament immunostain (47). Of greatest concern is differentiating plexiform schwannoma from a neurotropic melanoma. Neurotropic melanoma, a tumor favoring the skin and subcutaneous tissue of the head and neck area, grows as distinct fascicles and bundles of cells that involve peripheral nerves (45). Plexiform schwannomas may have a fascicular growth but

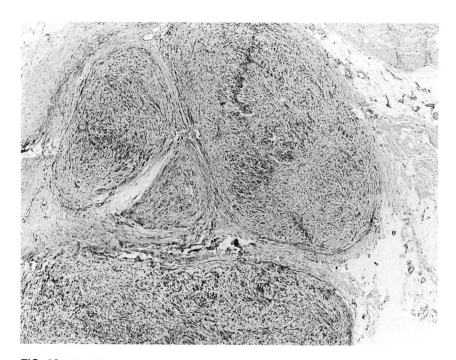

FIG. 16   Plexiform (multinodular) cutaneous schwannoma.

generally do not form cell bundles. Often in neurotropic melanoma there is an overlying lentigo-type in situ melanoma of the skin. Furthermore, the melanoma nuclei are larger, more irregular in shape, and uniformly prominently hyperchromatic. Characteristically, they also elicit a prominent desmoplastic reaction (29).

4.   Melanotic Schwannoma

Melanotic schwannoma, which is a rare form of schwannoma, has many confounding features (47). Like other forms of schwannoma, the tumor has the ultrastructure of differentiated Schwann cells and is S-100 protein–positive. Unlike others, the tumor is melanin-pigmented. There is a predilection for spinal nerves (21,30), but intestines or other viscera may also be affected (6). The peak incidence for this tumor is the fourth decade. Slightly more than 10% of melanotic schwannomas follow a malignant clinical course (6).

Grossly, one most often finds a circumscribed, ovoid, hard tumor enclosed by a thin fibrous membrane rather than by a distinct capsule. The cut surface commonly is pitch black and has the texture of dried tar. Infrequently pigment is noted only on microscopic examination. Bone erosion may be present, especially if the tumor is malignant.

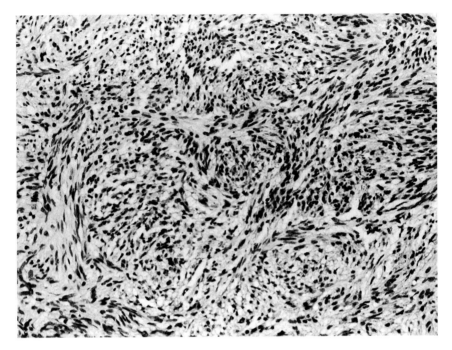

FIG. 17 Short fascicles of closely packed cells in a plexiform schwannoma can be misinterpreted as evidence of early malignant change, especially if mitotic figures are present.

Microscopically, melanotic schwannoma consists of plump spindle and epithelioid cells that are larger than those of conventional schwannoma (Fig. 18). Unlike in other forms of schwannoma, the nuclear membranes of cells in melanotic schwannoma are distinct. The cellular arrangement is fascicles, lobules, and nests. There is abundant cytoplasm that is eosinophilic to amphophilic and has a variable amount of brown–black pigment. The predominant pigment deposition is in melanophages. Often present are some cells with clear cytoplasm. Nuclei are round to ovoid, with delicate chromatin and a small distinct nucleolus. Occasional cells are multinucleated. Nucleoli may be enlarged and eosinophilic, a finding common in clinically malignant examples but not exclusive to such tumors.

The principal distinction is from metastatic melanoma. This is readily done in about 50% of the tumors because of the presence of psammoma bodies, a feature not found in melanomas. Psammomatous melanotic schwannoma (PMS) (6) by itself is fascinating because of an association in about half of cases with Carney's complex (5,6). Findings in this complex include lentiginous pigmentation; blue nevi; myxomas of the heart, skin, or breast; and endocrine overactivity (pigmented nodular adrenocortical disease with Cushing's syndrome; large-cell Ser-

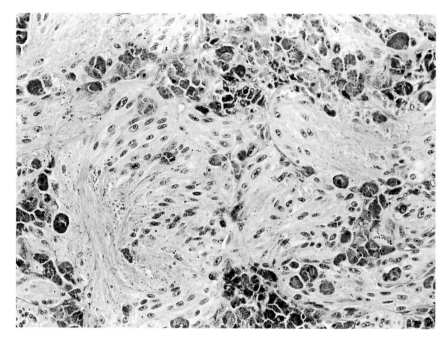

FIG. 18 Grossly black melanotic schwannoma. Nests of plump spindle cells with amphophilic cytoplasm and ovoid partly vesicular nuclei were found in this example that arose from a paraspinal sympathetic ganglion and metastasized to the lung. Note prominent melanin deposits.

toli cell tumor of the testis with sexual precocity; and pituitary adenoma with acromegaly). Distinction of the nonpsammomatous group of melanotic schwannoma and PMS with faint psammoma body formation from melanoma relies on two histologic features generally associated with melanotic schwannoma but not seen with metastatic melanoma. They are a dendritic appearance of the cells, and usually benign or only slightly atypical cytologic features.

B. Neurofibroma

Neurofibroma differs significantly from schwannoma in that its cellular composition is mixed, with the most common cell type being a Schwann cell, both associated and unassociated with axons (47). This is accompanied by the perineurial-like cell, fibroblast, and cells intermediate between these several cell types (47,53). The tumor assumes several gross forms (47,59): (a) localized cutaneous neurofibroma

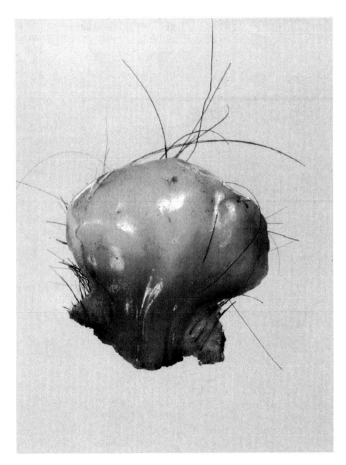

FIG. 19   Polypoid localized cutaneous neurofibroma. Cut surface of tumor is homogeneously tan–gray, noncystic, glistening, and firm to palpation.

(Fig. 19), (b) diffuse cutaneous neurofibroma, (c) localized intraneural neurofibroma (Fig. 20), (d) plexiform neurofibroma, and (e) massive diffuse soft-tissue neurofibroma (Fig. 21). Three of these forms of neurofibroma—localized cutaneous neurofibromas when multiple (Fig. 22), plexiform neurofibroma, and massive soft-tissue neurofibroma, are highly specific for type 1 neurofibromatosis (NF-1). Regardless of the form assumed, the cut surface of neurofibroma is homogeneously tan–gray, glistening, and firm. Microscopy reveals cells with short to slightly elongate gently curved dense nuclei about one third the size of schwannoma nuclei and inconspicuous cell cytoplasm. The cells are widely

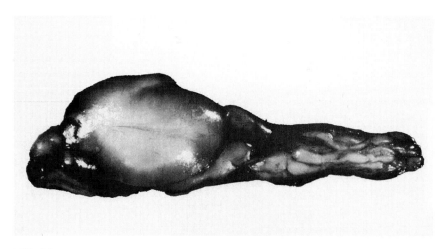

FIG. 20 Fusiform localized intraneural neurofibroma. The tumor is enclosed by a compressed epineurium, not by a true capsule.

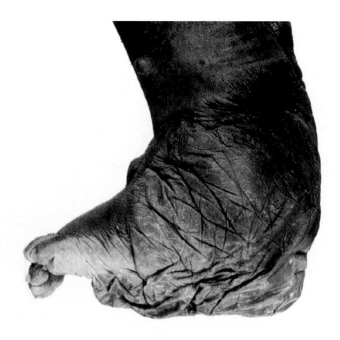

FIG. 21 Massive diffuse soft-tissue neurofibroma of the lower leg and foot of an individual with neurofibromatosis type 1. (Reprinted from Ref. 47.)

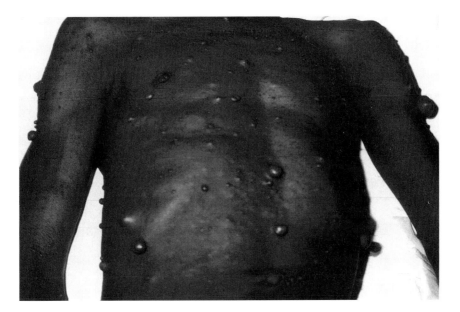

FIG. 22 Myriad cutaneous neurofibromas in a patient with neurofibromatosis type 1.

separated by a mucopolysaccharide matrix and a variable quantity of collagen fibers (Fig. 23).

1. Localized Cutaneous Neurofibroma

The most common form of neurofibroma, this presents as a polypoid or slightly elevated, firm nodule of the skin (Fig. 19). A patch of covering hyperpigmented epidermis (café-au-lait spot) is often present. The patch is tan in light-skinned individuals and dark brown in dark-skinned people. Grossly, a localized cutaneous neurofibroma can be confused with a common nevocytic nevus or neuronevus, but microscopically they are quite different. The widely separate curved nuclei and inapparent cytoplasm of neurofibroma cells contrast with cells of the nevus and neuronevus (47). The latter have ovoid nuclei, conspicuous cytoplasm, and sometimes multinucleated cells. Also, nevus cells are strongly and diffusely S-100 protein–reactive.

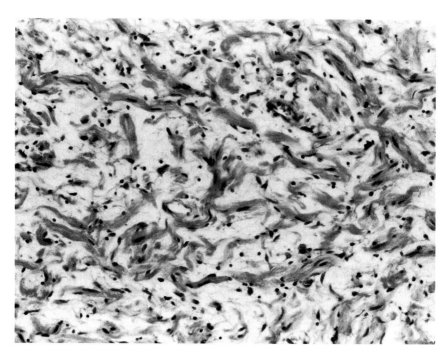

FIG. 23 Histology of neurofibroma with thin, slightly curved tumor nuclei enmeshed in a loose collection of collagen bundles. Presence of abundant collagen in this case is consistent with a localized intraneural neurofibroma. Tumor cell processes are not visible with the light microscope. In localized cutaneous neurofibromas, collagen fibers are generally inconspicuous.

2. Diffuse Cutaneous Neurofibroma

Characterized by a diffuse spread of tumor cells, diffuse cutaneous neurofibroma produces a localized thickening of the skin and subcutaneous tissue. Small nerve twigs in the tumor may be enlarged by neurofibromas. Because of the loose cellular arrangement of the neoplastic cells and their irregular permeation of subcutaneous fat (Fig. 24), the lesion may resemble dermatofibrosarcoma protuberans (DFSP). However, the nuclei of DFSP are larger and its cells are not reactive for S-100 protein. To further complicate the distinction, cells of DFSP commonly diffusely stain for CD34, a staining reaction seen in scattered cells of neurofibromas.

3. Localized Intraneural Neurofibroma

In this common form of the tumor, neurofibromatous growth is confined to a nerve and assumes a generally fusiform shape (47) (Fig. 20). There is remarkable vari-

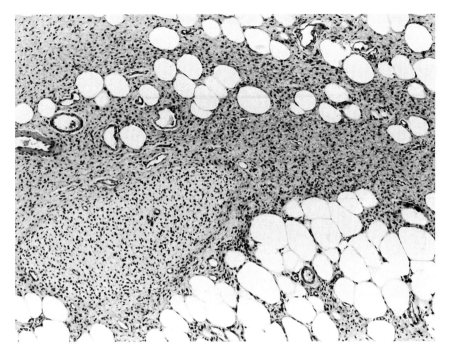

FIG. 24 Diffuse cutaneous neurofibroma with extension into subcutaneous tissue can simulate dermatofibrosarcoma protuberans.

ation in collagen fiber formation (Fig. 23), ranging from a layering of delicate collagen fibers to the presence of numerous thick collagen bundles imparting the appearance of shredded carrots. Residual nerve fibers are identified within the lesion, and tumor margins are sharp, consisting of a slightly thickened eosinophilic epineurium. Grossly and histologically localized intraneural neurofibroma may be confused with ganglioneuroma, especially when a neurofibroma involves a nerve ganglion and thus appears to contain ganglion cells. Ganglioneuromas, however, generally are pancake-shaped rather than fusiform. Microscopically, unlike neurofibroma, the cells of ganglioneuroma are associated with abundant nerve fiber formation, a feature readily apparent in sections stained for neurofilament proteins.

4. Plexiform Neurofibroma

Grossly and microscopically (Fig. 25), one sees multiple nodules involving a nerve plexus or, alternately, involving multiple fascicles of a single large nerve, such as the sciatic nerve. The nodules are smooth-surfaced and may be fusiform or polypoid. Extreme examples produce a tangle of irregularly sized nodules that

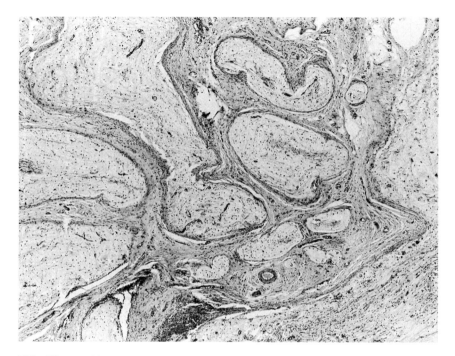

FIG. 25 Plexiform neurofibroma formed by neurofibromatous involvement of many small nerves of a nerve plexus.

can assume the appearance of a bag of worms (47). Because this form of neurofibroma is usually found only in individuals with NF-1, care must be taken in its diagnosis. The principal other plexiform nerve tumor for which plexiform neurofibroma may be mistaken is plexiform schwannoma. Unlike plexiform neurofibroma, plexiform schwannoma contains closely packed cells that are larger, with larger nuclei, and show a strong, diffuse immunoreactivity for S-100 protein. On the other hand, in contrast to plexiform schwannoma, plexiform neurofibroma often contains diffuse or pooled mucin and central linear arrays of residual nerve fibers.

5. Massive Soft-Tissue Neurofibroma

Rarest of the forms of neurofibroma, massive soft-tissue neurofibroma accounts for some of the clinically most dramatic examples. A body part is enlarged and distorted by a soft-tissue overgrowth of neurofibroma (Fig. 21), leading to the formation variously of a bulbous mass, redundant tissue folds, or a cape-like flap (47). Melanotic pigmentation of the overlying skin is common. Histologically,

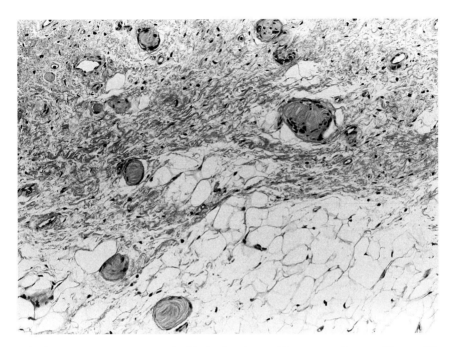

FIG. 26   Wagner-Meissner tactile-like bodies clustered in one area of a neurofibroma diffusely involving soft tissues. Bodies are composed of S-100 protein–reactive neoplastic Schwann cells.

neurofibroma cells diffusely infiltrate soft tissue (Fig. 26), including skeletal muscle. Wagner-Meissner tactile-like bodies (Fig. 26) are often present, whereas dispersed clusters of melanin pigmented cells are less frequently seen (47). This form of neurofibroma almost never undergoes malignant change, but may overly and obscure a solitary intraneural or plexiform neurofibroma of a medium-size or large nerve. The most worrisome histologic feature of the massive neurofibroma itself is the presence of hypercellular foci consisting of sheets of small hyperchromatic nuclei (47). These are readily misconstrued as evidence of malignant transformation. In actuality they represent neurofibroma nuclei that became closely aggregated in the absence of surrounding mucopolysaccharide matrix and collagen fibers.

C. Perineurioma

Perineurioma is a neoplasm composed entirely of cells having the ultrastructural and immunohistochemical features of perineurial cells (EMA-positive and S-100

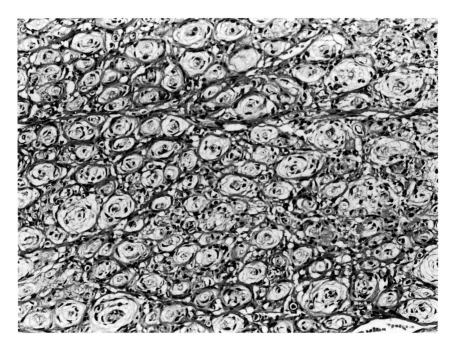

FIG. 27 Intraneural perineurioma. Tumor is characterized by sheets of pseudo-onion bulbs that predominantly stain for EMA.

protein–negative). Two distinctly different tumors fulfill this definition: intraneural perineurioma (Fig. 27) and soft-tissue perineurioma (Fig. 28). Both tumors have a monosomy of chromosome 22 (13,22).

1. Intraneural Perineurioma

Initially thought to be a hyperplasia and designated "localized hypertrophic neuropathy" (43), research demonstrating a chromosome 22 abnormality (13) supported reclassification as a neoplasm. Adolescents and young adults are affected, and about 30 cases have been reported. Almost always solitary, the lesion most commonly involves peripheral nerves of extremities. The leading clinical complaint is muscle weakness; muscle atrophy may or may not be present.

Pathologic findings include localized nerve enlargement, uncommonly extending for a distance of more than 10 cm. Seen histologically in longitudinal sections, the nerve enlargement is due to expansion of individual nerve fascicles by a distinctive cell proliferation. On cross-sections the cell proliferation is found to involve endoneurium and is characterized by concentric layers of perineurial cells

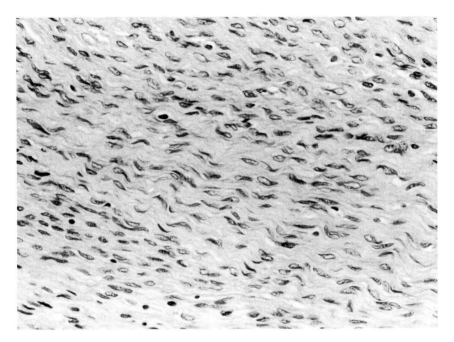

FIG. 28 Soft-tissue perineurioma. Aligned spindle cells with curved or wrinkled nuclei separated by linearly arranged fine collagen fibers is the dominant histologic feature on conventionally stained tissue. An EMA reaction should be positive.

encircling nerve fibers (Schwann cells and encased axons). Individual endoneurial spaces expanded by the proliferating cells have the appearance of pseudo-onion bulbs (Fig. 27). There is a resulting demyelination, and in some lesions demyelination and denervation may be extensive.

The only tumor that grossly and histologically simulates intraneural perineurioma is the localized hypertrophic neuropathy (62), a less common tumor bearing pseudo-onion bulbs similar to those seen in intraneural perineurioma. However, the proliferative cells are reactive for S-100 protein, not for EMA, and on electron microscopy they have the features of Schwann cells. Occasionally, focal areas of a lipofibromatous hamartoma of nerve may contain pseudo-onion bulbs, histologically simulating an intraneural perineurioma (47).

Intraneural perineuriomas are benign tumors and diagnosable on biopsy. Resection of the affected segment of nerve is to be avoided because removal of the tissue will not improve nerve function. Unfortunately, it is during an operation for examination of the affected nerve, when only a frozen section is available for pathologic guidance, that definitive treatment of the lesion may be attempted. For this reason, intraneural perineurioma should be included in the differential diagnosis of any segmentally enlarged nerve found in a young individual.

2.   Soft-Tissue Perineurioma

In contrast to intraneural perineurioma, soft-tissue perineurioma (STP) presents as a solitary soft-tissue tumor, usually unassociated with a nerve. Thus far, two forms have been recognized. First described was the form arising in subcutaneous and deep soft tissues of extremities and trunk (34); one such case has also been reported in the maxillary sinus (22). This form of perineurioma is nonsclerotic and affects mainly individuals of middle age, and preferentially females (4F:1M) (22). A second recently reported form, designated as sclerosing perineurioma, presents mainly in the dermis and subcutaneous tissue of the hands (fingers and palm) of young adult males (14M:5F) (16). Both forms of STP present as painless masses.

Grossly, perineuriomas are circumscribed firm to rubbery masses that on cut section are gray–white. No necrosis is present. Most STPs are relatively small, however, with those arising in sites away from the hand having a larger mean greatest dimension (mean 3.6 cm) than those removed from the fingers and palm (mean 1.5 cm).

The two forms of STP differ histologically. The first form simulates a fibroma (47). There is a generally solid growth of spindle cells arranged in distinct layers separated by collagen fibers (Fig. 28). Tumor cell nuclei vary from elongate with tapered ends to disk-shaped. Emanating from the nuclei are extremely long, thin, curved cell processes. Not uncommonly, areas of the tumor show tumor cells arranged in whorls (47). Nuclear pleomorphism and necrosis are absent, and mitotic figures are exceedingly rare. In contrast, STPs of the hands are sclerosing tumors of the dermis and subcutaneous tissue. Through the tumors wind strands and cords and even whirls of small epithelioid nuclei (47). Sometimes the nuclei are clustered. Because of the sclerosis, long cell processes are often difficult to demonstrate. Necrosis is not evident, and multinucleated cells and mitotic figures are rare.

The differential diagnosis of sclerosing perineurioma includes several lesions (16). Fibroma of tendon sheath, sclerotic fibroma, epithelioid neurofibroma, glomus tumor, tenosynovial giant cell tumor, epithelioid hemangioendothelioma, and benign sclerosed sweat gland tumor are among those tumors causing potential diagnostic problems. However, sclerosing perineurioma does not involve tendons and has a different immunoprofile from the tumors listed. Distinction from a sclerosed sweat gland tumor is especially difficult and may rest on an absence of keratin reactivity and ultrastructural demonstration of long, thin cell processes lined by basal lamina in perineurioma.

Treatment of STP consists of surgical removal. No recurrences have been reported.

D. Granular Cell Tumor

Granular cell tumor (GCT) consists of eosinophilic granular cells that are routinely PAS-positive and reactive for S-100 protein, and regarded as showing schwannian differentiation. An association of small nerves is sometimes seen. The tumor is uncommon and the vast majority of examples are benign.

There is a female predilection and all ages are affected, but the tumor is rare in children, who may have a congenital gingival granular cell tumor that histologically closely simulates GCT (49). The single most common site of origin of GCT is the tongue. Other common sites are skin and subcutaneous tissue of the head, trunk, breast, and extremities. Visceral examples are uncommon, although the larynx accounts for about 7% of cases (44).

Gross findings generally are a solitary nodule that in benign examples is usually not larger than 3 cm and in malignant cases is rarely smaller than 4 cm (47). The tumors may appear either circumscribed or infiltrative, but are routinely gray–white to yellow and firm to hard on sectioning (47). Malignant GCTs sometimes exhibit gross necrosis. Histologically, the cells grow in sheets, nests, and ribbons (32). One finds polyhedral and sometimes spindle cells with distinct granularity and cell membranes (Fig. 29). Cytoplasmic eosinophilic globules are common.

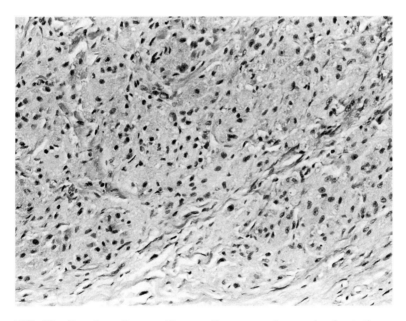

FIG. 29 Granular cell tumor. Tumor cells are coarsely granular due to the presence of large lysosomes. Presence of eosinophilic globules formed by large aggregates of lysosomes is a helpful histologic clue to the diagnosis.

Cytoplasmic granularity and eosinophilic globules, as well as rarer eosinophilic "angulate bodies," are histologic representations of large numbers of pleomorphic secondary lysosomes evident ultrastructurally. As a consequence, the cytoplasm avidly stains for PAS and KP-1 (CD68). Nuclei are commonly small, bland, or hyperchromatic. Frequently, especially with squamous mucosa and cutaneous lesions, the tumor elicits a pseudoepitheliomatous hyperplasia of the overlying epithelium. Histologically benign GCTs have bland cells and rarely contain mitotic figures. In contrast, GCTs deemed histologically malignant are reported to show at least three of the following: marked cellularity, pleomorphism, a high nuclear-to-cytoplasmic ratio, nucleolar prominence, readily identified mitotic figures, prominent tumor cell spindling, and foci of necrosis (15). The two sarcomas with which malignant GCT are most often confused histologically are granular cell leiomyosarcoma (distinguished by staining for muscle markers) and alveolar soft-part sarcoma (nonreactive for S-100 protein).

Distinction of benign from malignant GCT rests on histologic appearance or clinical behavior. Malignant GCTs are those that cause death by locally aggressive growth or that metastasize. Leading sites of metastases are lymph node and lung. Unfortunately, because the vast majority of clinically malignant GCTs are histologically benign, the predictive value of histologic features is low. This bears on treatment, which in all cases should be surgical excision with negative margins. Local recurrence after incomplete excision is common (1). If histologically malignant, the tumor should be treated by wide en bloc resection. More than 50% of individuals with clinically malignant GCTs have a fatal outcome (47).

E. Nerve Sheath Myxoma and Neurothekeoma

These tumors are in the first instance primarily a cutaneous tumor and in the second instance exclusively so. They are grouped together because of histologic similarities and an early assumption—no longer widely held (47)—that they are forms of the same lesion. Nerve sheath myxoma affects female adults preferentially (2F:1M), with the hand, followed by back, arm, and face/neck, the leading sites of involvement. Neurothekeomas show the same gender preference, but affected individuals are younger (children and young adults) and the leading sites are face, shoulder, and arm.

Grossly, both lesions are solitary, well-circumscribed, firm, and variously myxoid. Rarely do they exceed 3 cm in size. Histology varies and is the reason many regard the tumors as unrelated. The tumors are typically multilobular and the constituent cells either epithelioid or spindled, or both. However, nerve sheath myxoma generally is more sparsely cellular and extensively myxoid (Fig. 30), the cells more often spindled and stellate-shaped (Fig. 31). Furthermore, most nerve sheath myxoma cells are immunoreactive for S-100 protein, and peripherally located cells are expressive of EMA (47). Neurothekeoma is generally more

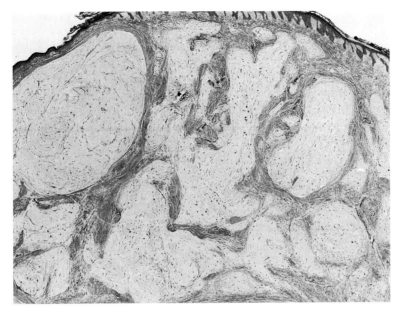

FIG. 30 Compartmentalized and lobulated cutaneous spindle cell myxoid tumor designated nerve sheath myxoma. Cells in rim of lobules may be EMA-positive. Cells in myxoid stroma, on the other hand, routinely stain for S-100 protein.

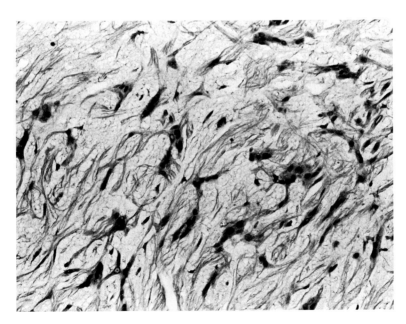

FIG. 31 Spindle cells in nerve sheath myxoma are commonly both multinucleate and stellate, features quite different from conventional schwannoma.

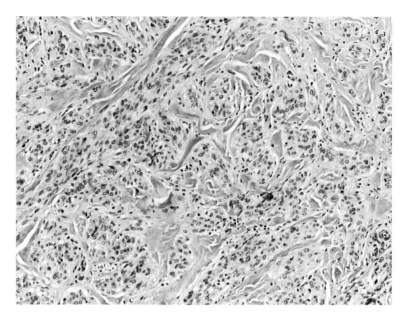

FIG. 32 Neurothekeoma, a dermal tumor characterized by irregular nests of epithelioid cells with faintly eosinophilic cytoplasm, enclosed by fibrous bands. Tumor cells are variously mono- and multinucleated and are nonreactive for S-100 protein.

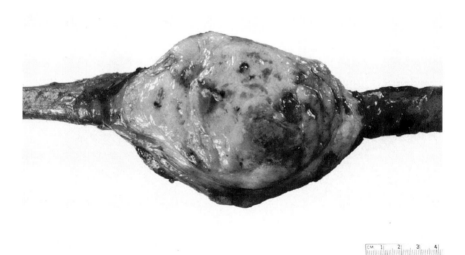

FIG. 33 Malignant peripheral nerve sheath tumor (MPNST) arising from the sciatic nerve on cut section is cream–tan, focally necrotic (*right*), and hard. Tumor invades skeletal muscle, forming a pseudocapsule.

cellular than nerve sheath myxoma and commonly is composed exclusively of epithelioid cells (Fig. 32). These are often multinucleated and consistently nonreactive for S-100 protein (47). Electron microscopy supports a Schwann cell differentiation for nerve sheath myxoma but not for neurothekeoma (47).

Both tumors are benign and are usually treated by surgical excision. Nerve sheath myxoma may be misinterpreted histologically for a low-grade myxofibrosarcoma, a misinterpretation resolved by an immunostain for S-100 protein. Cellular forms of neurothekeoma are easily confused with Spitz nevus.

F. Malignant Peripheral Nerve Sheath Tumor

Malignant peripheral nerve sheath tumor (MPNST) designates a malignant tumor previously referred to as malignant schwannoma or neurofibrosarcoma. Criteria that must be satisfied before a diagnosis is made is that the tumor is histologically malignant and is identified arising (a) from a peripheral nerve (Fig. 33); (b) from a neurofibroma (Figs. 34–36), schwannoma (61), ganglioneuroma Fig. 37)/ganglioneuroblastoma (46), or pheochromocytoma (41,42); (c) in a patient with NF-1 (23,57) and exhibiting the same histologic features as MPNSTs found originating

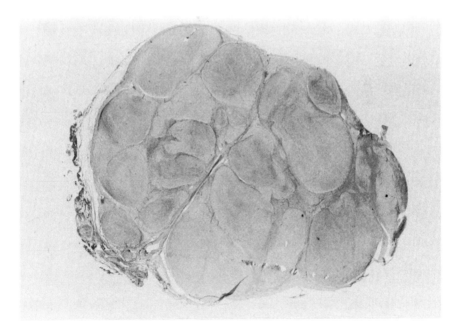

FIG. 34 MPNST arising from a plexiform neurofibroma. All fascicles in the cross-section of this markedly enlarged nerve are affected by tumor.

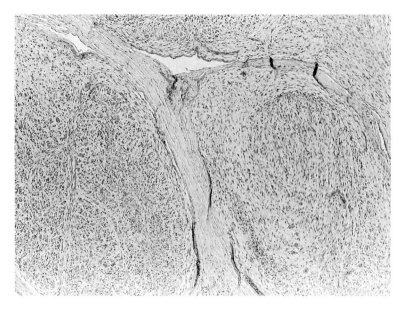

FIG. 35 Higher magnification of tumor in Fig. 34 showing malignant spindle cells replacing neurofibroma cells.

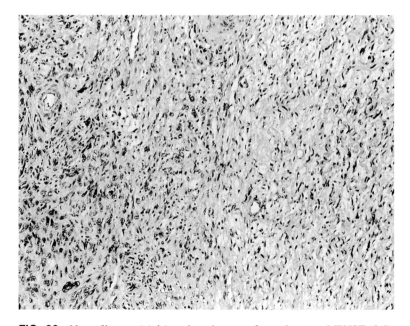

FIG. 36 Neurofibroma (*right*) undergoing transformation to a MPNST (*left*).

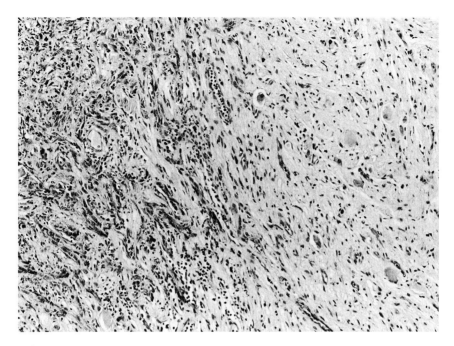

FIG. 37 MPNST arising from a ganglioneuroma. MPNST (*left*) arose by malignant transformation of neoplastic Schwann cells present in ganglioneuroma (*right*).

from a peripheral nerve; and (d) in a patient without NF-1 but having the same histologic features as that in item c as well as demonstrating immunoreactivity for S-100 protein. In 50–70% of cases, S-100 protein reactivity is found in scattered tumor cells (47,51). If dealing with a strongly and diffusely S-100 protein–reactive histologically malignant spindle or epithelioid cell tumor, melanoma rather than MPNST should be suspected.

Most MPNSTs present in persons between 20 and 50 years of age, and 50–60% of cases are NF-1-associated (47). There is a slight female predominance. Among individuals afflicted with NF-1 the incidence of MPNST is about 2% (48). Second in frequency are MPNSTs arising de novo from a peripheral nerve. About 11% are thought to be radiation-induced (10,20). The most common sites of origin are the buttock and thigh (26), brachial plexus, and paraspinal nerves (31). The sciatic is the most frequently affected nerve.

Gross findings are a solitary fusiform or globoid soft-tissue mass, estimated to arise from a neurofibroma in about 70% of cases (47), or from an otherwise unremarkable nerve (Fig. 33). Only rarely does a patient present with more than one MPNST (31). Surgeons dealing with possible MPNSTs should be aware that most

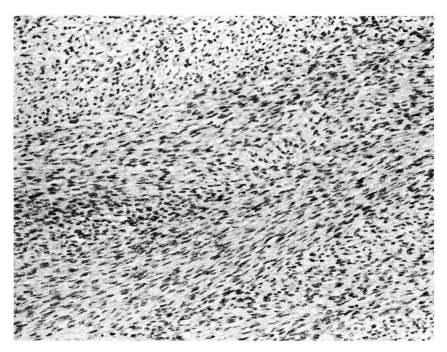

FIG. 38 Typical appearance of conventional fibrosarcoma-like fasciculated spindle cell MPNST.

extremity examples are aligned along the long axis of a limb. Excisions are tailored to this fact. Furthermore, MPNSTs invade surrounding soft tissue, forming pseudocapsules composed of a mixture of malignant cells and benign soft tissue, and on occasion measuring several centimeters thick. A frozen section from such an area may fail to confirm the presence of malignant tumor unless the biopsy penetrates the full thickness of the pseudocapsule (26). For this reason, resection with anticipated negative microscopic margins necessitates a wide en bloc resection outside the pseudocapsule, if surgically possible. On cut section MPNSTs are typically tan–creamy in color, hard, and partly to extensively necrotic.

Histologic findings vary. All but about 15% of MPNSTs consist of a fasciculated spindle cell tumor resembling a classical fibrosarcoma (Fig. 38) or, less frequently, one showing extensive fibrosis (47). Most of the tumors are histologically high grade, usually having a mitotic index of four or more mitoses per 10 high-power fields and commonly displaying geographic necrosis (26). A minority, usually those with extensive fibrosis, are low-grade lesions. Such conventional forms of MPNST must be distinguished from fibrosarcoma (S-100 protein–negative) and synovial sarcoma (usually keratin- or EMA-positive). Distinction from synovial sarcoma is further complicated by the recent report of some spindle cell MPNSTs immunoreactive for EMA and thought to show perineurial cell differentiation (25). In such a situation, distinction from synovial sarcoma may necessitate cytogenetic evaluation for the presence of an x/18 chromosomal translocation (50) or a molecular genetic study to identify the SYT-SSX fusion transcript of that tumor (19). This can be performed by reverse transcriptase– polymerase chain reaction assay on paraffin-embedded material (2). MPNSTs, in contrast to synovial sarcomas, do not show specific chromosomal transloca- tions (28,56).

The remaining 15% of MPNSTs exhibit unusual histologic features. These include MPNSTs composed predominantly of epithelioid cells (epithelioid MPNST) (Fig. 39) (9,33,35), but more often a divergent differentiation (11) such as rhabdomyosarcoma (57,60) and epithelial glands (55).

MPNSTs have a poor prognosis, with about 85% being histologically high- grade tumors and more than half of patients developing distant metastasis, com- monly to the lung. The overall 5- and 10-year survival rates are 34–39% and 23%, respectively (12,26). Survival is even worse for MPNSTs showing rhabdomyosar-

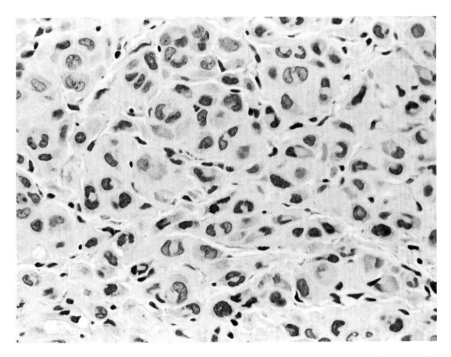

FIG. 39 Epithelioid MPNSTs such as seen here from the forearm of a child commonly arise de novo from nerve and are not associated with neurofibromatosis.

comatous (4) or angiosarcomatous differentiation (47). Treatment is the same as for a high-grade sarcoma, i.e., a wide en bloc surgical resection with adjuvant radiation or chemotherapy.

REFERENCES

1. Alessi DM, Zimmerman MC. Granular cell tumors of the head and neck. Laryngoscope 98:810–814, 1988.
2. Argani P, Zakowski MK, Klimstra DS, Rosai J, Ladanyi M. Detection of the SYT-SSX chimeric RNA of synovial sarcoma in paraffin-embedded tissue and its application in problematic cases. Mod Pathol 11:65–71, 1998.
3. Ariza A, Bilbao JM, Rosai J. Immunohistochemical detection of epithelial membrane antigen in normal perineurial cells and perineurioma. Am J Surg Pathol 12:678–683, 1988.
4. Brooks JJ, Freeman M, Enterline HT. Malignant Triton tumors. Natural history and immunohistochemistry of nine new cases with literature review. Cancer 55:2543–2549, 1985.
5. Carney JA, Gordon H, Carpenter PC, Shenoy V, Go VLW. The complex of myxomas, spotty pigmentation, and endocrine overactivity. Medicine 64:270–283, 1985.
6. Carney JA. Psammomatous melanotic schwannoma. A distinctive, heritable tumor with special associations, including cardiac myxoma and the Cushing's syndrome. Am J Surg Pathol 14:206–222, 1990.
7. Casadei GP, Scheithauer BW, Hirose T, Manfrini M, Van Houton C, Wood MB. Cellular schwannoma: a clinicopathologic, DNA flow cytometric and proliferation marker study of 71 cases. Cancer 75:1109–1119, 1990.
8. Deruaz JP, Janzer RC, Costa J. Cellular schwannoma of the intracranial and intraspinal compartment: morphological and immunological characteristics compared with classical benign schwannomas. J Neuropathol Exp Neurol 52:114–118, 1993.
9. Dicarlo EF, Woodruff JM, Bansal M, Erlandson RA. The purely epithelioid malignant peripheral nerve sheath tumor. Am J Surg Pathol 10:478–490, 1986.
10. Ducatman BS, Scheithauer BW. Post-irradiation neurofibrosarcoma. Cancer 51:1028–1033, 1983.
11. Ducatman BS, Scheithauer BW. Malignant peripheral nerve sheath tumors with divergent differentiation. Cancer 54:1049–1057, 1984.
12. Ducatman BS, Scheithauer BW, Piepgras DG, Reiman HM, Ilstrup DM. Malignant peripheral nerve sheath tumors. A clinicopathologic study of 120 cases. Cancer 57:2006–2021, 1986.
13. Emory TS, Sheithcauer BW, Hirose T, Wood M, Onofrio BM, Jenkins RB. Intraneural perineurioma: a clonal neoplasm associated with abnormalities of chromosome 22. Am J Clin Pathol 103:696–704, 1995.
14. Erlandson RA, Woodruff JM. Peripheral nerve sheath tumors: an electron microscopic study of 43 cases. Cancer 49:273–287, 1982.

15. Fanburg-Smith JC, Meis-Kindblom JM, Fante R, Kindblom LG. Malignant granular cell tumor of soft tissue. Diagnostic criteria and clinicopathologic correlation. Am J Surg Pathol 22:779–794, 1998.

16. Fetsch JF, Miettinen M. Sclerosing perineurioma. A clinicopathologic study of 19 cases of a distinctive soft tissue lesion with a predilection for the fingers and palms of young adults. Am J Surg Pathol 21:1433–1442, 1997.

17. Fletcher CDM, Davies SE. Benign plexiform (multinodular) schwannoma: a rare tumor unassociated with neurofibromatosis. Histopathology 10:971–980, 1986.

18. Fletcher CDM, Davies SE, McKee PH. Cellular schwannoma: a distinct pseudocarsomatous entity. Histopathology 11:21–35, 1987.

19. Fligman I, Lonardo F, Suresh CJ, Gerald WL, Woodruff JM, Ladanyi M. Molecular diagnosis of synovial sarcoma and characterization of a variant of SYT-SSX2 fusion transcript. Am J Pathol 147:1592–1599, 1995.

20. Foley KM, Woodruff JM, Ellis FT, Posner JB. Radiation-induced malignant and atypical PNST. Ann Neurol 7:311–318, 1980.

21. Font RL, Truong LD. Melanotic schwannoma of soft tissues. Electron-microscopic observations and review of the literature. Am J Surg Pathol 8:129–138, 1984.

22. Giannini C, Scheithauer BW, Jenkins RB, Erlandson RA, Perry A, Borell TJ, Hoda RS, Woodruff JM. Soft tissue perineurioma: evidence for an abnormality of chromosome 22, criteria for diagnosis, and review of the literature. Am J Surg Pathol 21:164–173, 1997.

23. Guccion JG, Enzinger FM. Malignant schwannoma associated with von Recklinghausen's neurofibromatosis. Virchows Arch A 383:43–57, 1979.

24. Harkin JC, Arrington JH, Reed RJ. Benign plexiform schwannoma. A lesion distinct from plexiform neurofibroma [Abstract]. J Neuropathol Exp Neurol 37:622, 1978.

25. Hirose T, Scheithauer BW, Sano T. Perineurial malignant peripheral nerve sheath tumor (MPNST): a clinicopathologic, immunohistochemical, and ultrastructural study of seven cases. Am J Surg Pathol 22:1368–1373, 1998.

26. Hruban RH, Shiu MH, Senie RT, Woodruff JM. Malignant peripheral nerve sheath tumors of the buttock and lower extremity: a study of 43 cases. Cancer 66:1253–1265, 1990.

27. Iwashita T, Enjoji M. Plexiform neurilemoma: a clinicopathological and immunohistochemical analysis of 23 tumors from 20 patients. Virchows Arch A 411:305–309, 1987.

28. Jhanwar SC, Chen Q, Li EP, Brennan MF, Woodruff JM. Cytogenetic analysis of soft tissue sarcomas: recurrent chromosomal abnormalities in malignant peripheral nerve sheath tumors (MPNST). Cancer Cytogenet 78:138–144, 1994.

29. Jain S, Allen PW. Desmoplastic malignant melanoma and its variants: a study of 45 cases. Am J Surg Pathol 13:358–373, 1989.

30. Killeen RM, Davy CL, Bauserman SC. Melanotic schwannoma. Cancer 62:174–183, 1988.

31. Kourea P, Bilsky MH, Leung DH, Lewis JJ, Woodruff JM. Subdiaphragmatic and intrathoracic paraspinal malignant peripheral nerve sheath tumor: a clinicopathologic study of 25 patients and 26 tumors. Cancer 82:2191–203, 1998.

32. Lack EE, Worsham GF, Callihan MD, et al. Granular cell tumor: a clinicopathologic study of 110 patients. J Surg Oncol 13:301–316, 1980.
33. Laskin WB, Weiss SW, Brathauer GL. Epithelioid variant of malignant peripheral nerve sheath tumor (malignant epithelioid schwannoma). Am J Surg Pathol 15:1136–1145, 1991.
34. Lazarus SS, Trombetta LD. Ultrastructural identification of a benign perineurial cell tumor. Cancer 41:1823–1829, 1978.
35. Lodding P, Kindblom L, Angervall LG. Epithelioid malignant schwannoma: a study of 14 cases. virchows Arch A 409:433–451, 1986.
36. Lodding P, Kindblom L-G, Angervall L, Stenman G. Cellular schwannoma: a clinicopathologic study of 29 cases. Virchows Arch A 416:237–248, 1990.
37. Lundborg G. Nerve regeneration and repair: a review. Acta Orthop Scand 58:145–169, 1987.
38. MacCollin M, Woodfin W, Kronn D, Short MP. Schwannomatosis: a clinical and pathologic study. Neurology 46:1072–1079, 1996.
39. Meis-Kindblom JM, Enzinger FM. Plexiform malignant peripheral nerve sheath tumor of infancy and childhood. Am J Surg Pathol 18:479–485, 1994.
40. Meis-Kindblom JM, Kindblom LG, Stenman G. Plexiform malignant peripheral nerve sheath tumor (MPNST) of infancy and childhood further characterized. Mod Pathol 11:12A, 1998.
41. Miettinen M, Saari A. Pheochromocytoma combined with malignant schwannoma: unusual neoplasm of the adrenal medulla. Ultrastruct Pathol 12:513–527, 1988.
42. Min KW, Clemens A, Bell J, Dick H. Malignant peripheral nerve tumor and pheochromocytoma: a composite tumor of the adrenal. Arch Pathol Lab Med 112:266–270, 1988.
43. Mitsumoto H, Wilbourn AJ, Goren H. Perineurioma as the cause of localized hypertrophic neuropathy. Muscle Nerve 3:403–412, 1980.
44. Peterson LJ. Granular cell tumor: review of the literature and report of a case. Oral Surg Oral Med Oral Pathol 37:728–735, 1974.
45. Reed RJ, Leonard DD. Neurotropic melanoma—a variant of desmoplastic melanoma. Am J Surg Pathol 3:301–311, 1979.
46. Ricci A Jr, Parham DM, Woodruff JM, Callihan T, Green A, Erlandson RA, et al. Malignant peripheral nerve sheath tumors arising from ganglioneuromas. Am J Surg Pathol 8:19–29, 1984.
47. Scheithauer BW, Woodruff JM, Erlandson RA. Tumors of the peripheral nervous system. Atlas of Tumor Pathology (Third Series). Washington, DC: Armed Forces Institute of Pathology, 1999.
48. Sorensen SA, Mulvihill JJ, Nielson A. Long-term follow-up of von Recklinghausen neurofibromatosis. N Engl J Med 314:1010–1015, 1986.
49. Torsiglieri AJ, Handler SD, Uri AK. Granular cell tumors of the head and neck in children: the experience at the Children's Hospital of Philadelphia. Int J Pediatr Otorhinolaryngol 21:249–258, 1991.
50. Turc-Carel C, Dal Cin P, Limon J, Li F, Sandberg AA. Translocation x:18 in synovial sarcoma. Cancer Genet Cytogenet 23:93, 1986.

51. Weiss SW, Langloss JM, Enzinger FM. Value of S-100 protein in the diagnosis of soft tissue tumors with particular reference to benign and malignant Schwann cell tumors. Lab Invest 49:299–308, 1983.
52. White W, Shiu MH, Rosenblum MK, Erlandson RA, Woodruff JM. Cellular schwannoma: a clinicopathologic study of 57 patients and 58 tumors. Cancer 66:1266–1275, 1990.
53. Woodruff JM. Pathology of major peripheral nerve sheath neoplasms. In: Weiss SW, Brooks JSJ, eds. Soft Tissue Tumors. Baltimore: Williams & Wilkins, 1996.
54. Woodruff JM. Cellular schwannoma and its necessary distinction from malignant peripheral nerve sheath tumors and sarcomas. Pathol Case Rev 3:118–122, 1998.
55. Woodruff JM, Christensen WN. Glandular peripheral nerve sheath tumors. Cancer 72:3618–3628, 1993.
56. Woodruff JM. Pathology of tumors of the peripheral nerve sheath in type 1 neurofibromatosis. Am J Med Genet (Semin Med Genet) 89:23–30, 1999.
57. Woodruff JM, Chernik N, Smith M, Millet W, Foote F. Peripheral nerve tumors with rhabdomyosarcomatous differentiation (malignant "Triton" tumors). Cancer 32:426–439, 1973.
58. Woodruff JM, Godwin TA, Erlandson RA, Susin M, Martini N. Cellular schwannoma: a variety of schwannoma sometimes mistaken for a malignant tumor. Am J Surg Pathol 5:733–744, 1981.
59. Woodruff JM, Marshall ML, Godwin TA, Funkhouser JW, Thompson NJ, Erlandson RA, et al. Plexiform (multinodular) schwannoma: a tumor simulating the plexiform neurofibroma. Am J Surg Pathol 7:691–697, 1983.
60. Woodruff JM, Perino G. Non germ cell or teratomatous malignant tumors showing additional rhabdomyoblastic differentiation, with emphasis on the malignant Triton tumor. Semin Diagn Pathol 11:69–81, 1994.
61. Woodruff JM, Selig AM, Crowley K, Allen PW. Schwannoma with malignant transformation: a rare distinctive peripheral nerve tumor. Am J Surg Pathol 18:882–895, 1994.
62. Yassini PR, Sauter K, Schochet SS, Kaufman HH, Bloomfield SM. A localized hypertropic mononeuropathy involving spinal roots and associated with sacral meningocele. J Neurosurg 79:774–778, 1993.

10
Smooth Muscle Neoplasms

Christian H. Hansen
St. Agnes Hospital
Baltimore, Maryland

Elizabeth Montgomery
The Johns Hopkins University
Baltimore, Maryland

Smooth muscle is widely distributed in the human body. The genitourinary, gastrointestinal, and respiratory tracts all possess a major component of smooth muscle that is directly involved in contractile function. Smooth muscle cells are also found in the skin, where they compose the dermal pilar erectile muscles. Functionally analogous smooth muscle is present in the nipple and the genitalia, particularly in the vulva and scrotum. Finally, a major component of smooth muscle exists in the medial layers of blood vessels throughout the body. Therefore, it is appreciable that smooth muscle neoplasms may arise in a variety of locations throughout the body, often corresponding to the normal smooth muscle distribution.

I. LEIOMYOMA

A. General Features

Benign smooth muscle neoplasms are relatively common tumors. Most occur in the female genital tract, arising from myometrial smooth muscle of the uterus. Less common sites include the gastrointestinal tract, the skin and subcutaneous tissues, the genitourinary tract, and the deep soft tissues.

Grossly, leiomyomas are typically well-circumscribed nodular tumors with a firm, gray to white cut surface. The cut surface often displays a whorled or lobulated appearance. Degenerative changes include hemorrhage with central brownish red softening, myxoid change with an hydropic gelatinous appearance, and cystic change. Calcification is common. The presence of significant hemorrhage and/or necrosis in a large tumor suggests potential malignancy.

B. Microscopic Features

Microscopic features of smooth muscle differentiation include spindle-shaped cells arranged as interlacing bundles or fascicles, which often intersect at right angles (Fig. 1). The nuclei are typically blunt-ended or "cigar-shaped" and often show nuclear membrane indentations. Juxtanuclear vacuoles containing glycogen, as demonstrated by periodic acid–Schiff (PAS) staining, are commonly seen. The cytoplasm contains longitudinally arranged myofilaments that are seen as eosinophilic striations and are highlighted by their fuchsinophilic staining with the Masson trichrome stain. A thin outer basal lamina is present between the cells that can be demonstrated by PAS or reticulin staining, or by immunohistochemical staining for collagen type IV.

The most characteristic microscopic pattern is that of intersecting fascicles of well-differentiated spindled smooth muscle cells. However, a diversity of other

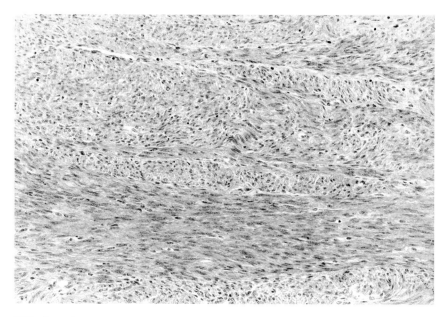

FIG. 1 Leiomyoma with typical spindle-shaped cells arranged in fascicles that often intersect at right angles.

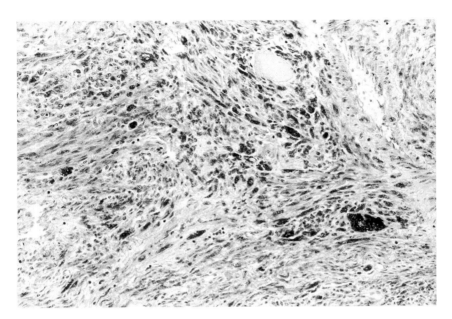

FIG. 2 Degenerative atypia (symplastic change) in a leiomyoma of longstanding duration, including enlarged, hyperchromatic, and pleomorphic nuclei and notable absence of
mitotic figures.

cytologic and architectural patterns may be encountered. Myxoid change with
prominent extracellular hyaluronic acid pooling, creating a separation of muscle
fibers, may impart a hypocellular appearance with a less obvious fascicular pattern. Similarly, tumors with extensive hyalinization due to the dense extracellular
collagen can also appear hypocellular. Nuclear palisading, resembling the so-
called Verocay bodies of benign nerve sheath tumors, is common. Longstanding
tumors may show focal calcification and, less frequently, metaplastic ossification.
Bizarre, enlarged, and hyperchromatic nuclei are sometimes present in tumors of
long duration (symplastic change) (Fig. 2). These nuclear changes may initially
appear alarming, but the lack of associated mitotic activity is often a clue to the degenerative nature of such pleomorphism. Occasionally, smooth muscle tumors are
composed of cytologically round cells with an epithelioid appearance (formerly
designated leiomyoblastoma) (1). Formalin fixation may cause artifactual perinuclear vacuolization. This epithelioid or clear cell morphology, more commonly
seen in the gastrointestinal tract, can present a diagnostic challenge and is further
addressed in the discussion of gastrointestinal stromal tumors.

C. Ultrastructural Features

Electron microscopic examination of leiomyomas reveals characteristic nuclear and cytoplasmic features. The nuclei commonly show prominent indentations of the nuclear membranes. Thin actin myofilaments (8–10 nm) are diffusely distributed throughout the cytoplasm. These myofilaments often aggregate into dense bodies or insert into electron-dense subplasmalemmal plaques (Fig. 3). Along the cytoplasmic membranes, pinocytotic vesicles are commonly seen. An external basal lamina is often prominent (2).

D. Immunohistochemical Findings

Immunohistochemical staining is often a useful adjunct to morphologic diagnosis. Expression of specific antigens may provide supportive evidence for a diagnosis when histologic findings are equivocal. Vimentin is a relatively nonspecific inter-

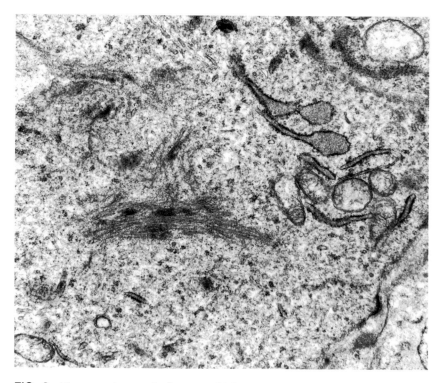

FIG. 3 Electron microscopic features of leiomyoma, including cytoplasmic, linearly aligned thin actin filaments with focal dense bodies and a subplasmalemmal dense plaque.

mediate filament associated with mesenchymal differentiation but may also be expressed in epithelial neoplasms. Leiomyomas consistently express vimentin. Desmin, another intermediate filament associated with myogenic differentiation, is commonly coexpressed with vimentin (3). More specific markers of myogenic differentiation include muscle-specific actin and smooth muscle actin. Muscle-specific actin is almost always expressed in leiomyomas (4,5). However, it is also expressed in skeletal and cardiac muscle as well as pericytes, myofibroblasts, myoepithelial cells, and decidual cells (6). Hence, its expression is not restricted to smooth muscle. Staining for more specific antibodies to α and γ isoforms of smooth muscle actin may also be performed. Normal smooth muscle, pericytes, myoepithelium, myofibroblasts, and most benign smooth muscle tumors will express smooth muscle actins (5).

E. Leiomyomas of the Skin and Subcutaneous Tissue

Leiomyomas of the skin and subcutaneous tissues (leiomyoma cutis) can be divided into three distinct subtypes. These include the superficial cutaneous (pilar) leiomyoma, the genital leiomyoma (including those arising in nipple, scrotum, and vulva), and the more deeply situated angioleiomyoma (vascular leiomyoma).

1. Cutaneous (Pilar) Leiomyoma

Superficial cutaneous leiomyomas usually present during early adulthood, occur with equal frequency in both sexes, and most commonly involve the extensor surfaces of the extremities. Other common locations include the trunk, face, and chest. Patients typically present with multiple, small, slow-growing tumor papules and nodules, which may be present individually or in groups. The grouped nodules may coalesce to form plaques in a linear or arciform distribution, often corresponding to a dermatome. More than one body site may be synchronously affected. Individual tumor nodules are small, usually less than 2–3 cm in diameter. The skin surface over the tumor nodules is often pink to red, but may appear yellow to brown. Occasionally, the nodules appear waxy, glistening, or semitranslucent. Telangiectatic vessels may be seen on the surface.

Burning, pinching, or stabbing pain that is exacerbated by fluctuations in temperature or application of pressure is frequently described. The pain may relate to the presence of nerve fibers within the tumor (7). Another possible mechanism of pain is ischemia, which would explain the exacerbation caused by exposure to cold temperatures, the reported change in color from red to white when painful (7), and the severe pain elicited by intratumoral injections of epinephrine (8). Pruritis has also been reported (7–9).

A family history of relatives with similar multifocal tumors may be elicited in some patients. Several reports have described a hereditary form of multiple leiomyomas of the skin. Pedigree analysis in these families suggests an autosomal dominant mode of inheritance. Familial multiple leiomyomas have also been described in association with dermatitis herpetiformis, familial adenomatous polyposis of the gastrointestinal tract (Gardner's syndrome), multiple uterine leiomyomas (Reed's syndrome), and multiple endocrine neoplasia type 1 (10–12).

Multifocal cutaneous leiomyomas are thought to arise from the arrectores pilorum muscle within the dermis. This hypothesis is supported by the occasional histologic finding of an arrectores pilorum muscle adjacent to or fused with the leiomyoma. Grossly, small firm nodular masses are present beneath the skin surface, which display a grayish white cut surface. Microscopically, a poorly circumscribed mass, composed of intersecting bundles of spindle-shaped cells with typical features of smooth muscle differentiation (see above), is seen within the reticular dermis. Infrequently, the tumor may encroach on the deeper subcutaneous fat. The smooth muscle bundles commonly show interdigitation of the fibers into the adjacent collagenous dermal stroma along the peripheral edge of the tumor, whereas the central portion of the tumor consists of solidly packed smooth muscle bundles. Above the tumor, a grenz zone of uninvolved papillary dermis separates the tumor from an often atrophic overlying epidermis (7,13). Importantly, mitotic activity is low and should be less than 1 mitotic figure per 10 high-power fields (hpf) (14). When the mitotic frequency equals or exceeds 1 mitotic figure per 10 hpf, the possibility of leiomyosarcoma should be considered, as discussed below. Solitary cutaneous leiomyomas occur less frequently than multifocal tumors. When they occur in nongenital sites, they are histologically similar to the multifocal lesions described above (13). The microscopic differential diagnosis of cutaneous pilar leiomyomas includes fibrous histiocytoma, cutaneous smooth muscle hamartoma, and accessory nipple.

Although malignant transformation does not occur, the multifocal nature of these lesions may render them difficult to excise. While surgical excision is the therapy of choice, total excision may be impossible, especially in cases where several coalescent grouped lesions are present. A high recurrence rate in these cases reflects such difficulties.

2. Genital Leiomyoma

Smooth muscle tumors classified as genital leiomyomas include those involving nipple, scrotum, and vulva. Although these tumors are often grouped together, published reports have identified distinguishing features at the different genital sites.

Leiomyoma of the nipple occurs in young adults and presents as a painful small nodular mass arising from the muscularis mamillae and areolae. These tumors are generally less than 1 cm in diameter. Microscopically, fascicles of well-differentiated, spindled smooth muscle cells are seen in the mid- to upper dermis. At the peripheral margin of the tumor, the fascicles interdigitate between the adjacent dermal collagen, creating an irregular margin. Hyperplasia of the superficial epidermis may be seen. Importantly, cytologic atypia and mitoses are not generally present. These smooth muscle tumors of the nipple are almost always benign and are considered analogous to cutaneous pilar leiomyomas (13,15,16). Extremely rare cases of leiomyosarcoma of the nipple have been reported (17,18).

Scrotal leiomyomas usually occur in middle-aged persons and are thought to arise from the dartos muscle of the scrotum. They are larger than other genital leiomyomas, with tumors as large as 14 cm reported in the literature. Clinically, they are usually painless lesions easily mistaken for benign epidermal inclusion cysts. Microscopically, fascicles of well-differentiated spindled smooth muscle cells are seen within the dermis and are surrounded by dartoic muscle fibers. As with cutaneous pilar and nipple leiomyomas, the peripheral margin typically shows an irregular, interdigitating, infiltrating border. Bizarre nuclei featuring nuclear enlargement, pleomorphism, hyperchromasia, macronucleoli, and multinucleation are occasionally present (19). These pleomorphic, bizarre nuclei are considered a degenerative phenomenon and are generally not an indication of malignancy. A grenz zone of uninvolved superficial papillary dermis is often present. Prominent lymphoid aggregates are frequently seen. Some scrotal smooth muscle tumors may show hypercellularity with numerous mitoses. The presence of any mitotic figures is indicative of malignancy and a diagnosis of leiomyosarcoma is appropriate (13,15,19).

Vulvar leiomyomas occur in early to middle adulthood. Clinically, these lesions often present as a painless lump on gynecologic examination and may be mistaken for a Bartholin's gland cyst. The labium majorum is the most common location. Although they vary in size, as a group they are generally smaller than scrotal leiomyomas. Microscopically, these tumors are composed of fascicles of well-differentiated spindled smooth muscle cells. In contrast to the other types of genital leiomyoma, these tumors are often well-circumscribed lesions. Infiltrating margins are not frequently seen and when present in combination with other unfavorable features (see below) may suggest a potentially malignant lesion. Myxoid change (especially common in pregnant patients) and hyalinization may be prominent. Criteria for defining malignancy have been difficult to establish with certainty. Although no single criterion has proven reliable alone, features suggesting potentially malignant behavior include tumors larger than 5 cm in diameter, 5 or more mitoses per hpf, and an infiltrating margin (15,20).

3. Angioleiomyoma (Vascular Leiomyoma)

Angioleiomyoma typically presents as a clinically painful, solitary nodular mass, most frequently located in the extremities. Another common location is the head and neck region. This tumor often occurs in middle-aged adults and is more common in females. Tactile pressure and exposure to cold temperatures exacerbate symptomatic pain, which may relate to vascular contraction with ischemia and/or

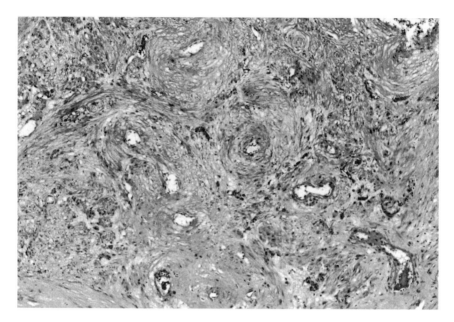

FIG. 4 Angioleiomyoma with prominent vascularity and proliferating smooth muscle bundles extending from vessel walls.

the occasional presence of intratumoral nerve fibers. The pain may worsen during pregnancy or menses. These tumors typically have been present for several years at the time of presentation and rarely recur following excision.

Grossly, these tumors are often small, firm, nodular, and well-circumscribed masses. Most tumors measure less than 2 cm in diameter. Upon sectioning, a gray-white or brown cut surface is seen. In contrast to the cutaneous leiomyomas of pilar origin, these tumors are located more deeply in subcutaneous tissue. Micro-scopically, these tumors comprise a mixture of smooth muscle and vascular elements (Fig. 4). Occasionally, a small component of adipose tissue and/or nerve is present. Myxoid and hyaline changes are common. Other occasional findings include calcification, hemosiderin, and lymphocytic inflammatory infiltrates. These lesions are essentially amitotic.

Three subtypes of angioleiomyoma have been described: solid, cavernous, and venous (50). Most tumors are of the solid type, with compact, spindled, smooth muscle bundles that surround and extend tangentially outward from small, slit-like vascular channels. The venous type is second in frequency, with less compact smooth muscle bundles surrounding venous vessels with thick muscular walls. Finally, the cavernous type comprises a smaller amount of smooth muscle that surrounds dilated vascular channels, sometimes containing luminal thrombi (7,21–23).

The microscopic differential diagnosis includes another painful lesion, the glomus tumor. Epithelioid, rounded cytology, a more abundant component of nerve fibers, and the classic subungual location (22–24) distinguish the glomus tumor, a tumor of pericytic differentiation.

F. Leiomyoma of Deep Soft Tissue

Benign smooth muscle neoplasms of the deep soft tissues are rare tumors with very few reported cases in the literature. They may occur at any age and with equal frequency in males and females. Clinically, these tumors often present as a painless mass, which may have been present for several years. They typically arise in the deep subcutaneous tissues or muscles of the extremities, the abdominal cavity, or the retroperitoneum.

Grossly, these are relatively large tumors, often greater than 5 cm in diameter, with an average reported size of 7.7 cm (25). Their larger size, as compared with leiomyomas at other sites, may reflect a long, clinically asymptomatic growth period. They are typically well-circumscribed and display a gray–white, whorled cut surface. Hemorrhage, cystic degeneration, and calcification may be present. Necrosis is notably absent.

Microscopically, these tumors are composed of intersecting fascicles of bland, spindled, smooth muscle cells with elongated, tapering eosinophilic cytoplasm. Most lack both significant nuclear pleomorphism and prominent nucleoli. However, cystic degeneration can be seen and may be associated with atypical, pleomorphic, bizarre nuclear morphology akin to that seen in the so-called ancient schwannoma (symplastic change). This nuclear atypia is considered a degenerative phenomenon associated with longstanding, slow-growing tumors. Other microscopic features include nuclear palisading, myxoid change, stromal hyalinization, dystrophic calcification, metaplastic ossification, and the presence of mature adipose tissue (lipoleiomyoma). Importantly, mitotic figures are notably scarce and should not be atypical. Quantitatively, they do not exceed 1 mitosis per 50 hpf and may even be absent.

Deep soft-tissue leiomyosarcomas far exceed leiomyomas in frequency. Therefore, histologic scrutiny, with particular emphasis on mitotic rate, is of utmost importance when making a benign diagnosis at this site. Although a specific threshold is difficult to establish, it has been suggested that when the mitotic rate exceeds 1 mitosis per 20 hpf, the potential for malignancy should be considered (25). Adequate sampling of tissue for thorough microscopic examination is required.

In females, it is also particularly important to note the precise location of tumors arising in the abdomen, as they may represent detachment of a pedunculated uterine leiomyoma. Mitotic rates in uterine tumors may be higher, and this may result in an erroneous diagnosis of deep soft-tissue leiomyosarcoma (25,26). Tumors arising in the vicinity of the pelvis in females should also be distinguished from the broad ligament, which may microscopically simulate a leiomyoma. Other soft-tissue neoplasms, such as fibrous histiocytoma, should also be considered in the differential diagnosis.

II. LEIOMYOSARCOMA

A. General Features

Malignant smooth muscle neoplasms occur less frequently than several other soft-tissue sarcomas, representing approximately 5–10% of all sarcomas (27). Although they may occur at any age, they are more common during adulthood and predominantly affect women. They arise at various locations and can bear a close resemblance to their benign counterparts upon gross inspection. Similar to leiomyomas, these malignant tumors display distinct, sharply marginated borders. They appear as solid, firm, nodular masses displaying a fleshy, gray–white to beige cut surface with a whorled or lobulated appearance. Cystic degeneration is occasionally prominent. However, in contrast to leiomyomas, malignant smooth muscle neoplasms are typically solitary, larger, and frequently display areas of hemorrhage and necrosis.

B. Microscopic Features

Microscopically, well-differentiated leiomyosarcomas show typical features of smooth muscle differentiation similar to those described above for leiomyomas. Increased mitotic activity is an important criterion in establishing a malignant diagnosis (Fig. 5). With lesser degrees of differentiation, atypical cytologic features are often present. Architecturally, moderately differentiated tumors are less orderly, with a more haphazard fascicular pattern. A greater degree of nuclear hyperchromasia and pleomorphism is seen, often with conspicuous nucleoli. The poorly differentiated tumors demonstrate an even greater degree of architectural disarray and nuclear anaplasia. Bizarre, pleomorphic, or multinucleated giant cells can be seen (Fig. 6). As is common with leiomyomas, nuclear palisading reminiscent of peripheral nerve sheath tumors may be prominent. Microscopic evidence of hemorrhage and/or necrosis is common, often corresponding to the gross appearance. A diagnostically important feature is the presence of mitotic figures. Mitotic figures are useful in establishing malignancy and are discussed below in the specific discussions of leiomyosarcoma at various sites.

Several microscopic variations from the usual well-differentiated smooth muscle pattern exist. One common variant, the "epithelioid" leiomyosarcoma (formerly designated leiomyoblastoma), is composed of round, rather than spindle, cells with central nuclei and abundant eosinophilic cytoplasm, imparting an epithelioid appearance (Fig. 7). The cytoplasm contains fewer myofilaments than the typical well-differentiated leiomyosarcoma. The epithelioid component is often

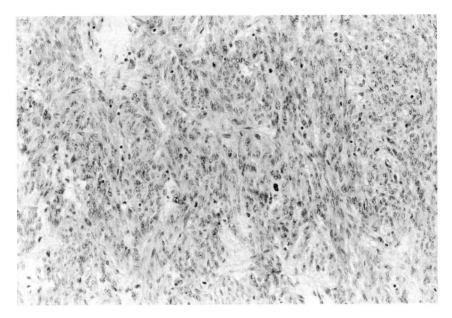

FIG. 5 Leiomyosarcoma with numerous mitotic figures.

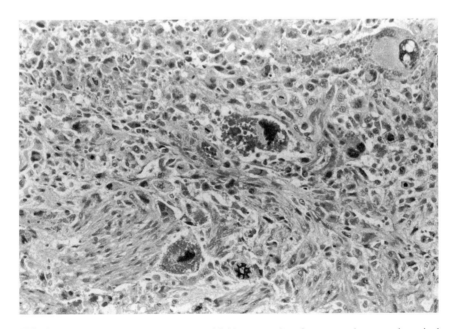

FIG. 6 Pleomorphic leiomyosarcoma with bizarre nuclear features and scattered atypical mitotic figures.

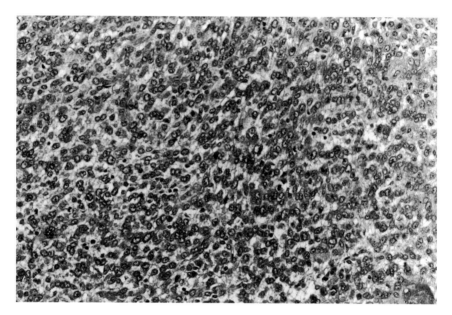

FIG. 7 Epithelioid leiomyosarcoma with more rounded rather than spindled cells and eosinophilic cytoplasmic staining.

admixed with a population of spindle cells showing typical features of smooth muscle differentiation. These epithelioid leiomyosarcomas commonly show artifactual cytoplasmic perinuclear clearing (vacuolar change) due to formalin fixation. This clear cell morphology can lead to difficulty in microscopically distinguishing these tumors from carcinoma, liposarcoma, melanoma, and other tumors. Importantly, these clear vacuoles do not stain for mucins, fat, or glycogen (1). Epithelioid leiomyosarcomas rarely occur in the soft tissues, but instead are commonly seen in the gastrointestinal tract. These tumors are described in further detail below in the discussion of gastrointestinal stromal tumors.

Other variant patterns include a myxoid pattern (Fig. 8), which may show microcystic change, a well-vascularized pericytomatous pattern, a "storiform" pattern reminiscent of fibrohistiocytic tumors, a hyalinized and often hypocellular pattern, and a "dedifferentiated" pattern with prominent nuclear enlargement, hyperchromasia, and pleomorphism. Granular leiomyosarcomas have also been described. Rare cases feature cytoplasmic hyaline globules. For further discussion and examples of these histologic patterns, the interested reader is referred to the selected references (27–33).

The histologic differential diagnosis of leiomyosarcoma includes other spindle cell neoplasms, such as fibrosarcoma, malignant peripheral nerve sheath tumor, hemangiopericytoma, synovial sarcoma, and malignant fibrous histiocy-

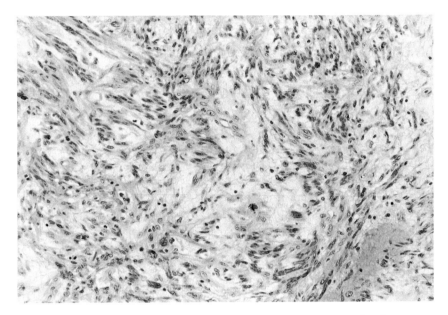

FIG. 8 Myxoid leiomyosarcoma with increased hyaluronic acid pooling between tumor cells.

toma. When evaluating cutaneous tumors, spindle cell melanoma, spindle cell squamous cell carcinoma, and atypical fibroxanthoma must be considered. Epithelioid tumors may be difficult to distinguish from carcinoma and melanoma. Clear cell (vacuolar) change may suggest a clear cell carcinoma or liposarcoma. Utilization of ancillary techniques, such as immunohistochemistry or electron microscopy, may be helpful in diagnostically challenging cases.

1. Ultrastructural Features

Well-differentiated leiomyosarcomas are ultrastructurally similar to leiomyomas, featuring prominent nuclear membranes indentations, diffusely distributed cytoplasmic myofilaments, scattered dense bodies, subplasmalemmal plaques, and membrane-bound pinocytotic vesicles. However, as these tumors become less differentiated, ultrastructural changes in malignant tumors include a decrease in myofilaments and pinocytotic vesicles, along with abundant rough endoplasmic reticulum, free ribosomes, and mitochondria (2).

2. Immunohistochemical Findings

As mentioned previously, immunohistochemistry can be extremely useful when the morphologic findings alone are insufficient for a definitive diagnosis. Similar to leiomyomas, vimentin will be consistently expressed by leiomyosarcomas. However, coexpression of vimentin and desmin is not as consistent in malignant smooth muscle tumors. In contrast to leiomyoma, desmin expression in leiomyosarcoma is often only focal or may be absent (3,34). One series reported a lack of desmin expression in almost half of the leiomyosarcomas examined (34). Muscle-specific actin is expressed in many leiomyosarcomas. However, its expression is not specific for leiomyosarcoma. Muscle-specific actin is also expressed in tumors of skeletal muscle, pericytic, and myofibroblastic differentiation (6,35). Nevertheless, its expression can provide supportive evidence for myogenic differentiation in morphologically difficult cases of leiomyosarcoma, especially when desmin expression is lacking (34). Leiomyosarcomas show variable expression of smooth muscle actins (4,5). The positive yield with smooth muscle actin antibodies may reflect the degree of differentiation within the tumor. When comparing desmin versus smooth muscle actin reactivity, positive staining may be seen more frequently with smooth muscle actin antibodies (36).

An interesting and important immunohistochemical feature of leiomyosarcoma is the occasional expression of epithelial antigens. One series documented both cytokeratin and epithelial membrane antigen staining in approximately half of the reported cases (37). The majority of these cases also showed coexpression of desmin and muscle-specific actin. This finding emphasizes the need to use a panel of several different antibodies when attempting to appropriately classify a tumor by immunohistochemistry. A variety of sarcomas (e.g., leiomyosarcoma, synovial sarcoma, epithelioid sarcoma, angiosarcoma) may express epithelial markers. Such expression should not by itself be construed as evidence of an epithelial neoplasm.

3. Criteria for Malignancy

Leiomyosarcomas of the soft tissues include those found in the deep soft tissues and retroperitoneum, skin and subcutaneous tissue, and blood vessels. An important concept to appreciate is that microscopically similar smooth muscle neoplasms arising at different sites do not always behave in the same manner. Hence, the establishment of criteria for malignancy has been difficult and has required correlation of site-specific pathologic findings with patient outcome. While several series report differing criteria for malignancy, they have provided important distinctions with regard to behavior of these tumors and their potential for malignancy at different sites. Criteria for malignancy, including tumor location, size, and mitotic rate, are discussed below for individual soft-tissue sites. Brief discussion of uterine leiomyosarcomas is provided to highlight the contrasting criteria for malignancy. Still, in some cases, it may not be possible to make a definitively malignant diagnosis and the designation of a tumor as "borderline" or "of uncertain malignant potential" may be appropriate. Smooth muscle neoplasms of the gastrointestinal tract (gastrointestinal stromal tumors) are discussed separately.

C. Deep Soft-Tissue/Retroperitoneal Leiomyosarcomas

Malignant smooth muscle neoplasms arising in the deep soft tissues and retroperitoneum can arise at any age, but most are diagnosed during middle age, between the ages of 40 and 70 (28–31,38–40). At the time of diagnosis, these tumors have been present for a period of weeks to several years (29,39). The majority of reports have shown a female predominance (28–31,38), especially among the retroperitoneal tumors (28). Within this deep soft-tissue and retroperitoneal subgroup, the retroperitoneal tumors occur most frequently. Of those arising in other deep soft tissues, the thigh is the most common site (29,38,40). Other sites include the omentum, mesentery, and serosal surfaces of visceral organs (27). Clinically, abdominal pain, nausea, vomiting, anorexia, weight loss, fatigue, and malaise are common presenting symptoms (31).

Correlation between size, mitotic rate, and clinical outcome attest to the fact that all smooth muscle neoplasms arising in these locations should be regarded with caution. While the average reported size of malignant tumors in several series ranged between 5 and 7.5 cm in diameter (28,29,31), recurrence has been described for tumors measuring as little as 1.5 cm (38). Similarly low thresholds for establishing malignancy apply when using mitotic index criteria. It has been suggested that tumors with 1–4 mitoses per 10 hpf should be regarded as potentially malignant, and those with 5 or more mitoses per 10 hpf considered malignant (27). However, it is important to remain aware that malignancy has been associated with as few as 1 mitotic figure per 10 hpf (31). Truly benign leiomyomas of the deep soft tissue are exceedingly rare, and such a diagnosis requires strict adherence to the mitotic index criterion. Any smooth muscle neoplasm of the deep soft tissue with greater than 1 mitotic figure per 20 hpf should be regarded as suspicious for malignancy (25). The presence of 1 mitosis per 10 hpf seems justifiably ample for a malignant designation. Thus, most tumors arising at these sites are best regarded as malignant, as small size and low mitotic activity do not necessarily predict a benign outcome. Metastases are most commonly found in the lungs and liver (28,29,31,38,41). Less common metastatic sites include other soft tissues (28,29,31), skin (28), gastrointestinal tract (31,41), bone (31), and lymph nodes (31,38).

D. Cutaneous/Subcutaneous Leiomyosarcomas

Superficial leiomyosarcomas typically occur in middle-aged to elderly adults (9,42–45). In contrast to those in the retroperitoneum and deep soft tissues, they are more common in males (9,42,44,45). The extremities are the most common sites of involvement, especially the proximal extensor surfaces of the lower extremities. Other common sites include hip, trunk, head and neck, and genital region (42–44). Patients clinically present with a raised nodular mass below the skin surface. Superficial cutaneous lesions display a pink, red, or brown discoloration of the skin surface, whereas subcutaneous tumors often do not show overlying discoloration. Irregular contours, pedunculation, umbilication, and skin ulceration may be seen (42,45). Pain is reported in the majority of cases. Other symptoms include pruritis, burning, and bleeding (46).

These superficial tumors have been subdivided into both cutaneous and subcutaneous leiomyosarcomas. This distinction reflects the hypothetical smooth muscle source from which these tumors arise. The more superficial cutaneous tumors are thought to arise from the arrectores pilorum muscle in the dermis or from superficial blood vessels, whereas the deeper subcutaneous tumors likely arise from deeper vessels (9). Two distinctly different growth patterns have been described (42–44). The cutaneous tumors arising from arrectores pilorum muscle show a diffuse growth pattern, characterized by a nonencapsulated, infiltrative proliferation of well-differentiated spindle cells, arranged in intersecting fascicles, extending into the adjacent collagen. They frequently display low cellularity, minimal cytologic atypia, lower mitotic rates, and a lack of tumor necrosis (43). In contrast, other tumors presumably of vascular origin, both cutaneous and subcutaneous, are characterized by a nodular growth pattern. These well-circumscribed neoplasms are more likely to show increased cellularity, nuclear pleomorphism, multinucleation, numerous mitoses, necrosis, and extension into the subcutaneous tissue (43).

As with smooth muscle neoplasms arising in the peripheral soft tissue and retroperitoneum, the clinical behavior of superficial leiomyosarcomas is often difficult to predict. Hence, criteria for establishing malignancy reflect such uncertainty. While there does appear to be some correlation between large size, high mitotic counts, and recurrence or metastasis (38,44), tumors with as few a 1 mitosis per 10 hpf (42,44) and as small as 0.8 cm (42) in diameter have demonstrated malignant behavior. Perhaps more importantly, the depth of these superficial tumors within the skin and subcutaneous tissue has prognostic significance. While cutaneous smooth muscle neoplasms have been reported to recur locally in 25–50% of cases, metastases are exceedingly rare (42,43,45,46). A single case of a dermal tumor that metastasized and eventually led to death of the patient has been reported. However, the location of the tumor in that case was described as "deep" dermis and was specifically distinguished from the location of more superficial cutaneous tumors in that series (45). In contrast, both recurrence (50–70% of cases) and metastases (30–40% of cases) have been reported more frequently with the deeper subcutaneous tumors (46). Therefore, any subcutaneous tumor should be regarded as having potential for recurrence or metastasis, whereas the cutaneous tumors are likely to only recur locally (43,46). In summary, the location, with specific regard to the depth of the tumor, may be most important in predicting behavior. Large tumor size and high mitotic rates are also useful, but these criteria alone are not always reliable indicators of malignancy. Any tumor with 1 or more mitotic figures per 10 hpf, regardless of location, should be considered potentially malignant. Metastases from these superficial leiomyosarcomas commonly involve the lungs, liver, and bone (38,42,44). Because both types of tumors may recur locally, wide surgical excision of these lesions is warranted and is the treatment of choice.

E. Vascular Leiomyosarcomas

Sarcomas arising in large blood vessels are rare neoplasms and include many different subtypes. Angiosarcomas arise from the endothelial vascular lining cells but rarely occur in large vessels. The so-called intimal sarcomas arise from the subendothelial mesenchymal cells and often manifest evidence of myofibroblastic differentiation. These intimal sarcomas frequently occur within large arterial vessels, particularly the great vessels such as the aorta and pulmonary artery. Leiomyosarcomas are derived from smooth muscle cells in the medial layer of blood vessels. In contrast, these tumors commonly occur in veins, most often the inferior vena cava (IVC) . Other locations, in order of frequency, are peripheral veins, pulmonary artery, and peripheral arterial vessels (47). Various types of vascular sarcomas, which are often difficult to classify, are rare and are reviewed elsewhere (48).

Leiomyosarcoma of the IVC typically presents during middle adulthood and predominantly occurs in women. Patients clinically present with symptoms that vary with the location of the tumor. Tumors arising in the middle portion of the IVC (infrahepatic/suprarenal) are most common (41.7%) and often present as a palpable abdominal mass with associated abdominal pain, weight loss, and occasional lower limb swelling. Clinically, the abdominal pain is often erroneously attributed to biliary tract disease. Evidence of renal dysfunction suggests extension into or obstruction of the renal vein. Those tumors involving the lower portion of the IVC (infrarenal) are next in frequency (34.0%), and patients more often present with a palpable abdominal mass, flank pain, and lower extremity edema. Finally, patients with tumors of the superior portion of the IVC (suprahepatic) (24.3%) can manifest symptoms of the Budd–Chiari syndrome (hepatic vein thrombosis) with associated jaundice, ascites, and hepatomegaly. Other general signs and symptoms in all groups include dyspnea, fever, night sweats, weakness, anorexia, nausea, vomiting, and increasing abdominal girth (49,50).

These leiomyosarcomas are relatively slow-growing tumors that are typically attached to the wall of the vena cava and exhibit extraluminal growth. Yet some do project into the lumen and are often associated with luminal thrombosis (49,51). Intraluminal tumor thrombi may extend into the renal veins, the hepatic vein, or even the right atrium. These tumors may also extend outward into the retroperitoneum. Reported cases range in size from 2 to 30 cm, with a mean diameter of 11 cm. Preoperatively, angiography, computed tomography (CT), and ultrasonography are important modalities for assessment of tumor size, location, and relationship to surrounding structures (50). Histologically, typical features of smooth muscle differentiation are present with varying degrees of cytologic atypia. Mitoses are often plentiful (52), but no specific mitotic threshold for malignant classification has been determined. As with other smooth muscle neoplasms of the retroperitoneum, a benign diagnosis in this location should be regarded with extreme caution. Necrosis may be present but does not necessarily imply a worse prognosis (51). Surgical resection seems to offer the only chance for survival. Location of the tumor determines the feasibility of successful resection. Tumors of the lower infrarenal segment of the IVC are most amenable to resection, whereas those of the upper suprahepatic segment are often inoperable (49,50,53). The rarity of this tumor precludes large clinical trials, but use of adjuvant chemotherapy and radiotherapy has been suggested. Thus far, the efficacy of such treatment appears limited (53,54). Overall postoperative survival is 27.9% and 14.2% at 5 and 10 years, respectively. The survival in patients with suprahepatic inoperable tumors, however, is dismal and averages 1 month (49). Half of all patients develop metastases. Common sites include lung, liver, kidney, pleura, chest wall, and bone (51).

Venous leiomyosarcomas of the extremities also occur in middle aged to elderly adults, but have an equal sex distribution. Peripheral veins of the lower extremities, including the iliac, femoral, popliteal, and saphenous veins, are most often involved. Clinically, the characteristic presentation is lower extremity edema. Hypervascularity of the tumor and compression of the adjacent artery within the confines of the conjunctiva vasorum (surrounding fibrous sheath) are both helpful in angiographic localization of the tumor (55). Projection into the vascular lumen with associated thrombosis is common. Reported cases vary in size, some measuring as large as 18 cm. Histologically, typical features of smooth muscle differentiation are seen, including interlacing fascicles of spindle cells, with variable mitotic rates and occasional hemorrhage and necrosis. Mitoses are generally frequent and do not appear useful in predicting outcome (52,56). Criteria for malignancy are not well defined. One series reported metastatic disease in all cases with variably sized tumors (55). Another series suggested that size might be an important predictor of outcome, as tumors smaller than 1.5 cm did not recur or metastasize (56). However, this contradicts a report in which a tumor as small as 1.5 cm metastasized (52). Therefore, prediction of behavior based on size and mitotic index criteria is precarious. As with IVC leiomyosarcomas, the distinction of benign from malignant neoplasms is difficult. Surgical excision is the treatment of choice. Common metastatic sites include lungs and liver (52,55).

Pulmonary artery leiomyosarcomas occur less frequently than intimal sarcomas, composing approximately 20% of all pulmonary artery sarcomas (57).

These tumors also arise in middle-aged adults with an approximately equal sex distribution. Clinically, symptoms include dyspnea, chest or back pain, cough, dizziness or syncope, hemoptysis, cyanosis, and evidence of right-sided heart failure. This combination of symptoms is often incorrectly attributed to pulmonary thromboembolism. Unfortunately, a correct diagnosis may not be made until time of autopsy. The tumors usually arise within the main pulmonary artery near the base of the heart with extension into the main pulmonary branches and sometimes into the lung. Angiography and CT are useful in both diagnosis and accurate localization. Pulmonary metastases are most common, but distant sites may be involved. The average survival from diagnosis is approximately 1 year (58,59).

Finally, leiomyosarcomas of peripheral arterial vessels are especially rare. The limited number of reported cases makes it difficult to formulate assumptions regarding their behavior. They also occur during middle adulthood with approximately equal sex distribution. The femoral artery appears to be the most common site. Clinically, they may be painful lesions with associated swelling of the involved extremity. Similar to leiomyosarcomas of peripheral veins, they also compress adjacent vessels, aiding in arteriographic diagnosis. Metastatic disease, especially to the lungs, is common (47,60).

F. Uterine Leiomyosarcomas

Smooth muscle tumors occur more frequently in the uterus than in the soft tissues. Hence, criteria for malignancy in uterine smooth muscle neoplasms have been more firmly established. Gross features suggesting malignancy include a large solitary nodule with foci of hemorrhage and necrosis. Cellularity, cytologic atypia, and mitotic activity are the most important histologic features to assess. Generally, tumors with fewer than 5 mitotic figures per 10 hpf are classified as leiomyomas. In contrast, leiomyosarcomas often have 10 or more mitoses per 10 hpf. Yet some tumors with 5–9 mitoses per 10 hpf, when associated with hypercellularity, cytologic atypia, or tumor cell necrosis, may also be classified as leiomyosarcoma. Those tumors with 5–10 mitotic figures per 10 hpf, but without significant cytologic atypia, are best classified as smooth muscle neoplasms of uncertain malignant potential (61).

Exceptions to these general guidelines include the mitotically active leiomyoma and tumors with prominent epithelioid or myxoid features. Mitotically active leiomyomas frequently occur in young females and do not recur or metastasize. Despite increased mitotic activity (often 5–15 per 10 hpf), these tumors are typically small and, by definition, lack any cytologic atypia or necrosis (62). Epithelioid smooth muscle tumors with 5 or more mitotic figures should be designated epithelioid leiomyosarcoma. Epithelioid tumors with 2–4 mitotic figures per 10 hpf with cytologic atypia, necrosis, or large size (>6 cm) should be classified as epithelioid smooth muscle neoplasm of uncertain malignant potential (63).

Myxoid leiomyosarcomas may demonstrate lower mitotic rates per unit area due to tumor cell separation by a background of myxoid matrix (64).

III. GASTROINTESTINAL STROMAL TUMORS (GIST)

Mesenchymal neoplasms arising within the muscular wall and connective tissues of the gastrointestinal tract occur infrequently in comparison with the more common neoplasms arising in the mucosal epithelium. These mesenchymal stromal tumors have been, and remain, the subject of controversy with regard to both their lineage of cellular differentiation and prediction of clinical behavior. Many demonstrate morphologic evidence of smooth muscle differentiation and are designated either leiomyomas or leiomyosarcomas. One particularly common cytomorphology is referred to as "epithelioid" or clear cell and, in the past, has been termed leiomyoblastoma (1). Less commonly, these mesenchymal tumors are classified as schwannomas (65) or gastrointestinal autonomic nerve tumors (66). But many show both morphologic and immunophenotypic features suggesting a mixture of smooth muscle, schwannian, and neural elements, or an even more primitive mesenchymal differentiation. As many do not demonstrate complete evidence of either pure smooth muscle or Schwann cell differentiation, they have collectively been termed gastrointestinal stromal tumors (GISTs).

More recently, speculation has focused on the interstitial cell of Cajal (ICC) as the cell of origin in GISTs. The ICCs are found in the muscular layers of the gastrointestinal tract and are considered "pacemaker" cells involved in gut motility. They possess ultrastructural features intermediate between fibroblasts and smooth muscle, but often favor myogenic differentiation. They are typically arranged in bundles, and are interspersed between and intimately associated with both enteric nerves (synapse-like contacts) and smooth muscle cells (gap junctions) of the muscular layers (67). Importantly, the tumor cells of GISTs possess similar ultrastructural morphologic features of incomplete smooth muscle differentiation (68,69). Furthermore, evaluation of GISTs and ICCs by immunohistochemistry and polymerase chain reaction for myosin heavy-chain isoform expression has revealed that both express the same embryonic isoform of the myosin heavy chain (70).

The interstitial cells of Cajal express the *c-kit* proto-oncogene, which encodes a transmembrane tyrosine kinase receptor (CD117). Stem cell factor is the endogenous ligand that binds the *c-kit* receptor (71). Interestingly, gastrointestinal stromal tumor cells have also been shown *c-kit* receptor (CD117). Other studies have found mutations in the *c-kit* proto-oncogene in stromal tumor cells. The mutations allow for activation of the *c-kit* receptor without ligand binding (gain-of-function mutations) (72,73). This finding implies that GISTs might be the result of activating mutations in the ICCs. One recent study has shown mutations specifically in exon 11 of the *c-kit* proto-oncogene predominantly in stromal tumors histologically designated as malignant, but only rarely in the benign tumors (73).

In summary, both benign and malignant tumors exhibiting either pure smooth muscle or pure Schwann cell differentiation exist and should appropriately be classified as such (e.g., leiomyoma, schwannoma). However, many tumors do not display pure features of either smooth muscle or schwannian differentiation; these have been designated gastrointestinal stromal tumors. Based on more recent studies, it now appears that many of these stromal tumors are derived from the interstitial cell of Cajal, an intermediate "pacemaker" cell with both myogenic and neural features. The term "gastrointestinal pacemaker cell tumor" (GI-PACT) has been proposed to replace "gastrointestinal stromal tumor" (GIST) (69).

A. General Features

Stromal tumors may arise at any location in the muscular wall of the gastrointestinal tract from the esophagus to the rectum, the stomach being the most common site of involvement (38,41,74). They typically present during middle to late adulthood and are more common in males (1,75). In younger patients, especially young females, they may be a manifestation of a clinical syndrome known as Carney's triad, which includes gastric epithelioid leiomyosarcomas, extra-adrenal paragangliomas, and pulmonary chondromas (76). Clinically, many patients with stromal tumors are asymptomatic when diagnosed (74,75). Others present with gastrointestinal bleeding, hematemesis, or melena due to ulceration of the overlying mucosa. Chronic blood loss may result in an iron deficiency anemia. Other symptoms include abdominal pain and weight loss (75).

B. Gross Features

Upon gross examination, most GISTs are well-circumscribed, solid, intramural, nodular masses. They may grow into the gastrointestinal lumen, often eroding the mucosal surface, or instead extend outward from the serosal surface. Occasionally, they grow in both directions and are described as having an "hour-glass" or "dumbbell" configuration. Tumors involving the external muscular layers may grow as pedunculated masses extending from the serosa (Fig. 9). Upon sectioning, the cut surface is gray, white, or tan, with a fleshy appearance. Hemorrhage, necrosis, and cyst formation may be seen (1,75).

C. Microscopic Features

Gastrointestinal stromal tumors are quite varied in their microscopic appearance and display many different cytologic and architectural patterns. Some show morphologic features of pure smooth muscle differentiation, as is common in the

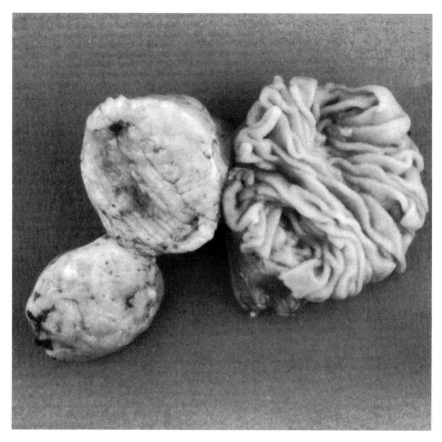

FIG. 9 Gastrointestinal stromal tumor growing as a pedunculated mass extending from the small-bowel serosal surface.

esophagus and rectum, and may be classified as leiomyoma or leiomyosarcoma. Others show pure Schwann cell differentiation and are classified as schwannoma (65). But the majority of cases show intermediate features or evidence of more primitive mesenchymal differentiation. Cytologically, either spindle cells or epithelioid round cells are seen, with many containing a mixture of both cell types. The spindle cells display features of smooth muscle differentiation, including fascicular architecture, elongated blunt-ended nuclei, and eosinophilic cytoplasm. In contrast, epithelioid cells are typically round cells with central nuclei and more abundant eosinophilic cytoplasm (Fig. 7). These epithelioid cells are often arranged in diffuse sheets or nests. Distinction of epithelioid tumors from carcinoma or melanoma can be difficult. Formalin fixation sometimes causes artifactual cytoplasmic perinuclear vacuolization (clear cell change) in the epithelioid cells. Clear cell change can similarly present a diagnostic challenge. The microscopic differential diagnosis may include clear cell or signet ring cell carcinoma, balloon cell melanoma, round cell liposarcoma, and myxoid chondrosarcoma, among many other clear cell neoplasms. Utilization of ancillary techniques, such as immunohistochemistry or electron microscopy, may be required. Other cytologic variants include tumors with granular, plasmacytoid, rhabdoid, or multinucleated cells. In addition to fascicular, diffuse, and nested architectural patterns, some tumors display "organoid," storiform, hemangiopericytomatous, or alveolar architecture. Nuclear palisading, reminiscent of Schwann cell differentiation, may be prominent. Other occasional microscopic findings include myxoid change, stromal hyalinization, extracellular eosinophilic globules ("skeinoid" fibers), cystic degeneration, hemorrhage, and necrosis. Some tumors appear well circumscribed, whereas others show an infiltrating margin that extends into the overlying mucosa or other adjacent structures (1,41,75,77–82).

Immunohistochemical staining may offer support in diagnostically difficult cases. Several large series have examined the immunophenotypic properties of stromal tumors (68,74,83–91), and thorough reviews of the literature have been published (79). Almost all stromal tumors express vimentin, an intermediate filament of limited specificity often associated with mesenchymal differentiation. Variable positive staining for desmin, muscle-specific actin, and smooth muscle actin often supports morphologic evidence of myogenic differentiation. Desmin may be expressed in up to 50% of cases, whereas muscle-specific actin and smooth muscle actin are expressed in approximately 68% and 57% of cases, respectively (79). Stromal tumors with features of schwannian or autonomic nerve differentiation may express S-100 protein or neuron-specific enolase. CD34, a marker of both endothelial and primitive hematopoietic stem cell differentiation, is expressed in many primitive or uncommitted fibroblastic mesenchymal neoplasms. Similarly, many stromal tumors exhibiting less morphologic and immunohistochemical evidence of myogenic or schwannian differentiation will express the CD34 antigen (91). As discussed above, many of these stromal tumors are now considered to be derived from gastrointestinal pacemaker cells. They express CD117, the *c-kit* receptor, in approximately 85% of cases. While coexpression of CD117 and muscle-specific actin may be seen in approximately one third of these cases, tumors with clear-cut morphologic features of leiomyoma or schwannoma often lack CD117 expression (68).

D. Criteria for Malignancy

Classification of a stromal tumor as benign or malignant can be a challenging task for the pathologist. Several series have compared pathologic findings with clinical outcome (1,41,75,77,78,92–94). The results of these series have been variable, and excellent literature reviews have been published (79,95). Despite the somewhat confusing and often conflicting data, general guidelines for determining malignancy can be extrapolated. Pathologic features of importance include tumor size, mitotic rate, cellularity, cytologic atypia, presence of tumor necrosis, and infiltration of mucosa or other adjacent tissues. Notably, no single feature alone is reliably predictive of clinical outcome. Collective evaluation of the pathologic findings is most appropriate. Significantly, tumor size and mitotic rate should be critically addressed. Franquemont, in an extensive review of the literature, concluded that mitotic rate and tumor size are most important in predicting aggressive behavior (95). In a similarly thorough review, Suster summarized the findings of many series and proposed a set of morphologic criteria for malignancy. These include tumor size greater than 5 cm, infiltration of adjacent structures, presence of tumor necrosis, increased nuclear-to-cytoplasmic ratio, mitotic rate of 1–5 per 10 hpf, and infiltration of overlying mucosa. Two or more of these criteria should be satisfied before a stromal tumor is classified as malignant (79). It is recognizably difficult to suggest a more specific mitotic threshold. The suggested range reflects the fact that many malignant tumors may have 2–5 or more mitoses per 10 hpf, but fatal cases have been described with only 1 mitosis per 10 hpf (78).

Although histopathologic evaluation is of critical importance, predictions regarding the behavior of these tumors on a purely morphologic basis are often unreliable. This has prompted a search for other possible indicators of malignancy. Several studies examining DNA ploidy status have found decreased survival in patients with tumors containing aneuploid cells (determined by flow cytometric cell cycle analysis) (84,96,97). Others have looked at nuclear proliferation markers, such as proliferating cell nuclear antigen (PCNA) and Ki-67 antigen, by immunohistochemical staining. Nuclear Ki-67 positivity in more than 10% of the total tumor cell population correlated with decreased long-term survival in one large series (84). Similarly, some series have shown a significant correlation between nuclear PCNA staining and decreased long-term survival (98,99). However, another examined both PCNA and Ki-67 antigen staining and failed to demonstrate significance in predicting survival (83). More recently, one series found mutations specific to exon 11 of the *c-kit* proto-oncogene that are present almost exclusively in the malignant stromal tumors (73). The finding of specific genetic mutations is certainly intriguing and may provide clues to the pathogenesis of these tumors. But the detection of specific genetic mutations and its utility as an aid to classification of stromal tumors requires further investigation before it can be reliably applied.

Tumor location within the gastrointestinal tract appears to have some prognostic significance. Many studies have shown decreased long-term survival in patients with small intestinal stromal tumors in comparison with those having the more common gastric tumors (74,83). A more recently published large case series focused specifically on the relationship between the anatomical location of stromal tumors and long-term patient survival. Stromal tumors arising in the esophagus were associated with the longest survival period, followed by those arising in stomach, colon, and small bowel (100).

In summary, combined factors must be considered when attempting to accurately predict clinical behavior. Careful histologic assessment is obviously critical. Location of the tumor also seems to have prognostic significance. Other ancillary techniques, including immunohistochemistry, ploidy analysis, proliferation marker staining, and genetic mutational analysis, may provide additional supportive information when morphologic findings are indeterminate. However, the predictive contribution of these nonmorphologic techniques requires further study and clarification before they can be incorporated into routine practice. Many cases will satisfy multiple fore-mentioned criteria for malignancy and can be classified as malignant. Other benign tumors will not meet any of these criteria. Unfortunately, still others may have both benign and malignant features. In such cases, application of these nonmorphologic techniques may be warranted if they are available. Oftentimes, a definitive classification is not possible and designation as "borderline" or "of uncertain malignant potential" is most appropriate.

IV. LEIOMYOMATOSIS PERITONEALIS DISSEMINATA

Leiomyomatosis peritonealis disseminata is a rare condition afflicting predominantly young women of childbearing age, characterized by the development of multiple smooth muscle nodules along the peritoneal surfaces of the abdominal cavity and pelvis. Common clinical associations include pregnancy and oral contraceptive use (101–103). Less often, it occurs in patients with hormone-producing neoplasms. In fact, the first report of this condition was in a patient with a granulosa cell tumor of the ovary, a neoplasm commonly associated with estrogen production (104). Concomitant endometriosis has also been described (102,105). Regression of these smooth muscle nodules may occur following delivery (post partum), during menopause, or following oophorectomy. These clinical associations indicate a hormonal pathogenesis, which has been substantiated by demonstration of both estrogen and progesterone receptors within the constituent smooth muscle cells (106). Specifically, a hormonally induced metaplasia of subperitoneal mesenchymal cells has been proposed (107). Furthermore, this metaplasia has been experimentally demonstrated in an animal model (108).

Recently, a small case series specifically examined clonality in these tumor nodules by X-chromosome inactivation analysis. In the four cases evaluated, the same parental X chromosome was nonrandomly inactivated in multiple nodules, indicating clonality in these tumors. In contrast to the prevailing theory of subperitoneal mesenchymal metaplasia, this finding suggests the possibility of multiple clonal metastatic tumor nodules. Another potential interpretation is that nonran-

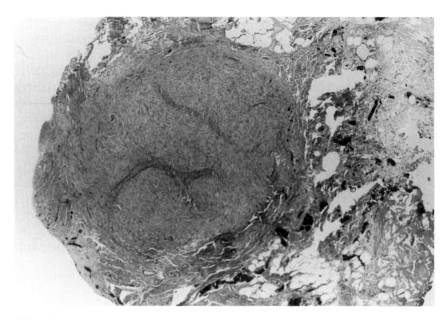

FIG. 10 Subperitoneal smooth muscle proliferation in a patient with leiomyomatosis peritonealis disseminata.

dom selection for an X-linked allele occurs in these tumors. Selection of such an allele may confer a predisposition to the development of leiomyomatosis perito-nealis disseminata in these patients. Future discovery of a specific genetic abnor-mality unrelated to the X chromosome in these tumors would allow for more spe-cific clonality studies. This could potentially resolve the pathogenetic controversy regarding metaplasia versus metastases (109).

Clinically, nonpregnant patients are more often symptomatic than preg-nant patients. They may present with abdominal or pelvic pain, dysmenorrhea, dyspareunia, urinary frequency, and constipation. Grossly, studding of the perito-neal surfaces with multiple, variably sized, gray to white firm nodules is typical. This presentation may be clinically and radiographically confused with peritoneal carcinomatosis. Microscopically, typical architectural and cytologic features of smooth muscle differentiation are seen (Fig. 10). An infiltrating growth pattern and cytologic atypia are generally lacking, and mitoses are infrequent. Other his-tologic findings include adjacent decidualized cells, especially in pregnant pa-tients, and areas of fibroblastic or myofibroblastic cells (101,103). These fibroblas-tic or myofibroblastic regions might represent intermediate stages of metaplasia between subperitoneal primitive mesenchyme and fully differentiated smooth muscle cells (107). Hyalinization can be seen, particularly in regressed nodules

(101,104). Ultrastructurally, an admixture of cells with fibroblastic, myofibroblastic, and smooth muscle features has been described, supporting the postulated metaplastic process (103).

The overwhelming majority of reported cases demonstrate benign behavior, often resolving following removal of hormonal stimulation (e.g., post partum). Following an initial surgical diagnosis, further therapy is often not necessary. Leuprolide acetate, a gonadotropin-releasing hormone agonist, has been shown to induce tumor nodule regression in a single reported case (110).

Rare cases of malignant transformation and subsequent metastases have been reported in the literature (111–113). Based on the limited number of malignant cases, it is difficult to determine features predictive of malignant behavior. Although one case involved increased cellularity and mitoses in some nodules (111,112), this has not always been a consistent finding (113). Adjuvant combination chemotherapy has been successful in one reported malignant case with a limited follow-up period but has not proven successful in other reported cases (112).

V. INTRAVENOUS LEIOMYOMATOSIS

Intravenous leiomyomatosis is a rare condition characterized by the presence of a benign smooth muscle proliferation in blood vessels. This process typically occurs in uterine vessels in the myometrium, but many cases also involve extrauterine vessels. Extrauterine involvement frequently involves veins of the broad ligament, uterus, ovary, and vagina. Infrequently, extension to the inferior vena cava, right atrium, and pulmonary vessels may occur. This intravenous proliferation is thought to arise either from the medial layer of blood vessels or from vascular invasion by a benign leiomyoma. Patients most often present during premenopausal adulthood (median age 44 years) with symptoms similar to and likely attributable to uterine leiomyomas, including pelvic pain, menorrhagia, abnormal vaginal bleeding, and uterine enlargement. Rare patients with right-sided cardiac involvement may manifest symptoms of congestive heart failure or hepatic dysfunction.

Patients typically have an enlarged leiomyomatous uterus. Intravenous extension of the uterine leiomyomas into myometrial or extrauterine vessels appears as coiled, convoluted, or plexiform worm-like intravascular plugs of tumor. These intravascular tumors may either be mobile or attached to the vessel wall. Microscopically, the tumors are composed of intravascular plugs of bland spindled cells arranged in intersecting fascicles with a superficial endothelial lining. These plugs of tumor may appear to arise from the vessel wall or may be contiguous with an extravascular leiomyoma. A wide variety of histologic changes seen in ordinary leiomyomas may be present, including hyalinization and hydropic change. Thick-walled blood vessels may be prominent in the intravascular tumor plugs, imparting an angiomatoid appearance. Cytologic atypia and mitotic activity are typically lacking. The mitotic rate should not exceed that of benign uterine leiomyomas (114,115–118). Other unusual histologic variants include cellular, epithelioid, clear cell, myxoid, lipoleiomyomatous, and symplastic variants (119). The histologic differential diagnosis includes leiomyoma surrounded by vessels with dilated vascular spaces, leiomyoma with vascular invasion, diffuse leiomyomatosis, leiomyosarcoma, and endometrial stromal sarcoma.

Hysterectomy with removal of any grossly visible extrauterine tumor is the recommended treatment. Postoperatively, approximately 70% of patients have no evidence of residual disease, whereas 30% experience symptoms related to persistent intravenous tumor growth. Recurrent disease may involve the iliac, pelvic, and hepatic veins, the inferior vena cava, the heart, and the lungs (114). Other therapeutic options include bilateral oophorectomy (surgical castration) or antiestrogenic therapy tamoxifen, as these tumors often express estrogen receptors (120).

VI. BENIGN METASTASIZING LEIOMYOMA

Benign metastasizing leiomyoma refers to the rare occurrence of a benign, well-differentiated extrauterine smooth muscle proliferation in a patient with a past history of uterine leiomyoma. The lung is the most common site, but these leiomyomatous proliferations are also seen in pelvic and periaortic lymph nodes, omentum, mesentery, mediastinum, inferior vena cava, right atrium, and soft tissues. Typically, patients are young to middle-aged women and are often asymptomatic. Pulmonary disease is frequently an incidental radiographic finding. Others present with symptoms related to pulmonary disease, including dyspnea, cough, and hemoptysis. Pulmonary function testing may suggest evidence of restrictive lung disease. Chest x-ray or CT scan often demonstrates multiple bilateral pulmonary nodules of variable size (121–129). Without therapeutic intervention, progressive pulmonary insufficiency may ensue and ultimately lead to death of the patient.

Microscopic examination of the metastatic nodules reveals bundles of well-differentiated spindled smooth muscle cells without significant cytologic atypia or mitotic activity (Fig. 11). With careful microscopic search, minimal mitotic activity can usually be identified (126), but most tumors average fewer than 1 mitotic figure per 10 hpf. Pulmonary interstitial replacement by the smooth muscle proliferation, with associated entrapment of airspaces and hyperplasia of alveolar epithelial cells, may impart a pseudoglandular or clefted appearance (126). Tumors presenting at other sites show similar bland cytologic features with few, if any, mitoses (122). Histologic review of the prior uterine resection specimen should reconfirm the diagnosis of benign leiomyoma.

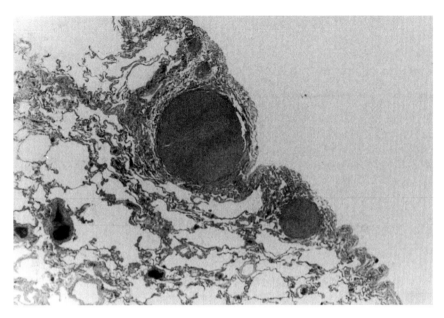

FIG. 11 "Benign metastasizing leiomyoma" of lung with well-differentiated smooth muscle within subpleural vascular spaces. This patient's previous hysterectomy revealed multiple uterine leiomyomata without evidence of malignancy.

The pathogenesis of these lesions has been a subject of controversy in the literature. Many speculate that these tumor nodules represent true metastatic lesions from an extremely low-grade leiomyosarcoma of the uterus. This hypothesis is supported by the often multifocal and bilateral pattern of distribution (125) and the presence of at least some mitotic activity in most lesions (126). Furthermore, ultrastructural variation in smooth muscle cell maturity was described in one series, with immature features used as evidence of a low-grade malignancy (126). Clinical and pathologic similarities between intravenous leiomyomatosis and benign metastasizing leiomyoma suggest that these two diseases may be closely related. A common unifying pathogenesis may involve vascular invasion by an otherwise histologically benign leiomyoma with subsequent metastases (129). Still others have reported cases with unusual patterns of tumor distribution and have suggested that benign metastasizing leiomyoma is due to development of multifocal primary tumors (124). This theory is conceptually similar to that proposed for leiomyomatosis peritonealis disseminata.

Therapeutic approaches described in the literature include surgery, hormonal manipulation, and cytotoxic chemotherapy. Hysterectomy is often performed to remove the theoretical source of the "primary" tumor. Thoracotomy with resection of "metastatic" pulmonary nodules has also been reported with successful outcome (130). Hormonal manipulation is based on demonstration of nuclear estrogen receptors within the tumor cells (123), decreased tumor growth in postmenopausal patients (125), and the observation of tumor regression during late pregnancy (125). Both oophorectomy (127) and the use of a luteinizing hormone–releasing hormone analog (128) have both been shown to be efficacious in reducing tumor size by decreasing endogenous estrogenic stimulation. In contrast, tamoxifen has been used to block estrogenic stimulation but has not proven useful (131). Finally, cytotoxic chemotherapy with high-dose ifosamide seems ineffective (131).

VII. IMMUNOSUPPRESSION-ASSOCIATED SMOOTH MUSCLE NEOPLASMS

Benign and malignant smooth muscle neoplasms have been described in association with immunosuppression. The typical clinical settings include both human immunodeficiency virus (HIV) infection (132–137) and posttransplantation therapeutic immunosuppression (138,139). The reported cases involving HIV-infected patients predominantly involve children and young adults, and show a peculiar predilection for visceral organs rather than the soft tissues. Common sites include lungs, gastrointestinal tract, and liver (132,133,136,137), but other sites have also been reported, including adrenal gland (134) and spleen (135).

Recently, several reports have demonstrated the presence of EBV in these tumors by in situ hybridization techniques (134,137–139). Importantly, adjacent uninvolved tissues did not show significant positivity for EBV viral sequences. Smooth muscle tumors in nonimmunocompromised patients were also negative for EBV viral sequences (137). These findings suggest a causal yet still unclarified role for EBV in the pathogenesis of these tumors (140).

Microscopically, well-differentiated smooth muscle features are seen, including spindle-shaped cells arranged in intersecting fascicles with variable nuclear pleomorphism and mitotic activity. Epithelioid histologic features are not typically seen in this setting (133). Criteria for establishing malignancy generally reflect those applied to smooth muscle neoplasms arising at the particular site in nonimmunocompromised patients. The designation of malignancy is particularly difficult in visceral organs, such as the liver, where criteria for malignancy are not well defined. In such cases, a designation of smooth muscle neoplasm of undetermined malignant potential may be appropriate (133,136). While multifocality might suggest malignant behavior with metastases, the association with Epstein-Barr virus (EBV) in these cases could also indicate multiple sites of primary involvement.

The differential diagnosis of these smooth muscle neoplasms includes those previously mentioned for smooth muscle tumors in general. However, in the setting of immunosuppression, this differential is expanded to include other spindle cell lesions, such as Kaposi's sarcoma and mycobacterial spindle cell pseudotumor. Kaposi's sarcoma, associated with human herpesvirus 8 (Kaposi's sarcoma–associated herpesvirus) infection (141), is histologically composed of a proliferation of small, angulated vascular spaces with a prominent population of adjacent spindle cells. PAS-positive hyaline globules, hemosiderin granules, and inflammatory infiltrates rich in plasma cells are frequently seen. Immunohistochemically, the spindle cells in Kaposi's sarcoma express vascular antigens, such as CD31, CD34, and factor VIII–related antigen (142).

Mycobacterial spindle cell pseudotumor is also seen in immunosuppressed patients and commonly involves the lymph nodes and spleen. Microscopically, these lesions are composed of a multinodular or diffuse proliferation of spindle cells with storiform architecture admixed with chronic inflammatory cells. The spindle cells represent histiocytic cells and contain numerous intracytoplasmic acid-fast bacilli (143). These organisms are easily demonstrated by Ziehl-Neelsen staining. Immunohistochemical staining should be interpreted with caution, as the histiocytic spindle cells may show desmin positivity (144).

REFERENCES

1. Stout AP. Bizarre smooth muscle tumors of the stomach. Cancer 15:400–409, 1962.
2. Ferenczy A, Richart RM, Okagaki T. A comparative ultrastructural study of leiomyosarcoma, cellular leiomyoma, and leiomyoma of the uterus. Cancer 28:1004–1018, 1971.
3. Evans DJ, Lampert IA, Jacobs M. Intermediate filaments in smooth muscle tumours. J Clin Pathol 36:57–61, 1983.
4. Schurch W, Skalli O, Seemayer TA, Gabbiani G. Intermediate filament proteins and actin isoforms as markers for soft tissue tumor differentiation and origin. I. Smooth muscle tumors. Am J Pathol 128:91–103, 1987.
5. Roholl PJM, Elbers HRJ, Prinsen I, Claessens JAJ, van Unnik JAM. Distribution of actin isoforms in sarcomas. An immunohistochemical study. Hum Pathol 21:1269–1274, 1990.
6. Tsukada T, Tippens D, Gordon D, Ross R, Gown AM. HHF35, a muscle-actin-specific monoclonal antibody. I. Immunocytochemical and biochemical characterization. Am J Pathol 126:51–60, 1987.
7. Montgomery H, Winkelmann RK. Smooth muscle tumors of the skin. Arch Dermatol 79:32–41, 1959.
8. Jansen LH, Driessen FML. Leiomyoma cutis. Br J Dermatol 70:446–451, 1958.
9. Stout AP. Solitary cutaneous and subcutaneous leiomyoma. Am J Cancer 29:435–469, 1937.

10. Kloepfer HW, Krafchuk J, Derbes V, Burks J. Hereditary multiple leiomyoma of the skin. Am J Hum Genet 10:48–52, 1958.
11. Auckland G. Hereditary multiple leiomyoma of the skin. Br J Dermatol 79:63, 1967.
12. Vellanki LS, Camisa C, Steck WD. Familial leiomyomata. Cutis 58:80–82, 1996.
13. Fisher WC, Helwig EB. Leiomyomas of the skin. Arch Dermatol 88:510–520, 1963.
14. Raj S, Calonje E, Kraus M, Kavanagh G, Newman PL, Fletcher CD. Cutaneous pilar leiomyoma: clinicopathologic analysis of 53 lesions in 45 patients. Am J Dermatopathol 19:2–9, 1997.
15. Newman PL, Fletcher CDM. Smooth muscle tumors of the external genitalia: clinicopathological analysis of a series. Histopathology 18:523–529, 1991.
16. Nascimento AG, Karas M, Rosen PP, Caron AG. Leiomyoma of the nipple. Am J Surg Pathol 3:151–154, 1979.
17. Hernandez FJ. Leiomyosarcoma of the male breast originating in the nipple. Am J Surg Pathol 2:299–304, 1978.
18. Lonsdale RN, Widdison A. Leiomyosarcoma of the nipple. Histopathology 20:537–539, 1992.
19. Slone S, O'Connor D. Scrotal leiomyomas with bizzare nuclei: a report of three cases. Mod Pathol 11:282–287, 1998.
20. Tavassoli F, Norris HJ. Smooth muscle tumors of the vulva. Ostet Gynecol 53:213–217, 1979.
21. Hachisuga T, Hashimoto H, Enjoji M. Angioleiomyoma. A clinicopathologic reappraisal of 562 cases. Cancer 54:126–130, 1984.
22. Magner D, Hill DP. Encapsulated angiomyoma of the skin and subcutaneous tissues. Am J Clin Pathol 35:137–141, 1961.
23. MacDonald DM, Sanderson KV. Angioleiomyoma of the skin. Br J Dermatol 91:161–168, 1974.
24. Ekestrom S. Comparison between glomus tumour and angioleiomyoma. Acta Pathol Microbiol Scand 27:86–93, 1950.
25. Kilpatrick SE, Mentzel T, Fletcher CDM. Leiomyoma of deep soft tissue. Clinicopathologic analysis of a series. Am J Surg Pathol 18:576–582, 1994.
26. Enzinger FM, Weiss SW. Benign tumors of smooth muscle. In: Soft Tissue Tumors. St. Louis: Mosby, 1995, pp. 467–490.
27. Enzinger FM, Weiss SW. Leiomyosarcoma. In: Soft Tissue Tumors. St. Louis: Mosby, 1995, pp. 491–510.
28. Wile AG, Evans HL, Romsdahl MM. Leiomyosarcoma of soft tissue: a clinicopathologic study. Cancer 48:1022–1032, 1981.
29. Hashimoto H, Daimaru Y, Tsuneyoshi M, Enjoji M. Leiomyosarcoma of the external soft tissues. A clinicopathologic, immunohistochemical, and electron microscopic study. Cancer 57:2077–2088, 1986.
30. Hashimoto H, Tsuneyoshi M, Enjoji M. Malignant smooth muscle tumors of the retroperitoneum and mesentery: a clinicopathologic analysis of 44 cases. J Surg Oncol 28:177–186, 1985.
31. Schmookler BM, Lauer DH. Retroperitoneal leiomyosarcoma. A clinicopathologic analysis of 36 cases. Am J Surg Pathol 7:269–280, 1983.
32. Suster S. Epithelioid leiomyosarcoma of the skin and subcutaneous tissue. Clinicopathologic, immunohistochemical, and ultrastructural study of five cases. Am J Surg Pathol 18:232–240, 1994.

33. Suster S, Rosen LB, Sanchez JL. Granular cell leiomyosarcoma of the skin. Am J Dermatopathol 10:234–239, 1988.

34. Azumi N, Ben-Ezra J, Battifora H. Immunophenotypic diagnosis of leiomyosarcomas and rhabdomyosarcomas with monoclonal antibodies to muscle-specific actin and desmin in formalin-fixed tissue. Mod Pathol 1:469–474, 1988.

35. Rangdaeng S, Truong LD. Comparative immunohistochemical staining for desmin and muscle specific actin. A study of 576 cases. Am J Clin Pathol 96:32–45, 1991.

36. Jones H, Steart PV, DuBoulay CEH, Roche WR. Alpha-smooth muscle actin as a marker for soft tissue tumours: a comparison with desmin. J Pathol 162:29–33, 1990.

37. Miettinen M. Immunoreactivity for cytokeratin and epithelial membrane antigen in leiomyosarcoma. Arch Pathol Lab Med 112:637–640, 1988.

38. Stout AP, Hill WT. Leiomyosarcoma of the superficial soft tissues. Cancer 11:844–854, 1958.

39. Phelan JT, Sherer W, Mesa P. Malignant smooth-muscle tumors (leiomyosarcomas) of soft tissue origin. N Engl J Med 266:1027–1030, 1962.

40. Gustafson P, Willen H, Baldetorp B, Ferno M, Akerman M, Rydholm A. Soft tissue leiomyosarcoma. A population-based epidemiologic and prognostic study of 48 patients, including cellular DNA content. Cancer 70:114–119, 1992.

41. Ranchod M, Kempson RL. Smooth muscle tumors of the gastrointestinal tract and retroperitoneum. A pathologic analysis of 100 cases. Cancer 39:255–262, 1977.

42. Fields JP, Helwig EB. Leiomyosarcoma of the skin and subcutaneous tissue. Cancer 47:156–169, 1981.

43. Kaddu S, Beham A, Cerroni L, Humer-Fuchs U, Salmhofer W, Kerl H, Soyer HP. Cutaneous leiomyosarcoma. Am J Surg Pathol 21:979–987, 1997.

44. Dahl I, Angervall L. Cutaneous and subcutaneous leiomyosarcoma, a clinicopathologic study of 47 patients. Pathol Eur 9:307–315, 1974.

45. Swanson PE, Stanley MW, Scheithauer BW, Wick MR. Primary cutaneous leiomyosarcoma. A histologic and immunohistochemical study of 9 cases, with ultrastructural correlation. J Cutan Pathol 15:129–141, 1988.

46. Wascher RA, Lee MYT. Recurrent cutaneous leiomyosarcoma. Cancer 70:490–492, 1992.

47. Kevorkian J, Cento DP. Leiomyosarcoma of large arteries and veins. Surgery 73:390–400, 1973.

48. Burke A, Virmani R. Tumors of the great vessels. In: Tumors of the Heart and Great Vessels. Washington, DC: Armed Forces Institute of Pathology, 1996, pp. 211–226.

49. Mingoli A, Feldhaus RJ, Cavallaro A, Stipa S. Leiomyosarcoma of the inferior vena cava: analysis and search of world literature on 141 patients and report of three new cases. J Vasc Surg 14:688–699, 1991.

50. Griffin AS, Sterchi JM. Primary leiomyosarcoma of the inferior vena cava: a case report and review of the literature. J Surg Oncol 34:53–60, 1987.

51. Burke AP, Virmani R. Sarcomas of the great vessels. A clinicopathologic study. Cancer 71:761–773, 1993.

52. Varela-Duran J, Oliva H, Rosai J. Vascular leiomyosarcoma. The malignant counterpart of vascular leiomyoma. Cancer 44:1684–1691, 1979.

53. Demers ML, Curley SA, Romsdahl MM. Inferior vena cava leiomyosarcoma. J Surg Oncol 51:89–93, 1992.

54. Fischer MG, Gelb AM, Nussbaum M, Haveson S, Ghali V. Primary smooth muscle tumors of venous origin. Ann Surg 196:720–724, 1982.

55. Berlin O, Stener B, Kindblom LG, Angervall L. Leiomyosarcoma of venous origin in the extremities. A correlated clinical, roentgenologic, and morphologic study with diagnostic and surgical implications. Cancer 54:2147–2159, 1984.

56. Leu HJ, Makek M. Intramural venous leiomyosarcoma. Cancer 57:1395–1400, 1986.

57. Nonomura A, Kurumaya H, Kono N, Nakanuma Y, Ohta G, Terahata S, Matsubara F, Matsuda T, Asaka T, Nishino T. Primary pulmonary artery sarcoma. Report of two autopsy cases studied by immunohistochemistry and electron microscopy, and review of 110 cases reported in the literature. Acta Pathol Jpn 38:883–896, 1988.

58. Baker PB, Goodwin RA. Pulmonary artery sarcomas. A review and report of a case. Arch Pathol Lab Med 109:35–39, 1985.

59. Eng J, Murday AJ. Leiomyosarcoma of the pulmonary artery. Ann Thorac Surg 53:905–906, 1992.

60. Leeson MC, Malaei M, Makley JT. Leiomyosarcoma of the popliteal artery. A report of two cases. Clin Orthop Rel Res 253:225–230, 1990.

61. Zaloudek CJ, Norris HJ. Mesenchymal tumors of the uterus. In: Kurman R, ed. Blaustein's Pathology of the Female Genital Tract, 4th ed. New York: Springer-Verlag, 1994, pp. 488–501.

62. Prayson RA, Hart WR. Mitotically active leiomyomas of the uterus. Am J Clin Pathol 97:14–20, 1992.

63. Kurman RJ, Norris HJ. Mesenchymal tumors of the uterus: VI. Epithelioid smooth muscle tumors including leiomyoblastoma and clear cell leiomyoma: a clinical and pathologic analysis of 26 cases. Cancer 37:1853–1865, 1976.

64. Prayson RA, Hart WR. Pathologic considerations of uterine smooth muscle tumors. Obstet Gynecol Clin N Amer 22:637–657, 1995.

65. Daimaru Y, Kido H, Hashimoto H, Enjoji M. Benign schwannoma of the gastrointestinal tract. A clinicopathologic and immunohistochemical study. Hum Pathol 19:257–264, 1988.

66. Lauwers GY, Erlandson RA, Casper ES, Brennan MF, Woodruff JM. Gastrointestinal autonomic nerve tumors. A clinicopathological, immunohistochemical, and ultrastructural study of 12 cases. Am J Surg Pathol 17:887–897, 1993.

67. Rumessen JJ, Thuneberg L. Pacemaker cells of the gastrointestinal tract: interstitial cells of Cajal. Scand J Gastroenterol 216 (Suppl):82–94, 1996.

68. Sarlomo-Rikala M, Kovatich AJ, Barusevicius A, Miettinen M. CD117: a sensitive marker for gastrointestinal stromal tumors that is more specific than CD34. Mod Pathol 11:728–734, 1998.

69. Kindblom LG, Remotti HE, Aldenborg F, Meis-Kindblom JM. Gastrointestinal pacemaker cell tumor (GIPACT). Gastrointestinal stromal tumors show phenotypic characteristics of the interstitial cells of Cajal. Am J Pathol 152:1259–1269, 1998.

70. Sakurai S, Fukasawa T, Chong JM, Tanaka A, Fukayama M. Embryonic form of smooth muscle myosin heavy chain (Smemb/MHC-B) in gastrointestinal stromal tumor and interstitial cells of Cajal. Am J Pathol 154:23–28, 1999.

71. Maeda H, Yamagata A, Nishikawa S, Yoshinaga K, Kobayshy S, Nishi K, Nishikawa S. Requirement of *c-kit* for development of intestinal pacemaker system. Development 116:369–375, 1992.

72. Hirota S, Isozaki K, Moriyama Y, Hashimoto K, Nishida T, Ishiguro S, Kawano K, Hanada M, Kurata A, Takeda M, Tunio GM, Matsuzawa Y, Kanakura Y, Shinomura Y, Kitamura Y. Gain-of-function mutations of *c-kit* in human gastrointestinal stromal tumors. Science 279:577–580, 1998.

73. Lasota J, Jasinski M, Sarlomo-Rikala M, Miettinen M. Mutations in exon 11 of *c-kit* occur preferentially in malignant versus benign gastrointestinal stromal tumors and do not occur in leiomyomas and leiomyosarcomas. Am J Pathol 154:53–60, 1999.

74. Ueyama T, Guo KJ, Hashimoto H, Daimaru Y, Enjoji M. A clinicopathologic and immunohistochemical study of gastrointestinal stromal tumors. Cancer 69:947–955, 1992.

75. Appelman HD, Helwig EB. Gastric epithelioid leiomyoma and leiomyosarcoma (leiomyoblastoma). Cancer 38:708–728, 1976.

76. Carney JA. The triad of gastric epithelioid leiomyosarcoma, functioning extra-adrenal paraganglioma, and pulmonary chondroma. Cancer 43:374–382, 1979.

77. Golden T, Stout AP. Smooth muscle tumors of the gastrointestinal tract and retroperitoneal tissues. Surg Gynecol Obstet 73:784–810, 1941.

78. Evans HL. Smooth muscle tumors of the gastrointestinal tract. A study of 56 cases followed for a minimum of 10 years. Cancer 56:2242–2250, 1985.

79. Suster S. Gastrointestinal stromal tumors. Semin Diagn Pathol 13:297–313, 1996.

80. Suster S, Fletcher CDM. Gastrointestinal stromal tumors with prominent signet ring cell features. Mod Pathol 9:609–613, 1996.

81. Suster S, Sorace D, Moran CA. Gastrointestinal stromal tumors with prominent myxoid matrix. Clinicopathologic, immunohistochemical, and ultrastructural study of nine cases of a distinctive morphologic variant of myogenic stromal tumor. Am J Surg Pathol 19:59–70, 1995.

82. Min KW. Small intestinal stromal tumors with skeinoid fibers. Clinicopathological, immunohistochemical, and ultrastructural investigations. Am J Surg Pathol 16:145–155, 1992.

83. Ma CK, DePeralta MN, Amin MB, Linden MD, Dekovich AA, Kubus JJ, Zarbo RJ. Small intestinal stromal tumors. A clinicopathologic study of 20 cases with immunohistochemical assessment of cell differentiation and the prognostic role of proliferation antigens. Am J Clin Pathol 108:641–651, 1997.

84. Rudolph P, Gloeckner K, Parwaresch R, Harms D, Schmidt D. Immunophenotype, proliferation, DNA ploidy, and biological behavior of gastrointestinal stromal tumors: a multivariate clinicopathological study. Hum Pathol 29:791–800, 1998.

85. Pike AM, Lloyd RV, Appelman HD. Cell markers in gastrointestinal stromal tumors. Hum Pathol 19:830–834, 1988.

86. Miettinen M. Gastrointestinal stromal tumors. An immunohistochemical study of cellular differentiation. Am J Clin Pathol 89:601–610, 1988.

87. Newman PL, Wadden C, Fletcher CDM. Gastrointestinal stromal tumours: correlation of immunophenotype with clinicopathologic features. J Pathol 164:107–117, 1991.

88. Franquemont DW, Frierson HF Jr. Muscle differentiation and clinicopathologic features of gastrointestinal stromal tumors. Am J Surg Pathol 16:947–954, 1992.

89. Ma CK, Amin MB, Kintanar E, Linden MD, Zarbo RJ. Immunohistologic characterization of gastrointestinal stromal tumors: a study of 82 cases compared with 11 cases of leiomyomas. Mod Pathol 6:139–144, 1993.

90. van de Rijn M, Hendrickson MR, Rouse RV. CD34 expression by gastrointestinal tract stromal tumors. Hum Pathol 25:766–771, 1994.

91. Miettinen M, Virolainen M, Rikala MS. Gastrointestinal stromal tumors—value of CD34 antigen in their identification and separation from true leiomyomas and schwannomas. Am J Surg Pathol 19:207–216, 1995.

92. Goldblum JR, Appelman HD. Stromal tumors of the duodenum. A histologic and immunohistochemical study of 20 cases. Am J Surg Pathol 19:71–80, 1995.

93. Tworek JA, Appelman HD, Singleton TP, Greenson JK. Stromal tumors of the jejunum and ileum. Mod Pathol 10:200–209, 1997.

94. Brainard JA, Goldblum JR. Stromal tumors of the jejunum and ileum. A clinicopathologic study of 39 cases. Am J Surg Pathol 21:407–416, 1997.

95. Franquemont DW. Differentiation and risk assessment of gastrointestinal stromal tumors. Am J Clin Pathol 103:41–47, 1995.

96. Cunningham RE, Federspiel BH, McCarthy WF, Sobin LH, O'Leary TJ. Predicting prognosis of gastrointestinal smooth muscle tumors, role of clinical and histologic evaluation, flow cytometry, and image cytometry. Am J Surg Pathol 17:588–594, 1993.

97. Cooper PN, Quirke P, Hardy GJ, Dixon MF. A flow cytometric, clinical, and histological study of stromal neoplasms of the gastrointestinal tract. Am J Surg Pathol 16:163–170, 1992.

98. Yu CC-W, Fletcher CDM, Newman PL, Goodlad JR, Burton JC, Levison DA. A comparison of proliferating cell nuclear antigen (PCNA) immunostaining, nucleolar organizer region (AgNOR) staining, and histological grading in gastrointestinal stromal tumors. J Pathol 166:147–152, 1992.

99. Amin MB, Ma CK, Linden MD, Kubus JJ, Zarbo RJ. Prognostic value of proliferating cell nuclear antigen index in gastric stromal tumors. Correlation with mitotic count and clincal outcome. Am J Clin Pathol 100:428–432, 1993.

100. Emory TS, Sobin LH, Lukes L, Lee DH, O'Leary TJ. Prognosis of gastrointestinal smooth-muscle (stromal) tumors. Dependence on anatomic site. Am J Surg Pathol 23:82–87, 1999.

101. Taubert HD, Wissner SE, Haskins AL. Leiomyomatosis peritonealis disseminata: an unusual complication of genital leiomyomata. Obstet Gynecol 25:561–574, 1965.

102. Valente PT. Leiomyomatosis peritonealis disseminata. A report of two cases and review of the literature. Arch Pathol Lab Med 108:669–772, 1984.

103. Tavassoli FA, Norris HJ. Peritoneal leiomyomatosis (leiomyomatosis peritonealis disseminata): a clinicopathologic study of 20 cases with ultrastructural observation. Int J Gynecol Pathol 1:59–74, 1982.

104. Willson JR, Peale RA. Multiple peritoneal leiomyomas associated with a granulosa cell tumor of the ovary. Am J Obstet Gynecol 64:204–208, 1952.

105. Kuo T, London SN, Dinh TV. Endometriosis occurring in leiomyomatosis peritonealis disseminata: ultrastructural study and histogenetic consideration. Am J Surg Pathol 4:197–204, 1980.

106. Due W, Pickartz H. Immunohistologic detection of estrogen and progesterone receptors in disseminated peritoneal leiomyomatosis. Int J Gynecol Pathol 8:46–53, 1989.

107. Parmley TH, Woodruff JD, Winn K, Johnson JWC, Douglas PH. Histogenesis of leiomyomatosis peritonealis disseminata (disseminated fibrosing deciduosis). Obstet Gynecol 46:511–516, 1975.

108. Fujii S, Nakashima N, Okamura H, Takenaka A, Kanzaki H, Okuda Y, Morimoto K, Nishimura T. Progesterone-induced smooth muscle-like cells in the subperitoneal nodules produced by estrogen. Experimental approach to leiomyomatosis peritonealis disseminata. Am J Obstet Gynecol 139:164–172, 1981.

109. Quade BJ, McLachlin CM, Soto-Wright V, Zuckerman J, Mutter GL, Morton CC. Disseminated peritoneal leiomyomatosis. Clonality analysis by X chromosome inactivation and cytogenetics of a clinically benign smooth muscle proliferation. Am J Pathol 150:2153–2166, 1997.

110. Hales HA, Peterson M, Jones KP, Quinn JD. Leiomyomatosis peritonealis disseminata treated with a gonadotropin-releasing hormone agonist. A case report. Am J Obstet Gynecol 167:515–516, 1992.

111. Akkersdijk GJM, Flu PK, Giard RWM, van Lent M, Wallenburg HCS. Malignant leiomyomatosis peritonealis disseminata. Am J Obstet Gynecol 163:591–593, 1990.

112. Raspagliesi F, Quattrone P, Grosso G, Cobellis L, Di Re E. Malignant degeneration in leiomyomatosis peritonealis disseminata. Gynecol Oncol 61:272–274, 1996.

113. Rubin SC, Wheeler JE, Mikuta JJ. Malignant leiomyomatosis peritonealis disseminata. Obstet Gynecol 68:126–129, 1986.

114. Clement PB. Intravenous leiomyomatosis of the uterus. Pathol Annu 23:153–183, 1988.

115. Norris HJ, Parmley T. Mesenchymal tumors of the uterus. V. Intravenous leiomyomatosis. A clinical and pathologic study of 14 cases. Cancer 36:2164–2178, 1975.

116. Harper RS, Scully RE. Intravenous leiomyomatosis of the uterus. A report of four cases. Obstet Gynecol 18:519–529, 1961.

117. Nogales FF, Navarro N, de Victoria JMM, Contreras F, Redondo C, Herraiz MA, Seco MA, Velasco A. Uterine intravascular leiomyomatosis: an update and report of seven cases. Int J Gynecol Pathol 6:331–339, 1987.

118. Mulvaney NJ, Slavin JL, Ostor AG, Fortune DW. Intravenous leiomyomatosis of the uterus: a clinicopathologic study of 22 cases. Int J Gynecol Pathol 13:1–9, 1994.

119. Clement PB, Young RH, Scully RE. Intravenous leiomyomatosis of the uterus. A clinicopathological analysis of 16 cases with unusual histologic features. Am J Surg Pathol 12:932–945, 1988.

120. Konrad P, Mellblom L. Intravenous leiomyomatosis. Acta Obstet Gynecol Scand 68:371–376, 1989.

121. Parenti DJ, Morley TF, Giudice JC. Benign metastasizing leiomyoma. A case report and review of the literature. Respiration 56:347–350, 1992.

122. Abell MR, Littler ER. Benign metastasizing uterine leiomyoma. Multiple lymph nodal metastases. Cancer 36:2206–2213, 1975.

123. Cramer SF, Meyer JS, Kraner JF, Camel M, Mazur MT, Tenenbaum MS. Metastasizing leiomyoma of the uterus. S-phase fraction, estrogen receptor, and ultrastructure. Cancer 45:932–937, 1980.

124. Cho KR, Woodruff JD, Epstein JI. Leiomyoma of the uterus with multiple extrauterine smooth muscle tumors: a case report suggesting multifocal origin. Hum Pathol 20:80–83, 1989.

125. Horstmann JP, Pietra GG, Harman JA, Cole NG, Grinspan S. Spontaneous regression of pulmonary leiomyomas during pregnancy. Cancer 39:314–321, 1977.

126. Wolff M, Kaye G, Silva F. Pulmonary metastases (with admixed epithelial elements) from smooth muscle neoplasms. Report of nine cases, including three males. Am J Surg Pathol 3:325–342, 1979.

127. Banner AS, Carrington CB, Emory WB, Kittle F, Leonard G, Ringus J, Taylor P, Addington WW. Efficacy of oophorectomy in lymphangioleiomyomatosis and benign metastasizing leiomyoma. N Engl J Med 305:204–209, 1981.

128. Hague WM, Abdulwahid NA, Jacobs HS, Craft I. Use of LHRH analogue to obtain reversible castration in a patient with benign metastasizing leiomyoma. Br J Obstet Gynaecol 93:455–460, 1986.

129. Canzonieri M, D'Amore ESG, Bartoloni G, Piazza M, Blandamura S, Carbonne A. Leiomyomatosis with vascular invasion. A unified pathogenesis regarding leiomyoma with vascular invasion, benign metastasizing leiomyoma, and intravenous leiomyomatosis. Virchows Arch 425:541–545, 1994.

130. Winkler TR, Burr LH, Robinson CLN. Benign metastasizing leiomyoma. Ann Thorac Surg 43:100–101, 1987.

131. Evans AJ, Wiltshaw E, Kochanowski SJ, MacFarlane A, Sears RT. Merastasizing leiomyoma of the uterus and hormonal manipulations. Case report. Br J Obstet Gynaecol 93:646–648, 1986.

132. Chadwick EG, Connor EJ, Hanson ICG, Joshi VV, Abu-Farsakh H, Yogev R, McSherry G, McClain K, Murphy SB. Tumors of smooth muscle origin in HIV-infected children. JAMA 263:3182–3184, 1990.

133. Van Hoeven KH, Factor SM, Kress Y, Woodruff JM. Visceral myogenic tumors. A manifestation of HIV infection in children. Am J Surg Pathol 17:1176–1181, 1993.

134. Zetler PJ, Filipenko JD, Bilbey JH, Schmidt N. Primary adrenal leiomyosarcoma in a man with acquired immune deficiency syndrome (AIDS). Further evidence for an increase in smooth muscle tumors related to Epstein-Barr infection in AIDS. Arch Pathol Lab Med 119:1164–1167, 1995.

135. Dugan MC. Primary adrenal leiomyosarcoma in acquired immunodeficiency syndrome. Arch Pathol Lab Med 120:797–798, 1996.

136. Ross JS, Del Rosario A, Bui HX, Sonbati H, Solis O. Primary hepatic leiomyosarcoma in a child with the acquired immunodeficiency syndrome. Hum Pathol 23:69–72, 1992.

137. McCain KL, Leach CT, Jenson HB, Joshi VV, Pollock BH, Parmley RT, DiCarlo FJ, Chadwick EG, Murphy SB. Association of Epstein-Barr virus with leiomyosarcomas in young people with AIDS. N Engl J Med 332:12–18, 1995.

138. Timmons CF, Dawson DB, Richards CS, Andrews WS, Katz JA. Epstein-Barr virus–associated leiomyosarcomas in liver transplantation recipients. Origin from either donor or recipient tissue. Cancer 76:1481–1489, 1995.

139. Lee ES, Locker J, Nalesnick M, Reyes J, Jaffe R, Alashari M, Nour B, Tzakis A, Dickman PS. The association of Epstein-Barr virus with smooth muscle tumors occurring after organ transplantation. N Engl J Med 332:19–25, 1995.

140. Leibowitz D. Epstein-Barr virus—an old dog with new tricks. N Engl J Med 332:55–57, 1995.

141. Cesarman E, Knowles DM. Kaposi's sarcoma-associated herpesvirus: a lympho-tropic human herpesvirus associated with Kaposi's sarcoma, primary effusion lym-phoma, and multicentric Castleman's disease. Semin Diagn Pathol 14:54–66, 1997.
142. Russell Jones R, Orchard G, Zelger B, Wilson Jones E. Immunostaining for CD31 and CD34 in Kaposi sarcoma. J Clin Pathol 48:1011–1016, 1995.
143. Chen KT. Mycobacterial spindle cell pseudotumor of lymph nodes. Am J Surg Pathol 16:276–281, 1992.
144. Umlas J, Federman M, Crawford C, O'Hara CJ, Fitzgibbon JS, Modeste A. Spindle cell pseudotumor due to mycobacterium avium-intracellulare in patients with ac-quired immunodeficiency syndrome (AIDS). Positive staining of mycobacteria for cytoskeleton filaments. Am J Surg Pathol 15:1181–1187, 1991.

11
Adult Skeletal Muscle Tumors

Phyllis R. Vezza
Our Lady of Fatima Hospital
North Providence, Rhode Island

Katherine E. Wolfe
Georgetown University Medical Center
Washington, DC

Pedram Argani
The Johns Hopkins Hospital and
The Johns Hopkins University
Baltimore, Maryland

I. INTRODUCTION

When soft-tissue tumors are considered in total, benign lesions outnumber malignant ones by a margin of more than 100 to 1 (1). The distribution is reversed, however, among skeletal muscle tumors, where malignant rhabdomyosarcoma (RMS) is 50-fold more common than benign rhabdomyoma. Most RMSs occur in the pediatric population, in which it is the most common soft-tissue sarcoma of children younger than 15 years. Hence, skeletal muscle tumors are quite uncommon in adults, limited to a small group of rhabdomyosarcomas and the rare rhabdomyomas. This chapter will delineate the clinicopathologic features of these lesions.

II. RHABDOMYOMA

Rhabdomyomas can be classified as follows:

1. Cardiac rhabdomyoma
2. Extracardiac rhabdomyoma
   a. Adult rhabdomyoma (AR)

   b.   Fetal rhabdomyoma (FR)
        (i)   Classic type
        (ii)   Intermediate type
   c.   Genital rhabdomyoma

This classification is not absolute in that there are isolated reports of tumors with composite features. These include tumors with features of both classic FR and AR (2,3), tumors with features of both classic and intermediate FR (4), and a cardiac rhabdomyoma with the histologic appearance of an AR (5). In addition, some have considered genital rhabdomyomas a subtype of fetal classic rhabdomyoma (6). Nonetheless, the majority of rhabdomyomas fall within one of these categories, so the classification has proven to be useful.

Historical Review

The term "rhabdomyoma" was first introduced by Zenker in 1864 (7). Pendl later described a case of rhabdomyoma arising in a male infant in 1897 (8). The sub-classification of rhabdomyomas, however, would have to wait for approximately 70 years. In the 1967 AFIP Soft Tissue Tumors fascicle, Stout and Lattes illustrated the histologic difference between FR and AR (9), but the first detailed description of the fetal type was by Dehner, Enzinger, and Font in 1972 (10). In 1980, diSant'Agnese and Knowles recognized the distinctive morphology and clinical presentation of the cellular variant of FR (6). Two years later, Konrad distinguished between FR and genital rhabdomyoma (11).

A.   Cardiac Rhabdomyoma

Although cardiac rhabdomyomas are the most common of all rhabdomyomas, they present almost exclusively in children. As their presentation only rarely involves adults (12), our discussion of them will be brief. These are not neoplastic but instead are considered hamartomatous lesions, and between 51% and 86% of cases are associated with tuberous sclerosis syndrome (13,14). This syndrome is characterized by a collection of hamartomatous lesions, including brain malformations, renal angiomyolipoma, epidermal nevi, and facial angiofibroma. Cardiac rhabdomyomas associated with the syndrome are congenital and frequently multiple. They often regress (15,16) but can cause life-threatening ventricular outflow obstruction and arrhythmias (12). Hence, surgery is indicated for symptomatic lesions, whereas clinical observation is indicated for the rest (17,18).

      These lesions most commonly involve the ventricle, and range from multiple microscopic lesions that are inapparent on gross examination (19) to larger solitary lesions measuring up to 9 cm. Microscopically, they are well demarcated and composed of uniformly vacuolated clear cells. Many contain a central vesicular nucleus from which radiate thin strands of pink cytoplasm extending to the cell membrane, separated by large cytoplasmic vacuoles; these are called "spider cells." The vacuolization is created by cytoplasmic glycogen, which can be demonstrated by positivity on periodic acid–Schiff (PAS) stains that disappears with diastase pretreatment. The cells have a myogenic immunophenotype, as they stain for desmin, actin, and myoglobin. Ultrastructurally, they demonstrate features of altered cardiac myocytes containing myofibrils, Z bands, and intercalated disks. Large pools of β-glycogen particles fill the cytoplasm.

B. Adult Rhabdomyoma

1. Clinical Features

Fewer than 100 cases of AR are reported in the literature (1). The mean age at the time of diagnosis is appoximately 50 years (7), with the reported age at presentation ranging from 2 to 82 years (20,21). The male-to-female ratio is approximately 4:1. Over 90% of all ARs occur in the head and neck region (6). The most common locations are the oropharyngeal cavity (base of the tongue, palate, floor of the mouth) and the larynx (22–27). The submandibular region (28) and soft tissues of the neck are also common sites of occurrence. Rare cases have been reported in the orbit (29), trigeminal nerve (20), and parotid gland (11). There are isolated reports of AR occurring outside of the head and neck region in such sites as stomach (30), mediastinum (31), heart (5), and prostate (32).

The most common presentation of AR is that of a unicentric mass that has been growing slowly over many years. One case involving the sternohyoid muscle was present for at least 55 years, eventually growing to a length of 10 cm (33). ARs have occasionally been discovered incidentally during surgery or at autopsy. When tumors grow submucosally, they may form polypoid lesions that obstruct the upper aerodigestive tract, leading to such symptoms as progressive hoarseness, dysphagia, foreign-body sensation, or dyspnea with stridor (22). Only rare tumors are truly multicentric, though approximately 25% are composed of multiple grossly contiguous nodules (see below). Spontaneous regression has not been documented.

2. Gross Features

ARs are usually encapsulated, well-circumscribed, unifocal lesions. Approximately 25% of tumors are grossly multinodular (34). The median size is 3 cm, with reported sizes ranging from 0.5 to 10 cm (1). The cut surface is typically uniform, tan–brown, and rubbery. Necrosis is absent, though the surface of polypoid submucosal tumors can undergo erosion (22).

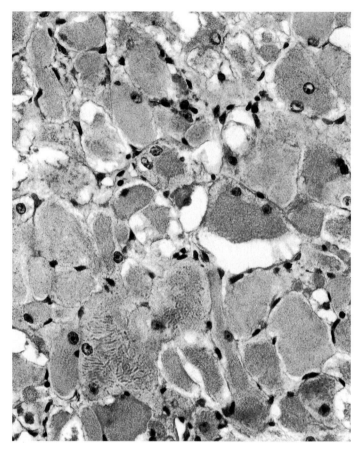

FIG. 1 Adult rhabdomyoma. Note the large, polygonal cells and the dense eosinophilic cytoplasm.

3. Microscopic Features

Histologically, these lesions have a lobular architecture and characteristically contain closely packed large polygonal cells with abundant eosinophilic granular cytoplasm, and usually peripherally placed nuclei (Fig. 1). The deeply eosinophilic cytoplasm of the cells reflects their prominent myofibril content, which is concordant with their differentiated skeletal muscle nature. However, since the myofibrils are typically haphazardly oriented, cross-striations are only occasionally evident through the light microscope, and typically within scattered elongated "strap" cells. A consistent feature is the presence of haphazardly arranged, rod-like, intracytoplasmic crystals. These structures, termed "match stick" or "jack-straw" crystals, actually represent clusters of randomly oriented, elongated, hypertrophic Z bands. Both cross-striations and jack-straw crystals are readily highlighted with phosphotungstic acid–hematoxylin (PTAH) stain. Cytoplasmic vacuoles containing variable amounts of glycogen and lipid can be identified, though only few cells will show enough vacuolization to produce the spider cell morphology typical of cardiac rhabdomyomas. Glycogen can be demonstrated by showing granular staining with PAS that disappears upon pretreatment with diastase, whereas lipid can be demonstrated using oil red O stains. Nuclei are usually small and round, with vesicular chromatin and variably prominent nucleoli. Intranuclear inclusions are occasionally identified. Variations in cell size can occur, with larger cells ranging up to 150 μm in diameter and containing two or three peripherally located nuclei (11). The stromal background is scant, consisting of delicate bands of collagen and small blood vessels. Mitotic figures, necrosis, and significant nuclear atypia are not characteristic of these lesions and should suggest alternative diagnoses.

4. Ancillary Studies

Immunohistochemical staining is useful for confirming the presence of myogenic differentiation, which helps exclude other lesions in the histologic differential diagnosis of AR. Desmin, muscle-specific actin, and myoglobin stains are usually strongly positive. Cytokeratin, epithelial membrane antigen, glial fibrillary acidic protein (GFAP), CD68, and leukocyte common antigen stains are consistently negative. Variable results have also been obtained with S-100 protein, Leu-7, and vimentin. Of interest, several antigens that are normally restricted to fetal muscle have been detected in AR. These include fetal myosin (35) and CD56 (neural cell adhesion molecule) (36), which is expressed strongly in fetal muscle at 18 weeks gestation but weakly at 35 weeks. In addition, focal staining for α-smooth muscle actin, which is postulated to be transiently expressed in fetal skeletal muscle development (37), has been documented in AR (34). These findings indicate that AR may in fact be less differentiated than their appearance would suggest.

Electron microscopy shows the characteristic features of skeletal muscle differentiation, specifically the presence of alternating thick (135–150 nm diameter, or myosin) and thin (50–70 nm diameter, or actin) myofilaments. Hypertrophied Z bands are prominent and easily discernible, correlating with the abnormal rod-like crystalline structures (jack straws) that are visible by light microscopy. These hypertrophied structures resemble the structurally modified Z disks characteristic of the rod myopathies, such as congenital nemaline myopathy (38). Numerous mitochondria of variable morphologies are typically present. Some are swollen, elongated, and contain lamellar and crystalline inclusions, whereas others contain electron-dense material in their cristae (11). Variable collections of glycogen and occasionally lipid are easily recognized. The small nuclei may contain intranuclear inclusions (11). A thin, continuous basement membrane surrounds each tumor cell. Intercellular junctions are absent (7).

5.   Histogenesis

In their textbook, Enzinger and Weiss point out the remarkable fact that there is no record of an AR arising in the musculature of the limbs, where skeletal muscle is so abundant. The predilection for the head and neck may relate to the fact that the skeletal muscle in this area is distinct embryologically; it is derived from the third and fourth branchial arches, unlike the peripheral musculature, which is derived from myotomes (1). The nature of ARs is unclear. While the name suggests that they are benign neoplasms, most believe that they represent degenerative (39) or malformative (hamartomatous or choristomatous) (20) lesions. However, the theory that they represent neoplasms was recently supported by a report of a single case that comprised a clonal cytogenetic abnormality. In this report, the tissue sent for karyotyping was from the second recurrence of a parapharyngeal rhabdomyoma. A reciprocal translocation, t(15;17)(q24;p13), was detected in 60% of evaluated metaphases. A minor clone was also characterized involving the long arm of chromosome 10 (36). If clonality is equated with neoplasia, this report suggests that at least some ARs are neoplastic. Further cytogenetic analyses of AR (particularly primary tumors) and/or molecular analyses of clonality will be needed to confirm this hypothesis.

6.   Treatment and Prognosis

ARs are invariably benign, as complete excision is thought to be curative and metastases have never been reported. However, like other benign lesions, ARs can recur if incompletely excised. The recurrence rate has ranged from 16% to 42% of cases (34,36). It is not entirely clear if the multinodular tumors tend to recur more often (34,40). Recurrence may be seen after many years due to the extremely slow growth rate; one reported case recurred 35 years after the original excision (31).

7.   Differential Diagnosis

The differential diagnosis for AR centers on other lesions composed of large pink polygonal cells that occur in the head and neck area. These include granular cell tumors, alveolar soft-part sarcoma (ASPS), hibernoma, the recently described crystal-storing histiocytosis, paraganglioma, and rhabdomyosarcoma.

    Granular cell tumors (Abrikossoff's tumor) were originally thought to be of myogenic origin and hence were termed *granular cell myoblastoma*. They are now thought to show Schwann cell differentiation, and many are intimately associated with small peripheral nerves. Like AR, these tumors consist of nests of round to polygonal cells with an eosinophilic granular cytoplasm and small nuclei. However, the cytoplasmic granularity corresponds not to myofilaments but to the accumulation of secondary lysosomes containing lipid breakdown products (38). This accounts for their granular PAS positivity that resists diastase treatment, in contrast to the glycogen of rhabdomyomas, which is diastase-sensitive. No cross-striations are appreciated. The cells stain uniformly for S-100 protein, as is consistent with schwannian differentiation, and CD68, which indicates the presence of lysosomes. They are negative for myogenic markers such as desmin and muscle-specific actin. Granular cell tumors are classically associated with pseudoepitheliomatous hyperplasia of their overlying mucosa, whereas the epithelium most often associated with polypoid submucosal ARs is atrophic.

ASPS is a rare malignant tumor of uncertain histogenesis. The head and neck is a common location, particularly in children. These tumors often grow exceedingly slowly, which belies their malignant nature. Like ARs, ASPS consists of large eosinophilic cells, and approximately 50% of cases can stain for desmin, albeit focally. However, the architecture of ASPS is distinctive. The tumor cells are arranged in nests separated by thin capillary septa, with central degeneration of tumor cells creating an alveolar pattern. PAS staining reveals diagnostic diastase-resistant crystalloid rods that correspond ultrastructurally to membrane-bound filamentous crystals. Many patients show vascular invasion and present with lung metastases, which are never seen in ARs.

Hibernomas are tumors of brown fat typically found in the axilla, neck, or scapular region of patients under 40 years of age. They are composed of adipocytes with discrete borders and a granular or finely vacuolated eosinophilic cytoplasm. These vacuoles contain lipid and lipofuscin pigment. The cells are generally smaller than those of ARs, have a less densely eosinophilic cytoplasm, and do not express muscle markers immunohistochemically.

Kapadia et al. (41) have reported three cases of crystal-storing histiocytosis associated with lymphoplasmacytic lymphoma that were initially mistaken for AR. These lesions result from the accumulation of phagocytosed crystalline monoclonal immunoglobulin within the cytoplasm of the histiocytes, resulting in enlarged cells with granular pink cytoplasm. Parallel arrays of these proteins can mimic cross-striations, but true cross-striations do not occur. The presence of an adjacent atypical lymphoplasmacytic infiltrate (often with Dutcher bodies) is the best clue as to the nature of this process (Fig. 2). Immunohistochemical stains also are distinctive, showing positivity for CD68 and negativity for all myogenic markers.

Paragangliomas are common in the head and neck region, have a nested architecture, and often have abundant granular cytoplasm that raises the differential diagnosis of AR. Immunohistochemical stains can readily make this distinction. Paragangliomas are negative for muscle markers and instead stain for neuroendocrine markers such as chromogranin, synaptophysin, and neuron-specific eno-

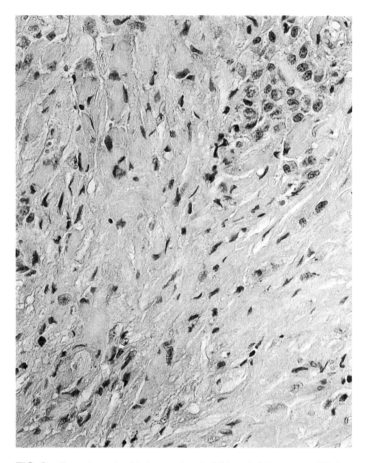

FIG. 2 Crystal-storing histiocytosis mimicking rhabdomyoma. Histiocytes bearing dense cytoplasmic crystalline inclusions mimic skeletal muscle cells. A cluster of neoplastic plasma cells is present at the upper right.

lase. The presence of an S-100 protein–positive population of sustentacular cells surrounding the nests is characteristic of paraganglioma.

Rhabdomyosarcoma must be included in the differential diagnosis of any lesion showing skeletal muscle differentiation, given the comparative infrequency of benign skeletal muscle lesions. Given the typical adult age at presentation and differentiated appearance of AR, pleomorphic rhabdomyosarcoma would be the major consideration. The absence of mitoses, necrosis, and pleomorphism in AR usually makes this distinction readily apparent. Another cause for confusion on morphologic grounds is the occasional case of treated embryonal rhabdomyosarcoma, in which chemotherapy seems to obliterate the actively dividing tumor cells and to effect differentiation in the remainder, leading to a differentiated rhabdo-myomatous appearance (42). Attention to the younger age of the patient and the clinical history of therapy can avoid this potential pitfall.

C. Fetal Rhabdomyoma

FRs are even rarer than ARs. They are so named because their histopathology re-capitulates the normal histology of developing fetal skeletal muscle. As such, they pose significant potential for confusion with rhabdomyosarcoma. Like ARs, these tumors occur most commonly in the head and neck region. An association with the basal cell nevus syndrome, which includes odontogenic keratocysts of the jaw, rib abnormalities, and macrocephaly in addition to the predisposition to basal cell carcinoma and other neoplasms, has been described (1,43–47). FRs are often di-vided into two types: the classic (or *myxoid*) type and the intermediate (also known as *cellular* or *juvenile*) type. As mentioned above, this distinction is not absolute, since some tumors show overlapping morphologic features. Because their mor-phology and their clinical presentation is somewhat distinct, we will discuss these features separately. As their characteristics on ancillary studies and their differen-tial diagnosis are essentially the same, these aspects will be discussed together.

Classic Type

1. Clinical Features

The classic FR has a predilection for children younger than 1 year, though the re-ported age spectrum ranges from birth to 59 years (48). The male-to-female ratio is approximately 3:1. While the head and neck is the favored site, rare cases have involved the chest wall (6), abdominal wall (11), and retroperitoneum (45). Within the head and neck region, they specifically target the periauricular region. The usual presentation is that of a slowly growing mass. Up to 25% are congenital (4).

2. Gross Features

Classic FRs are unencapsulated but well-demarcated, noninfiltrative lesions (Fig. 3). The usual size range is 2–6 cm, with reported sizes ranging up to 12.5 cm (4). They are almost always unifocal. Importantly, tumors are usually located su-perficial to the underlying musculature, often in the subcutaneous tissue or sub-mucosa. On cut section, tumors are gray, often mucoid in texture, and do not show necrosis.

3. Microscopic Features

The histopathology of classic FR resembles normal developing fetal musculature of 6–12 weeks gestation. The stroma is highly abundant and mucoid, composed of mucopolysaccharides that stain positively with Alcian blue (Fig. 4). Two cell

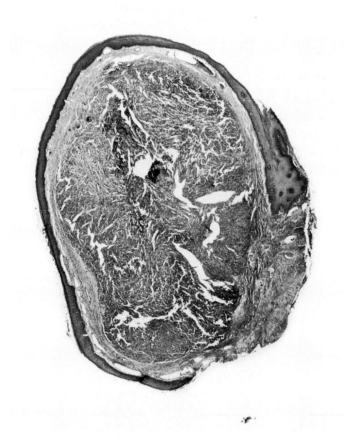

FIG. 3 Low power view of a fetal rhabdomyoma of the tongue. Note the circumscribed nature of the lesion underlying squamous mucosa.

types are loosely arranged in this matrix. First is a population of oval- to spindle-shaped primitive mesenchymal cells with indistinct cytoplasm, analogous to the primitive fibroblastic cells of developing skeletal muscle. Second is a population of immature elongated skeletal muscle fibers that resemble fetal myotubes. The latter are scattered haphazardly as single cells within the lesion, though they tend to be more abundant at its perimeter (10). They contain centrally placed oval nuclei with fine chromatin and inconspicuous nucleoli, and tapered, thin, often bipolar cell processes. The cytoplasm is pale pink and in most cases cross striations can be identified (though a thorough search is often required). Mitoses and pleomorphism are not present.

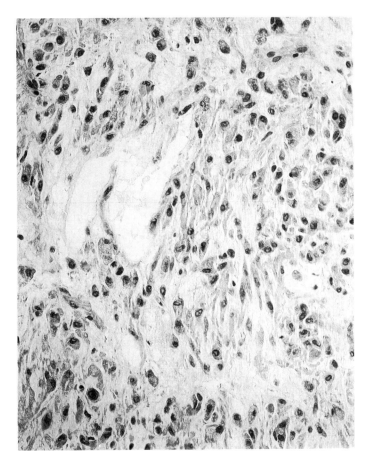

FIG. 4 Fetal rhabdomyoma, myxoid type. Note the myxoid background and the primitive appearance of the spindle cells, resembling that of fetal myotubes.

Intermediate Type

1. Clinical Features

The intermediate variant of FR also most frequently presents in the head and neck region. In contrast to the classical variant, adults are more commonly affected. The documented age range falls between 2.5 and 60 years with a male-to-female preponderance of approximately 3:1 (1,4,6,49). They also usually present as slowly growing, asymptomatic masses. While the classical FR tends to be superficially located, intermediate FRs are often found in the deep tissues of the head and neck and often are submucosal. Typical sites of occurrence include tongue (6), cheek

(49), larynx (50), and nasopharynx (4,6). Cases have also been reported in thigh (6), upper arm (51), and stomach (6).

2. Gross Features

Like the classic type, these tumors are well circumscribed but usually unencapsulated (4). Reported sizes range from 1.0 to 5.0 cm (4,6). The cut surface reveals firm light tan to gray–white tissue without hemorrhage or necrosis.

3. Microscopic Features

Intermediate FR shows a degree of rhabdomyoblastic differentiation that is greater than that of classic FR and approaches but does not reach the level of AR. Hence, it is "intermediate" in its level of differentiation. In contrast to the classic type of FR, the intermediate type shows minimal to no myxoid matrix and only scattered primitive mesenchymal cells. The lesion is dominated instead by tightly packed, elongated spindled muscle fibers (hence the alternative name *cellular*). These cells are often strap-shaped, with central vesicular nuclei with variably prominent nucleoli and deeply eosinophilic cytoplasm with frequent cross-striations (Figs. 5 and 6). They are larger than the primitive myotubes of classic FR, and the cytoplasmic and nuclear features reflect more advanced muscular differentiation. These fibers are arranged somewhat haphazardly, but often as intersecting fascicles. Occasionally, a herringbone or plexiform pattern can be appreciated. Some cells show vacuolization due to intracellular glycogen, but only rare cells are large and rounded like those of AR. Some cases may display mild pleomorphism, and occasional mitoses can be present. However, abundant mitotic figures and extreme pleomorphism are not attributes of this lesion and suggest instead the diagnosis of rhabdomyosarcoma.

4. Ancillary Features

The immunohistochemical staining pattern of FRs of both classic and intermediate types is generally similar to that of ARs. Tumors express myoglobin, desmin, and muscle-specific actin. Variable staining is reported with vimentin, S-100 protein, smooth muscle actin, and GFAP. Cytokeratin, epithelial membrane antigen, CD68, and Leu-7 are negative (4).

Electron microscopic examination of FRs reveals organized bundles of alternating thick and thin myofilaments with Z bands in the cytoplasm of the eosinophilic spindle cells, features that are characteristic of skeletal muscle differentiation. Unlike ARs, hypertrophic Z bands are an uncommon finding. FRs also contain fewer mitochondria and lack the mitochondrial inclusions that are typical of ARs (38). Glycogen is usually identified in the cytoplasm, and the cells are coated by basal lamina. The primitive mesenchymal cells identified light microscopically show no distinctive evidence of differentiation ultrastructurally.

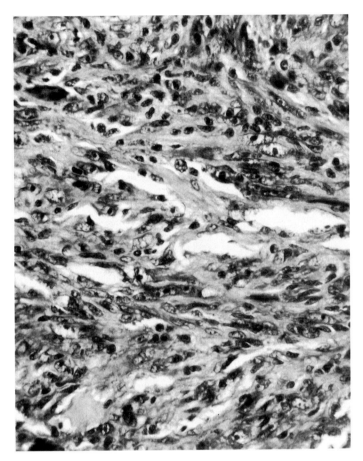

FIG. 5 Fetal rhabdomyoma, intermediate type. This cellular lesion is composed of spindle cells with prominent nucleoli, and minimal myxoid material in the background.

5. Histogenesis

FRs are postulated to be hamartomatous lesions, based on their morphologic resemblance to developing fetal skeletal muscle. Their occurrence as congenital lesions supports this concept, as does their association with the malformative basal cell nevus syndrome. Their occasional association with peripheral nerves has raised the possibility of a relationship to neuromuscular hamartoma.

6. Treatment and Prognosis

FRs are usually cured by complete excision; only rare recurrences and no metastases of well-characterized lesions have been reported (52). Their benign nature is

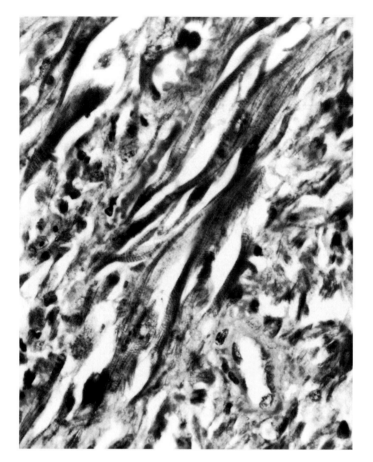

FIG. 6 Fetal rhabdomyoma. Cross-striations are evident at high power.

questioned only by isolated, somewhat controversial case reports of an association with rhabdomyosarcoma (see below).

7. Differential Diagnosis

The distinction of FR from rhabdomyosarcoma is most crucial because a misdiagnosis of rhabdomyosarcoma will trigger unnecessary and potentially harmful chemotherapy. Embryonal rhabdomyosarcoma, particularly its well-differentiated spindle cell variant, poses the main consideration. The intermediate type of FR, being more cellular and having occasional mitoses and mild pleomorphism, is more likely to cause confusion. Both architectural and cytologic features can be helpful in this differential diagnosis. In contrast to FR, rhabdomyosarcomas are usually situated deeper in the soft tissue and have an infiltrative border. While submucosal rhabdomyosarcomas may show a cambium layer, FRs do not. Cytologically, rhabdomyosarcomas show pleomorphism in the form of enlarged, hyperchromatic, angulated nuclei beyond that which is acceptable in FR. On careful examination, rhabdomyosarcomas usually show more than the scattered mitoses that are acceptable in FR. Necrosis is often present in rhabdomyosarcoma but absent in FR.

Two cases reported in the literature have raised the possibility that FR may rarely undergo malignant transformation. One patient reported by Kodet et al. (53) was an 18-month-old infant who had a lesion of the tongue resected and diagnosed as a fetal cellular rhabdomyoma, only to develop a first recurrence that was mitotically active and a second recurrence that was diagnostic of mixed embryonal/alveolar rhabdomyosarcoma. While it is possible that this was an FR that transformed into a rhabdomyosarcoma, some features of the initial tumor were not typical of cellular FR. First, the lesion had an infiltrative border, and it seems likely from the report that the surgical margins of the first two biopsies were microscopically positive. Second, the lesion presented in an infant, not the usual adult affected by cellular FR. Could this lesion have been a well-differentiated rhabdomyosarcoma from the start in which further sampling of the incompletely excised initial lesions might have shown diagnostic pleomorphism and mitoses? Given the well-known ability of spindle cell rhabdomyosarcomas to mimic benign rhabdomyoma, such a scenario seems possible. A second case, reported in Enzinger and Weiss's *Soft Tissue Tumors* (1), was that of a 3-week-old whose initial biopsy show FR but whose subsequent biopsy at 23 weeks showed rhabdomyosarcoma. Illustrations of this case were not provided. The potential for rare cases of FR to undergo malignant transformation remains unresolved at this point. Given these two reports, any case of presumed FR with atypical features should most certainly be examined carefully to exclude sarcoma. Careful clinical follow-up of such patients may be in order. Regardless, these isolated reports do not negate the fact that the usual FR behaves in a benign fashion.

Infantile fibromatosis invading normal skeletal muscle can also mimic FR, as the infiltrating lesional fibroblasts of the fibromatosis simulate the primitive cells of FR and the damaged, regenerative native skeletal muscle fibers simulate the differentiating myotube-like cells of FR. The infiltrative nature of fibromatosis, often best appreciated when it incorporates neighboring stromal elements such as adipose tissue, is the most useful distinctive feature (1). Furthermore, fibromatoses are usually more deeply situated than FR.

D. Genital Rhabdomyoma

1. Clinical Features

Genital rhabdomyomas present as slow-growing, polypoid masses in the genital tract of middle-aged women. The average age of occurrence is approximately

38 years (11,54–57). Tumors most commonly involve the vulva or vagina, but rarely have involved the cervix. Most are asymptomatic, though some lesions cause vaginal bleeding and/or dyspareunia (11,55–59). There are no reports of recurrence or malignant transformation.

2. Gross Features

Genital rhabdomyomas are polypoid lesions that usually measure less than 3 cm in diameter. They are usually covered by a smooth, intact epithelial surface. They are unencapsulated and composed of gray to pink, homogeneous, firm tissue.

3. Microscopic Features

The characteristic histology is that of scattered, highly mature skeletal muscle fibers set in an abundant hypocellular submucosal stroma. The fibers range from long, thin, spindle cells to strap cells, with dense eosinophilic cytoplasm containing easily discernible cross-striations. Neither cytoplasmic vacuoles nor crystalline inclusions are demonstrated, and mitoses are absent. The cells usually have one central round nucleus with a prominent nucleolus, but pleomorphism is not present. Nuclei are sometimes peripherally located, as is seen in mature skeletal muscle. The stroma is variably fibrous and myxoid, and contains thin-walled blood vessels (11). The overlying mucosa is intact, and subepithelial condensations of muscle fibers (cambium layer) are not present.

4. Ancillary Features

Immunohistochemically, the muscle fibers express desmin, myoglobin, actin, and myosin. Ultrastructurally, these lesions show a greater degree of myofilament organization than either AR or FR. Well-organized sarcomeric units that contain thick and thin fibers with regularly spaced Z bands are usually identified (7,38,58). This appearance is highly reminiscent of normal adult skeletal muscle and accounts for the ease with which cross-striations can usually be detected microscopically. Hypertrophic Z bands as are seen in AR are not found.

5. Histogenesis

Whether these are hamartomatous, reactive, or neoplastic lesions remains controversial. Some have not considered genital rhabdomyomas to be a distinct entity, instead classifying them as mere FRs affecting the vulvovaginal area (6). Given their site-specific occurrence, the fact that they affect a different age group and gender, and their distinctive histopathology, we favor their being distinctive.

6. Treatment and Prognosis

As with all types of rhabdomyoma, local excision is curative. Rhabdomyomas do not recur and follow a benign course.

7. Differential Diagnosis

Embryonal rhabdomyosarcoma involving the vulvovaginal area is the most crucial differential diagnostic consideration. This form of rhabdomyosarcoma characteristically undermines the native mucosa to form multiple polypoid nodules that grossly resemble a bunch of grapes; hence, the descriptive name "sarcoma botryoides." The stroma of these polyps may be largely myxoid and hypocellular, and contain only scattered rhabdomyoblasts, causing confusion with rhabdomyoma. However, both clinical and pathologic features can reliably distinguish these entities. Embryonal rhabdomyosarcoma typically occurs in younger patients; approximately 90% of patients are younger than 5 years. Rhabdomyosarcomas are often grossly larger than the usual genital rhabdomyoma and usually are more infiltrative of normal tissues. Microscopically, the cells are more primitive, mitotically active, and form subepithelial condensations (cambium layer), none of which is seen in genital rhabdomyomas.

Benign fibroepithelial stromal polyps of the vulva and vagina is the main clinical differential diagnosis. These can be seen at any age but also usually affect middle-aged women. The composition of their stroma is varied, ranging from nondescript bland spindle cells to pleomorphic multinucleated cells with pink cytoplasm that can simulate rhabdomyoblasts. However, true cross-striations are not identified. While the stromal cells are usually immunoreactive for desmin, curiously they often are nonimmunoreactive for actin stains. They also typically stain for estrogen and progesterone receptors, which may explain the association of these polyps with pregnancy (60).

III. RHABDOMYOSARCOMA

Rhabdomyosarcomas (RMSs) presenting in adults fall within two categories. The first, pleomorphic RMSs, is an entity that appears specific to adults but for which the diagnostic criteria have evolved significantly over the past 50 years. We will discuss this entity in detail following a brief historical overview. The second category is formed by the occasional presentation of pediatric (embryonal and alveolar) RMSs in adults. As these pediatric lesions are thoroughly covered in the chapter by Parham, our discussion of them will be limited to the distinctive features of their adult presentation.

A. Pleomorphic Rhabdomyosarcoma

1. Historical Review

Pleomorphic RMS was first described by Arthur Purdy Stout in 1946 as the classic form of RMS (61). In his landmark article, he described the tumor cells as those that "have some of the characteristics of rhabdomyoblasts, and which have arisen in skeletal muscle . . . or immediately adjacent to them." Pleomorphic RMS was soon after accepted as one of the more common adult pleomorphic sarcomas. In 1958, Horn and Enterline included pleomorphic RMS in their histologic classification of RMS, along with the embryonal, botryoid, and alveolar types (62). This classification was adopted in 1969 by the World Health Organization (WHO) Classification of Soft Tissue Tumors (63). The introduction of the concept of malignant fibrous histiocytoma (MFH) in the 1970s and its subsequent acceptance by pathologists as the most common pleomorphic sarcoma in adults dramatically changed the view of pleomorphic RMS. Many pleomorphic sarcomas previously accepted as pleomorphic RMS were retrospectively reclassified as MFH (64,65). Pleomorphic RMS became an extremely uncommon diagnosis, and in the 1980s several papers expressed skepticism about the existence of pleomorphic RMS (66–68).

The concept of pleomorphic RMS has recently been revisited and is slowly regaining acceptance. Reasons for this are twofold. First, the concept of MFH has come under critical review, perhaps triggered by the realization that the original concept of MFH as a histiocytic malignancy that can show fibroblastic features was wrong (69). MFH is now considered to be a pleomorphic fibrosarcoma (70); however, some pathologists had used nonspecific evidence of "histiocytic differentiation" to classify tumors as MFH (68). Other pathologists had used MFH as a wastebasket term for any pleomorphic sarcoma with a storiform pattern. On critical review, the possibility that specific entities like RMS might be hidden under the category of MFH became apparent. Second, objective ancillary techniques that can prove skeletal muscle differentiation have become available, rendering the criterion of demonstrating cross-striations by light microscopy unnecessary. These include specific immunohistochemical markers and ultrastructural findings. This section will define these criteria and the clinicopathologic features of the tumors that meet them.

2. Clinical Features

Pleomorphic RMS accounts for 5–7% of all pleomorphic adult soft-tissue sarcomas. In a recent review by Schürch examining 325 pleomorphic adult sarcomas (71), 18 (5%) pleomorphic RMS were found; the age range of this group was 28–84 years with a mean age of 61 years. Pleomorphic RMS accounted for 46% of all RMS in adulthood. In 1993, Gaffney and colleagues reported a 6.8% incidence of pleomorphic RMS following review of all the pleomorphic sarcomas at their institutions since 1980 (72). The age range in this series was 27–84 years with a mean age of 56 years. Of note, cases of pleomorphic RMS in children were not identified in either series.

Pleomorphic RMS usually arises in the large skeletal muscles of the extremities, most commonly in the thigh. Well-characterized lesions have also been reported in the retroperitoneum (71), breast (71), larynx (73), salivary gland (74), bladder (75), kidney (76), uterus (77), neck (78), and mediastinum (79). Males appear to be afflicted more frequently than females. Patients usually present with a painless but rapidly growing soft-tissue mass. Metastases to the lungs are not uncommonly seen at the time of initial presentation and reflect the aggressive nature of these tumors.

3. Gross Features

Pleomorphic RMSs are usually unicentric, large (greater than 10 cm) tumors that are centered within the deep skeletal muscle. The sizes ranged from 6 to 25 cm in one study (72). The tumors are usually well circumscribed, with a fleshy, gray-pink cut surface. Extensive necrosis is nearly universal while cystic change and focal hemorrhage is not uncommon.

4. Microscopic Features

The presence of bizarre rhabdomyoblasts featuring dense eosinophilic cytoplasm and pleomorphic vesicular nuclei with prominent nucleoli is the hallmark feature of pleomorphic RMS. These rhabdomyoblasts take on numerous shapes, most of which were described in Stout's original delineation of the entity (Fig. 7). Rounded cells feature concentrically arranged filaments surrounding a central nucleus. The strap-shaped cell is a thin spindled one containing multiple nuclei arranged in tandem. Racquet (tadpole)– shaped cells have one larger rounded end bearing the nucleus and one tapered end containing only cytoplasm (61). "Spider cells" are polygonal and vacuolated due to the presence of extensive intracellular glycogen. While these cell shapes are similar to those of the rhabdomyoblasts of embryonal RMS, their nuclei are far more pleomorphic. More nondescript cells are commonly present, including cells with hyaline intracytoplasmic inclusions simulating rhabdoid tumor, and cells with foamy cytoplasm. While these cells can be focally arranged in fascicular patterns suggestive of leiomyosarcoma (Fig. 8) or storiform patterns suggestive of MFH, the tumor cells of pleomorphic RMS are most commonly haphazardly arranged. Their stroma is most commonly fibrous, but can be focally myxoid and is frequently infiltrated by lymphocytes and histiocytes. Mitoses are typically abundant, and necrosis is always present.

While the morphologic appearances can be highly suggestive of pleomorphic RMS, the diagnosis cannot be proven on routine histology without the presence of cross-striations. However, cross-striations are infrequently found, even with use of the PTAH stain. Hence, ancillary studies are generally needed to make this diagnosis.

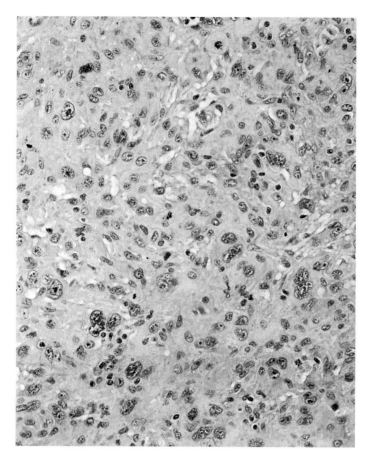

FIG. 7 Pleomorphic rhabdomyosarcoma. Large pleomorphic tumor cells with dense eosinophilic cytoplasm are haphazardly arranged.

5. Ancillary Features

Immunohistochemical stains serve several roles in the diagnosis of pleomorphic RMS. The first is to confirm the diagnosis of sarcoma and demonstrate generic muscular differentiation. Pleomorphic RMSs are almost always cytokeratin-negative and S-100 protein–negative, which helps exclude carcinoma and melanoma from the differential diagnosis and place the lesion in the pleomorphic sarcoma category. Multiple markers of muscular differentiation are available. The 53-kd muscle cell intermediate filament desmin is perhaps the most specific and reliable in paraffin-embedded tissue, and is consistently expressed in RMS

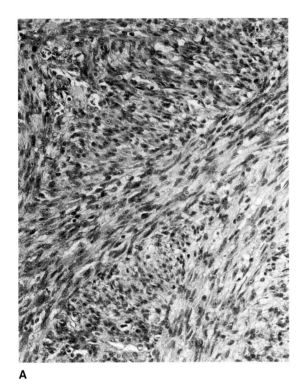

A

FIG. 8 (A) Spindle cell
rhabdomyosarcoma of
adult. This tumor grows
n an intersecting fascicular pattern usually associated with leiomyosarcoma.
(B) Immunohistochemi-
cal stain for MyoD1
demonstrates intense nu-
clear positivity, confirming the diagnosis of
rhadbomyosarcoma.

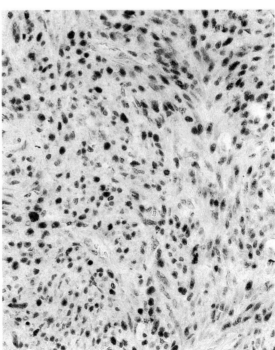

B

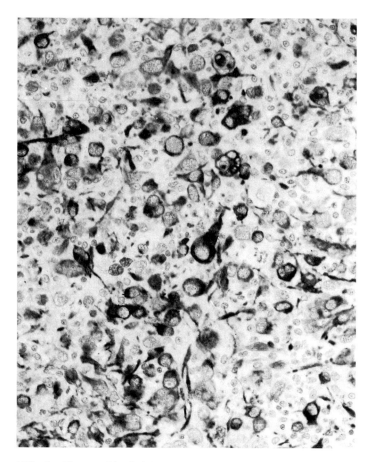

FIG. 9 Pleomorphic rhabdomyosarcoma, immunohistochemical stain for desmin. Intensely positive cells have rounded and racquet (tadpole) shapes.

(Fig. 9). Stains for muscle-specific actin (HHF35) and α-sarcomeric actin are also consistently positive. However, none of these stains is specific for skeletal muscle differentiation. Desmin is expressed in normal smooth muscle cells and myofibroblasts; not surprisingly, it is also expressed consistently in leiomyosarcomas and occasionally in MFH. Even "sarcomeric-specific" actins can stain smooth muscle and myofibroblasts, and hence lack specificity for skeletal muscle. This is not a problem in the pediatric age group, in which leiomyosarcoma and MFH are vanishingly rare. In a child, evidence of myogenic differentiation in a poorly differentiated tumor can be taken as strong evidence for the diagnosis of RMS. For adult lesions, in which high-grade leiomyosarcoma and MFH are always in the differential, proof that a lesion is an RMS requires more specific immunohisto-chemical markers.

Two categories of specific immunohistochemical markers of sarcomeric differentiation are currently available (80). Markers of the first type detect skeletal muscle–specific cytoplasmic proteins. The best characterized marker in this category is myoglobin, an oxygen-binding heme protein found in skeletal and cardiac muscles. In normal striated muscle development, myoglobin is expressed relatively late, after proteins like desmin, and its concentration increases with maturation (81,82). This pattern of expression is paralleled in RMS, in which consistent staining is present only in well-differentiated tumors that feature cells with abundant cytoplasm (83). Unfortunately, staining can be focal or completely negative in poorly differentiated tumors, and hence the sensitivity of myoglobin stains is limited. Furthermore, several pitfalls exist in the interpretation of myoglobin stains. It is well known that myoglobin is readily released by damaged skeletal muscle; this accounts for the myoglobinuria frequently experienced by trauma patients. What is less well known is that when a nonmyogenic tumor infiltrates and damages skeletal muscle, the infiltrating tumor cells can take up released myoglobin, leading to false-positive myoglobin staining (84). In addition, the currently available antisera to this marker are somewhat challenging to optimize for paraffinized tissue. All of the above make the interpretation of stains for myoglobin challenging.

The other category of marker of skeletal muscle differentiation is the family of myogenic transcription factors (85). These include MyoD1, myogenin, myf-5, and mrf-4 (herculin). MyoD1 is perhaps the best characterized of these markers. MyoD1 is a 45-kd nuclear phosphoprotein that mediates the commitment of primitive mesenchymal cells to the skeletal muscle phenotype. By binding to their enhancer regions, MyoD1 is thought to transactivate genes for muscle structural proteins such as desmin, myosin, and actin (86). Antibodies to MyoD1 have shown great utility in the diagnosis of primitive pediatric RMS (87). Several studies have demonstrated the usefulness of this antigen in diagnosing RMS in adults (85,88). It appears to be extremely sensitive and specific, and is complimentary to myoglobin in that it stains less differentiated cells reliably (Fig. 8B). Like anti-myoglobin antibodies, however, the antisera against MyoD1 have been somewhat challenging to apply to paraffinized tissue. Care must be taken to accept only nuclear staining as positive, as cytoplasmic staining has been documented in other tumors like alveolar soft-part sarcoma (86,89). The development of new monoclonal antibodies to MyoD1 and the use of heat-induced antigen retrieval methods holds promise for making this stain more easily applicable in everyday practice. Newer antibodies to myogenin are proving to be easily applicable and highly effective in the diagnosis of pediatric-type RMS (87,90). The utility of these antibodies in the diagnosis of pleomorphic RMS has yet to be determined and will require further study.

Despite all of the caveats, however, convincing staining for either MyoD1 or myoglobin is excellent specific evidence of skeletal muscle differentiation. In a tumor with a compatible morphologic appearance and staining for other reliable muscle markers like desmin, myoglobin or MyoD1 immunoreactivity is generally considered sufficient evidence to render the diagnosis of pleomorphic RMS.

Electron microscopy is the other tool that can confirm the diagnosis of pleomorphic RMS. Alternating thick (15-nm) and thin (6-nm) filaments and Z disks are usually identified in more differentiated rhabdomyoblasts but may not be seen in poorly differentiated tumors. With this in mind, Erlandson sought the minimal ultrastructural criterion for the diagnosis of RMS (91) and defined it as ribosome/myosin complexes. These consist of parallel bundles of rigid, thick, 15-nm myosin filaments associated with ribosomes arranged in single file. These structures are identical to those found in the earliest stages of normal myofibrillogenesis (91). It is significant that myosin/ribosome complexes generally form before immunoreactivity for markers like desmin (which coincides temporally with the formation of Z disks) can be demonstrated. Hence, electron microscopy can be more sensitive than immunohistochemistry for detecting muscle differentiation in some cases. However, sampling error can limit the sensitivity of ultrastructural analysis.

6. Histogenesis

The predominance of pleomorphic RMS in the extremities would perhaps suggest that this tumor originates from the skeletal muscle that is so abundant there. However, this theory cannot account for the existence of this tumor in such sites as uterus and kidney, which are normally devoid of skeletal muscle. Instead, pleomorphic RMS, like other RMS, is thought to arise from primitive mesenchymal cells in a variety of sites that differentiate along rhabdomyoblastic lines.

7. Treatment and Prognosis

This variant of RMS is a high-grade sarcoma with an extremely poor prognosis. It has a rapid growth rate and there is a high incidence of regional and distant metastases at initial diagnosis. Most metastases involve the regional lymph nodes, lungs, or brain. In two recent studies that used strict criteria for diagnosis of pleomorphic RMS, the poor prognosis of this tumor was substantiated (71,72). In Gaffney's study of 11 pleomorphic RMS, 7 of 8 patients with follow-up had died within 2–28 months of diagnosis. In 2 of these patients, the cause of death was not determined, but 5 patients died of widespread disease (72). In Schürch's study of 18 patients pleomorphic RMS, 8 of 15 with follow-up died with either local recurrance or distant metastasis (71). Several authors feel that the prognosis of RMS is appreciably worse than that of other pleomorphic sarcomas and that this justifies the special studies needed to distinguish them. Combined treatments of surgical resection, chemotherapy, and radiation treatments have been utilized.

8. Differential Diagnosis

The differential diagnosis of pleomorphic RMS is extremely broad. Once mimics of neoplasia, such as regenerating skeletal muscle (92) and myositis, are eliminated, the differential diagnosis comes down to that of pleomorphic malignant neoplasms. Carcinomas and melanomas are numerically far more common than sarcomas and merit serious consideration in each case. Negativity for cytokeratins and S-100 protein excludes these entities. The potential for anaplastic large-cell lymphoma to present as a soft-tissue mass is being recognized, and this entity should also be considered particularly given the radical difference in its therapy. Negativity for CD30 and ALK1 antibodies is helpful here. As alluded to above, other pleomorphic sarcomas, such as MFH, pleomorphic liposarcoma, and pleomorphic leiomyosarcoma, can be virtually indistinguishable from pleomorphic RMS on light microscopy. While MFH and pleomorphic leiomyosarcoma typically feature storiform and fascicular patterns, respectively, compared with the usual nondescript patterns of RMS, these features are not uniform. The presence of pleomorphic lipoblasts characterizes liposarcoma, but nonspecific vacuolization can occur in any anaplastic cell. Since the morphologic features can overlap, ancillary studies (myoglobin or MyoD1 immunostaining or electron microscopy) are generally needed to prove sarcomeric differentiation.

Once a malignant tumor has been shown to demonstrate rhabdomyoblastic differentiation, other entities must be excluded before the diagnosis of pleomorphic RMS can be accepted. Heterologous rhabdomyosarcomatous differentiation occurs in a broad range of neoplasms, many of which are more common than RMS. These include carcinosarcomas from a variety of sites, malignant mixed mullerian tumor of the uterus and ovary, ovarian Sertoli-Leydig cell tumor, malignant peripheral nerve sheath tumor (malignant Triton tumor), malignant ectomesenchymoma (containing ganglion cells and neuroblasts), malignant mesenchymoma (containing liposarcomatous or osteoid/cartilagaginous elements), and Wilms' tumor. Attention to the clinical presentation and thorough sampling will help distinguish these entities. For example, a primary renal tumor in a child with the appearance of pleomorphic RMS is statistically more likely to be an anaplastic Wilms' tumor. Thorough sampling of such tumors can reveal other elements (blastema, tubules) or clues (nephrogenic rests) that confirm the diagnosis of Wilms' tumor. In the visceral organs of adults where carcinomas predominate, the morphologic appearance of pleomorphic RMS most likely represents a part of a carcinosarcoma, and further sampling may disclose an epithelial component. Finally, it has become apparent that pediatric-type RMS can have anaplastic areas that mimic the appearance of pleomorphic RMS. The younger age of these patients and the presence of well-defined classic embryonal or alveolar histology in other areas of these tumors help make this distinction (80).

B. Juvenile Rhabdomyosarcoma in Adults

Although classically tumors of childhood, both embryonal rhabdomyosarcoma (ERMS) and alveolar rhabdomyosarcoma (ARMS) occasionally present in adults. The reader is referred to Chapter 15 for the main pathologic and genetic features of these tumors. Their presentation and differential diagnosis are somewhat different in adults. ARMS accounts for a greater proportion of these cases, which is not surprising given that its peak age incidence (adolescents and young adults) is higher that that of ERMS. In adults, ERMS involves the head and neck region less frequently than in children, instead affecting the extremities more often (93). In contrast, ARMS in adults commonly involves the head and neck region, particularly the nasopharynx and nasal cavity (94). A vast potential for misdiagnosis exists in this setting, where the differential diagnosis for a small round blue cell tumor like ARMS includes porly differentiated carcinoma, lymphoma, small-cell neuroendocrine carcinoma, melanoma, and olfactory neuroblastoma. All of these lesions are far more common in adults than ARMS, and with a small biopsy the diagnosis of ARMS may not be considered. Further confusion is created when an ARMS contains abundant cytoplasmic glycogen; here the potential for misdiagnosis as clear cell carcinoma is present (95).

While there has been no systematic comparison of the survival of adults and children with RMS, several studies have demonstrated a trend toward diminished survival in adults. In a review of 110 ARMSs from the AFIP, the median survival was slightly shorter in patients older than 20 years (96), and only 1 in 6 adults with ARMS in another study was free of disease on follow-up (94). The 5-year survival in a series of adult ERMS was only 21%, though this correlated with the presence of advanced stage (93). In addition, the spindle cell variant of ERMS, which is associated with paratesticular location and excellent prognosis in children, is likely not prognostically favorable in adults. Two adult patients with tumors of this morphology died of progressive disease in a recent study (97).

ACKNOWLEDGMENTS

We thank Bruce Wenig, MD (New York), Cyril Fisher MD (London), and Russel L. Corio, DDS (Baltimore) for generously providing cases of these rare lesions for our illustrations. Dr. Corio generously granted permission to publish Figs. 3, 5, and 6. We thank Dr. Wenig for reviewing the manuscript. We thank Norman Barker and Pete Lund for giving photographic assistance and Lisa Madden for typing the manuscript.

REFERENCES

1. Enzinger FM, Weiss SW. Soft Tissue Tumors, 3rd ed. St. Louis: Mosby, 1995.
2. Whitten RO, Benjamin DR. Rhabdomyoma of the retroperitoneum. A report of a tumor with both adult and fetal characteristics: a study by light and electron microscopy, histochemistry, and immunochemistry. Cancer 59:818–824, 1987.
3. Sangueza O, Sangueza P, Jordan J, White CRJ. Rhabdomyoma of the tongue. Am J Dermatopathol 12:492–495, 1990.
4. Kapadia SB, Meis JM, Frisman DM, Ellis GL, Heffner DK. Fetal rhabdomyoma of the head and neck: a clinicopathologic and immunophenotypic study of 24 cases. Hum Pathol 24:754–765, 1993.
5. Yu GH, Kussmaul WG, DiSesa VJ, Lodato RF, Brooks JS. Adult intracardiac rhabdomyoma resembling the extracardiac variant. Hum Pathol 24:448–451, 1993.
6. di Sant'Agnese PA, Knowles DM. Extracardiac rhabdomyoma: a clinicopathologic study and review of the literature. Cancer 46:780–789, 1980.
7. Willis J, Abdul-Karim FW, di Sant'Agnese PA. Extracardiac rhabdomyomas. Semin Diagn Pathol 11:15–25, 1994.
8. Pendl F, Ober EN. Uber ein congenitales rhabdomyom der zung. Ztsch Neilkund 18:457–468, 1897.
9. Stout AP, Lattes R. Rhabdomyoma. In: Firminger HI, ed. Tumors of the Soft Tissue. Atlas of Tumor Pathology, Fascicle 1, Series 2. Washington, DC: Armed Forces Institute of Pathology, 1967, pp. 64–66.
10. Dehner LP, Enzinger FM, Font RL. Fetal rhabdomyoma. An analysis of nine cases. Cancer 30:160–166, 1972.
11. Konrad EA, Meister P, Hubner G. Extracardiac rhabdomyoma: report of different types with light microscopic and ultrastructural studies. Cancer 49:898–907, 1982.
12. Enbergs A, Borggrefe M, Kurlemann G, Fahrenkamp A, Scheld HH, Jehle J, Breithardt G. Ventricular tachycardia caused by cardiac rhabdomyoma in a young adult with tuberous sclerosis. Am Heart J 132:1263–1265, 1996.
13. Harding CO, Pagon RA. Incidence of tuberous sclerosis in patients with cardiac rhabdomyoma. Am J Med Genet 37:443–446, 1990.
14. Webb DW, Osborne JP. Incidence of tuberous sclerosis in patients with cardiac rhabdomyoma. Am J Med Genet 42:754–755, 1992.
15. Smythe JF, Dyck JD, Smallhorn JF, Freedom RM. Natural history of cardiac rhabdomyoma in infancy and childhood. Am J Cardiol 66:1247–1249, 1990.
16. Nir A, Tajik AJ, Freeman WK, Seward JB, Offord KP, Edwards WD, Mair DD, Gomez MR. Tuberous sclerosis and cardiac rhabdomyoma. Am J Cardiol 76:419–421, 1995.
17. Jacobs JP, Konstantakos AK, Holland FW, Herskowitz K, Ferrer PL, Perryman RA. Surgical treatment for cardiac rhabdomyomas in children. Ann Thorac Surg 58:1552–1555, 1994.
18. Black MD, Kadletz M, Smallhorn JF, Freedom RM. Cardiac rhabdomyomas and obstructive left heart disease: histologically but not functionally benign. Ann Thorac Surg 65:1388–1390, 1998.
19. Grellner W, Henssge C. Multiple cardiac rhabdomyoma with exclusively histological manifestation. Forensic Sci Int 78:1–5, 1996.

20. Zwick DL, Livingston K, Clapp L, Kosnik E, Yates A. Intracranial trigeminal nerve rhabdomyoma/choristoma in a child: a case report and discussion of possible histogenesis. Hum Pathol 20:390–392, 1989.

21. Goldman RL. Multicentric benign rhabdomyoma of skeletal muscle. Cancer 16: 1609–1613, 1963.

22. Roberts DN, Corbett MJ, Breen D, Jonathan DA, Smith CE. Rhabdomyoma of the larynx: a rare cause of stridor. J Laryngol Otol 108:713–715, 1994.

23. Johansen EC, Illum P. Rhabdomyoma of the larynx: a review of the literature with a summary of previously described cases of rhabdomyoma of the larynx and a report of a new case. J Laryngol Otol 109:147–153, 1995.

24. Modlin B. Rhabdomyoma of the larynx. Laryngoscope 92:580–582, 1982.

25. Imperatori CJ. Rhabdomyoma of the larynx: report of a case. Laryngoscope 43:945–948, 1933.

26. Metheetrairut C, Brown DH, Cullen JB, Dardick I. Pharyngeal rhabdomyoma: a clinico-pathological study. J Otolaryngol 21:257–261, 1992.

27. Wood GS, Brammer R, Durham JC, Dichtel W. Adult rhabdomyoma of the larynx. Ear Nose Throat J 72:296–298, 1993.

28. Murrell GL, Barnes M, Langford FP, Kenan PD. Submandibular rhabdomyoma. Ear Nose Throat J 71:663–664, 1992.

29. Knowles DM, Jakobiec FA. Rhabdomyoma of the orbit. Am J Ophthalmol 80:1011–1018, 1975.

30. Tuazon R. Rhabdomyoma of the stomach. Report of a case. Am J Clin Pathol 52:37–41, 1969.

31. Box JC, Newman CL, Anastasiades KD, Lucas GW, Latouff OM. Adult rhabdomyoma: presentation as a cervicomediastinal mass (case report and review of the literature). Am Surg 61:271–276, 1995.

32. Morra MN, Manson AL, Gavrell GJ, Quinn AD. Rhabdomyoma of prostate. Urology 39:271–273, 1992.

33. Parson HG, Puro HE. Rhabdomyoma of skeletal muscle. Report of a case. Am J Surg 89:1187–1190, 1955.

34. Kapadia SB, Meis JM, Frisman DM, Ellis GL, Heffner DK, Hyams VJ. Adult rhabdomyoma of the head and neck: a clinicopathologic and immunophenotypic study. Hum Pathol 24:608–617, 1993.

35. Eusebi V, Ceccarelli C, Daniele E, Collina G, Viale G, Mancini AM. Extracardiac rhabdomyoma: An immunocytochemical study and review of the literature. Appl Pathol 6:197–207, 1988.

36. Gibas Z, Miettinen M. Recurrent parapharyngeal rhabdomyoma. Evidence of neoplastic nature of the tumor from cytogenetic study. Am J Surg Pathol 16:721–728, 1992.

37. Skalli O, Gabbiani G, Babai F, Seemayer TA, Pizzolato G, Schurch W. Intermediate filament proteins and actin isoforms as markers for soft tissue tumor differentiation and origin. II. Rhabdomyosarcomas. Am J Pathol 130:515–531, 1988.

38. Erlandson RA. Diagnostic Transmission Electron Microscopy of Tumors. New York: Raven Press, 1994.

39. Blaauwgeers JL, Troost D, Dingemans KP, Taat CW, Van den Tweel JG. Multifocal rhabdomyoma of the neck. Report of a case studied by fine-needle aspiration, light

and electron microscopy, histochemistry, and immunohistochemistry. Am J Surg Pathol 13:791–799, 1989.

40. Zachariades N, Skoura C, Sourmelis A, Liapi-Avgeri G. Recurrent twin adult rhabdomyoma of the cheek. J Oral Maxillofac Surg 52:1324–1328, 1994.

41. Kapadia SB, Enzinger FM, Heffner DK, Hyams VJ, Frizzera G. Crystal-storing histiocytosis associated with lymphoplasmacytic neoplasms. Report of three cases mimicking adult rhabdomyoma. Am J Surg Pathol 17:461–467, 1993.

42. d'Amore ES, Tollot M, Stracca-Pansa V, Menegon A, Meli S, Carli M, Ninfo V. Therapy associated differentiation in rhabdomyosarcomas. Mod Pathol 7:69–75, 1994.

43. Dahl I, Angervall L, Save-Soderbergh J. Foetal rhabdomyoma. Case report of a patient with two tumours. Acta Pathol Microbiol Scand 84:107–112, 1976.

44. Gorlin RJ. Nevoid basal-cell carcinoma syndrome. Medicine 66:98–113, 1987.

45. DiSanto S, Abt AB, Boal DK, Krummel TM. Fetal rhabdomyoma and nevoid basal cell carcinoma syndrome. Pediatr Pathol 12:441–447, 1992.

46. Klijanienko J, Caillaud JM, Micheau C, Flamant F, Schwaab G, Avril MF, Ponzio-Prion A. Basal-cell nevomatosis associated with multifocal fetal rhabdomyoma. A case. Presse Med 17:2247–2250, 1988.

47. Hardisson D, Jimenez-Heffernan JA, Nistal M, Picazo ML, Tovar JA, Contreras F. Neural variant of fetal rhabdomyoma and naevoid basal cell carcinoma syndrome. Histopathology 29:247–252, 1996.

48. Gardner DG, Corio RL. Fetal rhabdomyoma of the tongue, with a discussion of the two histologic variants of this tumor. Oral Surg Oral Med Oral Pathol 56:293–300, 1983.

49. Crotty PL, Nakhleh RE, Dehner LP. Juvenile rhabdomyoma. An intermediate form of skeletal muscle tumor in children. Arch Pathol Lab Med 117:43–47, 1993.

50. Granich MS, Pilch BZ, Nadol JB, Dickersin GR. Fetal rhabdomyoma of the larynx. Arch Otolaryngol. 109:821–826, 1983.

51. Osgood PJ, Damron TA, Rooney MT, Goldschmidt AM, Sullivan TJ. Benign fetal rhabdomyoma of the upper extremity. A case report. Clin Orthop 200–204, 1998.

52. Smith NM, Thornton CM. Fetal rhabdomyoma: two instances of recurrence. Pediatr Pathol Lab Med 16:673–680, 1996.

53. Kodet R, Fajstavr J, Kabelka Z, Koutecky J, Eckschlager T, Newton WAJ. Is fetal cellular rhabdomyoma an entity or a differentiated rhabdomyosarcoma? A study of patients with rhabdomyoma of the tongue and sarcoma of the tongue enrolled in the intergroup rhabdomyosarcoma studies I, II, and III. Cancer 67:2907–2913, 1991.

54. Chabrel CM, Beilby JO. Vaginal rhabdomyoma. Histopathology 4:645–651, 1980.

55. Gold JH, Bossen EH. Benign vaginal rhabdomyoma: a light and electron microscopic study. Cancer 37:2283–2294, 1976.

56. Ceremsak RJ. Benign rhabdomyoma of the vagina. Am J Clin Pathol 52:604–606, 1969.

57. Gad A, Eusebi V. Rhabdomyoma of the vagina. J Pathol 115:179–181, 1975.

58. Leone PG, Taylor HB. Ultrastructure of a benign polypoid rhabdomyoma of the vagina. Cancer 31:1414–1417, 1973.

59. Gee DC, Finckh ES. Benign vaginal rhabdomyoma. Pathology 9:263–267, 1977

60. Nucci MR, Fletcher CDM. Pathol Case Rev 3:151–157, 1998.

61. Stout AP. Rhabdomyosarcoma of the skeletal muscles. Ann Surg 123:447–472, 1946.
62. Horn RC, Enterline HT. Rhabdomyosarcoma: a clinicopathological study and classification of 39 cases. Cancer 11:181–199, 1958.
63. Enzinger FM, Lattes R, Torloni H. Histologic Typing of Soft Tissue Tumors. An International Classification of Tumors. Geneva: World Health Organization, 1969.
64. Weiss SW, Enzinger FM. Malignant fibrous histiocytoma: an analysis of 200 cases. Cancer 41:2250–2266, 1978.
65. Kearney MM, Soule EH, Ivins JC. Malignant fibrous histiocytoma: a retrospective study of 167 cases. Cancer 45:167–178, 1980.
66. Seidal T, Kindblom LG, Angervall L. Rhabdomyosarcoma in middle-aged and elderly individuals. APMIS 97:236–248, 1989.
67. Miettinen M. Rhabdomyosarcoma in patients older than 40 years of age. Cancer 62:2060–2065, 1988.
68. Molenaar WM, Oosterhuis AM, Ramaekers FC. The rarity of rhabdomyosarcomas in the adult. A morphologic and immunohistochemical study. Pathol Res Pract 180:400–404, 1985.
69. Fletcher CD. Pleomorphic malignant fibrous histiocytoma: fact or fiction? A critical reappraisal based on 159 tumors diagnosed as pleomorphic sarcoma. Am J Surg Pathol 16:213–228, 1992.
70. Erlandson RA, Woodruff JM. Role of electron microscopy in the evaluation of soft tissue neoplasms, with emphasis on spindle cell and pleomorphic tumors. Hum Pathol 29:1372–1381, 1998.
71. Schürch W, Begin LR, Seemayer TA, Lagace R, Boivin JC, Lamoureux C, Bluteau P, Piche J, Gabbiani G. Pleomorphic soft tissue myogenic sarcomas of adulthood. A reappraisal in the mid-1990s. Am J Surg Pathol 20:131–147, 1996.
72. Gaffney EF, Dervan PA, Fletcher CD. Pleomorphic rhabdomyosarcoma in adulthood. Analysis of 11 cases with definition of diagnostic criteria. Am J Surg Pathol 17:601–609, 1993.
73. Da Mosto MC, Marchiori C, Rinaldo A, Ferlito A. Laryngeal pleomorphic rhabdomyosarcoma. A critical review of the literature. Ann Otol Rhinol Laryngol 105:289–294, 1996.
74. Lin J, Yip KM, Chow LT. Pleomorphic rhabdomyosarcoma of the submandibular salivary gland. Otolaryngol Head Neck Surg 116:545–547, 1997.
75. Lauro S, Lalle M, Scucchi L, Vecchione A. Rhabdomyosarcoma of the urinary bladder in an elderly patient. Anticancer Res 15:627–629, 1995.
76. Grignon DJ, McIsaac GP, Armstrong RF, Wyatt JK. Primary rhabdomyosarcoma of the kidney. A light microscopic, immunohistochemical, and electron microscopic study. Cancer 62:2027–2032, 1988.
77. Ordi J, Stamatakos MD, Tavassoli FA. Pure pleomorphic rhabdomyosarcomas of the uterus. Int J Gynecol Pathol 16:369–377, 1997.
78. de Jong AS, Kessel-van Vark M, Albus-Lutter CE. Pleomorphic rhabdomyosarcoma in adults: immunohistochemistry as a tool for its diagnosis. Hum Pathol 18:298–303, 1987.

79. Suster S, Moran CA, Koss MN. Rhabdomyosarcomas of the anterior mediastinum: report of four cases unassociated with germ cell, teratomatous, or thymic carcinomatous components. Hum Pathol 25:349–356, 1994.

80. Hollowood K, Fletcher CD. Rhabdomyosarcoma in adults. Semin Diagn Pathol 11: 47–57, 1994.

81. Eusebi V, Ceccarelli C, Gorza L, Schiaffino S, Bussolati G. Immunocytochemistry of rhabdomyosarcoma. The use of four different markers. Am J Surg Pathol 10:293–299, 1986.

82. Kagen LJ, Christian CL. Immunologic measurements of myoglobin in human adult and fetal skeletal muscle. Am J Physiol 211:656–660, 1966.

83. de Jong AS, van Vark M, Albus-Lutter CE, van Raamsdonk W, Voute PA. Myosin and myoglobin as tumor markers in the diagnosis of rhabdomyosarcoma. A comparative study. Am J Surg Pathol 8:521–528, 1984.

84. Eusebi V, Bondi A, Rosai J. Immunohistochemical localization of myoglobin in non-muscular cells. Am J Surg Pathol 8:51–55, 1984.

85. Tallini G, Parham DM, Dias P, Cordon-Cardo C, Houghton PJ, Rosai J. Myogenic regulatory protein expression in adult soft tissue sarcomas. A sensitive and specific marker of skeletal muscle differentiation. Am J Pathol 144:693–701, 1994.

86. Gomez JA, Amin MB, Ro JY, Linden MD, Lee MW, Zarbo RJ. Immunohistochemical profile of myogenin and MyoD1 does not support skeletal muscle lineage in alveolar soft part sarcoma. Arch Pathol Lab Med 123:503–507, 1999.

87. Wang NP, Marx J, McNutt MA, Rutledge JC, Gown AM. Expression of myogenic regulatory proteins (myogenin and MyoD1) in small blue round cell tumors of childhood. Am J Pathol 147:1799–1810, 1995.

88. Wesche WA, Fletcher CD, Dias P, Houghton PJ, Parham DM. Immunohistochemistry of MyoD1 in adult pleomorphic soft tissue sarcomas. Am J Surg Pathol 19:261–269, 1995.

89. Wang NP, Bacchi CE, Jiang JJ, McNutt MA, Gown AM. Does alveolar soft-part sarcoma exhibit skeletal muscle differentiation? An immunocytochemical and biochemical study of myogenic regulatory protein expression. Mod Pathol 9:496–506, 1996.

90. Cui S, Hano H, Harada T, Takai S, Masui F, Ushigome S. Evaluation of new monoclonal anti-MyoD1 and anti-myogenin antibodies for the diagnosis of rhabdomyosarcoma. Pathol Int 49:62–68, 1999.

91. Erlandson RA. The ultrastructural distinction between rhabdomyosarcoma and other undifferentiated "sarcomas." Ultrastruct Pathol 11:83–101, 1987.

92. Guillou L, Coquet M, Chaubert P, Coindre JM. Skeletal muscle regeneration mimicking rhabdomyosarcoma: a potential diagnostic pitfall. Histopathology 33:136–144, 1998.

93. Lloyd RV, Hajdu SI, Knapper WH. Embryonal rhabdomyosarcoma in adults. Cancer 51:557–565, 1983.

94. Nakhleh RE, Swanson PE, Dehner LP. Juvenile (embryonal and alveolar) rhabdomyosarcoma of the head and neck in adults. A clinical, pathologic, and immunohistochemical study of 12 cases. Cancer 67:1019–1024, 1991.

95. Chan JK, Ng HK, Wan KY, Tsao SY, Leung TW, Tse KC. Clear cell rhabdomyosarcoma of the nasal cavity and paranasal sinuses. Histopathology 14:391–399, 1989.
96. Enzinger FM, Shiraki M. Alveolar rhabdomyosarcoma. An analysis of 110 cases. Cancer 24:18–31, 1969.
97. Rubin BP, Hasserjian RP, Singer S, Janecka I, Fletcher JA, Fletcher CD. Spindle cell rhabdomyosarcoma (so-called) in adults: report of two cases with emphasis on differential diagnosis. Am J Surg Pathol 22:459–464, 1998.

12

Vascular Anomalies and Neoplasms

Salwa S. Sheikh
Dhahran Health Center
Dhahran, Saudi Arabia

Elizabeth Montgomery
The Johns Hopkins University
Baltimore, Maryland

Classification systems of any tissue proliferation include hamartomas, malformations, hyperplasias, and neoplasms. Classification of vascular lesions is difficult as conceptual confusion persists between vascular malformations, hyperplasias, and neoplasms. For example, infantile hemangiomas are characterized by proliferation of vessels but often undergo spontaneous regression, thus having features of both neoplasia and hyperplasia. Despite the inherent difficulty in applying such classification systems to vascular lesions, they are generally understood and remain the convention.

An abbreviated overview of nontumorous vascular lesions follows before discussion of neoplasms.

I. HAMARTOMAS

A. Phakomatosis Pigmentovascularis

Phakomatosis pigmentovascularis represents a combination of both vascular and melanocytic nevi. Most cases have been reported in the Japanese literature. The disease is divided into four different types depending on the vascular/melanocytic lesion involved, with each type further subdivided into isolated cutaneous or systemic forms. The most commonly accepted opinion regarding pathogenesis of phakomatosis pigmentovascularis is that it results from developmental abnormalities of the neural crest–derived vasomotor nerves and melanocytes (1). Histopathologically, the nevus flammeus/skin lesions associated with phakomatosis pigmentovascularis are indistinguishable from port-wine stains, consisting of ectatic vessels in the affected site (see below under "Nevus Flammeus").

B. Eccrine Angiomatous Hamartoma

The rare cutaneous hamartoma eccrine angiomatous hamartoma (EAH) features proliferation of both capillaries and eccrine glands. EAH usually appears at birth or during early childhood with slow growing, painful solitary or multiple lesions. Lesions typically affect acral surfaces, although other areas can also be involved.
    Several congenital malformations have been associated with EAH.

II. VASCULAR MALFORMATIONS

Malformations refer to aberrant embryologic development. Vascular malformations can be either functional as in nevus anemicus, or can be structural involving capillaries, larger vessels, or lymphatics.

A. Functional Malformations

Nevus Anemicus

Nevus anemicus is an uncommon macular lesion that usually involves the upper chest of women. It has irregular margins and is usually surrounded by satellite macules. The pathogenesis is believed to involve either increased sensitivity to vasoconstrictor stimuli or decreased sensitivity to vasodilator stimuli. Lesions are usually asymptomatic and require no treatment.

B. Anatomical Malformations

In general, the diagnosis of these lesions is best made on clinical and radiologic grounds as their features may be essentially indistinguishable on histologic examination.

1. Capillary Malformations

a. Cutis Marmorata Telangiectatica Congenita   Cutis marmorata telangiectatica congenita is a reticulated localized or generalized bluish-appearing cutaneous lesion present at birth. It differs from cutis marmorata, which represents a physiologic response to cold more prominent in neonates. When the lesion is localized, it usually has a sharp midline demarcation, typically diminishing with time and, in some cases, disappearing completely. In 50% of patients, various congenital malformations have been described.

b.   Nevus Flammeus   Nevus flammeus is a term that usually encompasses congenital vascular malformations commonly involving the head and neck region (1). In fact, about 25–40% of newborns have red macular lesions of the head and neck. *Salmon patches* are small lesions seen on the forehead that often disappear during childhood. *Port-wine stain*, which is usually unilateral and nuchal, tends to persist into adult life. *Sturge-Weber syndrome* refers to large port-wine stains in the distribution of the ophthalmic branch of trigeminal nerve along with ipsilateral leptomeningeal angiomatosis. *Klippel-Trenaunay syndrome* includes nevus flammeus of a limb with or without hypertrophy of that limb secondary to deep vascular malformations. Histologically, nevus flammeus shows increased dilated and thin-walled blood vessels, commonly in the papillary and reticular dermis, although subcutaneous fat can be involved.

c.   Hyperkeratotic Vascular Stains   Most of the lesions associated with hyperkeratotic vascular stains fall under the rubric of angiokeratoma (see below). However, some authors restrict application of the term angiokeratoma to acquired hyperkeratotic lesions resulting from ectasia of preexisting blood vessels in the papillary dermis. Hyperkeratotic vascular stains, on the other hand, represent ectasia of vascular malformations involving the dermis and subcutaneous tissue.

2.   Venous and Arterial Malformations

Venous malformations are often misdiagnosed as cavernous hemangiomas although venous lesions should feature an abundance of smooth muscle in the abnormal vessel walls rather than thin ectatic channels on histologic examination. Venous malformations appear as blue-purple single or multiple nodules and are often associated with thrombophlebitis in adjacent regions. These lesions may be associated with other anomalies:

Mafucci's syndrome consists of multiple vascular malformations and diffuse asymmetrical enchondromatosis along with other musculoskeletal malformations (2,3). Many patients with Maffucci's syndrome have spindle cell hemangioendotheliomas/hemangiomas (further described below).

Klippel-Trenaunay syndrome consists of vascular malformations, congenital varicose veins, and hypertrophy of the involved (most commonly lower) limb.

Blue rubber bleb nevus syndrome (further discussed below) is a rare syndrome associated with venous malformations of the skin and gastrointestinal tract. Most patients complain of nocturnal pain in the lesions, and gastrointestinal lesions may bleed. Histologically there are ectatic, irregular, thin-walled blood vessels (4).

3. Lymphatic Malformations

a. Cutaneous Lymphatic Malformations   On biopsies, cutaneous lymphatic malformations are frequently incorrectly diagnosed as lymphangiomas or lymphangioma circumscriptum. They are often present at birth and commonly involve the shoulder, axillary folds, and head and neck region. Characteristically, lesions appear as groups of multiple vesicle-like lesions with irregular margins. Microscopic examination reveals ecstatic vascular channels with associated haphazard bundles of smooth muscle surrounded by loose stroma. Ki-67 (a proliferation marker) staining of these lesions shows minimal activity, leading some authors to suggest that their growth is secondary to engorgement by chyle and inflammation rather than neoplastic proliferation (5).

b. Lymphangiomatosis   Lymphangiomatosis is characterized by diffuse or multifocal abnormal lymphatic channels involving soft tissue, viscera, and/or bone. The lesions appear at birth or during early childhood as sponge-like progressive swelling of the involved area, which is usually the limb.

   Histologically, the lesion shows dilated interconnecting lymphatic channels forming lobules involving the dermis, subcutaneous fat, soft tissue, and/or bone.

III. DILATATION OF PRE-EXISTING VESSELS

A. Spider Angiomas

Spider angiomas are present in 10–15% of the normal population, including children. They are more common among those with chronic liver disease and during pregnancy. Clinically, they are characterized by radiating blood vessels emanating from red, elevated puncta. When biopsied, the microscopic lesions consist of central arterioles from which thin arterioles branch and radiate.

B. Telangiectasia

Telengiectasias are characterized by dilatation of terminal vessels, most commonly venules, but sometimes arterioles and capillaries. Although these frequently accompany collagen vascular diseases, they may also be seen in patients with sun damage and chronic graft-versus-host disease. *Osler-Rendu-Weber disease* is a condition in which telangectasias present early in childhood and may involve skin, mucous membranes, and internal organs.

   Histologically, lesions are characterized by dilated vascular channels, which are often surrounded by lymphocytes.

C. Angiokeratomas

Angiokeratoma is a term that encompasses acquired lesions with hyperkeratotic telengiectasias that may arise singly or multiply (1). *Angiokeratoma of Fordyce* consists of multiple dark papules involving the vulva or scrotum. *Angiokeratoma corporis diffusum* is seen either as an idiopathic condition or in association with various other diseases, including *Fabry's disease.*

  Histologically, there are dilated thin-walled vessels in the papillary dermis with overlying hyperkeratosis.

D. Lymphangiectasia

These are the lymphatic counterparts of angiokeratomas with acquired dilatation of lymphatics secondary to obstruction, clinically appearing as multiple translucent vesicles that leak milky fluid if punctured.

IV. HYPERPLASIAS/REACTIVE VASCULAR LESIONS

This group includes vascular proliferations that result from infectious processes, immunologic disturbances, or host response to a variety of other causes, including trauma.

A. Bacillary Angiomatosis

Bacillary (epithelioid) angiomatosis (BA) is a pseudoneoplastic vascular proliferation, first described in 1983 by Stoler et al. in HIV-infected individuals (6). The disease has a predilection for, but is not restricted to, immunocompromised patients (7,8). The causative organisms are of the genus *Bartonella*, formerly called Rochalimaea (9–11). Two species of *Bartonella* are responsible: *B. quintana* (12) and *B. henselae* (13–15). These organisms are susceptible to antibiotics, including erythromycin, rifampin, and doxycycline, which often must be administered for a 4- to 6-week course to avoid relapse. Although cutaneous lesions are the most frequently recognized manifestation of this disease, a systemic infection typically ensues in the immunosuppressed host with involvement of almost any site, including lymph nodes, bone marrow, viscera, and soft tissue. In immunocompetent individuals, lesions are believed to remain localized to the inoculation site (16).

  Histologically the lesions of bacillary angiomatosis consist of a lobulated proliferation of capillary-sized vessels lined by "activated" or mildly atypical endothelium (Fig. 1). Aggregates of neutrophils, leukocytoclastic debris, and granular flocculent material are present both in the vascular lobules and in the adjacent

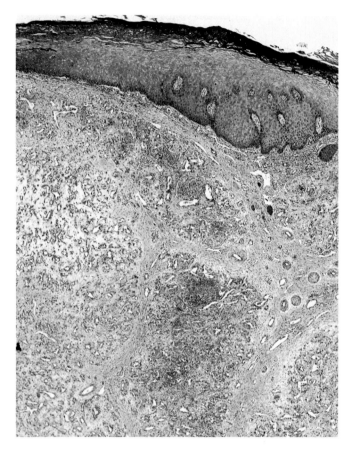

FIG. 1 Bacillary angiomatosis consists of a lobulated proliferation of capillaries with necroinflammatory zones.

soft tissue. The infectious agent is $0.5–1.0$ μm in length and appears as clumps of small curved rods when stained with Warthin-Starry (Fig. 2).

The differential diagnosis of bacillary angiomatosis primarily includes three entities: pyogenic granuloma, Kaposi's sarcoma, and *Carrión's disease*. A detailed discussion of the latter is presented in the following section and will not be reiterated here, other than to note that Carrión's disease is rarely seen outside of its endemic areas in South America.

Dermal examples of bacillary angiomatosis bear a superficial resemblance to *pyogenic granuloma* (lobular capillary hemangioma). In fact, some reports in the earlier literature of "disseminated pyogenic granuloma" may actually refer to

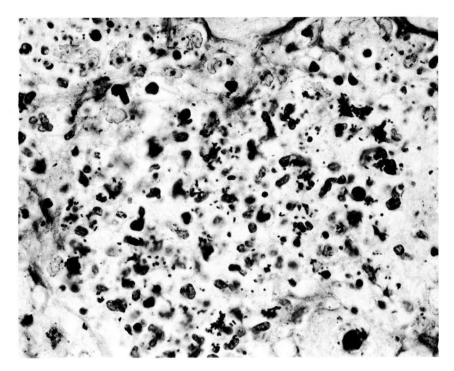

FIG. 2   On Warthin-Starry (silver) staining, the etiologic agent, *Bartonella henselae*, appears as black coccobacilli.

examples of BA (8,17). However, in contrast to pyogenic granuloma, BA contains vessels lined by plumper, more atypical-appearing endothelial cells and it exhibits acute inflammatory foci, even in the absence of surface ulceration.

Kaposi's sarcoma (KS) enters into the differential diagnosis of BA because both processes have a predilection for immunosuppressed, especially HIV-positive individuals and both are frequently characterized by the presence of multiple cutaneous lesions. However, KS has predominantly spindle cells with slit-like vascular channels and lacks the lobulated proliferation of BA. KS also differs by featuring a lymphoplasmacytic, rather than polymorphonuclear, inflammatory reaction. Periodic acid–Schiff–positive, diastase-resistant hyaline globules, especially when present in a clustered, grape-like arrangement, are a well-recognized feature of the plaque and nodular stages of KS.

BA can prove fatal if left untreated and therefore should be at the forefront of the pathologist's differential diagnosis when evaluating vascular proliferations arising in immunocompromised patients, especially if leukocytoclastic debris or acute inflammation is present.

B. Verruga Peruana/Carrión's Disease/Oroya Fever

During construction of a railway between Lima and La Oroya, Peru, at least 7000 individuals died from a severe febrile illness that later came to be known by Peruvian doctors as Oroya fever (18). The condition is also referred to as Carrión's disease, after Daniel A. Carrión, a medical student who established the relationship between the febrile condition and cutaneous lesions, designated "verruga peruana nodules," that may subsequently develop. In endemic areas, the term *la verruga* is used to encompass both manifestations of this biphasic disease. The etiologic agent is *Bartonella bacilliformis*, a gram-negative bacteria. Humans are the only reservoirs of Carrión's disease, which is transmitted by a nocturnal sandfly called *Lutzomyia (Phlebotomus) verrucarum.*

It is a life-threatening disease with an incubation period of approximately 3 weeks. Patients develop fever and an acute, severe, hemolytic anemia, with parasitization of circulating erythrocytes by the microorganism. Infiltration of the reticuloendothelial system leads to hepatosplenomegaly and lymphadenopathy. A tissue phase, which signals improvement in the patient's condition, appears approximately 2 months after the hematic phase and is characterized by the development of verruga peruana nodules primarily involving the face and extremities (Fig. 3). In endemic areas, where more than 60% of asymptomatic individuals have

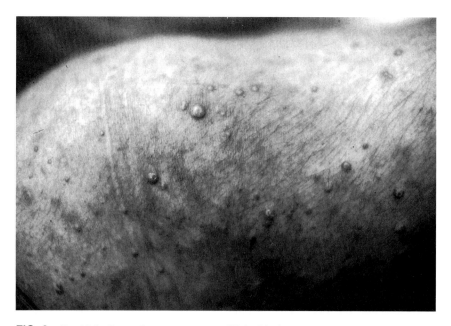

FIG. 3 Carrión's disease/verruga peruana. Clinical lesion.

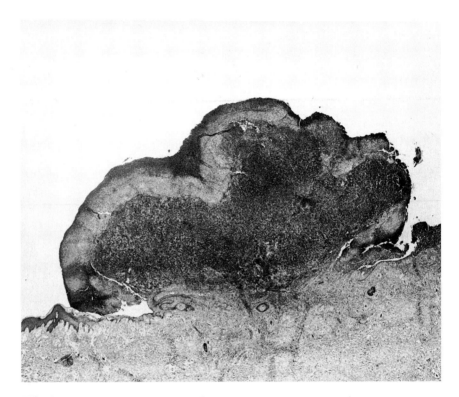

FIG. 4   Nodular lesion of Carrión's disease.

antibodies to *B. bacilliformis*, infections may follow a shorter course, and healthy individuals harboring the organism have been identified.

Histologically, the lesions can be classified as *miliary*, when small and confined to the papillary dermis; *nodular* (Fig. 4), when small to medium-sized and present in the reticular dermis or subcutis; or *mular*, when large and involving both skin and subcutaneous tissue (19). All have a lobulated vascular proliferation lined by plump atypical endothelial cells ("verruga cells"), commonly admixed with inflammatory cells. Superficial lesions generally resolve over a period of 4–6 weeks, whereas deeper nodules may persist for up to 4 months. The identification of granular structures, Rocha-Lima inclusions, assists in confirming the diagnosis (Fig. 5). These are best seen when tissues are stained with special stains, e.g., Giemsa, Warthin-Starry, and PAS/D stains. When inclusions are not found, the diagnosis rests on clinicopathologic correlation.

Superficial examples may be polypoid and, when accompanied by well-formed vessels with patent lumina, may bear resemblance to *pyogenic granuloma*

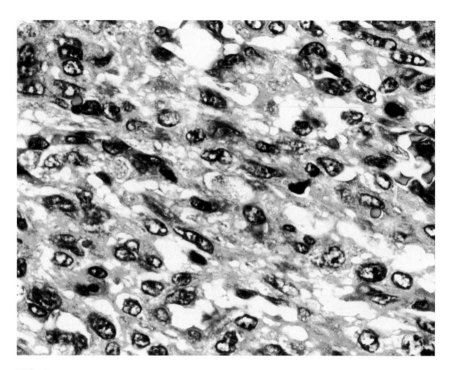

FIG. 5 Granular intracytoplasmic bodies may be identified in endothelial cells in Carrión's disease and occasionally pale-staining bacteria forms can be seen on Giemsa stains (center of field).

or *bacillary angiomatosis*. However, the epidemiologic context should allow for differentiation as *B. bacilliformis* is almost entirely restricted to endemic areas. Lesions that arise in less distensible tissues may exhibit more solid "angioblastic" growth suggestive of a neoplastic process (20).

C. Papillary Endothelial Hyperplasia/ Masson's Pseudoangiosarcoma

The benign reactive process known as papillary endothelial hyperplasia (PEH, also called Masson's pseudoangiosarcoma) represents an unusually exuberant form of organizing vascular thrombus (21). PEH may occur at any age and involve virtually any vessel (22–24), including those of neoplastic processes and vascular malformations (4). However, in "pure" form, they present as solitary, superficial, firm, bluish or erythematous masses, involving the fingers, head and neck, or anorectal region. PEH may even involve the superior vena cava, leading to superior vena cava syndrome (25); may mimic Stewart-Treves syndrome with lymphedema of the limb post therapy for breast carcinoma (26), or may be associated with paroxysmal nocturnal hemoglobinuria resulting in venous thrombosis and PEH (27). Multiple lesions have also been recently reported, which, when localized to a single anatomical site, makes its distintion from angiosarcoma even more critical (28). Commonly, physical examination reveals limited mobility of the process about its longitudinal axis. Gross examination may reveal confinement of the process to the lumen of a dilated vessel, usually a vein.

Histologically, this intravascular lesion manifests papillary fronds with cores of fibrin or hyalinized collagen, lined by a single layer of endothelial cells that lack significant atypia and mitotic activity (21,29–32) (Figs. 6 and 7). Occasionally, the fronds appear to be "free-floating" within the vessel lumen. Extravascular extension may occasionally be seen, although it is usually not extensive.

The following features help differentiate PEH from *angiosarcoma*, a tumor with which it has occasionally been confused: (a) the frequent confinement of the process to a vascular lumen, (b) lack of cellular pleomorphism, (c) the typical ar-

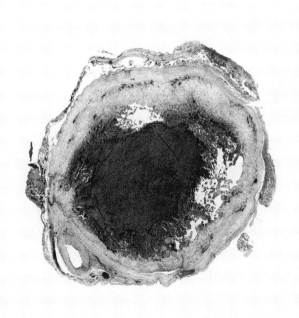

FIG. 6   In this thrombosed vessel, an intraluminal papillary proliferation is present to the right of and above the thrombus.

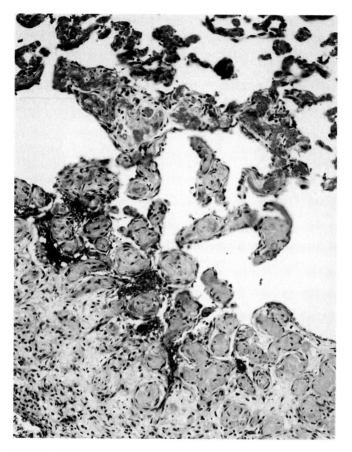

FIG. 7 At higher magnification of the papillary area in Fig. 6, hyalinized fibrin cores are surrounded by a coating of endothelial cells.

rangement of the endothelium in a monolayer, (d) low mitotic rate, and (e) paucity of cellular necrosis.

D. Intravascular Fasciitis

Nodular fasciitis is a well-characterized reactive pseudosarcomatous myofibroblastic proliferation that usually arises in the superficial fascia, subcutis, or muscle. In these locations, it generally evolves into a relatively well-circumscribed 2- to 3-cm mass after initial rapid growth. Similar proliferations may also develop in other sites, such as the periosteum (parosteal fasciitis) and within blood ves-

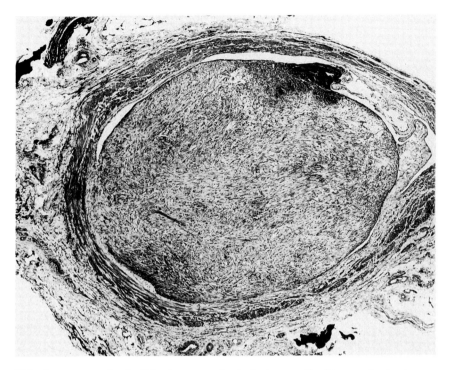

FIG. 8 Intravascular fasciitis. As a general rule, lesions confined to vascular lumina are benign.

sels (intravascular fasciitis) (33). Recurrence following simple local excision is uncommon.

Intravascular fasciitis can be seen at any age and has no gender predilection. However, it occurs most frequently in children and young adults, where it favors the upper extremities and head and neck region (33–35).

Gross examination reveals one or more masses with either a circumscribed or a somewhat infiltrative appearance. Close scrutiny sometimes reveals the intimate association with one or more vessels, usually veins. Intravascular fasciitis shares many histologic features with nodular fasciitis, the key distinction being the former's association with vasculature (Fig. 8). A solitary round or oval mass, a serpentine growth, or a multinodular or plexiform proliferation may be noted, depending on the extent of the process and the number and type of vessels involved. The intima, media, and adventitia of the vessel wall, as well as the juxtaposed soft tissue, are often involved by the loose "feathery" proliferation of myofibroblastic cells. Extravasated erythrocytes and scattered lymphocytes are usually present. Osteoclast-like giant cells, cystic degeneration, and keloid-like collagen are additional features that may be noted.

Ganglion-like myofibroblasts, a characteristic feature of *proliferative fasciitis* and proliferative myositis, are typically absent. Mitoses may be numerous, and this feature, in conjunction with focal cellularity or a history of rapid growth, may lead to an incorrect diagnosis of *sarcoma*. However, intravascular fasciitis usually is small, circumscribed, and of bland nuclear morphology.

In contrast to *vascular smooth muscle tumors*, intravascular fasciitis is less likely to exhibit a fascicular growth pattern. Also, smooth muscle cells are usually somewhat larger than myofibroblasts due to more abundant eosinophilic cytoplasm and more frequently feature blunt-ended nuclei and juxtanuclear vacuoles. Finally, longitudinal cytoplasmic striations, as demonstrated with Masson's trichrome stain, are a characteristic feature of smooth muscle but are infrequently seen and less developed in myofibroblasts.

E.   Angiolymphoid Hyperplasia with Eosinophilia (Epithelioid Hemangioma)

In 1969, Wells and Whimster published a group of nine lesions under the descriptive designation "angiolymphoid hyperplasia with eosinophilia" (ALHE) (36). All of the lesions arose in the head and neck region and were predominantly located in the subcutaneous tissues. "Epithelioid hemangioma" and "histiocytoid hemangioma" are other designations proposed later that encompass these benign vascular lesions. Still, ALHE is probably the most appropriate term for this entity as it is well established in the literature.

Clinically, ALHE is characterized by nodules or papules predominantly located in the head and neck region. The lesions may be multifocal and associated with regional lymphadenopathy and, occasionally, peripheral eosinophilia (37).

Kimura's disease, a disease almost exclusively seen in the Far East, also has predilection for the head and neck region and may also be multifocal with regional adenopathy and peripheral blood eosinophilia (38). However, while adenopathy and peripheral eosinophilia may be seen in both, they are less common in ALHE. The latter also typically presents as a smaller mass that is almost invariably unilateral (38).

Histologically ALHE (36,39,40,37,43,44) is easily distinguished from Kimura's disease. It is characterized by a proliferation of benign capillary-sized vessels lined by plump epithelioid endothelial cells, and there is usually an associated infiltrate of lymphocytes and eosinophils (Fig. 9). Many lesions in soft tissue are associated with a large vessel showing mural damage (45) (Fig. 10). The process is well marginated and often surrounded by lymphoid follicles. Dermal examples of ALHE, as opposed to subcutaneous ones, are less well marginated, generally

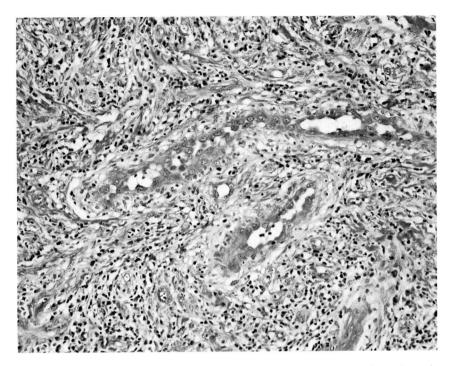

FIG. 9 At higher magnification, epithelioid hemangioma consists of well-formed vessels with plump endothelial cells in an inflammatory background.

are not associated with medium-sized vessels, and less commonly have lymphoid follicles.

ALHE is considered a reactive or quasi-neoplastic condition. Features that suggest that at least some examples of ALHE are reactive in nature include (a) predilection for superficial sites with minimal soft-tissue padding; (b) history of trauma in some instances; (c) localized, relatively marginated and symmetrical arrangement about a medium-sized vessel, in many subcutaneous examples; (d) evidence of damage to involved larger vessels; (e) identification of features consistent with intralesional maturation (i.e., a transition from "immature" small vessels without patent lumina to vessels with well-defined lumina, sometimes without epithelioid endothelium); and (f) a pronounced inflammatory reaction.

Local recurrence has been noted in up to one third of patients. Multiple lesions have been described. This seems more attributable to multicentricity than evidence of metastases because there are no reported deaths attributable to this process.

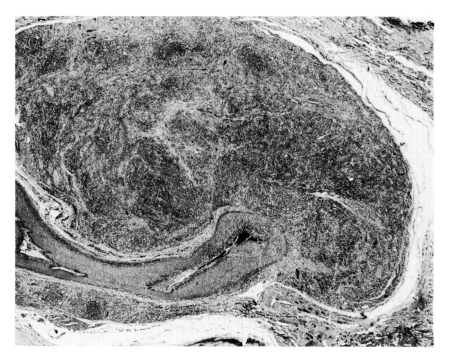

FIG. 10 Epithelioid hemangioma/angiolymphoid hyperplasia with eosinophilia. This well-circumscribed lesion emanates from a medium-sized artery, as can be seen on this Movat stain. Note the prominent internal elastic lamina of the affected vessel.

V. BENIGN VASCULAR TUMORS

For the pathologist, the following general morphologic features in a vascular tumor support a benign diagnosis: (a) zonated or lobular growth; (b) bland morphology with minimal mitotic activity; (c) arrangement of the endothelium in a monolayer; and (d) presence of a "mature" vascular pattern with appropriate supporting elements or evidence of intralesional maturation (46).

A. Pyogenic Granuloma

The term *pyogenic granuloma* is a misnomer; the lesion was first believed to be infectious (47,48). Currently it is considered as an exaggerated vascular hyperplasia with granulation tissue-like features or a variant of capillary hemangioma (49,50).

The lesions may involve mucosal, cutaneous, subcutaneous, or even intravascular sites (51,52), most often involving the gingiva, fingers, and mouth. It is more common in males under the age of 18. From 18 to 40 years of age women are more commonly affected, and after the age of 40 both sexes are affected equally (53). A history of trauma is reported in approximately one third of cases (54,55). Local recurrence has been reported in up to 16% of cases treated by simple excision. Tumors of the oral and nasal mucosa show a marked predilection for women in their reproductive years (54,56), especially during the first trimester of pregnancy when they are referred to as granuloma gravidarum, epulis, or gingival tumor of pregnancy.

On histologic examination, there is proliferation of mitotically active capillary-sized vessels that may be associated with larger feeder vessels and arrangement in a multilobular pattern (Figs. 11 and 12). The surface of these lesions if frequently ulcerated, especially in mucosal sites. Fibromyxoid stroma and/or inflammatory cells may also be seen in the deeper portions.

The differential diagnosis of pyogenic granuloma includes vascular tumefactions that result from treatable infections (i.e., bacillary angiomatosis, and *Carrión's disease* which is localized to endemic regions). *Bacillary angiomatosis* dif-

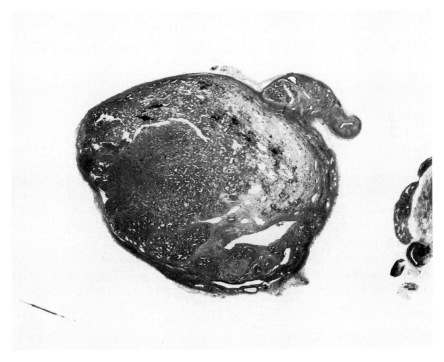

FIG. 11 Lobular capillary hemangioma/pyogenic granuloma. This well-circumscribed tumor has a "feeder vessel" seen at the upper right.

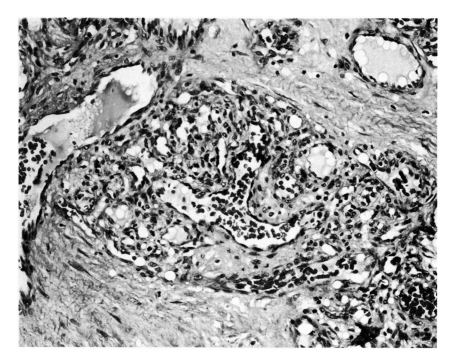

FIG. 12 All varieties of capillary hemangioma are characterized by small vessels budding from larger ones in a lobular configuration.

fers from pyogenic granuloma by containing scattered foci of necrosis with flocculent material, neutrophils, and leukocytoclastic debris.

Pyogenic granuloma must be also be distinguished from malignant vascular tumors, such as angiosarcoma and the nodular stage of Kaposi's sarcoma. *Angiosarcoma* differs from pyogenic granuloma by exhibiting more infiltrative growth with interanastomosing vascular channels lined by plump, atypical endothelial cells. Necrosis and atypical mitoses are also commonly present.

A single nodular lesion of *Kaposi's sarcoma* can bear a close clinical resemblance to pyogenic granuloma. However, Kaposi's disease, in contrast to pyogenic granuloma, is frequently a multifocal process associated with immunosuppression and has an increased incidence in certain ethnic groups. The nodular lesions of Kaposi's sarcoma are dominated by spindle cells with slit-like vascular spaces. Intracytoplasmic, PAS-positive/diastase-resistant, eosinophilic hyaline globules and a peripheral plasma cell response are additional features characteristically present at this stage of Kaposi's sarcoma but are not seen in pyogenic granuloma.

B. Capillary Hemangioma

Capillary hemangiomas are common and are the most common tumor of infancy, seen in about 10–20% of babies (64,65). They may on rare occasion be associated with congenital malformations (66). There is a distinct female preponderance, with a F/M ratio of up to 3 : 1. In children, capillary hemangiomas are typically cellular and have been referred to as infantile hemangioendothelioma, juvenile hemangioma, strawberry nevus, and cellular capillary hemangioma (67).

These lesions most commonly involve the skin or subcutis of the head and neck region, although any site may be involved (68). Rarely, they may attain large size and may even have life-threatening consequences. In large lesions, the increased capillary surface can cause platelet trapping, thrombocytopenia, and a coagulopathy known as Kasabach-Merritt syndrome (69).

Capillary hemangiomas typically have a clinical course characterized by proliferation in the first few months of life, followed by regression and, in many instances, virtually complete involution without any treatment by age 7 years (70). The rare patients with life-threatening or severely disfiguring consequences have in recent years been treated, with varying degrees of success, by selective embolization, laser resection, amd other means (71–74). Capillary hemangiomas are the predominant form of intramuscular hemangiomas.

Histologically, capillary hemangiomas are characterized by highly cellular, mitotically active, and poorly canalized vessels proliferating in a well-circumscribed, lobulated growth pattern. Superficial capillary hemangioma (strawberry nevus or hemangioma) must be differentiated from vascular stains. The term *nevus flammeus* has been used to encompass a wide variety of congenital macular stains. These macular stains are very common, occurring in a third or more of newborn infants (75–77). Those located in the center of the face commonly disappear by age 1 year, whereas nape lesions fade more slowly and often incompletely. Port-wine stains (nevus venosus), on the other hand, occur far less frequently. They consist of larger macules with irregular borders that tend to enlarge in proportion to the growth of the child and generally do not fade (78,79). They are typically flat in infancy and childhood but may become elevated and nodular later in life. Unlike capillary hemangiomas, congenital macular stains are not characterized by endothelial proliferation (80) and, as such, are not associated with the Kasabach-Merritt syndrome. In fact, when biopsied early in life, they typically reveal minimal or no apparent histologic abnormality (79,81).

C. Cavernous Hemangioma

Cavernous hemangiomas are common vascular tumors in both children and adults, with an equal male-to-female ratio (82,83). Although there appears to be a strong

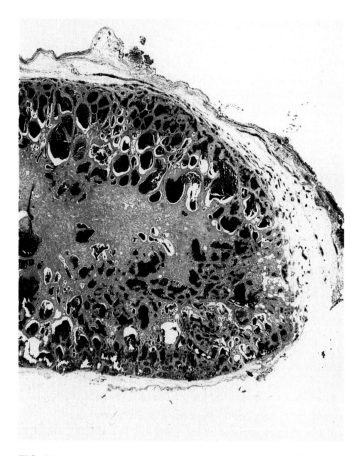

FIG. 13 Cavernous hemangioma showing numerous ectatic vessels.

predeliction for the upper half of the body, any site can be involved (84,85). Unlike capillary hemangiomas, cavernous hemangiomas do not frequently regress. Rarely, large, deep-seated examples may be associated with the Kasabach-Merritt consumptive coagulopathy syndrome.

Cutaneous cavernous hemangiomas are soft, elevated, dark blue or purplish masses that compress easily and blanch with pressure. Deep-seated examples may be clinically inapparent.

The histology is characterized by either a lobulated or a poorly marginated collection of engorged thin-walled vascular channels lined by flattened endothelium (Fig. 13).

Cavernous hemangiomas have been described as part of various syndromes (66,86). *Maffucci's syndrome* is a congenital but nonhereditary syndrome of dyschondroplasia and hemangiomata, with no sex predilection (2,3). The osseous lesions are enchondromas that eventually give rise to chondrosarcomas in approximately 15% of patients (87). While the vascular lesions in some reports seem to represent cavernous hemangiomas, many appear to be examples of spindle cell hemangioendothelioma/hemangioma. *Blue rubber bleb nevus syndrome* consists of multiple small dome-shaped vascular lesions involving the skin and internal organs, especially the gastrointestinal tract (4).

D. Deep Angiomatous Lesions

Benign deep vascular lesions represent a disease spectrum with considerable clinicopathologic overlap. All share the capacity to be infiltrative and therefore may be difficult to cure with local surgical excision. Acknowledging these points and given evidence suggesting that the predominant vessel pattern and anatomical location seem to have little influence on the recurrence rate, it has been proposed that the intramuscular tumors be grouped under the generic designation of "angioma" (88). The lesions that come under this category include intramuscular hemangioma, arteriovenous malformations, and venous hemangiomas.

Intramuscular hemangiomas are relatively uncommon and most likely present in the first three decades; congenital examples are well described. The most common site of involvement is the lower extremity. On histologic examination, intramuscular hemangiomas consist of poorly marginated proliferations of vessels intermixed with varying amounts of supporting elements, such as adipose and fibroconnective tissue (88,89) (Fig. 14). The presence of extensive overgrowth of fat in intramuscular hemangiomas often leads to misdiagnoses of intramuscular lipomas. *Arteriovenous malformations* can be either congenital or acquired. The diagnosis is best made by clinical and radiologic studies as opposed to histologic findings. Although they are often obvious on angiograms, extensive histologic sampling may be required to identify direct arteriovenous anastamoses or to confirm the presence of arterialized veins (90,91). *Venous hemangiomas* involve deep structures and are often thrombosed due to sluggish blood flow. Histologically, there are blood filled endothelial-lined channels with prominent muscular walls with a paucity of elastic tissue (92).

E. Glomeruloid Hemangioma

Glomeruloid hemangioma is rare and occurs as a component of the POEMS syndrome (93,94) which is characterized by the following features: *p*olyneuropathy, *o*rganomegaly (hepatosplenomegaly and lymphadenopathy), *e*ndocrinopathy (amenorrhea, gynecomastia, hypothyroidism, adrenal insufficiency, and glucose intolerance), *m*onoclonal protein (marrow plasmacytosis, paraproteinemia), and *s*kin lesions. The latter include glomeruloid and cherry angiomas, acanthosis, hy-

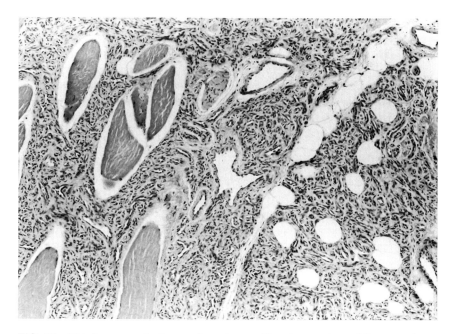

FIG. 14 This intramuscular hemangioma is a capillary hemangioma. Like many intramuscular hemangiomas, this one has admixed fat.

perpigmentation, and hypertrichosis. Glomeruloid hemangiomas are commonly
multifocal, mostly appearing as small papules involving skin of the trunk or proximal extremities. Histologic examination reveals dilated, ectatic vessels with intraluminal capillary conglomerates, architecturally resembling renal glomeruli.
Occasionally, the stromal cells between the vessels contain PAS-positive, diastase-
resistant globules that are believed to represent phagocytized immunoglobulin.

    Due to the presence of multiple cutaneous vascular lesions, some har-
boring eosinophilic globules, the possibility of *Kaposi's sarcoma* may come to
mind. However, glomeruloid hemangioma is easily distinguished by its restricted
intravascular growth, well-formed vascular channels, and lack of a spindled
component.

F. Angioblastoma (Acquired Tufted Angioma, Progressive Capillary Hemangioma)

Angioblastomas are typically slow-growing, painful lesions mostly presenting
before the age of 10 years, most commonly during the first year of life (95–97).
On histologic examination, lesions consist of irregular nodules (cannonballs) of

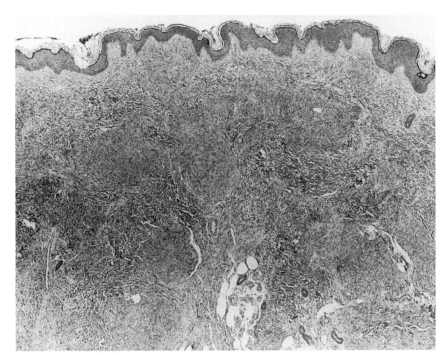

FIG. 15 Angioblastoma. Multiple nodules are seen in the dermis.

capillary-sized vessels growing within the dermis (Fig. 15). The vascular nodules protrude into vascular spaces giving the appearance of intravascular "tufts" (Fig. 16). The morbidity of these lesions is predominantly cosmetic; metastases have not been recorded despite frequent recurrences.

G. Targetoid Hemosiderotic Hemangioma

Recognition of this rare benign vascular lesion by pathologists is primarily of importance because its histology overlaps somewhat with that of Kaposi's sarcoma (98–100). However, its clinical presentation is distinctive. It typically occurs as a solitary lesion on the trunk or extremities of young adults, mainly males. These lesions usually have a central violaceous or brown–black papule, bordered by an inner pale zone and a more peripherally situated ecchymotic ring. As such, these lesions resemble a target.

The histology of targetoid hemosiderotic hemangioma (THH) is characterized by ectatic thin-walled vascular channels situated in the superficial dermis. Intraluminal papillary endothelial projections and fibrin thrombi may be present.

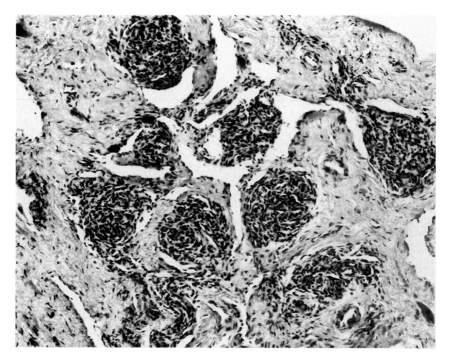

FIG. 16 Angioblastoma/tufted hemangioma. Note the spindle cell proliferations (tufts), which compress the associated capillaries into crescent shapes.

Deeper vessels, located in the reticular dermis, have an angulated, irregular, and slit-like appearance with permeative growth pattern.

The most important differential diagnosis is with *Kaposi's sarcoma*, which differs histologically by containing apoptotic endothelial cells, clusters of intracytoplasmic eosinophilic hyaline globules, and a plasma cell infiltrate.

Of note, cutaneous lesions with a targetoid appearance may also be observed in erythema multiforme, erythema chronicum migrans of Lyme disease, and within cherry angiomas in patients with primary amyloidosis. However, the clinical features and histology of these disease processes are substantially different from those of THH.

VI. LESIONS OF INDETERMINATE BIOLOGICAL POTENTIAL

The three lesions described below under vascular tumors of indeterminate biological potential are rare tumors that are not obviously malignant but have the tendency of either aggressive local behavior or distant metastasis. Although spindle cell hemangioendothelioma has been included with this group, accumulating evidence suggests that the lesion is, in fact, benign.

A. Spindle Cell Hemangioendothelioma (Hemangioma)

Spindle cell hemangioendothelioma typically presents as a superficial slow growing painless mass involving the dermis and/or subcutis (101–103). These lesions may develop at any age, may be single or multifocal, and most commonly involve the hands and feet. A small number of cases have been associated with other disease processes, such as Maffucci's syndrome, Klippel-Trenaunay syndrome, and an early onset of varicose veins. The lesions tend to grow in "crops" on the affected distal extremity site but do not metastasize.

The histology of spindle cell hemangioendothelioma is highly characteristic, with a well-marginated lesion showing two components: (a) cavernous vascular spaces, similar to those seen in a cavernous hemangioma, lined by epithelioid endothelial cells with occasional intracytoplasmic lumina, frequently associated with phleboliths (Fig. 17), and (b) a spindle cell proliferation vaguely reminiscent of *Kaposi's sarcoma* (Fig. 18). Lack of hyaline globules, epithelioid endothelial cells with intracytoplasmic lumina, and no known association with HIV status aid in distinguishing this entity from Kaposi's sarcoma. Although these lesions were initially believed to be low-grade angiosarcomas, additional experience with large numbers of patients has led to the belief that they are probably benign, and these may ultimately be reclassified as spindle cell hemangiomas (103a).

B. Endovascular Papillary Angioendothelioma (Dabska's Tumor) and Retiform Hemangioendothelioma

The Dabska tumor is an exceedingly rare lesion, first described in children, that is capable of regional lymph node metastasis (104). The tumors tend to be superficial, primarily involving the skin and subcutis, and are composed of proliferations of capillary-sized vessels lined by cuboidal or columnar endothelial cells occasionally forming intraluminal tufts (Fig. 19). Lymphocytes are commonly seen intravascularly and surrounding the capillary proliferation. Epithelioid endothelial cells with intracytoplasmic lumina are often seen in Dabska's tumors, a feature also seen in other vasoformative processes such as *spindle cell hemangioendothelioma*, *epithelioid hemangioendothelioma*, and *epithelioid hemangioma*. Another tumor, *retiform hemangioendothelioma*, seems to be either similar or identical to the Dabska tumor; the latter has been described in adults (second to fourth decade) as distinctive form of *low-grade angiosarcoma* of the skin that recurs frequently but has a very low metastatic rate (119,153,154). Since two tumors from Dabska's original series are now known to have caused the patients' death after a long interval, the Dabska tumors are probably best classified as low-grade sarcomas.

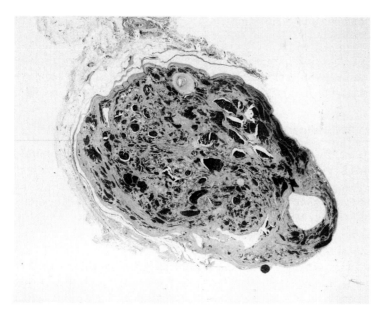

FIG. 17 Spindle cell hemangioendothelioma/hemangioma. A hyalinized vessel with a phlebolith is present at the top center portion of this well-circumscribed tumor.

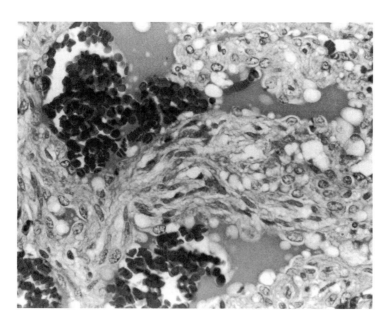

FIG. 18 Spindle cell hemangioendothelioma/hemangioma. Spindle cells are adjacent to ectatic vascular spaces. Intracytoplasmic lumina may sometimes be seen in the spindle cells.

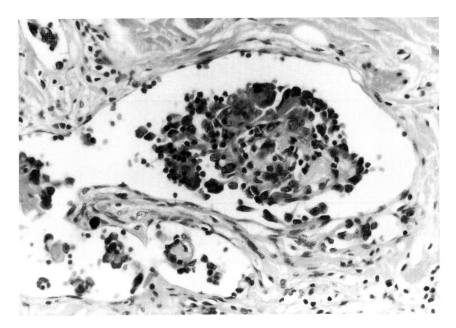

FIG. 19 Dabska's tumor.

The lesions are located preferentially on the lower and upper limbs, although any site can be involved. Clinically the lesions present as slow-growing exophytic masses or plaque-like skin nodules. Histologically, typical described features are long arborizing vessels reminiscent of normal rete testes lined by monomorphic "hobnail" endothelial cells, a prominent lymphocytic infiltrate, and focal intraluminal papillary projections similar to those seen in Dabska's tumor. By immunohistochemistry, the endothelial cells are positive for factor VIII–related antinen, CD31, CD34, and Ulex europaeus I lectin. The presence of staining with vascular endothelial-related growth factor 3 (VEGFR3) has recently led to the suggestion that these display features of lymphatic vessels and confirmed that these tumors may occur in adults (104a).

C. Kaposiform Infantile Hemangioendothelioma

Kaposiform infantile hemangioendothelioma (KIH) is a rare vascular tumor that primarily affects infants and children manifesting as a large retroperitoneal mass frequently associated with consumptive coagulopathy (Kasabach-Merritt syndrome) (106,107). The tumor is reported to have an association with lymphangiomatosis and is sometimes complicated by intestinal obstruction, jaundice, and he-

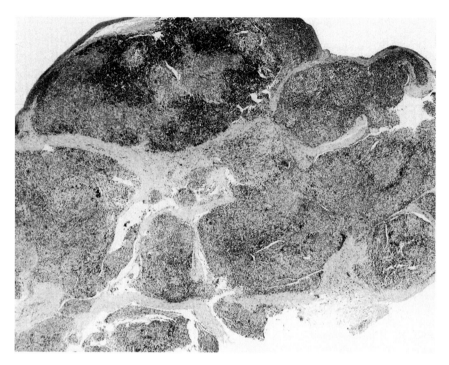

FIG. 20 Kaposiform hemangioendothelioma of infancy. Despite the alarming cellularity, the lesion retains a lobular architecture.

moperitoneum. In the majority of cases, the tumor is lethal due to aggressive local behavior although distant metastases have not been reported.

The tumors are characterized histologically by infiltrative, lobular growth of well-formed capillaries, sometimes containing fibrin thrombi, admixed with short fascicles of spindle cells with slit-like spaces (Figs. 20 and 21).

The differential diagnosis includes other pediatric vascular tumors such as *cellular capillary hemangioma*, which lacks the spindle cells with slit-like spaces. The lobulated growth pattern, lack of a prominent interanastomosing vascular pattern, and paucity of significant cytologic atypia aid in distinguishing this tumor from *angiosarcoma*.

Features that distinguish kaposiform infantile hemangioendothelioma from *Kaposi's sarcoma* include the young age of the patient, lack of an association with HIV status, confinement of the process to one general site or location (usually deep-seated), lobulated architecture of the vascular proliferation, less pronounced lymphoplasmacytic response, and infrequent hyaline globules.

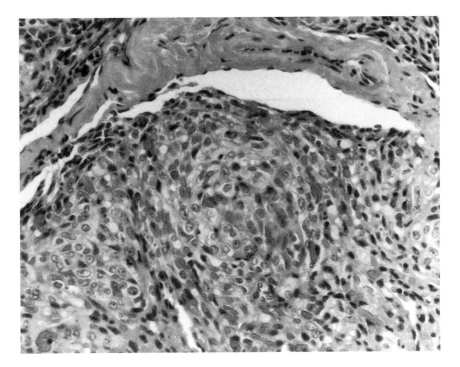

FIG. 21 Kaposiform hemangioendothelioma of infancy.

VII. MALIGNANT VASCULAR TUMORS

A. Epithelioid Hemangioendothelioma

Epithelioid hemangioendothelioma (EHE) is a low-grade vascular neoplasm that can occur at any age. There is no sex predilection and the predominant sites of involvement are the soft tissues, lungs, liver, and bone (45,108–111). The tumors typically present as a superficial or deep solitary mass, or occasionally multiple masses, with a predilection for the extremities. Lesions in the soft tissue are frequently associated with a vessel, most commonly a vein. In the largest soft-tissue series reported, the local recurrence rate was about 15%, and the metastasis rate was 31%, mostly to regional lymph nodes; 13% of patients died of disease. Features that may correlate with more aggressive biological behavior include mitotic counts of greater than 1 mitosis per 10 high-power fields, spindled tumor cell morphology, the presence of necrosis, and prominent cytologic atypia.

When EHE occurs within the lung, it has been referred to as intravascular bronchioloalveolar tumor (IVBAT) (112,113). IVBAT is more common in women, characteristically presenting as multiple and bilateral 1-cm nodules. Extensive disease at the time of presentation, peripheral lymphadenopathy with or without metastasis, and hepatic metastasis are associated with poor outcome in pulmonary epithelioid hemangioendothelioma. Hepatic involvement is also commonly seen in women presenting with multifocal and bilobar masses (114). Before diagnosing a primary pulmonary or hepatic EHE, patients should be thoroughly evaluated for evidence of an extrapulmonary primary tumor.

Grossly the tumor, regardless of the site, is well marginated, firm, rubbery, and has cartilaginous consistency. Calcifications may be seen. Microscopically the tumor is commonly angiocentric and composed of short cords and nests of epithelioid endothelial cells with eosinophilic cytoplasm, occasionally showing intracellular vacuoles/lumina, embedded in myxohyaline matrix (Figs. 22 and 23). The intracytoplasmic vacuoles may contain intraluminal erythrocytes, a sign of "primitive" vasoformative differentiation.

The differential diagnosis includes a number of entities ranging from metastatic *adenocarcinoma* with infiltrating cells showing intracytoplasmic va-

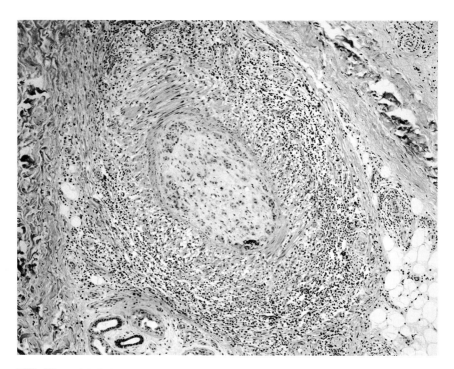

FIG. 22 Epithelioid hemangioendothelioma. Although this tumor appears confined to a vessel, in other foci, it infiltrated the surrounding tissue.

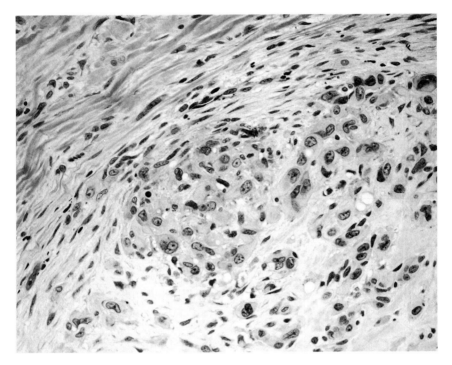

FIG. 23 Epithelioid hemangioendothelioma. Intracytoplasmic lumina are apparent in some of the cells and can be confused with mucin vacuoles. Distinguishing these tumors from adenocarcinomas is usually easily accomplished by immunohistochemical staining.

coules or signet ring cells to high-grade sarcomas. Carcinoma is not vasocentric, and different areas may show obvious gland formation. The vacuoles are also mucicarmine-positive and the neoplastic cells are positive for antibodies against cytokeratin and negative for vasular markers by immunohistochemistry. A panel approach is recommended as occasionally EHE may show some cytokeratin positivity. *Melanoma* also comes into the differential diagnosis as it is a great mimicker and may appear as infiltrating epithelioid cells with eosinophilic cytoplasm. Close attention should be paid to melanin pigment, intranuclear inclusions, binucleation, and prominent intranuclear inclusions. By immunohistochemistry, melanoma cells are usually positive for S-100 protein and HMB-45 and negative for vascular markers and keratin. *Epithelioid angiosarcoma* is distinguished in most instances by its paucity of myxohyaline matrix and its tendency for more atypia, cellularity, mitotic activity, and necrosis. Interanastomosing vascular channels with prominent melanoma-like intranuclear inclusions are also more prevalent in angiosarcoma.

Features that distinguish epithelioid hemangioendothelioma from *epithelioid hemangioma* are the infiltrative growth pattern, less pronounced inflammatory response, more primitive vascular pattern of the former as opposed to well-formed vessels and inflammatory background of the latter. *Epithelioid sarcoma*, which has a strong predilection for the tendons and aponeuroses, also enters the differential diagnosis. It differs histologically by featuring a rather distinctive geographic or granulomatous growth pattern with central necrosis. *Chondrosarcoma*, like epithelioid hemangioendothelioma, contains sulfated acid mucins. However, in contrast to chondrosarcoma, the neoplastic cells of EHE typically lack S-100 protein expression.

Two uncommon considerations in the differential diagnosis are also worth brief mention. First, epithelioid hemangioendothelioma exhibiting pleural or peritoneal extension can grow in an organ encasing manner and produce a pattern reminiscent of *malignant mesothelioma*. Second, osseous epithelioid hemangioendothelioma, especially if multifocal, can be confused histologically with *myeloma* since both tumors may feature coarse granular nuclear chromatin and hyaline-like eosinophilic cytoplasm. However, correlation with appropriate clinical parameters (e.g., asbestos exposure, paraproteinemia, etc.) and a battery of histochemical and/or immunohistochemical studies lead to the correct diagnosis.

B. Kaposi's Sarcoma

Kaposi's sarcoma (KS) was first described as "idiopathic multiple pigmented sarcoma of the skin" in 1872 (115). There are different epidemiologic subgroups that are at high risk for KS (116).

(1) *Classic or European form.* This subtype classically affects elderly men, with an increased incidence in Ashkenazic Jews and people of Mediterranean descent (117–119). The disease has an indolent course, with lesions involving predominantly the lower legs. Secondary malignancies have been reported in more than 30% of cases, mostly of hematopoietic origin (120).

(2) *African or Endemic form.* This variant has had its highest incidence in Zaire and Uganda (121,122). The disease has been subsequently subdivided in two groups: young to middle-aged adults with mostly benign nodular disease, and children with fulminant lymphadenopathic disease (typically fatal in 2–3 years).

(3) *Iatrogenic form associated with immunosuppression.* This subtype is descibed in transplant patients. KS may assume a chronic or aggressive course. It is usually more aggressive than the classic form, although regression may follow discontinuation of immunosuppression (123,124).

(4) *AIDS-Associated or Epidemic form.* The risk of developing KS is 300 times greater in the AIDS population than in other immunosuppressed patients (125). It is more common in homosexual men with AIDS practicing oroanal and anal intercourse. Epidemiologic evidence suggests involvement of an infectious

agent in the origin of KS. Cytomegalovirus (CMV) has been postulated as a cofactor in the pathogenesis of this disease, although no consistent association has been established. The CMV genome does not appear to integrate into KS cells (126), and CMV is so ubiquitous in the population at risk for KS that its mere presence may reflect nothing more than a coexisting generalized infection (127,128). Other viral etiologies have been proposed, including herpes simplex, hepatitis A, hepatitis B, and herpesvirus 16. More recently, a new human herpesvirus (HSV-8) has been implicated as a possible etiologic agent, the DNA sequence of which is seen in more than 90% of specimens from KS patients (119,129).

Three clinical disease patterns of KS have been recognized (121): (a) nodular, (b) aggressive, and (c) generalized. *Nodular disease* is characterized by the presence of circumscribed cutaneous or subcutaneous nodules. It usually pursues an indolent course, although internal involvement, which is frequently asymptomatic, is often present at the time of death. The *aggressive form* of KS generally arises from a background of preexisting nodular disease. It is characterized by extensive exophytic and ulcerative or deep infiltrative growth usually involving the extremities. Osseous and visceral involvement are commonly present but may be clinically silent. The *generalized form* of KS includes lymphadenopathic disease with or without systemic involvement and occurs primarily in children. AIDS-associated KS may appear at any stage but usually affects those with advanced immune suppression and CD4 T-cell counts of less than 500 cells/mm^3. In contrast to the classic form, AIDS-associated KS lesions are often seen on the chest and face.

KS is a vascular/lymphatics-related process with endothelial and vascular-derived supporting cells being the key elements (130,131). Flow cytometric analyses of Kaposi's lesions show diploid results (132,133).

Histologically there are no well-defined differences between the four subtypes of KS. The earliest or the *patch lesions* occur in the upper dermis. The changes appear very inconspicous and may be easily dismissed as an inflammatory condition.

Characteristically in early lesions there is proliferation of thin-walled jagged capillaries around preexisting dermal vessels and adnexa. When these proliferations cause protrusion into the lumen of a preexisting larger dermal vessel, the resulting appearance has been called the "promontory sign." Some endothelial cells may contain apoptotic nuclei. Variable numbers of inflammatory cells dominated by lymphocytes and plasma cells are usually seen along with extravasated erythrocytes, hemosiderin deposition, and intracytoplasmic PAS-positive hyaline globules (134). As KS progresses to involve the full thickness of the dermis, it becomes palpable, clinically recognized as *plaque stage*, and has more prominent spindle cell component dispersed among the dermal collagen, forming slit-like spaces that frequently contain erythrocytes. *Nodular lesions* (Fig. 24) of KS represent further development and grossly appear well circumscribed, violaceous, and dome-shaped

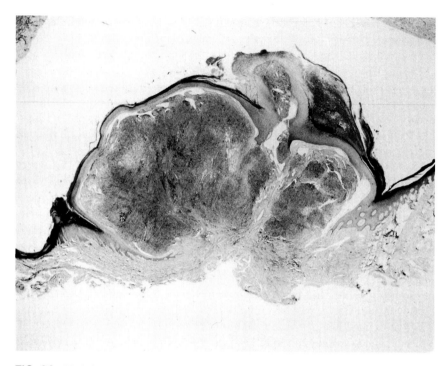

FIG. 24 Nodular Kaposi's sarcoma. This lesion appears remarkably similar to Carrión's disease (see Fig. 4).

or polypoid. The spindle cells dominate, forming fascicles and sheets with scattered extravasated erythrocytes, hemosiderin-laden macrophages, hyaline globules, and inflammatory cells (Fig. 25). Although prominent cytologic atypia and abundant mitotic figures are not usually present, they are sometimes seen. Rarely *lymphangioma-like variants* may occur which appear as ectatic lymphatic-like channels with absence of or minimal accompanying secondary features (135). From a histogenetic point of view, current evidence suggests that KS is a proliferation of vessels. Whether this represents endothelium of blood vessels or lymphatics has sparked some controversy (130,131). More recently, it is thought to be closely related to vascular smooth muscle cells (119).

As noted above, there are no well-defined morphologic or immunohistochemical differences between the classical, endemic, iatrogenic (immunosuppressive), and AIDS-associated forms of KS. While the histologic diagnosis of well-developed nodular or plaque lesions is generally not difficult, early patch (macular) lesions may have sufficiently subtle morphology that a definite diagnosis cannot be rendered. In the latter instance, little is usually lost by adopting a conservative

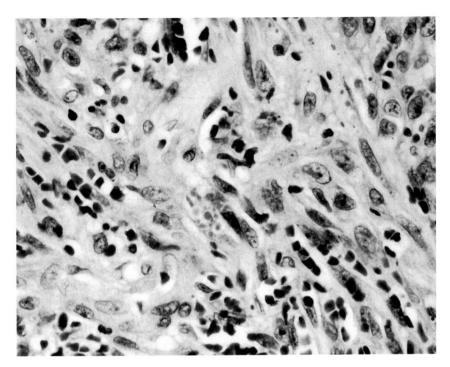

FIG. 25 Hyaline globules, which are erythrophagolysosomes, are a constant feature of Kaposi's sarcoma and can be seen in the center of this field.

stance, providing supportive medical management, and rebiopsying the patient at a later date when more typical lesions are present.

Pleomorphic or anaplastic change ("malignant transformation") has been reported in KS. Lesions with this morphology are believed capable of true metastases. In some instances, the morphology is indistinguishable from a spindled or poorly differentiated angiosarcoma. Other examples have been likened to fibrosarcoma or undifferentiated malignancies (118,121,137).

Clinically, the lymphangioma-like variant of classic KS (135,138,139) does not appear to vary substantially from more typical cases. However, its histology differs by featuring a predominance of ectatic lymphatic-like channels that permeate the dermis. Associated inflammation is minimal, but hemosiderin deposition is seen. A minor, ill-defined, spindle cell component may be present, but it is not usually intermingled with the vascular clefts as in more typical Kaposi's lesions.

KS may involve lymph nodes (140–143), either as an initial, sometimes isolated, manifestation, or as a later component of disseminated disease. Like cutaneous examples, it is readily recognized when the disease is fully established but is difficult to characterize in its initial stages. Early changes include subcapsular sinus ectasia and intrasinusoidal vascular proliferation. Step sectioning may be required to identify a spindle cell component. Caution is advised when diagnosing early nodal KS, especially when clinical details are not at hand, since other intranodal vascular proliferations may exhibit morphologic overlap (i.e., vascular transformation of sinuses/nodal angiomatosis) (144,145). Intranodal palisaded myofibroblastoma, a recently characterized benign myofibroblastic proliferation that occurs predominantly in the inguinal lymph nodes of adults, also shares some morphologic resemblance to advanced intranodal KS (146–148).

The clinical differential of KS is quite long due to the various stages through which the disease passes. It includes (acro-)angiodermatitis, bacillary angiomatosis, pyogenic granuloma, melanoma, cutaneous lymphoma, blue nevus, dermatofibroma, hemangioma, cicatrix, postinflammatory pigmentation, and a number of other conditions (149). The challenge lies in recognizing early stages of the disease as well as unusually aggressive examples. An accurate diagnosis in these instances is dependent on a high index of suspicion and appropriate clinicopathologic correlation.

Pseudo-Kaposi's sarcoma (9) is an unfortunate term that includes (*acro-*) *angiodermatitis* (150), which refers to skin lesions on lower extremities of patients with chronic venous insufficiency, and *Stewart-Bluefarb syndrome*, which consists of an arteriovenous malformation that clinically resembles KS. Both types resemble KS clinically but are distinct histologically. In acrodermatitis, the histopathologic changes are those of stasis dermatitis with an increased number of thick-walled blood vessels lined by plump endothelial cells, hemosiderin deposition, and extravasated red blood cells. In Stewart-Bluefarb syndrome an arteriovenous shunt may be identified. *Targetoid hemosiderotic hemangioma* (THH), addressed above, may mimic KS histologically, but the clinical presentation is quite different. *Acquired progressive lymphangioma* (benign lymphangioendothelioma) has not been described in immunocompromised patients (151,152). This lesion presents as a solitary macule or plaque that enlarges slowly and is cured by local excision. Histologically, there are interanastomosing endothelial-lined vascular clefts lacking erythrocytes, with a collagen dissecting pattern. *Bacillary angiomatosis* enters into the differential diagnosis since it has both a predilection for immunosuppressed patients and is typically a multifocal or generalized process. In fact, in the AIDS population, it is not uncommon for this disease to coexist with KS. Its proper distinction is important because it is the result of a treatable infection, which, if unmanaged, can prove fatal.

Nodular KS features a prominent spindled component that commonly contains areas with a fascicular growth pattern. As a result, *soft-tissue sarcomas*, including fibrosarcoma and leiomyosarcoma, may be considered in the differential diagnosis. All three tumors contain cells capable of reacting with immunohistochemical antibodies directed against muscle-specific and smooth muscle actins.

Although longitudinal cytoplasmic fibrillations may also be seen in all three, they are much more prevalent and better defined in leiomyosarcoma. The latter entity differs further from the other two by featuring blunt-ended nuclei and more abundant eosinophilic cytoplasm. The plasma cell infiltrate, slit-like vascular spaces, degree of red blood cell extravasation, and hyaline globules in KS set it apart from both leiomyosarcoma and fibrosarcoma. Although a variety of vascular proliferations have been described as primary intranodal processes, *vascular transformation of sinuses* is probably the most likely to be mistaken for KS (145). It is believed to be due to complete occlusion of the efferent lymphatic channels with or without coexisting partial occlusion of the nodal veins. Four major vascular patterns are described, i.e., cleft-like, rounded or oval, solid, and plexiform patterns. There is frequently associated fibrosclerosis and red blood cell extravasation. The intervening lymphoid parenchyma may be mildly or markedly depleted depending on the extent of the sinusoidal expansion.

C. Angiosarcoma

In this chapter, angiosarcoma is used in a generic sense to encompass fully malignant neoplasms of endothelial derivation whether originating from lymphatics (lymphangiosarcoma) or blood vessels (hemangiosarcoma). Angiosarcoma is a rare tumor, estimated to compose less than 1% of all sarcomas (155). It can occur in a variety of clinical settings involving any site, but there is a particularly strong predilection for the skin and subcutis (119,156,157). In this superficial location angiosarcoma occurs in three distinct clinical settings: (a) face and scalp of the elderly (158–161); (b) extremities of patients with chronic lymphedema (162–164); and (c) at sites previously subjected to radiation therapy (165–171). Angiosarcomas may develop in association with foreign bodies (172,173), defunctionalized arteriovenous fistulas (174), and also are seen with increased frequency in patients with neurofibromatosis (175–177). Other carcinogenic agent exposures have also been implicated, particularly in hepatic tumors, e.g., thorotrast, arsenic compounds, and vinyl chloride (178).

1. Angiosarcoma of Face and Scalp
   (Wilson Jones Angiosarcoma)

Cutaneous angiosarcoma of the face and scalp affects predominantly elderly patients and is usually found on the scalp and upper forehead. It is more common in men than women, with no predisposing factors. Most cases are multifocal. Clinically, the lesion appears as an ill-defined bruise-like area, occasionally starting as erythema and edema. More advanced cases appear as indurated plaques/nodules, which may ulcerate, with or without small satellite nodules in the vicinity. Tumors grow slowly and centrifugally in a relatively short period. The single most important prognostic factor is tumor size, and the prognosis is poor (158,159).

2.   Lymphedema-Associated Angiosarcoma
     (Stewart-Treves Syndrome)

Lymphedema-associated angiosarcoma now bears the eponym of Stewart and
Treves, who first described this condition in patients with breast carcinoma status
post radical mastectomy with or without radiation (179). The average interval between the onset of postmastectomy lymphedema and the appearance of angiosarcoma is approximately 5–10 years (45). Angiosarcomas have subsequently been
described in areas of lymphedema secondary to a variety of other mechanisms.
Patients with congenital lymphedema tend to develop a superimposed angiosarcoma at an earlier age than their postmastectomy counterparts, and lymphedema
has usually been present for 20 years or more. The latter patients have a somewhat
longer mean survival time (45,180). Gross examination typically reveals pit-
ting, indurated skin with red or bluish purple macular, papular, polypoid, or fungating lesions. The tumors may be either solitary or multicentric, sometimes
with an appearance of a dominant mass with satellite nodules. The prognosis of
lymphedema-associated angiosarcoma is as dismal as that of other forms of conventional angiosarcomas.

3.   Postirradiation Angiosarcoma

Postirradiation angiosarcomas have a predilection for the skin and subcutis, although they occasionally arise in more deep-seated sites. Affected individuals can
be subdivided into two groups, based on whether radiotherapy was given for a benign disorder, such as hemangioma or eczema, or for a malignancy, such as gynecologic or breast cancers (165–169, 181). The mean interval to angiosarcoma
is shorter in the group treated for a malignancy, i.e., approximately 11 years vs.
22 years for benign conditions. This difference could be due to the use of higher
irradiation dosages in the malignant group.

4.   Angiosarcoma of Deep Soft Tissue

Angiosarcoma of the deep tissue is rare and information about it is limited. Most
cases involve the extremities or trunk, and many are poorly differentiated. In general, these tumors behave as high-grade sarcomas. Some deep-seated tumors appear to originate from medium-size to large vessels. Epithelioid morphology is
well documented in this group and may lead to an erroneous diagnosis of carcinoma or melanoma (182,182a).

5.   Angiosarcoma of the Breast Parenchyma

Angiosarcomas arising in the breast account for about less than 0.1% of malignant neoplasms in the breast, characteristically occurring in young women in their

twenties or thirties. The most common presentation is that of a diffusely enlarged breast with a painless, soft mass with blue, red, or black discoloration of the overlying skin. The outcome in general is poor and most patients expire within 2 years.

In contrast to the case of angiosarcomas of the skin and subcutaneous tissue, grading is prognostically significant (45,183–185).

The differential diagnosis for primary angiosarcoma of the breast parenchyma includes a variety of hemangioma types (186,187). *Hemangiomas* tend to be small and are often an incidental microscopic finding.

Histopathologically, angiosarcoma has a broad morphologic spectrum. At one extreme, the tumor may consist entirely of well-developed hemangioma or lymphangioma-like vasculature in which the only clues of malignancy are the interanastomosing and infiltrative nature of the process, the presence of mild nuclear hyperchromasia, and occasional crowding or piling up of the endothelium, sometimes forming small papillations (Fig. 26). The opposite end of the spectrum includes both a spindle cell pattern reminiscent of fibrosarcoma or Kaposi's sarcoma

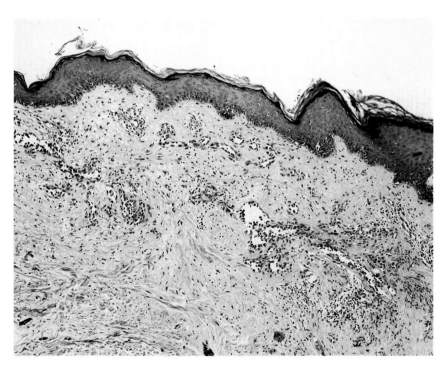

FIG. 26 The diagnosis of angiosarcoma can be difficult when cytologic atypia is not prominent. In this lesion, enlarged endothelial cells aid in the diagnosis, but the haphazard arrangement of the vascular channels is also a clue.

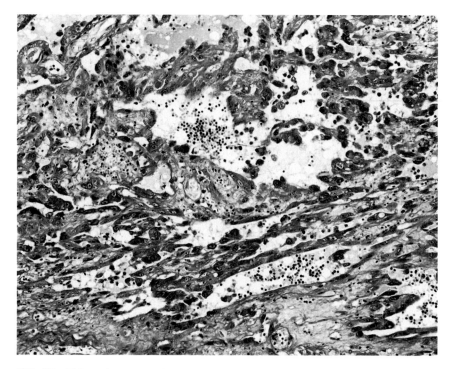

FIG. 27   This angiosarcoma displays large atypical epithelioid endothelial cells. Vascular channels are obvious in this field, but when they are inapparent, distinction from carcinoma and melanoma may require application of immunohistochemical stains.

and an "undifferentiated" pattern consisting of plump epithelioid neoplastic cells (Fig. 27) with prominent nucleoli and diffuse sheet-like growth, suggestive of carcinoma or melanoma. A high index of suspicion, knowledge of the clinical findings, and thorough tumor sampling are essential to establish the correct diagnosis at these morphologic extremes. When well-developed vessels are not apparent, the presence of cytoplasmic vacuolization consistent with early lumen development and a red blood cell or hemosiderin-rich milieu may serve as important clues that point in the direction of a vascular tumor. A reticulin stain can help highlight tube-like vascular growth, which may be inapparent in hematoxylin-eosin-stained sections.

   Immunohistochemistry can prove invaluable when vasoformative architecture is minimal or absent. The endothelial cells stain positive with factor VIII–related antigen, CD34, CD31, and *Ulex europaeus*. However, a panel approach is recommended because poorly differentiated tumors may not express all the vascular markers and epithelioid variants may stain positive with epithelial cell markers such as cytokeratin.

VIII. DISORDERS ERRONEOUSLY CONSIDERED AS VASCULAR NEOPLASMS

A. Angioendotheliomatosis

Angioendotheliomatosis is a broad term that has been used to describe intravascular proliferations frequently associated with systemic manifestations (188). It encompasses two different processes: "malignant angioendotheliomatosis," which is an intravascular form of malignant lymphoma, and "benign or reactive" angioendotheliomatosis, which is a self-limited intravascular proliferation of endothelial cells that occurs in the skin as a response to a variety of stimuli (119). Both benign and malignant clinical courses have been recognized, but the morphologic distinction between these subgroups was not fully appreciated until the advent of immunohistochemistry (189).

Malignant angioendotheliomatosis/intravascular lymphomatosis is a rapidly fatal, aggressive disease generally associated with progressive clinical manifestations leading to death within 1 year. The disease most commonly affects older adults, mostly involving the skin and/or central nervous system (190–192). Cutaneous lesions consist of tender erythematous or purple nodules and plaques on the trunk. Telangiectasia, hemorrhage, and ulceration may be present in these areas. The most common central nervous system manifestation is progressive dementia, although other findings can include decreased visual acuity, blindness, and speech disturbances. Approximately one third of patients exhibit serologic abnormalities (i.e., rheumatoid factor, antinuclear antibodies) that postdate the onset of disease. Secondary involvement of other organs, including lymph nodes, spleen, and gastrointestinal tract, may be demonstrable in 25% or more of cases. However, the bone marrow is typically uninvolved.

On histologic examination, intravascular lymphomatosis features dilated blood vessels that are filled by highly atypical cells with hyperchromatic nuclei and abundant mitoses (Fig. 28). Occasionally, the tumor cells are enmeshed within fibrin thrombi. The malignant infiltrate sometimes spills over into the surrounding tissues, and regional necrosis may be present. The neoplastic cells are typically immunoreactive with antileukocyte common antigen, as well as B- or, rarely, T-cell subset markers.

Benign (reactive) angioendotheliomatosis is usually limited to skin and is characterized by activated immune status (119,189,193), either as a result of an ongoing infection (i.e., bacterial endocarditis, tuberculosis) or an allergic/hypersensitivity reaction. The anatomical distribution and clinical appearance of these le-

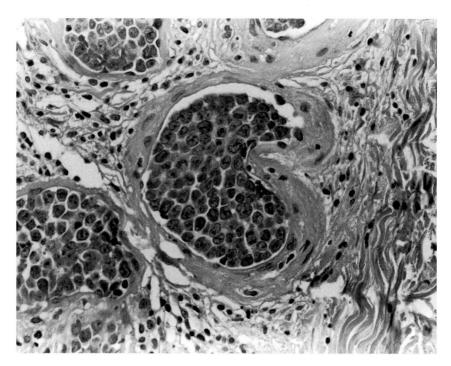

FIG. 28 Intravascular lymphoma.

sions overlaps with the findings in intravascular lymphomatosis. However, patients with benign angioendotheliomatosis do not exhibit profound neurologic manifestations and typically improve spontaneously or following treatment (i.e., antibiotics, steroids) directed at the underlying cause of the immunologic derangement.

Benign angioendotheliomatosis features a proliferation of endothelial cells in dilated blood vessels with a mild perivascular inflammatory infiltrate. The endothelial cells show no atypia or mitoses but often occlude the vessel lumina with associated fibrin thrombi. Occasionally, recanalized vessels with a "glomeruloid" architecture may be present. The proliferating endothelial cells are immunoreactive with vascular markers.

B. Kimura's Disease

Kimura's disease appears almost exclusively in the Far East, where it presents as a massive subsutaneous swelling, primarily in the head and neck region (194). Although confusion with angiolymphoid hyperplasia with eosinophilia (epithelioid

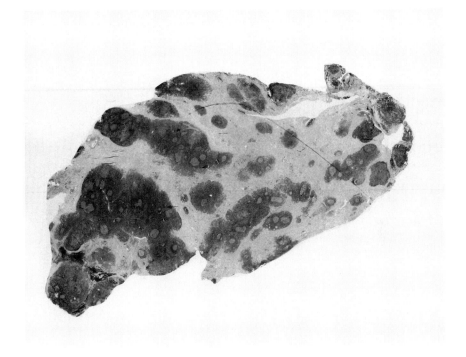

FIG. 29 Kimura's disease is predominantly a fibroinflammatory rather than a vascular lesion, despite confusion in the literature. Lymphoid follicles, fibrosis, and eosinophilic microabscesses are features of this disease.

hemangioma) exists in the literature, these disorders are currently viewed as two separate and distinct entities (119,195–198). It is an inflammatory disorder that consists of proliferations of lymphoid and angiomatous tissue accompanied by lymphadenopathy, peripheral blood eosinophilia, and elevated IgE levels. The masses may be multifocal or bilateral. The lesion is considered to be the result of an aberrant immunologic response to an as yet undetermined antigenic stimulus.

The condition is characterized histologically by a poorly marginated fibro-inflammatory mass predominantly involving the subcutaneous tissue (Fig. 29). There are prominent germinal center formation, variable amount of fibrosis depending on the stage of the lesion, and infiltration of eosinophils. In contrast to *angiolymphoid hyperplasia* with eosinophilia (epithelioid hemangioma), the vessels in Kimura's disease are typically well canalized, lack epithelioid morphology, and for the most part tend to be a relatively minor or inconspicuous component of the process (Fig. 30).

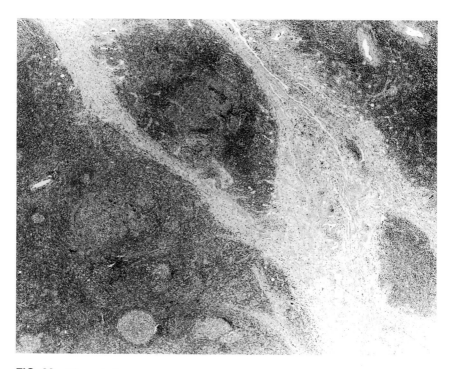

FIG. 30   Kimura's disease.

REFERENCES

1. Requena L, Sangueza O. (1997) Cutaneous vascular anomilies. Part I. Hamarto-
    mas, malformations, and dilatation of preexisting vessels. J Am Acad Dermatol 37,
    523–49.
2. Umansky A. (1946) Dyschondroplasia with hemangiomata (Maffuci's syndrome).
    Report of a case with mild osseous manifestations. Bull Hosp Joint Dis 7, 59–68.
3. Fanburg J, Meis J, Rosenberg A. (1993) Maffuci's syndrome: multiple enchondromas
    and spindle cell hemangioendothelioma. Mod Pathol 6, 6A.
4. Fine R, Derbes V, Clark W. (1961) Blue rubber bleb nevus. Arch Dermatol 84,
    144–147.
5. Mahle C, Schwartz M, Popek E, Bocklage T. (1997) Intraabdominal lymphangiomas
    in children and adults. Assessment of proliferative activity. Arch Pathol Lab Med 121,
    1055–1062.
6. Stoler MH, Bonfiglio TA, Steigbigel RT. (1983) An atypical subcutaneous infec-
    tion associated with acquired immune deficiency syndrome. Am J Clin Pathol 80,
    714–718.

7. LeBoit PE, Berger TG, Egbert BM, et al. (1989) Bacillary angiomatosis. The histopathology and differential diagnosis of a pseudoneoplastic infection in patients with human immunodeficiency virus disease. Am J Surg Pathol 13, 909–920.

8. Cockerell CJ, LeBoit PE. (1990) Bacillary angiomatosis: a newly characterized, pseudoneoplastic, infectious, cutaneous vascular disorder. J Am Acad Dermatol 22, 501–12.

9. Requena L, Sangueza O. (1997) Cutaneous vascular proliferations. Part II. Hyperplasias and benign neoplasms. J Am Acad Dermatol 37, 887–920.

10. Nosal J. (1997) Review. Bacillary angiomatosis, cat-scratch disease, and Bartonellosis: what's the connection. Int J Dermatol 36, 405–411.

11. Smith D. (1997) Cat-scratch disease and related clinical syndromes. Am Family Physician 55, 1783–1789.

12. Brenner SA, Rooney JA, Manzewitsch P, Regnery RL. (1977) Isolation of Bartonella (Rochalimea) henselae: effects of methods and blood collecting and handling. J Clin Microbiol 35, 544–547.

13. Relman DA, Loutit JS, Schmidt TM, et al. (1990) The agent of bacillary angiomatosis: an approach to the identification of uncultured pathogens. N Engl J Med 323, 1573–1580.

14. Relman DA, Falkow S, LeBoit PE, et al. (1991) The organism causing bacillary angiomatosis, peliosis hepatis, and fever and bacteremia in immunocompromised patients. N Engl J Med 324, 1514 (letter).

15. Reed JA, Brigati DJ, Flynn SD, et al. (1992) Immunocytochemical identification of *Rochalimea henselae* in bacillary (epithelioid) angiomatosis, parenchymal bacillary peliosis, and persistent fever with bacteremia. Am J Surg Pathol 16, 650–657.

16. Cockerell CJ, Bergstresser PR, Myrie-Williams C, et al. (1990) Bacillary epithelioid angiomatosis occurring in an immunocompetent individual. Arch Dermatol 126, 787–790.

17. Nappi O, Wick MR. (1986) Disseminated lobular capillary hemangioma (pyogenic granuloma): a clinicopathologic study of two cases. Am J Dermatopathol 8, 379–385.

18. Howe C. (1943) Carrión's disease: immunologic studies. Arch Intern Med 72, 147–167.

19. Arias-Stella J, Lieberman PH, Erlandson RA, et al. (1986) Histology, immunohistochemistry, and ultrastructure of the verruga in Carrión's disease. Am J Surg Pathol 10, 595–610.

20. Arias-Stella J, Lieberman PH, Garcia-Caceres U, et al. (1987) Verruga peruana mimicking malignant neoplasms. Am J Dermatopathol 9, 279–291.

21. Masson P. (1923) Hémangioendotheliome végétant intravasculaire. Bull Soc Anat Paris 93, 517–523.

22. Tosios K, Koutlas I, Papanicolaou S. (1994) Intravascular papillary endothelial hyperplasia of the oral soft tissues: Report of 18 cases and review of the literature. J Oral Maxillofac Surg 52, 1263–1268.

23. Axiotis C, Merino M, Ain K, Norton J. (1991) Papillary endothelial hyperplasia in the thyroid following Fine-Needle Aspiration. Arch Pathol Lab Med 115, 240–242.

24. Kristof R, Roost D, Wolf H, Schramm J. (1997) Intravasular papillary endothelial hyperplasia of the sellar region. J Neurosurg 86, 558–563.

25. Park J, Chung-Park M, Snow N. (1990) Intravascular papillary endothelial hyperplasia of superior vena cava: a rare cause of the superior vena cava syndrome. Thorax 46, 272–273.

26. Romani J, Puig L, Costa I, Morgas J. (1997) Masson's intravascular papillary endothelial hyperplasia mimicking Stewart-Treves syndrome: report of a case. Cutis 59, 148–150.

27. Dunphy C, Sotelo-Avila C, Luisiri A, Chu J. (1994) Paroxysmal nocturnal hemoglobinuria associated with venous thrombosis and papillary endothelial hyperplasia presenting as ulcerated duodenal mass. Arch Pathol Lab Med 118, 837–840.

28. Stewart M, Smoller B. (1994) Multiple lesions of intravascular papillary endothelial hyperplasia (Masson's lesions). Arch Pathol Lab Med 118, 315–316.

29. Hashimoto H, Daimaru Y, Enjoji M. (1983) Intravascular papillary endothelial hyperplasia: a clinicopathologic study of 91 cases. Am J Dermatopathol 5, 539–546.

30. Kuo T, Sayers PM, Rosai J. (1976) Masson's "vegetant intravascular hemangioendothelioma": a lesion often mistaken for angiosarcoma. Study of seventeen cases located in the skin and soft tissues. Cancer 38, 1227–1236.

31. Clearkin KP, Enzinger FM. (1976) Intravascular papillary endothelial hyperplasia. Arch Pathol Lab Med 100, 441–444.

32. Amerigo J, Berry CL. (1980) Intravascular papillary endothelial hyperplasia in the skin and subcutaneous tissue. Virchows Archiv A Pathol Anat Histopathol 387, 81–90.

33. Patchefsky AS, Enzinger FM. (1981) Intravascular fasciitis. A report of 17 cases. Am J Surg Pathol 5, 29–32.

34. Kahn MA, Weathers DR, Johnson DM. (1987) Intravascular fasciitis: a case report on an intraoral location. J Oral Pathol 16, 303–306.

35. Freedman PD, Lumerman H. (1986) Intravascular fasciitis: a report of two cases and review of the literature. Oral Surg Oral Med Oral Pathol 62, 549–554.

36. Wells GC, Whimster IW. (1969) Subcutaneous angiolymphoid hyperplasia with eosinophilia. Br J Dermatol 81, 1–15.

37. Tsanh WYW, Chan JKC. (1993) The family of epithelioid vascular tumors. Histol Histopathol 8, 187–212.

38. Urabe A, Tsuneyoshi M, Enjoji M. (1987) Epithelioid hemangioma versus Kimura's disease: a comparative clinicopathologic study. Am J Surg Pathol 11, 758–766.

39. Enzinger FM, Weiss SW. (1988) Benign tumors and tumorlike lesions of blood vessels. In: Soft Tissue Tumors, 2nd ed. Philadelphia: Mosby, pp. 489–532.

40. Rosai J. (1982) Angiolymphoid hyperplasia with eosinophilia of the skin. Its nosological position in the spectrum of histiocytoid hemangioma. Am J Dermatopathol 4, 175–184.

41. Rosai J, Ackerman LR. (1974) Intravenous atypical vascular proliferation. Arch Dermatol 109, 714–717.

42. Allen PW, Ramakrishna B, MacCormac LB. (1992) The histiocytoid hemangiomas and other controversies. Pathol Annu 27, 51–87.

43. Olsen TG, Helwig EB. (1985) Angiolymphoid hyperplasia with eosinophilia: a clinicopathologic study of 116 patients. J Am Acad Dermatol 12, 781–796.

44. Fetsch JF, Weiss SW. (1991) Observations concerning the pathogenesis of epithelioid hemangioma (angiolymphoid hyperplasia). Mod Pathol 4, 449–455.

45. Weiss S, Sobin L. (1994) Classification of Tumors. Histological Types of Soft Tissue Tumors, 2nd ed. New York: Springer-Verlag.

46. Weiss SW. (1989) Vascular tumors: a deductive approach to diagnosis. Surg Pathol 2, 185–201.

47. Poncet MM, Dor, L. (1897) De la botyromycose humaine. Rev Chir (Paris) 18, 996–997.

48. Hartzell MB. (1904) Granuloma pyogenicum (botryomycosis of French authors). J Cutan Dis 22, 520–525.

49. Mills SE, Cooper PH, Fechner RE. (1980) Lobular capillary hemangioma: the underlying lesion of pyogenic granuloma: a study of 73 cases from the oral and nasal mucus membranes. Am J Surg Pathol 4, 471–479.

50. Cooper PH, Mills SE. (1982) Subcutaneous granuloma pyogenicum-lobular capillary hemangioma. Arch Dermatol 118, 30–33.

51. Cooper PH, McAllister HA, Helwig EB. (1979) Intravenous pyogenic granuloma: A study of 18 cases. Am J Surg Pathol 3, 221–228.

52. Ulbright TM, Santa Cruz DJ. (1980) Intravenous pyogenic granuloma. Cancer 45, 1646–1652.

53. Michelson HE. (1925) Granuloma pyogenicum: A clinical and histologic review of twenty nine cases. Arch Dermatol 12, 495–505.

54. Leyden JJ, Master GH. (1979) Oral cavity pyogenic granuloma. Arch Dermatol 108, 226–228.

55. Kerr DA. (1951) Granuloma pyogenicum. Oral Surg 4, 158–176.

56. McDonald RH. (1956) Granuloma gravidarum: pregnancy tumor of the gingiva. Am J Obstet Gynecol 72, 1132–1136.

57. Nichols GE, Gaffey MJ, Mills SE, et al. (1992) Lobular capillary hemangioma: an immunohistochemical study including steroid hormone receptor status. Am J Clin Pathol 97, 770–775.

58. Strohal R, Gillitzer R, Zonzits E, et al. (1991) Localized vs generalized pyogenic granuloma. Arch Dermatol 127, 856–861.

59. Pembroke AC, Grice K, Levantine AV, et al. (1978) Eruptive angiomata in malignant disease. Clin Exp Dermatol 3, 147–156.

60. Foldvari F. (1935) Post-traumatic angioma. Br J Dermatol 47, 463–467.

61. Zaynoun ST, Juljulian HH, Kurban AK. (1974) Pyogenic granuloma with multiple satellites. Arch Dermatol 109, 689–691.

62. Taira JW, Hill TL, Everett MA. (1992) Lobular capillary hemangioma (pyogenic granuloma) with satellitosis. J Am Acad Dermatol 27, 197–300.

63. Amerigo J, Gonzalez-Campora R, Galera H, et al. (1983) Recurrent pyogenic granuloma with multiple satellites: Clinicopathological and ultrastructural study. Dermatologica 166, 117–121.

64. Holmdahl K. (1955) Cutaneous hemangiomas in premature and mature infants. Acta Paediatr Scand 44, 370–379.

65. Amir J, Metzker A, Krikler R, et al. (1986) Strawberry hemangioma in preterm infants. Pediatr Dermatol 3, 331–332.

66. Burns AJ, Kaplan LC, Mulliken JB. (1991) Is there an association between hemangiomas and syndromes with dysmorphic features? Pediatrics 88, 1257–1267.

67. Gonzalez-Crussi F, Reyes-Mugica M. (1991) Cellular hemangiomas of infancy ("hemangioendotheliomas"). Light microscopic, immunohistochemical, and ultrastructural observations. Am J Surg Pathol 15, 769–778.

68. Hughes R, Oates J. (1997) Capillary haemangioma of the parotid in an adult: an unusual case and a review of the literature. J Laryngol Otol 111, 588–589.

69. Kasabach HH, Merritt KK. (1940) Capillary Hemangioma with extensive purpura: report of a case. Am J Dis Child 59, 1063–1070.

70. Bowers RE, Graham EA, Tomlinson KM. (1960) The natural history of the strawberry nevus. Arch Dermatol 82, 667–680.

71. Folkman J. (1989) Successful treatment of angiogenic disease. N Engl J Med 320, 1211–1212.

72. Enjolras O, Riche MC, Merland JJ, et al. (1990) Management of alarming hemangiomas of infancy: a review of 25 cases. Pediatrics 85, 491–498.

73. Apfelberg DB, Lane B, Marx MP. (1991) Combined (team) approach to hemangioma management: arteriography with superselective embolization plus YAG laser/sapphire tip resection. Plast Reconstr Surg 88, 71–82.

74. Ezekowitz RA, Mulliken JB, Folkman J. (1992) Interferon alfa-2a therapy for life-threatening hemangiomas of infancy. N Engl J Med 326, 1456–1463.

75. Osburn K, Schosser RH, Everett MA. (1987) Congenital pigmented and vascular lesions in newborn infants. J Am Acad Dermatol 16, 788–792.

76. Margileth AM, Museles M. (1965) Current concepts in diagnosis and management of congenital cutaneous hemangiomas. Pediatrics 36, 410–416.

77. Pratt AG. (1953) Birthmarks in infants. Arch Dermatol Syph 67, 302–305.

78. Barsky SH, Rosen S, Geer DE, et al. (1980) The nature and evolution of port wine stains: a computer-assisted study. J Invest Dermatol 74(3), 154–157.

79. Smoller BR, Rosen S. (1986) Port wine stains. A disease of altered neural modulation of blood vessels. Arch Dermatol 122, 177–179.

80. Mulliken JB, Glowacki J. (1982) Hemangiomas and vascular malformations in infants and children: a classification based on endothelial characteristics. Plast Reconstr Surg 70, 48–51.

81. Lever WF, Schaumberg-Lever G. (1983) In: Histopathology of the Skin, 6th ed. Philadelphia: JB Lippincott, pp. 623–651.

82. Coffin CM, Dehner LP. (1993) Vascular tumors in children and adolescents: a clinicopathologic study of 228 tumors in 222 patients. Pathol Annu 1, 97–120.

83. Johnson WC. (1976) Pathology of cutaneous vascular tumors. Int J Dermatol 15, 239–270.

84. Escada P, Capucho C, Silva J, Ruah C, Vital J, Penha R. (1997) Cavernous hemangioma of the fascial nerve. J Laryngol Otol 111, 858–861.

85. Borum, M. (1997) Cavernous colorectal hemangioma. Dig Dis Sci 42, 2468–2470.

86. Smith DW. (1982) Recognizable Patterns of Human Malformations, 3rd ed. Philadelphia: WB Saunders.

87. Lewis RJ, Ketcham A. (1973) Maffucci's syndrome: functional and neoplastic significance. J Bone Joint Surg 55A, 1465–1479.

88. Beham A, Fletcher CDM. (1991) Intramuscular angioma: a clinicopathological analysis of 74 cases. Histopathology 18, 53–59.

89. Allen PW, Enzinger FM. (1972) Hemangiomas of skeletal muscle: an analysis of 89 cases. Cancer 29, 8–23.

90. Szilagyi DE, Elliot JP, DeRusso FJ, et al. (1965) Peripheral congenital arteriovenous fistulas. Surgery 57, 61–81.

91. Zelch MG, Geisinger MA. (1990) Arteriography of the extremities, In: Radiology. Diagnosis–Imaging–Intervention, vol 2. Taveras JM, Ferrucci JT, Buonocore E, eds. Lippincott, St. Louis, chap. 142, pp. 1–16.

92. Niechaje IA, Sternby NH. (1983) Diagnostic accuracy and pathology of vascular tumors and tumor-like lesions. Chir Plastica 7, 153–161.

93. Shimpo S, Nishitani H, Tsunemura T. (1968) Solitary plasmacytoma with polyneuritis and endocrine disturbance. Nippon Rinsho 26, 2444–2456.

94. Ishikawa O, Nihei, Ishikawa H. (1987) The skin changes of POEMS syndrome. Br J Dermatol 117, 523–526.

95. Nakagawa K. (1949) Case report of angioblastoma of the skin. Hifuka Seibyoka Zasshi 59, 92–94.

96. Wilson Jones E. (1976) Dowling oration 1976. Malignant vascular tumors. Clin Exp Dermatol 1, 287–312.

97. Leaute-Labreze C, Bioulac-Sage P, Labbe L, Meraud J, Taieb A. (1997) Tufted angioma associated with platlet trapping syndrome: response to aspirin. Arch Dermatol 133, 1077–1079.

98. Santa Cruz DJ, Aronberg J. (1988) Targetoid hemosiderotic hemangioma. J Am Acad Dermatol 19, 550–558.

99. Rapini RP, Golitz LE. (1990) Targetoid hemosiderotic hemangioma. J Cutan Pathol 17, 233–235.

100. Vion B, Frenk E. (1992) Targetoid hemosiderotic hemangioma. Dermatology 184, 300–302.

101. Weiss SW, Enzinger FM. (1986) Spindle cell hemangioendothelioma: a low grade angiosarcoma resembling a cavernous hemangioma and Kaposi's sarcoma. Am J Surg Pathol 10, 521–530.

102. Scott GA, Rosai J. (1988) Spindle cell hemangioendothelioma: report of seven additional cases of a recently described vascular neoplasm. Am J Dermatopathol 10, 281–288.

103. Fletcher CDM, Beham A, Schmid C. (1991) Spindle cell haemangioendothelioma: a clinicopathological and immunohistochemical study indicative of a non-neoplastic lesion. Histopathology 18, 291–301.

103a. Perkins P, Weiss SW. (1996) Spindle cell hemangioendothelioma. An analysis of 78 cases with reassessment of its pathogenesis and biologic behavior. Am J Surg Pathol 20, 1196–1204.

104. Dabska M. (1969) Malignant endovascular papillary angioendothelioma of the skin in childhood. Clinicopathologic study of six cases. Cancer 24, 503–510.

104a. Fanburg-Smith JC, Michal M, Partanen TA, Alitalo K, Miettinen M. (1999) Papillary intralymphatic angioendothelioma (PILA). A report of 12 cases of a distinctive vascular tumor with phenotypic features of lymphatic vessels. Am J Surg Pathol 23, 1004–1010.

105. Patterson K, Chandra RS. (1985) Malignant endovascular papillary angioendothelioma. Cutaneous borderline tumor. Arch Pathol Lab Med 109, 671–673.
106. Zukerburg LR, Nickoloff BJ, Weiss SW. (1993) Kaposiform hemangioendotheloma of infancy and childhood. An aggressive neoplasm associated with Kasabach-Merritt syndrome and lymphangiomatosis. Am J Surg Pathol 17, 321–328.
107. Vin-Christian K, McCalmont T, Frieden I. (1997) Kaposiform hemangioendothelioma. An aggressive, locally invasive vascular tumor that can mimic hemangioma of infancy. Arch Dermatol 133, 1573–1578.
108. Weiss SW, Enzinger FM. (1982) Epithelioid hemangioendothelioma: a vascular tumor often mistaken for a carcinoma. Cancer 50, 970–981.
109. Weiss SW, Ishak KG, Dail DH, et al. (1986) Epithelioid hemangioendothelioma and related lesions. Semin Diagn Pathol 3, 259–287.
110. Zelger B, Wambacher B, Steiner H, Zelger B. (1997) Cutaneous epithelioid hemangioendothelioma, epithelioid cell histiocytoma and spitz nevus. Cutan Pathol 24, 641–647.
111. Begbie S, Bell D, Nevell D. (1997) Mediastinal epithelioid hemangioendothelioma in a patient with type IV Ehler-Danlos syndrome: a case report and review of the literature. Am J Clin Oncol 20, 412–415.
112. Dail DH, Liebow AA, Gmelich JT. (1983) Intravascular, bronchiolar, and alveolar tumor of lung: an analysis of twenty cases of a peculiar sclerosing endothelial tumor. Cancer 51, 452–464.
113. Azumi N, Churg A. (1981) Intravascular sclerosing bronchiolo-aveolar tumor. Am J Surg Pathol 5, 587–596.
114. Ishak KG, Sesterhenn IA, Goodman ZG, et al. (1984) Epithelioid hemangioendothelioma of the liver: a clinicopathologic and follow up study of 32 cases. Hum Pathol 15, 839–852.
115. Kaposi M. (1872) Idiopathic multiple pigmented sarcoma of the skin. (Translated from German in CA–A Cancer Journal for Clinicians 1982; 32:342–347.) Arch F Dermatol Syph 4, 265–273.
116. Krown S. (1997) Acquired immunodeficiency syndrome-associated Kaposi's sarcoma. Biology and management. Med Clin North Am 81, 471–494.
117. Reynolds WA, Winkelmann RK, Soule EH. (1965) Kaposi's sarcoma: a clinicopathologic study with particular reference to its relationship to the reticuloendothelial system. Medicine 44, 419–443.
118. Cox FH, Helwig EB. (1959) Kaposi's sarcoma. Cancer 12, 289–298.
119. Requena L, Sangueza O. (1998) Cutaneous vascular proliferations. III. Malignant neoplasms, other cutaneous neoplasms with significant vascular component, and disorders erroneously considered as vascular neoplasms. J Am Acad Dermatol 38, 143–175.
120. Safai B, Mike V, Giraldo G, et al. (1980) Association of Kaposi's sarcoma with second primary malignancies: possible etiopathogenic implications. Cancer 45, 1472–1479.
121. Templeton AC. (1981) Kaposi's sarcoma. Pathol Annu 2, 315–336.
122. Kestens L, Melbye M, Biggar RJ, Stevens WJ, Piot P, BeMuynck A, Taelman H, De Feyter M, Paluku L, Gigase PL. (1985) Endemic African Kaposi's sarcoma is not associated with immunodeficiency. Int J. Cancer 36, 49–54.

123. Penn I. (1983) Kaposi's sarcoma in immunosuppressed patients. J Clin Lab Immunol 12, 1–10.

124. Penn I. (1997) Kaposi's sarcoma in transplant recipients. Transplantation 64, 669–673.

125. Beral V, Peterman TA, Berkelman RL, Jaffee HW. (1990) Kaposi's sarcoma among persons with AIDS: a sexually transmitted infection. Lancet 335, 123–128.

126. Drew WL, Conant MA, Miner RC, et al. (1982) Cytomegalovirus and Kaposi's sarcoma in young homosexual men. Lancet 2, 125–127.

127. Giraldo G, Beth E, Henle G, et al. (1978) Antibody patterns to herpesviruses in Kaposi's sarcoma. II. Serological association of American Kaposi's sarcoma with cytomegalovirus. Int J Cancer 22, 126–131.

128. Giraldo G, Beth E, Huang E-S. (1980) Kaposi's sarcoma and its relationship to cytomegalovirus (CMV). III. CMV DNA and CMV early antigens in Kaposi's sarcoma. Int J Cancer 26, 23–29.

129. Moore P, Chang Y. (1998) Kaposi's sarcoma (KS), KS-associated Herpesvirus, and the criteria for causality in the age of molecular biology. Am J Epidemiol 147, 217–221.

130. Beckstead J, Wood G, Fletcher V. (1985) Evidence for the origin of Kaposi's sarcoma from lymphatic endothelium. Am J Pathol 119, 294–300.

131. McNutt NS, Fletcher V, Conant MA. (1983) Early lesions of Kaposi's sarcoma in homosexual men. An ultrastructural comparison with other vascular proliferations in skin. Am J Pathol 111, 62–77.

132. Bisceglia M, Bosman C, Quirke P. (1992) A histologic and flow cytometric study of Kaposi's sarcoma. Cancer 69, 793–798.

133. Fukunaga M, Silverberg SG. (1990) Kaposi's sarcoma in patients with acquired immune deficiency syndrome. A flow cytometric DNA analysis of 26 lesions in 21 patients. Cancer 66, 758–764.

134. Chor PJ, Santa Cruz DJ. (1992) Kaposi's sarcoma: a clinicopathologic review and differential diagnosis. J Cutan Pathol 19, 6–20.

135. Leibowitz MR, Dagliotto M, Smith E, et al. (1980) Rapidly fatal lymphangioma-like Kaposi's sarcoma. Histopathology 4, 559–566.

136. Reed WB, Kamath HM, Weiss L. (1974) Kaposi sarcoma, with emphasis on internal manifestations. Arch Dermatol 110, 115–118.

137. Smith KJ, Skelton HG, James WD, et al. (1991) Angiosarcoma arising in Kaposi's sarcoma (pleomorphic Kaposi's sarcoma) in a patient with human immunodeficiency disease. J Am Acad Dermatol 24, 790–792.

138. Gange RW, Wilson-Jones E. (1979) Lymphangioma-like Kaposi's sarcoma: a report of three cases. Br J Dermatol 100, 327–334.

139. Ronchese F, Kern AB. (1957) Lymphangioma-like Kaposi's sarcoma. Arch Dermatol 75, 418–427.

140. Bhana D, Templeton AC, Master SP, Kyalwazi SK. (1970) Kaposi's sarcoma of lymph nodes. Br J Cancer 24, 464–470.

141. Ramos W, Taylor HB, Hernandez BA, et al. (1976) Primary Kaposi's sarcoma of lymph nodes. Am J Clin Pathol 66, 998–1003.

142. O'Connell KM. (1977) Kaposi's sarcoma of lymph nodes: histologic study of lesions in 16 cases in Malawi. J Clin Pathol 30, 696–703.

143. Amazon K, Rywlin AM. (1979) Subtle clues to diagnosis by conventional microscopy: lymph node involvement in Kaposi's sarcoma. Am J Dermatopathol 1, 173–176.
144. Chan JKC, Frizzera G, Fletcher CDM, et al. (1992) Primary vascular tumors of lymph nodes other than Kaposi's sarcoma. Analysis of 39 cases and delineation of two new entities. Am J Pathol 16, 335–350.
145. Chan JKC, Warbke RA, Dorfman R. (1991) Vascular transformation of sinuses of lymph nodes. A study of its morphologic spectrum and distinction from Kaposi's sarcoma. Am J Surg Pathol 15, 732–743.
146. Weiss SW, Gnepp DR, Bratthauer GL. (1989) Palisaded myofibroblastoma. A benign mesenchymal tumor of lymph node. Am J Surg Pathol 13, 341–346.
147. Suster S, Rosai J. (1989) Intranodal hemorrhagic spindle cell tumor with amianthoid fibers. Report of six cases of a distinctive mesenchymal neoplasm of the inguinal region that simulated Kaposi's sarcoma. Am J Surg Pathol 13, 347–357.
148. Fletcher CDM, Starling RW. (1990) Intranodal myofibroblastoma presenting in the submandibular region: evidence of a broader clinical and histologic spectrum. Histopathology 16, 287–294.
149. Blumenfeld W, Egbert BM, Sagebiel RW. (1985) Differential diagnosis of Kaposi's sarcoma. Arch Pathol Lab Med 109, 123–127.
150. Mali JWH, Kuiper JP, Hamers AA. (1965) Acro-angiodermatitis of the foot. Arch Dermatol 92, 515–518.
151. Watanabe M, Kishiyama K, Ohkawara A. (1983) Acquired progressive lymphangioma. J Am Acad Dermatol 8, 663–667.
152. Wilson Jones E, Winkelmann RK, Zachary CB, et al. (1990) Benign lymphangioendothelioma. J Am Acad Dermatol 23, 229–235.
153. Calonje E, Fletcher D, Wilson-Jones E. (1994) Retiform hemangioendothelioma. A distinctive form of low-grade angiosarcoma delineated in a series of 15 cases. Am J Surg Pathol 18, 115–125.
154. Sanz-Trelles A, Rodrigo-Fernandez I, Ayala-Carbonero A, Contreras-Rubio F. (1997) Retiform hemangioendothelioma. A new case in a child with diffuse endovascular papillary endothelial proliferation. J Cutan Pathol 24, 440–444.
155. Bardwil JM, Mocega EE, Butler JJ, Russin DJ. (1968) Angiosarcomas of the head and neck region. Am J Surg 116, 548–553.
156. Nielsen G, Young R, Prat J, Scully R. (1997) Primary angiosarcoma of the ovary. A report of seven cases and review of the literature. Int J Gynecol Pathol 16, 378–382.
157. Mordkin R, Dahut W, Lynch J. (1997) Renal angiosarcoma: a rare primary genitourinary malignancy. South Med J 90, 1159–1160.
158. Maddox JC, Evans HL. (1981) Angiosarcoma of skin and soft tissue: a study of 44 cases. Cancer 48, 1907–1921.
159. Holden CA, Spittle MF, Jones EW. (1987) Angiosarcoma of the face and scalp: prognosis and treatment. Cancer 59, 1046–1057.
160. Haustein U-F. (1991) Angiosarcoma of the face and scalp. Int J Dermatol 30, 851–856.
161. Sordillo PP, Chapman R, Hajdu SI, et al. (1981) Lymphangiosarcoma. Cancer 48, 1674–1679.

162. Woodward AH, Ivins JC, Soule EH. (1972) Lymphangiosarcoma arising in chronic lymphedematous extremities. Cancer 30, 562–572.
163. McSwain B, Whitehead W, Bennett L. (1973) Angiosarcoma: report of three cases of postmastectomy lymphangiosarcoma and one of hemangiosarcoma. South Med J 66, 102–106.
164. Benda JA, Al-Jurf AS, Benson III AB. (1987) Angiosarcoma of the breast following segmental mastectomy complicated by lymphedema. Am J Clin Pathol 87, 651–655.
165. Goett DK, Detlefs RL. (1985) Postirradiation angiosarcoma. J Am Acad Dermatol 12, 922–926.
166. Chen KTK, Hoffman KD, Hendricks EJ. (1979) Angiosarcoma following therapeutic irradiation. Cancer 44, 2044–2048.
167. Nanus DM, Kelson D, Clark GC. (1987) Radiation-Induced Angiosarcoma. Cancer 60, 777–779.
168. Moskaluk CA, Merino MJ, Danforth DN, Medeiros LJ. (1992) Low-grade angiosarcoma of the skin of the breast: a complication of lumpectomy and radiation therapy for breast carcinoma. Hum Pathol 23, 710–714.
169. McCarthy WD, Pack GT. (1950) Malignant blood vessel tumors. A report of 56 cases of angiosarcoma and Kaposi's sarcoma. Surg Gynecol Obstet 91, 465–482.
170. Amendola BE, Amendola MA, McClatchey KD, Miller CH. (1989) Radiation-associated sarcoma: a review of 23 patients with postradiation sarcoma over a 50-year period. Am J Clin Oncol 12, 411–415.
171. Cancellieri A, Eusebi V, Mambelli V, et al. (1991) Well-differentiated angiosarcoma of the skin following radiotherapy. Pathol Res Pract 187, 301–306.
172. Weiss WM, Riles TS, Gouge TH, Mizrachi HH. (1991) Angiosarcoma at the site of a dacron vascular prosthesis: a case report and literature review. J Vasc Surg 14, 87–91.
173. Hayman J, Huygens H. (1983) Angiosarcoma developing around a foreign body. J Clin Pathol 36, 515–518.
174. Keane MM, Carney DN. (1993) Angiosarcoma arising from a defunctionalized arteriovenous fistula. J Urol 149, 364–365.
175. Brown RW, Tornos C, Evans HL. (1992) Angiosarcoma arising from malignant schwannoma in a patient with neurofibromatosis. Cancer 70, 1141–1144.
176. Chauduri B, Ronan SG, Manaligod JR. (1980) Angiosarcoma arising in a plexiform neurofibroma. Cancer 46, 605–610.
177. Riccardi VM, Wheeler TM, Pickard LR, King B. (1984) The pathophysiology of neurofibromatosis: II. Angiosarcoma as a complication. Cancer Genet Cytogenet 12, 275–280.
178. Popper H, Thomas LB, Telles NC, et al. (1978) Development of hepatic angiosarcoma in man induced by vinyl-chloride, thorotrast and arsenic. Am J Pathol 92, 349–376.
179. Stewart FW, Treves N. (1948) Lymphangiosarcoma in postmastectomy lymphedema. A report of six cases in elephantiasis chururgica. Cancer 1, 64–81.
180. Mackenzie DH. (1971) Lymphangiosarcoma arising in chronic congenital and idiopathic lymphoedema. J Clin Pathol 24, 524–529.

181. Edeiken S, Russo DP, Knecht J, et al. (1992) Angiosarcoma after tylectomy and radiation therapy for carcinoma of the breast. Cancer 70, 644–647.

182. Fletcher CDM, Beham A, Bekir S, et al. (1991) Epithelioid angiosarcoma of deep soft tissue: a distinctive tumor readily mistaken for an epithelial neoplasm. Am J Surg Pathol 15, 915–924.

182a. Meis-Kindblom JM, Kindblom LG. (1998) Angiosarcoma of Soft Tissue: a Study of 80 cases. Am J Surg Pathol 22, 683–697.

183. Donnell RM, Rosen PP, Lieberman PH, et al. (1981) Angiosarcoma and other vascular tumors of the breast: pathologic analysis as a guide to prognosis. Am J Surg Pathol 5, 629–642.

184. Rosen PP, Kimmel M, Ernsberger D. (1988) Mammary angiosarcoma. The prognostic significance of tumor differentiation. Cancer 62, 2145–2151.

185. Chen KTK, Kirkgaard DD, Bocian JJ. (1980) Angiosarcoma of the breast. Cancer 46, 368–371.

186. Rosen PP, Jozefczyk MA, Boram LH. (1985) Vascular tumors of the breast. IV. Venous hemangioma. Am J Surg Pathol 9, 659–665.

187. Jozefczyk MA, Rosen PP. (1985) Vascular tumors of the breast. II. Perilobular hemangiomas and hemangiomas. Am J Surg Pathol 9, 491–503.

188. Person JR. (1977) Systemic angioendotheliomatosis: a possible disorder of a circulating angiogenic factor. Br J Dermatol 96, 329–331.

189. Wick MR, Rocamora A. (1988) Reactive and malignant "angioendotheliomatosis": a discriminant pathologic study. J Cutan Pathol 15, 260–271.

190. Bhawan J, Wolff SM, Ucci AO, et al. (1985) Malignant lymphoma and malignant angioendotheliomatosis: one disease. Cancer 55, 570–576.

191. Sheibani K, Battifora H, Winberg CD, et al. (1986) Further evidence that "malignant angioendotheliomatosis" is an angiotropic large cell lymphoma. N Engl J Med 314, 943–948.

192. Ferry JA, Harris NL, Picker LJ, et al. (1988) Intravascular lymphomatosis (malignant angioendotheliomatosis): A B-cell neoplasm expressing surface homing receptors. Mod Pathol 1, 444–452.

193. Martin S, Pitcher D, Tschen J, et al. (1980) Reactive angioendotheliomatosis. J Am Acad Dermatol 2, 117–123.

194. Kimura T, Yoshimura S, Ishikawa E. (1948) Abnormal granuloma with proliferation of lymphoid tissue. Nippon Byori Gakkai Kaishi 37, 179–180.

195. Chan JKC, Hui PK, Ng CS, et al. (1989) Epithelioid hemangioma (angiolymphoid hyperplasia with eosinophilia) and Kimura's disease in Chinese. Histopathology 15, 557–574.

196. Googe PB, Harris NL, Mihm MC. (1987) Kimura's disease and angiolymphoid hyperplasia with eosinophils: Two distinct histopathological entities. J Cutan Pathol 14, 263–271.

197. Hui PK, Chan JKC, Ng CS, et al. (1989) Lymphadenopathy of Kimura's disease. Am J Surg Pathol 13, 177–186.

198. Kung ITM, Gibson JB, Bannatyne PM. (1984) Kimura's disease: a clinicopathological study of 21 cases and its distinction from angiolymphoid hyperplasia with eosinophilia. Pathology 16, 39–44.

13
Cartilage- and Bone-Forming Tumors Originating in Soft Tissue

John X. O'Connell
Surrey Memorial Hospital
Surrey, British Columbia, Canada

I. INTRODUCTION

Apart from sesamoid bones, which reside within tendons and ligaments, the somatic soft tissues are typically devoid of bone and cartilage. Although the specialized mesenchymal cells that form bone and cartilage are not normally found in soft tissue, in a variety of circumstances the anomalous production of these matrices occurs at this site. The conditions that give rise to this "heterotopic" matrix span the spectrum from reactive processes to benign and malignant neoplasms. In virtually all of these, the matrix-producing cells are derived from undifferentiated fibroblast-like cells that reside normally within the soft tissues. Under appropriate stimuli, these "inducible osteoprogenitor cells" are transformed into osteoblasts and chondrocytes (1). The circumstances that produce these changes within mesenchymal cells are varied and often incompletely understood; however, several distinct clinicopathologic syndromes are recognized. These will be discussed under the following headings.

1. Predominantly osseous masses of soft tissue
2. Predominantly cartilaginous masses of soft tissue
3. Other matrix-containing soft-tissue tumors

II. PREDOMINANTLY OSSEOUS MASSES OF SOFT TISSUE

A. Myositis Ossificans

1. General and Clinical Features

Myositis ossificans (MO) is a nonneoplastic bone-forming reactive "pseudo-tumor" occurring in soft tissue (2–6). The term myositis ossificans is intrinsically misleading because the process is not primarily inflammatory, nor is it always confined to muscle. Histologically and clinically identical forms may occur in tendons and aponeuroses (4,6,7). Some authors recognize two distinct forms, termed "posttraumatic" and "pseudomalignant," representing circumstances in which there is, or is not, a history of preceding trauma (3,4,6,8). The clinical and pathologic features (apart from the history of trauma) are essentially identical in each of these (2,5,7). MO can thus be considered a single entity, in which there may or may not be a recalled history of injury (2,5,7,9). MO is commonest in the second and third decades of life (2–7,10). There is no sex predilection (2,3,5,6). The masses most commonly arise in the large skeletal muscles of the proximal extremities; the quadriceps and the brachialis are affected in approximately 80% of cases (6,7). Patients present with a short history (usually less than 3 months) of pain and swelling in the affected region. There may be localized erythema and heat, suggesting an infectious process, particularly in younger patients (7). In early lesions (within the first 3 weeks), radiographs demonstrate only a soft-tissue mass (9,11,12). Typically, soft-tissue calcification is evident only after approximately 6 weeks (9,11,12). Mature lesions of MO appear as ossified soft-tissue nodules (Fig. 1). Magnetic resonance imaging (MRI) of early lesions, which often present as nonspecific soft-tissue masses, reveals inhomogeneous signal intensity with intense surrounding soft-tissue edema. MO usually measures less than 5 cm (2,3). Resection results in cure. Local recurrence is extremely uncommon, even if resection margins are positive (2–6).

2. Microscopic Features

Since MO is a reactive process that occurs secondary to soft-tissue injury, the histologic appearance of an individual lesion depends on the part of the mass that is examined and the time at which it is excised (2–8). In general, the quantity of bone formed and its degree of maturity increase with time (2–8). One of the defining microscopic features of MO is a reproducible transition from cellular sheets of spindle cells in the center of the mass to a less cellular bone-rich periphery (2,7). This phenomenon, which is virtually pathoneumonic of MO, is termed "zoning" (2,7). The central aspect of MO consists of intersecting fascicles of plump spindle cells (Fig. 2). These cells demonstrate central elongated nuclei and visible nucleoli. Mitotic figures are readily found; however, marked nuclear atypia is not seen. The spindle cells gradually merge with thin trabeculae of woven bone that appear

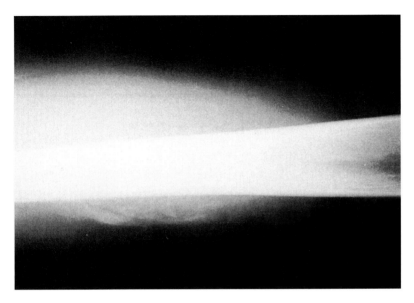

FIG. 1   A mature mineralized myositis ossificans in the soft tissues of the thigh adjacent to the femur.

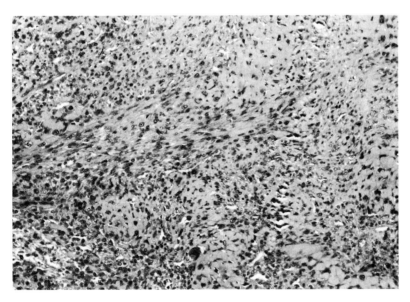

FIG. 2   Intersecting fascicles of plump spindle cells typical of the central aspect of myositis ossificans. There is no bone present in this field.

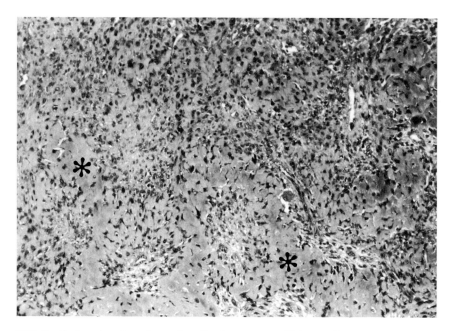

FIG. 3   Early trabeculae of nonmineralized woven osteoid (*asterisk*).

to arise directly from the stroma (Fig. 3). As the trabeculae become more defined, prominent surface layers of osteoblasts become evident, i.e., so-called osteoblastic rimming (Fig. 4). These intersecting trabeculae of woven bone demonstrate a gradual transition to mature lamellar bone at the periphery of the mass. Microscopic foci of hypercellular reactive callus-like cartilage may also be found (5,6). The skeletal muscle may show edema and degenerative changes. Although injury, either recognized or occult, is the initiating mechanism for MO, necrotic skeletal muscle is not usually found within the mass. Lesions that are resected earlier in their evolution demonstrate a greater predominance of spindle cells with relatively less mineralized bone, whereas more "mature" lesions are dominated by bone. Ultimately, if a mass is not resected, a soft-tissue nodule of mature lamellar cortical and cancellous bone will ensue (Fig. 5) (13,14). These nodules will even contain normal bone marrow (14).

3.   Differential Diagnosis

A variety of other ossifying soft-tissue masses may clinically and pathologically be considered in the differential diagnosis of MO. Fibrodysplasia (myositis) ossificans progressiva is a rare inherited condition characterized by multifocal soft-tissue and para-articular ossification. It affects children and is discussed in detail

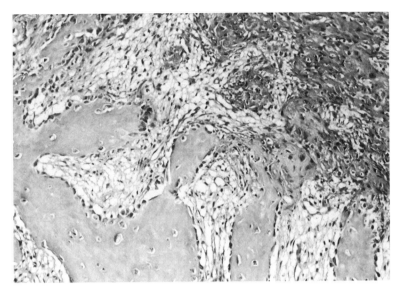

FIG. 4   More mature bone towards the periphery of a lesion demonstrating "osteoblastic rimming."

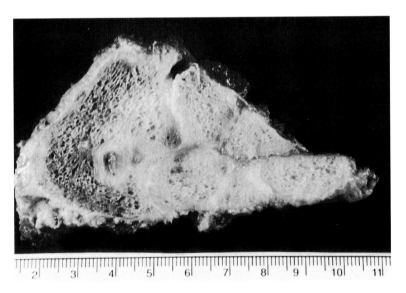

FIG. 5   Gross photograph of the cut section of a completely mature mass of myositis ossificans. The central aspect is composed of grossly "normal" cancellous bone with hematopoietic (*dark*) and fatty (*light*) bone marrow.

in later sections. Soft-tissue osteosarcoma, which is one of the most important differential diagnostic considerations, is discussed in detail below. Soft-tissue masses entirely composed of mature lamellar cortical and cancellous bone have been termed soft-tissue osteomas (14); however, it is likely that these represent completely mature masses of previously unrecognized MO. Ossifying fibromyxoid tumor and synovial sarcoma may also present as intramuscular ossified soft-tissue masses. The clinical and histologic features that allow their separation from MO are discussed in separate sections. Heterotopic bone formation within skeletal muscle, often in a para-articular location, is a common consequence following central nervous system injury and occasionally occurs following severe burns and total joint arthroplasty (15–18). In these circumstances, the bone formation usually develops within 1–3 months following the injury. Other reactive pseudotumors, such as nodular fasciitis and proliferative fasciitis, may also be associated with heterotopic reactive bone formation similar to MO (19–22). In these circumstances, the masses usually arise within subcutaneous tissue, typically are smaller than MO, and the bone that is formed lacks the characteristic zonal architecture. Fibro-osseous pseudotumor is the name applied to a reactive bone and cartilaginous mass that occurs in the digits. It is discussed in detail in a later section.

B. Fibrodysplasia (Myositis) Ossificans Progressiva

1. General and Clinical Features

Fibrodysplasia ossificans progressiva (FOP) is an extremely rare (less than one person per million affected) autosomal dominant inherited condition characterized by extensive soft-tissue ossification at multiple sites (23,24). The progressive nature of the process results in severe disability (23,24). Affected patients have a variety of skeletal abnormalities, particularly affecting the digits and cervical spine. The most common and virtually diagnostic finding is the presence of short great toes (23–25). Fibrodysplasia ossificans progressiva affects males and females equally. The soft-tissue ossification typically begins in the first decade of life. Trauma, either accidental or surgical, often initiates the process and the children present with painful swollen soft tissues at the affected site (23–25). There is progressive stiffness and loss of function of the muscles in the area (23–27). Development of soft-tissue calcification and ossification ensues in 2–3 months (23–27). Although any tissue site may be affected, the ossifying process is usually worst in the paraspinal region, especially in the cervical musculature. Soft-tissue ossification tends to be progressive. The cause of FOP is unknown; however, mutations in the genes encoding for bone morphogenetic protein are the most likely cause (24,27). Surgical intervention should be avoided in this disease, since excision of a mass of heterotopic bone results in rapid recurrence with accelerated ossification (24). Most patients with FOP do not have affected family members, suggesting that virtually all cases represent sporadic mutations (24).

2. Microscopic Features

Since FOP is essentially a reactive process in which there is uncontrolled inappropriate soft-tissue ossification, the histologic appearance varies depending on the time course of the process (23–28). In this regard it is similar to MO (23–28); however, several differences between the two conditions are evident. Unlike MO, which clinically and pathologically presents as a single soft-tissue mass, FOP presents as a confluence of multiple nodules. The morphology of an individual lesion depends on its stage of development (23–28). Early lesions, which radiologically are unmineralized, typically show an intramuscular proliferation of uniform mitotically active spindle-shaped fibroblasts embedded in myxoid extracellular ground substance (23–28). The cells and myxoid material "infiltrate" between skeletal myocytes (23–28). This appearance closely resembles infantile fibromatosis, frequently resulting in misdiagnosis without appropriate clinical information (23–28). As lesions develop there is increasing production of cartilage and bone matrix. The latter may arise via an intramembranous mechanism or secondary to endochondral ossification (26,27). In either form, the bone and cartilage, like that in MO, is often hypercellular and architecturally primitive (26,27). With time, complete maturation to lamellar bone occurs. Late lesions are composed entirely of lamellar cortical and cancellous bone and may contain bone marrow.

3. Differential Diagnosis

The most important differential diagnoses for FOP are infantile fibromatosis and soft-tissue sarcoma, such as infantile fibrosarcoma or embryonal rhabdomyosarcoma (see relevant sections). The clinical scenario is extremely important in this regard because small biopsy samples of early lesions may closely simulate fibromatosis. Attention to clinical details and consideration of examination of the child's feet for the characteristic short great toes is useful. Distinction of FOP from soft-tissue sarcoma is based on recognition of the bland proliferating cells that are present in this disorder, unlike the atypical, cytologically malignant cells that are present in the soft-tissue sarcomas. FOP differs from MO by demonstrating a multinodular growth and lacking the zonal microscopic qualities of the latter entity. MO is rare in the first decade of life.

C. Fibro-osseous Pseudotumor of Digits

1. General and Clinical Features

Fibro-osseous pseudotumor of digits, also referred to as florid reactive periostitis, is a nonneoplastic reactive bone- and cartilage-rich mass that occurs within the soft tissues of the distal extremities, predominantly affecting the digits of the hands (29–32). It can be considered as being the distal soft-tissue equivalent of MO. This condition affects males and females equally and is most common in the second and third decade of life (29,30). Patients characteristically present with a short history of a painful or painless digital swelling (29,30,32). Less than half of the patients give a history of trauma to the site (30). In a minority there is localized erythema (29,30). Radiographs demonstrate soft-tissue swelling of the affected digit and, in a minority, linear "periosteal" bone formation on the underlying phalanx. The majority of the masses lack detectable mineralization at presentation (29,30). Most fibro-osseous pseudotumors measure less than 3.0 cm and are described as firm or rubbery at the time of excision (Fig. 6) (29). Local excision results in cure. Recurrence is unusual even though the masses are typically removed with positive surgical margins (29,30).

2. Microscopic Findings

Many of the histologic features of MO are found in fibro-osseous pseudotumor of digits. Specifically, this condition is characterized by considerable hypercellularity, an often high mitotic rate, and bone formation that varies in its degree of histologic maturity depending on the stage at which the lesion is removed and examined. A transition from fascicles of spindle cells to progressively mature bone resulting in a "zonal" appearance similar to MO is found in a minority of cases (30,31). Like the other reactive proliferations discussed above, cellular immature

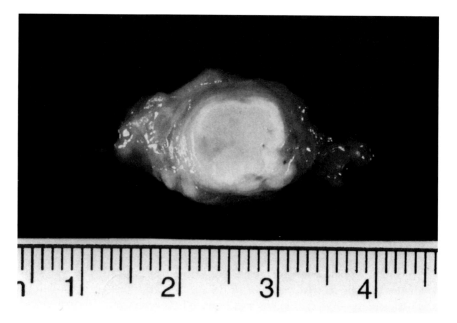

FIG. 6   Resection specimen of an intact fibro-osseous pseudotumor. The mass contains abundant reactive cartilage explaining the pale cut surface.

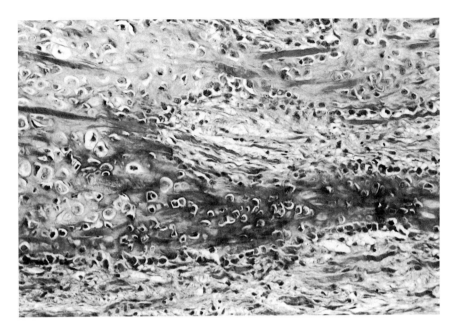

FIG. 7   Immature woven bone with prominent osteoblastic rimming.

cartilage tissue is often a component of fibro-osseous pseudotumor of digits (29,30). Overall, the tissue closely resembles fracture callus (Figs. 7 and 8).

3.   Differential Diagnosis

The differential diagnosis of fibro-osseous pseudotumor includes all of the previously discussed entities, in addition to soft-tissue osteosarcoma, discussed below. These masses also should be distinguished from fracture callus occurring in association with phalangeal fracture. Finally, fibro-osseous pseudotumor has many similarities to bizarre periosteal osteochondromatous proliferation and subungual exostosis (33,34). However, both of the latter conditions demonstrate radiographically detectable attachment to the underlying phalanx and pathologically lack the callus-like appearance of fibro-osseous pseudotumor.

D.   Soft-Tissue Osteosarcoma

1.   General and Clinical Features

Soft-tissue osteosarcomas are rare malignant neoplasms, accounting for less than 1% of soft-tissue sarcomas (35–37). In contrast to conventional osseous osteosarcoma that typically affects young adults in the second and third decades, soft-

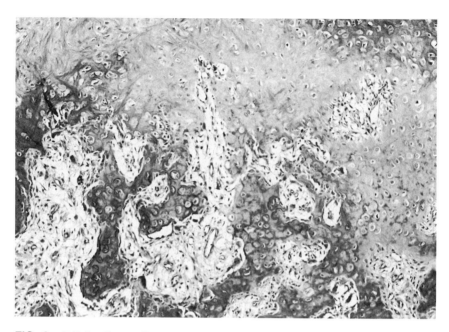

FIG. 8 Cellular fibrocartilage exhibiting enchondral ossification. A typical finding in fibro-osseous pseudotumor.

tissue osteosarcoma occurs in older patients, predominantly in the fifth and sixth decades (35–40). A minority of affected patients have a history of prior radiation therapy (35–38). The tumors typically arise in the proximal extremities and present as a painless or minimally tender mass (35–39). Most measure greater than 5.0 cm in size (Fig. 9) (35–39). Some patients claim a history of recent or remote trauma to the affected site. Radiographs usually show only a soft-tissue mass without calcification (35–39). The underlying skeleton appears normal. Soft-tissue osteosarcomas are high-grade malignant tumors, and up to 85% of patients develop metastases and ultimately die of tumor (35–39). Treatment of the primary tumor requires wide local excision and/or amputation with cytotoxic chemotherapy, depending on clinical circumstances.

2. Microscopic Features

The majority of soft-tissue osteosarcomas are high-grade malignant tumors composed of pleomorphic spindle cells. All of the histologic subtypes of osseous osteosarcoma occur in the soft tissues (35–39). Therefore, tumors can be classified as osteoblastic, chondroblastic, fibroblastic, small-cell, telangiectatic, or resembling malignant fibrous histiocytoma. The latter is the most common. In these, the

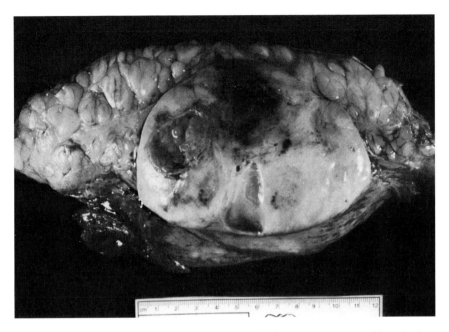

FIG. 9   Large fleshy soft-tissue mass typical of soft-tissue osteosarcoma. Note the heterogeneous appearance of the cut surface of the tumor, which is a typical feature of high-grade sarcomas.

majority of the tumor resembles a high-grade undifferentiated pleomorphic sarcoma, such as storiform pleomorphic malignant fibrous histiocytoma. As such, the tumor cells exhibit marked variation is size and shape in addition to demonstrating extreme nuclear pleomorphism (35–39). Mitotic figures are readily found, and atypical forms may be seen. Spontaneous necrosis is common (35–39). The neoplastic bone matrix may be minimally or completely unmineralized. It outlines individual tumor cells in a lace-like manner (Fig. 10). Bone matrix production is also typically patchy. Large expanses of tumor may be devoid of recognizable bone or osteoid (Fig. 11). This can result in diagnostic error on small biopsy samples. In chondroblastic tumors, pleomorphic chondrocytes embedded in irregular hyaline cartilage matrix are found admixed with other high-grade foci of tumor (35–40). The small-cell and telangiectatic variants of osteosarcoma are the rarest subtypes to be found in the soft tissues (35–40). In the former, the tumor is composed of undifferentiated "small blue" cells similar to those found in Ewing's sarcoma/primitive neuroectodermal tumor (PNET). However, the small cells are associated with lace-like neoplastic bone production in osteosarcoma, in contrast to Ewing's sarcoma. In the telangiectatic variant of soft-tissue osteosarcoma, blood-filled

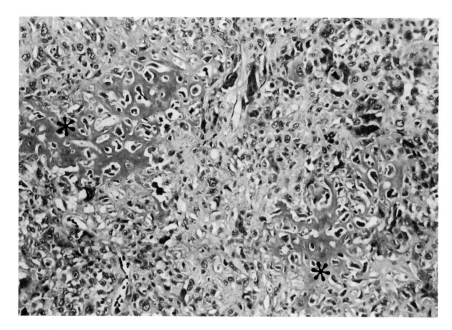

FIG. 10 Irregular lace-like aggregates of neoplastic bone matrix (*asterisk*) surrounding pleomorphic tumor cells.

spaces that lack an endothelial lining are present in the tumor. Histologically low-grade soft-tissue osteosarcomas are extremely uncommon. Only a single case has been reported (41).

3. Differential Diagnosis

Soft-tissue osteosarcoma closely resembles other pleomorphic high-grade soft-tissue sarcomas, such as malignant fibrous histiocytoma, pleomorphic liposarcoma, and high-grade leiomyosarcoma. It is distinguished from these by the presence of neoplastic bone and osteoid matrix and the absence of other lines of differentiation. One of the most important differential diagnostic considerations is myositis ossificans. Soft-tissue osteosarcoma demonstrates consistently greater cytologic atypia than myositis ossificans. The zoning phenomenon that is the histologic hallmark of myositis ossificans is not present in osteosarcoma. In addition, while myositis ossificans occurs in a similar anatomical distribution as soft-tissue osteosarcoma, it affects a distinctly different age group of patients.

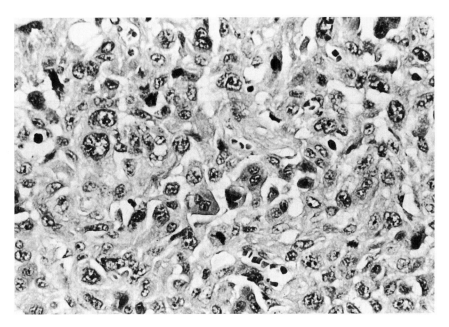

FIG. 11   No neoplastic osteoid is present in this photomicrograph. The tumor is histologically indistinguishable from high-grade undifferentiated soft-tissue sarcoma (MFH) in fields such as this one.

III. PREDOMINANTLY CARTILAGINOUS MASSES OF SOFT TISSUE

A. Soft-Tissue Chondroma

1.   General and Clinical Features

Soft-tissue chondromas are benign cartilage neoplasms that predominantly occur in adults in the fourth through seventh decades of life (42–45). There is a slight male predominance (45). A soft-tissue chondroma most commonly arises in the superficial soft tissues of the distal extremities, particularly on the volar aspect of the wrist where it presents as a painless soft-tissue nodule (42–46). Radiographs often reveal calcification that shows the typical arrangement of rings and arcs characteristic of hyaline cartilage (Fig. 12) (43,45,47). The tumors frequently show attachment to deep structures, such as tendon sheath, joint capsule, or periosteum (42,43). During removal, they often "pop out" because of their well-circumscribed outline. Most soft-tissue chondromas measure less than 3.0 cm (42,43,45). Size greater than 5.0 cm is exceptional (45). Soft-tissue chondromas are treated by lo-

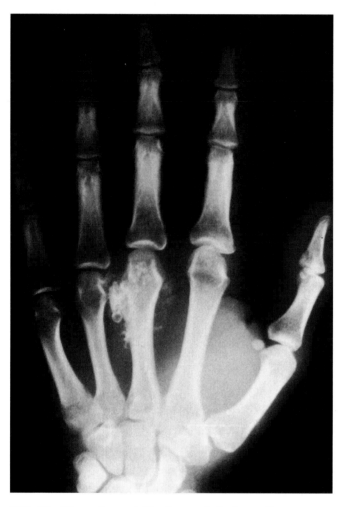

FIG. 12   Ring and arc calcifications typical of a cartilage tumor are present in this dorsally located soft-tissue chondroma adjacent to the third metacarpal.

cal resection only. Recurrence develops in 10–15% of patients following excision (42,43,45).

2.   Microscopic Features

Soft-tissue chondromas are well-circumscribed neoplasms composed of hyaline cartilage in the majority of instances (42–47). Within an individual tumor there

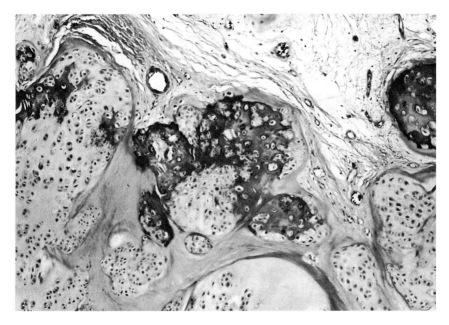

FIG. 13   Compressed lobules of hyaline cartilage embedded in a fibrous background. Note the patchy calcification of the cartilage matrix.

are multiple compressed lobules of cartilage that are separated by collagen bands (Figs. 13 and 14). The lobules exhibit relative hypercellularity and clusters of chondrocytes (42–47). Individual cells often demonstrate enlarged nuclei and visible nuclcoli. However, mitoses are rare. Overall, the degree of cellularity and cytologic atypia that is present in soft-tissue chondroma equals or exceeds that found in low-grade intraosseous chondrosarcoma. This is a feature that, although characteristic for soft-tissue chondroma, may cause diagnostic confusion. The hyaline cartilage matrix often undergoes calcification and ossification accounting for the radiographic findings (42–47). The calcifications appear as purple granules that frequently outline individual chondrocytes in a lace-like manner. A minority of soft-tissue chondromas are composed of myxoid cartilage as opposed to hyaline cartilage. In these tumors, the chondrocytes lie within flocculent granular extracellular matrix and lack well-developed lacunes (42,43,45). A cellular giant cell–rich infiltrate may be found at the periphery of these tumors, accounting for their occasional designation as giant cell chondromas (42,43,45). Immunohistochemical staining demonstrates that the chondrocytes of soft-tissue chondroma stain positively for S-100 protein and vimentin.

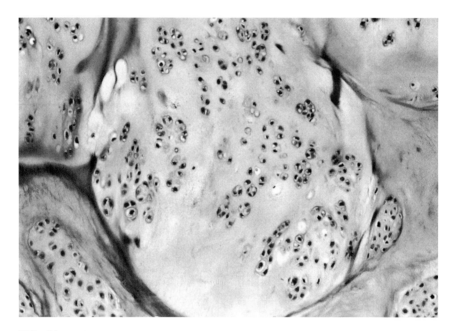

FIG. 14 A single nodule of tumor demonstrating the hyaline cartilage matrix, the relative hypercellularity and the clustering of the chondrocytes that is typical of soft-tissue chondroma.

3. Differential Diagnosis

Soft-tissue chondroma should be distinguished from soft-tissue chondrosarcomas of myxoid and mesenchymal types, which are discussed in detail below. Foci of cellular hyaline cartilage may be found in reactive bone-producing conditions such as myositis ossificans, fibrodysplasia ossificans progressiva, and fibro-osseous pseudotumor of digits (all discussed in detail above). Primary skeletal chondrosarcoma with soft-tissue extension may simulate soft-tissue chondroma. Knowledge of the clinical circumstances and radiographic findings of an underlying intraosseous cartilage tumor should prevent misdiagnosis. Invasive destructive growth, which is characteristically present in the soft-tissue extension of osseous chondrosarcoma, is not present in soft-tissue chondroma.

B. Extraskeletal Myxoid Chondrosarcoma

1. General and Clinical Features

Extraskeletal myxoid chondrosarcomas (EMCs) are rare soft-tissue sarcomas that predominantly occur in adulthood (48–51). There is a slight male predilection

(48,49,51). The tumors most commonly occur in the deep soft tissues of the extremities (48–51). They usually present as a painless or minimally tender slow-growing mass. Most of the tumors measure greater than 5.0 cm in size (Fig. 15). In the original series outlining the behavior of EMC, the tumor was considered to be of relatively low grade, with a low incidence of metastasis and an indolent clinical course (48). More recent experience with series of patients followed for longer periods have shown a high rate of metastases and tumor-related death, suggesting that this tumor should be considered a high-grade neoplasm (49,51). The risk of metastasis appears to be increased among patients who have inadequate resection of the primary tumor. Cytogenetic analysis of EMC demonstrates a consistent translocation between chromosomes 9 and 22, t(9;22)(q22-31;q11-12), which serves as a diagnostic marker for this neoplasm (52,53).

2. Microscopic Features

Extraskeletal myxoid chondrosarcomas are lobulated myxoid tumors that characteristically demonstrate low cellularity (48–51,54). The individual tumor cells are small, oval, and have minimal amounts of eosinophilic cytoplasm surrounding the nucleus. The nuclei are central, dark staining, and usually lack visible nucle-

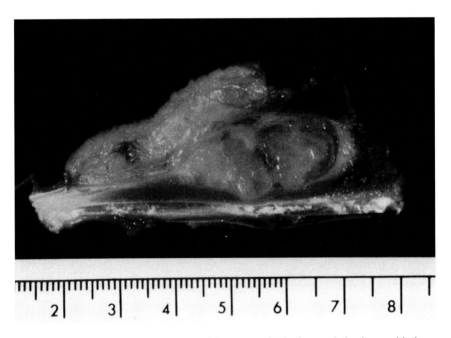

FIG. 15 A lobulated gelatinous myxoid tumor typical of extraskeletal myxoid chondrosarcoma.

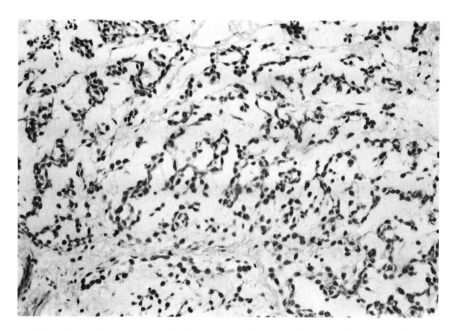

FIG. 16 Short intersecting cords of relatively uniform small tumor cells present in a pale myxoid ground substance.

oli. Tumor cells are arranged in linear arrays that appear as straight lines or curves (Fig. 16). Mitotic figures are usually inconspicuous. The tumor cells are embedded in a basophilic flocculent matrix that is relatively hypovascular. Like most cartilage neoplasms, a distinctly nodular/lobular growth is evident. The lobules are separated by strands of eosinophilic collagen. In low-grade tumors the degree of cellularity is low, whereas higher grade tumors typically show greater cellularity with less extracellular matrix. Hyaline cartilage is not found in EMC. Rarely dedifferentiation occurs in EMC (54,55). In these tumors, conventional low-grade EMC is associated with a high-grade undifferentiated sarcoma lacking recognizable cartilaginous differentiation (54,55). This phenomenon is analogous to dedifferentiation that occurs in skeletal chondrosarcoma and soft-tissue low-grade liposarcoma. It usually implies an aggressive clinical course. Immunohistochemical stains demonstrate positive staining for vimentin and S-100 protein in the chondrocytes in EMC (in the majority of cases).

3. Differential Diagnosis

Extraskeletal myxoid chondrosarcoma should be distinguished from soft-tissue chondroma. The latter typically is a smaller neoplasm that occurs in the distal extremities. True hyaline cartilage that occurs in soft-tissue chondroma is not present in EMC. A variety of other myxoid soft-tissue tumors may be confused with EMC. Principal among these are intramuscular myxoma, myxoid liposarcoma, myxofibrosarcoma (myxoid malignant fibrous histiocytoma) and benign and malignant peripheral nerve sheath tumors (see relevant sections).

C.   Mesenchymal Chondrosarcoma

1.   General and Clinical Features

Mesenchymal chondrosarcoma (MC) is the rarest of the primary cartilaginous tumors of soft tissue (56). This tumor also arises in the skeleton. In fact, skeletal MC is more common than the soft-tissue variant (57). Males and females are equally affected (57). The tumors occur in all age groups; however, the majority are diagnosed in patients in the second through fourth decades (56,57). Any soft-tissue site may be affected; however, MC has a distinct predilection to involve the soft tissues of the craniospinal axis (57,58). The meninges account for the single most common soft-tissue site (57). The presenting symptoms depend on the location of the tumor. Central nervous system MCs often present with headache, seizures, or other site-specific deficits (58–60). Deep soft-tissue tumors of the extremities have nonspecific symptoms related to the presence of a mass (57). Radiographs demonstrate mineralization in the majority of cases (56,57). Treatment of MC involves wide local resection and cytotoxic chemotherapy; however, these tumors demonstrate an aggressive clinical course, with up to 50% patients dying of disease within 5 years (56–58).

2.   Microscopic Features

Mesenchymal chondrosarcoma is dominated by a noncartilaginous population of small blue cells, similar to those that compose Ewing's sarcoma/PNET (Fig. 17) (57–61). These cells are typically arranged as sheets and cohesive clusters supported by a branching capillary network. The latter vessels usually show acute-angle branching resembling that seen in hemangiopericytoma. Individual tumor cells are oval to spindle in shape and demonstrate high nuclear to cytoplasmic ratios. The visible cytoplasm is eosinophilic to clear. Mitotic figures are readily found, and necrosis in pretreatment biopsies is often present. Islands of cellular hyaline and fibrocartilage are found randomly within the background of small blue cells (Fig. 18) (57–61). These vary in size but usually measure less than 1.0 mm. In these foci the chondrocytes lie in recognizable lacunes. They usually demonstrate only mild cytologic atypia. These cartilaginous foci that form the diagnostic feature of MC may be scant; small biopsy fragments may not demonstrate them. Immunohistochemical staining reveals that the undifferentiated small blue cells

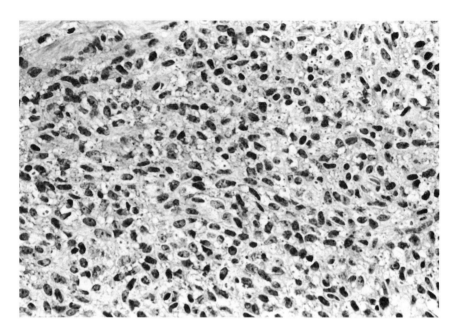

FIG. 17 Small uniform oval to slightly spindle cells typical of mesenchymal chondrosarcoma. In this field the tumor resembles a Ewing's sarcoma/primitive neuroectodermal tumor.

stain positively for CD99 and vimentin (61). The cartilage cells label for vimentin and S-100 protein (61).

3.   Differential Diagnosis

The differential diagnosis of MC is principally that of other small blue cell tumors of soft tissue. As such, this includes Ewing's sarcoma/PNET, rhabdomyosarcoma, malignant lymphoma, and small-cell osteosarcoma. The first two of these are discussed in detail in other sections. Malignant lymphomas rarely present as primary masses within soft tissue. The presence of the hyaline cartilage nests allows correct diagnosis because these never occur in malignant lymphoma. In small biopsy specimens that lack cartilage, immunohistochemical investigation allows appropriate classification of the tumor. The distinction of MC from small-cell osteosarcoma revolves around the recognition of neoplastic bone production by the small-cell component of the tumor. This phenomenon does not occur in MC and, if present, defines the tumor as a small-cell osteosarcoma. As has been stated above, small-cell osteosarcoma is the rarest histologic variant of extraskeletal osteosarcoma.

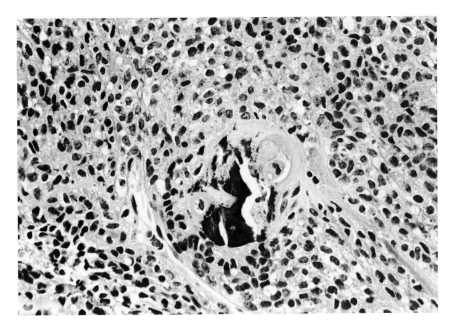

FIG. 18 Small nodule of partially mineralized hyaline cartilage within background of undifferentiated "blue cells."

IV. OTHER MATRIX-CONTAINING SOFT-TISSUE TUMORS

A. Aneurysmal Cyst of Soft Tissue

1. General and Clinical Features

Primary soft-tissue "tumors" histologically identical to osseous aneurysmal bone cyst have been designated aneurysmal cysts of soft tissue (62). These are extremely rare lesions; fewer than 10 have been reported (62–66). They occur in all age groups (62–66). There is no sex predilection. Patients present with symptoms related to an enlarging soft-tissue mass, usually of short duration (62–66). The underlying skeleton is normal. Local resection results in cure; there have been no cases of local recurrence. Soft-tissue aneurysmal cyst most likely is an unusual manifestation of a posttraumatic reactive process, similar to myositis ossificans (62).

2. Microscopic Features

Aneurysmal cyst of soft tissue demonstrates all of the histologic features of aneurysmal bone cyst (62–66). These lesions contain blood-filled cystic spaces that

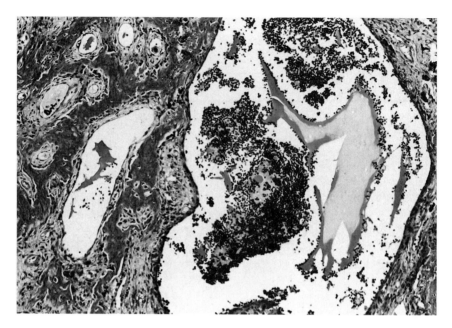

FIG. 19   A partially blood-filled cystic space characteristic of aneurysmal cyst of soft tissue. Note the reactive woven bone adjacent to the wall of the cystic space.

lack endothelial lining (Fig. 19). The solid components between the cysts are composed of a confluence of moderately cellular spindle cell nodules, often with abundant osteoclast-like giant cells (Fig. 20). These solid foci, in addition to the septae that divide the cysts, contain linear streamers of woven bone that typically demonstrate osteoblastic rimming. Aggregates of moderately cellular basophilic "chondroid" material may also be present (62). The latter appears relatively specific for aneurysmal cysts of bone and soft tissue.

3.   Differential Diagnosis

Soft-tissue aneurysmal cysts should principally be distinguished from myositis ossificans and soft-tissue osteosarcoma. Both of these are discussed in detail above. Briefly, aneurysmal cysts of soft tissue lack the orderly zoning that characterizes myositis ossificans. Multiple blood-filled cystic spaces that lack endothelial lining, which are the defining feature of the aneurysmal cyst, are not present in myositis ossificans. The high-grade atypia and disordered bone matrix production that are prominent features of the majority of soft-tissue osteosarcomas are not present in aneurysmal cysts of soft tissue.

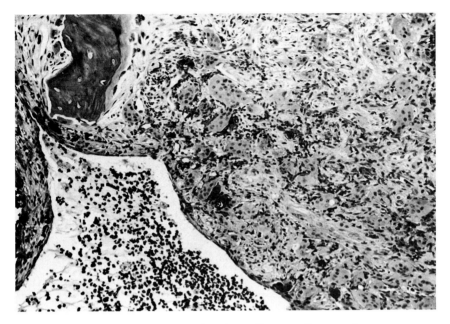

FIG. 20   A more solid nodule resembling giant cell tumor adjacent to the cyst space.

B. Giant Cell Tumor of Soft Tissue

1. General and Clinical Features

Giant cell tumors of soft tissue are primary soft-tissue neoplasms that are histo-logically identical to osseous giant cell tumor (63). Approximately half of these lesions are associated with metaplastic bone production that may be present in the tumor or surround it in a shell-like manner (67,68). Soft-tissue giant cell tumor demonstrates a spectrum of histologic appearance and clinical behavior that ex-tends from benign to highly malignant. At the latter end of the spectrum, the tu-mors are often classified as giant cell malignant fibrous histiocytomas (69–71). These tumors have a high incidence of metastases and tumor-related mortality (69–71). On the other hand, the histologically benign lesions typically demon-strate an indolent clinical course with a low incidence of recurrence, even follow-ing incomplete excision (63,67,68). Giant cell tumors of soft tissue affect males and females equally and are most common in the fourth and fifth decades of life (63,67–71). In general, the histologically benign tumors measure less than 5.0 cm and are superficial, whereas the malignant variants are often larger and deeper (63,67–71). Any tissue site can be affected.

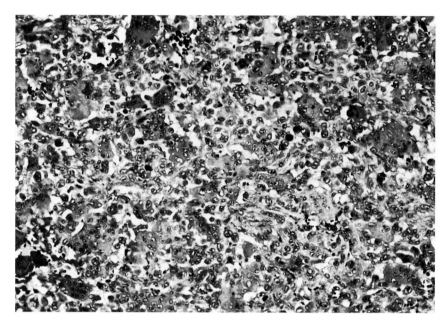

FIG. 21 Evenly distributed osteoclast-like giant cells embedded in a background of bland spindled mononuclear cells. The nuclear morphology of the latter closely resembles that within the multinucleated cells.

2. Microscopic Features

Soft-tissue giant cell tumor, like its intraosseous counterpart, is composed of an admixture of mononuclear cells and multinucleated osteoclast-like giant cells (63,67,68). The latter are evenly distributed among mononuclear cells that vary in morphology from spindled to oval. In benign tumors, the mononuclear cells demonstrate central oval to spindled nuclei with vesicular chromatin and small eosinophilic nucleoli. Typically, the mononuclear cell nuclei are identical to the nuclei of the osteoclast-like giant cells (Fig. 21). Mitotic counts are quite variable but may be as high as 10 per 10 high-power fields examined. Necrosis and cystic change may also be present in both benign and malignant variants. In malignant giant cell tumors, the mononuclear cells exhibit greater degrees of nuclear atypia, including hyperchromatism, irregular macronucleoli, and atypical mitotic figures (Fig. 22) (69–71). The osteoclast-like giant cells appear similar in both benign and malignant forms (63,67–71). In both types of tumor metaplastic bone may be present. This is typically woven, and may be distributed at the periphery of the mass or as sheets and/or trabeculae within the tumor proper (Fig. 23). Foci of vascular invasion at the periphery of the tumor nodules may be seen in both benign and ma-

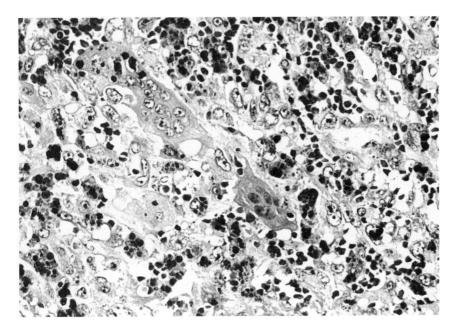

FIG. 22   In this malignant giant cell tumor of soft tissue, the mononuclear cells exhibit marked nuclear pleomorphism in contrast to the benign variants.

lignant tumors, similar to the angioinvasion often seen in osseous giant cell tumor. By immunohistochemistry the multinucleated osteoclast-like giant cells demonstrate strong reactivity for CD68 supporting their histiocytic origin (67). The mononuclear cells demonstrate focal staining for CD68, HAM-56, and muscle actin. This staining profile is identical to that of osseous giant cell tumor (67).

3.   Differential Diagnosis

Soft-tissue giant cell tumor should be distinguished from soft-tissue recurrence of conventional osseous giant cell tumor. This is readily accomplished by obtaining an appropriate clinical history and radiographs. Histologically, benign soft-tissue giant cell tumor should be distinguished from giant cell tumor of tendon sheath, which has many similar clinical and pathologic features (see above). Briefly, in giant cell tumor of tendon sheath, the osteoclast-like giant cells are frequently clustered, the mononuclear cells are more uniformly oval or "histiocyte-like" and the nodules often contain bands of hyalinized collagen. In addition, an attachment to a synovial sheath is frequently present in giant cell tumor of tendon sheath. Metaplastic bone that is commonly present in soft-tissue giant cell tumor is only rarely a feature of giant cell tumor of tendon sheath. Some aneurysmal cysts of soft tis-

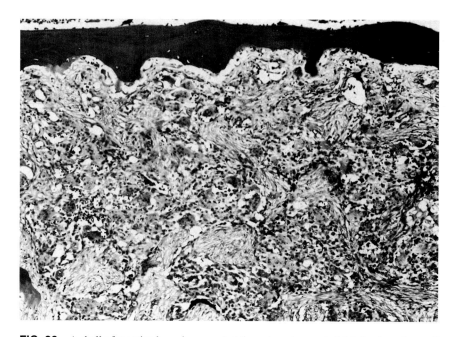

FIG. 23 A shell of reactive bone is present at the external aspect of this benign giant cell tumor of soft parts.

sue demonstrate large numbers of osteoclasts that may result in a close resemblance to soft-tissue giant cell tumor. In general, the aneurysmal cysts demonstrate greater histologic variability, and by definition these lesions are predominantly cystic whereas the giant cell tumors are predominantly solid. Malignant soft-tissue giant cell tumors are essentially identical to the so-called giant cell variant of malignant fibrous histiocytoma (see above). The malignant tumors that contain metaplastic bone should, however, be distinguished from soft-tissue osteosarcoma. In giant cell tumors, including the malignant forms, the bone that is present is histologically benign. As such, it exhibits mature architecture and is associated with cytologically benign osteoblasts and osteocytes. This is in contrast to soft-tissue osteosarcoma in which direct bone and osteoid production by cytologically high-grade sarcoma cells is found. In general, the neoplastic matrix in soft-tissue osteosarcoma is immature and disorganized (see above).

REFERENCES

1. Ekelund A, Brosjo O, Nilsson OS. Experimental induction of heterotopic bone. Clin Orthop Rel Res 263:102–112, 1991.

2. Ackerman LC. Extra-osseous localized non-neoplastic bone and cartilage formation (so-called myositis ossificans). Clinical and pathological confusion with malignant neoplasms. J Bone Joint Surg A 40:279–298, 1958.
3. Angervall L, Stener B, Stener I, Ahren C. Pseudomalignant osseous tumour of soft tissue. A clinical, radiological and pathological study of five cases. J Bone Joint Surg B 51:654–663, 1969.
4. Lagier R, Cox JN. Pseudomalignant myositis ossificans. A pathological study of eight cases. Hum Pathol 6:653–665, 1975.
5. Sumiyoshi K, Tsuneyoshi M, Enjoji M. Myositis ossificans. A clinicopathologic study of 21 cases. Acta Pathol Jpn 35:1109–1122, 1985.
6. Ogilvie-Harris DJ, Fornasier VL. Pseudomalignant myositis ossificans: heterotopic new-bone formation without a history of trauma. J Bone Joint Surg A 62:1274–1283, 1980.
7. Nuovo MA, Norman A, Chumas J, Ackerman LV. Myositis ossificans with atypical clinical, radiographic, or pathologic findings: a review of 23 cases. Skeletal Radiol 21:87–101, 1992.
8. Heinrich SD, Zembo MM, MacEwen GD. Pseudomalignant myositis ossificans. Orthopedics 12:599–602, 1989.
9. Kransdorf MJ, Meis JM, Jelinek JS. Myositis ossificans: MR appearance with radiologic-pathologic correlation. Am J Roentgenol 157:1243–1248, 1991.
10. Clapton WK, James CL, Morris LL, Davey RB, Peacock MJ, Byard RW. Myositis ossificans in childhood. Pathology 24:311–314, 1992.
11. Shirkhoda A, Armin A, Bis KG, Makris J, Irwin RB, Shetty AN. MR imaging of myositis ossificans: variable patterns at different stages. J Magnet Reson Imaging 5:287–292, 1995.
12. Cvitanic O, Sedlak J. Acute myositis ossificans. Skeletal Radiol 24:139–141, 1995.
13. Mody BS, Patil SS, Carty H, Klenerman L. Fracture through the bone of traumatic myositis ossificans. J Bone Joint Surg B 76:607–609, 1994.
14. Schweitzer ME, Greenway G, Resnick D, Haghighi P, Snoots WE. Osteoma of soft parts. Skel Radiol 21:177–180, 1992.
15. Garland DE. Surgical approaches for resection of heterotopic ossification in traumatic brain-injured adults. Clin Orthop Rel Res 263:59–70, 1991.
16. Garland DE. A clinical perspective on common forms of acquired heterotopic ossification. Clin Orthop Rel Res 263:13–29, 1991.
17. Ahrengart L. Periarticular heterotopic ossification after total hip arthroplasty. Risk factors and consequences. Clin Orthop Rel Res 263:49–58, 1991.
18. Kjaersgaard-Andersen P, Sletgard J, Gjerloff C, Lund F. Heterotopic bone formation after noncemented total hip arthroplasty. Location of ectopic bone and the influence of postoperative antiinflammatory treatment. Clin Orthop Rel Res 252:156–162, 1990.
19. Allen PW. Nodular fasciitis. Pathology 4:9–26, 1972.
20. Hutter RVP, Stewart FW, Foote FW. Fasciitis. A report of 70 cases with follow-up proving the benignity of the lesion. Cancer 15:992–1003, 1962.
21. Stout AP. Pseudosarcomatous fasciitis in children. Cancer 14:1216–1222, 1961.
22. Wasman JK, Willis J, Makley J, Abdul-Karim FW. Myositis ossificans-like lesion of nerve. Histopathology 30:75–78, 1997.

23. Smith R, Athanasou NA, Vipond SE. Fibrodysplasia ossificans progressiva: clinico-pathologic features and natural history. Q J Med 89:445–456, 1996.

24. Bridges AJ, Kou-Ching H, Singh A, Churchill R, Miles J. Fibrodysplasia ossificans progressiva. Semin Arth Rheum 24:155–164, 1994.

25. Heidelberger KP, DiPietro M. Fibrodysplasia ossificans progressiva. Ped Pathol 7: 105–109, 1987.

26. Cramer SF, Ruehl A, Mandel MA. Fibrodysplasia ossificans progressiva: a distinctive bone-forming lesion of the soft tissue. Cancer 48:1016–1021, 1981.

27. Kaplan FS, Tabas JA, Gannon FH, Finkel G, Hahn GV, Zasloff MA. The histopathology of fibrodysplasia ossificans progressiva: an enchondral process. J Bone Joint Surg A 75:220–230, 1993.

28. Maxwell WA, Spicer SS, Miller RL, Halushka PV, Westphal MC, Setser ME. Histochemical and ultrastructural studies in fibrodysplasia ossificans progressiva (myositis ossificans progressiva). Am J Pathol 87:483–498, 1977.

29. Dupree WB, Enzinger FM. Fibro-osseous pseudotumor of the digits. Cancer 58: 2103–2109, 1986.

30. Spjut HJ, Dorfman HD. Florid reactive periostitis of the tubular bones of the hands and feet: a benign lesion which may resemble osteosarcoma. Am J Surg Pathol 5: 423–433, 1981.

31. Ostrowski ML, Spjut HJ. Lesions of the bones of the hands and feet. Am J Surg Pathol 21:676–690, 1997.

32. Craver RD, Correa-Gracian H, Heinrich S. Florid reactive periostitis. Hum Pathol 28:745–747, 1997.

33. Meneses MF, Unni KK, Swee RG. Bizarre parosteal osteochondromatous proliferation of bone (Nora's lesion). Am J Surg Pathol 17:691–697, 1993.

34. Miller-Breslow A, Dorfman HD. Dupytren's (subungual) exostosis. Am J Surg Pathol 12:368–378, 1988.

35. Lee JSY, Fetsch JF, Wasdhal DA, Lee BP, Pritchard DJ, Nascimento AG. A review of 40 patients with extraskeletal osteosarcoma. Cancer 76:2253–2259, 1995.

36. Chung EB, Enzinger FM. Extraskeletal osteosarcoma. Cancer 60:1132–1142, 1987.

37. Sordillo PP, Hajdu SI, Magill GB, Golbey RB. Extraosseous osteogenic sarcoma: a review of 48 patients. Cancer 51:727–734, 1983.

38. Jensen ML, Schumacher B, Jense OM, Nielsen OS, Keller J. Extraskeletal osteosarcomas: a clinicopathologic study of 25 cases. Am J Surg Pathol 22:588–594, 1998.

39. Bane BL, Evans HL, Ro JY, Carrasco CH, Grignon DJ, Benjamin RS, Ayala AG. Extraskeletal osteosarcoma: a clinicopathologic review of 26 cases. Cancer 66:2762–2770, 1990.

40. Dubec JJ, Munk PL, O'Connell JX, Lee MJ, Janzen D, Connell D, Masri B, Logan PM. Soft tissue osteosarcoma with telangiectatic features: MR imaging findings in two cases. Skel Radiol 26:732–736, 1997.

41. Yi ES, Shmookler BM, Malawer MM, Sweet DE. Well-differentiated extraskeletal osteosarcoma: a soft-tissue homologue of parosteal ostesarcoma. Arch Pathol Lab Med 115:906–909, 1991.

42. Humphreys S, Pambakian H, McKee PH, Fletcher CDM. Soft tissue chondroma—a study of 15 tumours. Histopathology 10:147–159, 1986.

43. Chung EB, Enzinger FM. Chondroma of soft parts. Cancer 41:1414–1424, 1978.
44. Fletcher CDM, Krausz T. Cartilaginous tumours of soft tissue. Appl Pathol 6:208–220, 1988.
45. Dahlin DC, Salvador AH. Cartilaginous tumors of the soft tissues of the hands and feet. Mayo Clin Proc 49:721–726, 1974.
46. DelSignore JL, Torre BA, Miller RJ. Extraskeletal chondroma of the hand: Case report and review of the literature. Clin Orthop Rel Res 254:147–152, 1990.
47. Bansal M, Goldman AB, DiCarlo EF, McCormack R. Soft tissue chondromas: diagnosis and differential diagnosis. Skel Radiol 22:309–315, 1993.
48. Enzinger FM, Shiraki M. Extraskeletal myxoid chondrosarcoma: an analysis of 34 cases. Hum Pathol 3:421–435, 1972.
49. Saleh G, Evans HL, Ro JY, Ayala AG. Extraskeletal myxoid chondrosarcoma: a clinicopathologic study of ten patients with long term follow-up. Cancer 70:2827–2830, 1992.
50. Abromovici LC, Steiner GC, Bonar F. Myxoid chondrosarcoma of soft tissue and bone: A retrospective study of 11 cases. Hum Pathol 26:1215–1220, 1995.
51. Jambhekar NA, Baraniya J, Baruah R, Joshi U, Badwar R. Extraskeletal myxoid chondrosarcoma: clinicopathologic, histochemical, and immunohistochemical study of 10 cases. Int J Surg Pathol 5:77–82, 1997.
52. Sciot R, Dal Cin P, Fletcher C, Samson I, Smith M, De Vos R, Van Damme B, Van den Berghe H. t(9;22)(q22-31;q11-12) is a constant marker of extraskeletal myxoid chondrosarcoma: evaluation of three cases. Mod Pathol 8:765–768, 1995.
53. Brody RI, Ueda T, Hamelin A, Jhanwar SC, Bridge JA, Healey JH, Huvos AG, Gerald WL, Ladanyi M. Molecular analysis of fusion of EWS to an orphan nuclear receptor gene in extraskeletal myxoid chondrosarcoma. Am J Pathol 150:1049–1058, 1997.
54. Antonescu CR, Argani P, Erlandson RA, Healey JH, Ladanyi M, Huvos AG. Skeletal and extraskeletal myxoid chondrosarcoma: a comparative clinicopathologic, ultrastructural, and molecular study. Cancer 83:1504–1521, 1998.
55. Ramesh K, Gahukamble L, Sarma NH, Al Fituri OM. Extraskeletal myxoid chondrosarcoma with dedifferentiation. Histopathology 27:381–382, 1995.
56. Kransdorf MJ, Meis JM. Extraskeletal osseous and cartilaginous tumors of the extremities. Radiographics 13:853–884, 1993.
57. Nakashima Y, Unni KK, Shives TC, Swee RG, Dahlin DC. Mesenchymal chondrosarcoma of bone and soft tissue: a review of 111 cases. Cancer 57:2444–2453, 1986.
58. Rushing J, Armonda RA, Ansari Q, Mena H. Mesenchymal chondrosarcoma: a clinicopathologic and flow cytometric study of 13 cases presenting in the central nervous system. Cancer 77:1884–1891, 1996.
59. Bagachi M, Husain N, Goel MM, Agrawal PK, Bhatt S. Extraskeletal mesenchymal chondrosarcoma of orbit. Cancer 72:2224–2226, 1993.
60. Jacobs JL, Merriam JC, Chadburn A, Garvin J, Housepian E, Hilal SK. Mesenchymal chondrosarcoma of the orbit: report of three new cases and review of the literature. Cancer 73:399–405, 1994.
61. Granter SR, Renshaw AA, Fletcher CDM, Bhan AK, Rosenberg AE. CD99 reactivity in mesenchymal chondrosarcoma. Hum Pathol 27:1273–1276, 1996.

62. Rodriguez-Peralto JL, Lopez-Barea F, Sachez-Herrera S, Atienza M. Primary aneur-ysmal cyst of soft tissues (extraosseous aneurysmal cyst). Am J Surg Pathol 18:632–636, 1994.

63. Salm R, Sissons HA. Giant-cell tumours of soft tissues. J Pathol 107:27–39, 1972.

64. Petrik PK, Fidlay JM, Sherlock RA. Aneurysmal cyst, bone type, primary in an artery. Am J Surg Pathol 17:1062–1066, 1993.

65. Lopez-Barea F, Roriguez-Peralto JL, Burgos-Lizaldez E, Alvarez-Linera J, Sanchez-Herrera S. Primary aneurysmal cyst of soft tissue. Report of a case with ultrstructural and MRI studies. Virchows Arch 428:125–129, 1996.

66. Shannon P, Bedard Y, Bell R, Kandel R. Aneurysmal cyst of soft tissue: report of a case with serial magnetic resonance imaging and biopsy. Hum Pathol 28:255–257, 1997.

67. Wehrli BM, Nielsen GP, Rosenberg AE, O'Connell JX. Soft tissue giant cell tumor: a clinicopathologic study of 16 benign and malignant variants. Mod Pathol 12:15a, 1999 (abstract).

68. Oliveira AM, Dei Tos AP, Fletcher CDM, Nascimento AG. Giant cell tumor of soft tissues: a clinicopathologic analysis of 21 cases. Mod Pathol 12:14a, 1999 (abstract).

69. Guccion JG, Enzinger FM. Malignant giant cell tumor of soft parts: an analysis of 32 cases. Cancer 29:1518–1529, 1972.

70. Alguacil-Garcia A, Unni KK, Goellner JR. Malignant giant cell tumor of soft parts: an ultrastructural study of four cases. Cancer 40:244–253, 1977.

71. Angervall L, Hagmar B, Kindblom LG, Merck C. Malignant giant cell tumor of soft tissues: a clinicopathologic, cytologic, ultrastructural, angiographic and microangio-graphic study. Cancer 47:736–747, 1981.

14

Synovial-Related Tumors and Tumors of Uncertain Histogenesis

William B. Laskin
Northwestern University Medical School and
Northwestern Memorial Hospital
Chicago, Illinois

Cyril Fisher
The Royal Marsden NHS Trust
London, England

I. SYNOVIAL-RELATED TUMORS

The synovial membrane lines diarthrodial joints, tendons, and bursae. Its cells synthesize hyaluronic acid, a major component of the synovial fluid, exhibit phagocytic and antigen processing activity, and facilitate transfer of solutes between the synovial fluid and blood (1,2).

By light microscopy, the lining cell of the synovial membrane assumes a flat to columnar shape depending on the local mechanical forces and possesses an oval nucleus and lightly eosinophilic cytoplasm with an indistinct cell border. The cells are arranged in one to three poorly defined layers. They do not reside on a basement membrane but blend into the underlying stroma, which may be composed of fibroconnective tissue, fat, or skeletal muscle (3,4).

Ultrastructural analysis has shown that the more superficially located cells of the synovial membrane (B cells) possess features of fibroblasts and synthesize hyaluronic acid. The underlying layers consist of an admixture of B cells and cells that appear to exhibit phagocytic properties (A cells). The presence of cells with ultrastructural features common to both A and B cells indicate that these cellular elements form a morphologic continuum, modulating back and forth depending on functional demands (4).

A variety of benign and neoplastic processes arise from the stromal elements of the tenosynovium. These include fibroma of tendon sheath, synovial chondromatosis, soft-tissue chondroma, synovial lipoma and hemangioma, and, rarely, synovial chondrosarcoma. However, only the members of the tenosynovial giant cell tumor family most accurately recapitulate the cytomorphology of the synovial lining and will be discussed in this chapter.

The two major forms of the tenosynovial giant cell tumor, the localized or nodular variant (nodular tenosynovitis) and the diffuse variant (intra-articular pigmented villonodular synovitis and the extra-articular diffuse giant cell tumor), demonstrate overlapping cytoarchitectural features yet exhibit different growth characteristics that seem to depend on their site of origin (5,6). The localized or nodular variant initially grows into the tenosynovial channel pursues a direction into the soft tissue and away from the channel that restricts its growth. Here external forces and pressure applied by the enveloping tendon sheath and overlying fascia and skin result in a circumscribed tumor. Localized lesions may also develop within small joint spaces of the hands or feet where tight bony confines similarly restrict growth. Tumors arising in large joints, such as knee or bursa, tend to demonstrate a sheet-like and villonodular growth pattern within open spaces that offer little resistance.

The true etiohistogenesis of the tenosynovial giant cell tumor is still uncertain. Jaffe et al. (5) proposed that all tenosynovial giant cell tumors are reactive, inflammatory processes based primarily on histologic assessment. A history of antecedent trauma can be elicited in some cases. Synovial proliferations resulting from intra-articular deposition of blood or foreign material (including material from orthopedic prostheses) share some histologic features with tenosynovial giant cell tumor but do not completely reproduce the histopathology of the latter (7,8). Conversely, evidence supporting a neoplastic cause includes the paucity of inflammation within the lesions, the capability of diffuse lesions to demonstrate autonomous growth, the potential of the tumor to recur, and rare documentation of cases that have undergone malignant transformation and metastatic spread (see Sec. I.C, "Malignant Tenosynovial Giant Cell Tumor").

Cytogenetic and molecular analyses of tenosynovial giant cell tumors have shed new light on the controversy that surrounds the histogenesis of the tumor. The demonstration of simple karyotypic abnormalities and DNA aneuploidy in a few examples of tenosynovial giant cell tumor tends to favor a true neoplasm (9). However, a recent study showing a polyclonal population of cells from digital and diffuse giant cell tumors by preferential X chromosome inactivation analysis has more convincingly demonstrated that this group of tumors most likely represents a nonneoplastic proliferation of synovial lining cells (10).

A. Localized Tenosynovial Giant Cell Tumor (Nodular Tenosynovial Giant Cell Tumor)

1. Clinical Findings and Outcome

The localized or nodular variant of the tenosynovial giant cell tumor (L-TGCT) is exceedingly more common than the diffuse form and represents, next to the ganglion cyst, the most frequently encountered tumor affecting the hand (11). The lesion has a peak incidence between 30 and 50 years of age. Tumors involving the hand occur more commonly in males, whereas an equal sex distribution has been reported for tumors arising in the toes (12). The tumor less frequently develops in the knee, ankle, wrist, and elbow. Polyarticular involvement by L-TGCT is an exceedingly rare event.

In the digit, L-TGCT usually presents as a slow-growing, painless mass with discomfort or pain reported in only about 20% of tumors (6,11). Tumors arising in the knee are more often associated with tenderness or a locking or snapping sensation with joint movement. On physical examination, the lesion is nonfluctuant and usually not attached to the overlying skin. However, tumors developing in the distal aspect of the finger or toe may become adherent to the skin and ulcerate. Plain radiographs of the lesion show cortical erosion of the underlying bone in 10% (13) to around 50% (14) of cases, especially with tumors involving the toes.

Due to the tumor's limited growth potential, the outcome of L-TGCT is excellent, with only a 10–20% recurrence rate (1). Recurrences more commonly occur with an inadequate primary excision of the tumor that leaves minute "satellite" nodules behind in the adjacent soft tissue. Thus, a complete (local) excision, including a rim of normal tissue, is the preferred surgery (1). Increased mitotic activity and cellularity, features more commonly observed early in the evolution of the process, have been associated with a higher rate of recurrence (15).

2. Gross Findings

At surgery, a lobulated mass with a fibrous pseudocapsule and an attachment to the underlying synovium is the usual finding. Occasionally, the tumor does not have a synovial attachment and presents as a "loose body" floating free within the joint space.

At gross examination, L-TGCT appears as a firm, well-circumscribed, lobulated mass. Tumors of the digits are small and typically measure between 0.5 and 4 cm (1). Lesions arising in the wrist, ankle, and, especially, knee are generally larger and show more variability in shape. The tumor has a firm consistency and the cut surface is gray–white. The presence of yellow foci in the tumor represents aggregates of xanthoma cells, whereas brown pigment indicates hemosiderin deposition.

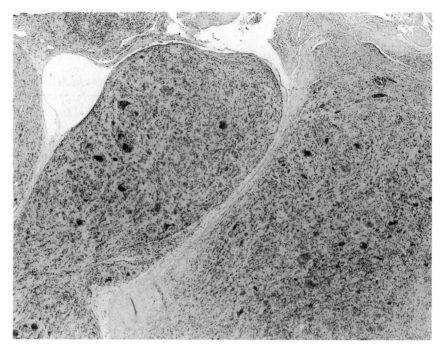

FIG. 1 Localized tenosynovial giant cell tumor. Fibrous synovial-derived tissue surrounds and focally invaginates the substance of the tumor (*upper right*), resulting in a lobulated but well-delineated contour.

3. Microscopic Findings

At low magnification, the L-TGCT is a well-circumscribed, partially encapsulated mass. This fibrous capsule, which is probably derived from native tenosynovium, sends traversing bands into the substance of the tumor, resulting in a lobulated mass (Fig. 1). The L-TGCT consists of an admixture of polygonal and spindled mononuclear cells, xanthoma cells, and multinucleated giant cells set in a collagenous, variably hyalinized stroma that is punctuated by rounded and cleft-like spaces. The overall cellularity and the distribution and relative proportions of these cellular elements characteristically vary throughout a given lesion. The central portion of the tumor tends to be more cellular than the well-marginated periphery of the nodule where the cells become smaller, aggregates of xanthoma cells and hemosiderin-laden cells are usually present in greater abundance, and stroma is more densely collagenized ("peripheral maturation") (Fig. 2).

The chief proliferating element is a mononuclear cell with a polygonal or short spindled shape, a scanty amount of pale to eosinophilic cytoplasm, and a

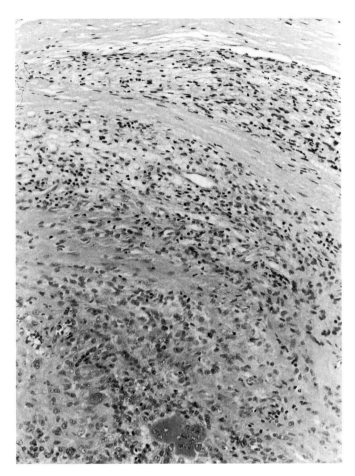

FIG. 2 A histologic feature that is helpful in differentiating tenosynovial giant cell tumor from malignant processes is the presence of "peripheral maturation." At the smoothly contoured periphery of a tumor nodule (*top*), the cells possess smaller nuclei and are predominantly xanthomatous.

centrally-positioned, oval to reniform-shaped nucleus which often possesses a longitudinal groove (Fig. 3). These cells grow in a sheet-like configuration or within tightly aggregated nests invested by collagen. Mitotic activity varies but is typically higher in more cellular tumors. Rao and Vigorita (12) reported 3 or more mitoses per 10 high-power fields in more than 10% of the nodular variants in their study.

Other cellular components include osteoclast-like giant cells that possess several to more than 50 closely aggregated nuclei (Fig. 3). The close morphologic

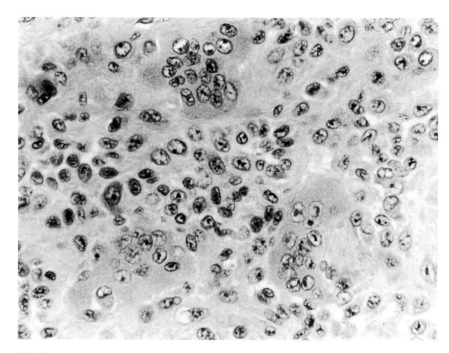

FIG. 3   The principal cell of the tenosynovial giant cell tumor has a polygonal shape, clear to eosinophilic cytoplasm, and a bland-appearing oval to reniform-shaped nucleus. Osteoclast-like giant cells with multiple nuclei are cytologically similar to the nuclei of the accompanying mononuclear cells.

resemblance of the nuclei of the giant cells to the nuclei of the surrounding mononuclear cells suggests that the giant cell forms from fusion of the mononuclear cells. Cells containing lipid (foamy or xanthomatous cells) and hemosiderin deposits are present in the majority of cases. Touton giant cells are occasionally observed.

Cleft-like, "pseudoglandular" spaces are characteristic of tenosynovial giant cell tumor and are more commonly observed in tumors arising in association with larger joints, such as the knee and ankle (6) (Fig. 4). Some of these elongated spaces are partially lined by synovial-like cells and probably represent native synovium engulfed by the advancing tumor. In time, these spaces lose their cellular lining. The spaces may be empty or contain xanthoma cells.

The amount and type of stromal collagen depends partially on the cellularity of the lesion. Tumors studied early in their evolution are generally more cellular and have relatively small quantities of delicate collagen. In older, less cellular lesions, thick bands of dense collagen and extensively hyalinized collagen remi-

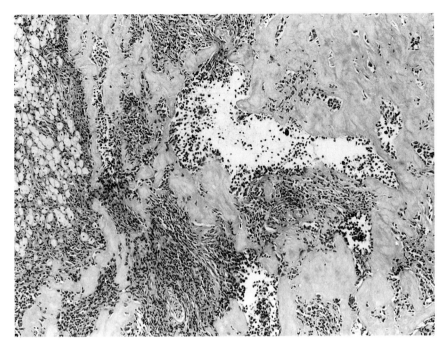

FIG. 4 A cleft-like, "pseudoglandular" space forms in hyalinized collagen of a localized tenosynovial giant cell tumor. Some of these spaces probably originate from invaginations of synovium. Gradually the synovial lining is lost, resulting in a space partially lined by tumor cells.

niscent of osteoid (pseudo-osteoid) prevail (Fig. 4). Unusual histologic findings include cartilaginous or osseous metaplasia (1). Inflammation is sparse, but scattered collections of lymphocytes may be identified. Occasionally, a nodular giant cell tumor may undergo infarct leaving only a peripheral rim of viable tissue.

Immunohistochemically, both reactive synovial lining cells and the cells of the tenosynovial giant cell tumor demonstrate monocytic/histiocytic differentiation. Along with vimentin, the mononuclear cells express macrophage-related antigens CD68 (KP1), HAM-56, and α_1-antichymotrypsin (16,17). Antivimentin, CD68 (KP1), α_1-antichymotrypsin, and leukocyte common antigen (LCA) decorate the multinucleated giant cells (16,17). Both components variably express the dendritic fibroblast marker factor XIIIa (18).

4. Differential Diagnosis

Granulomatous processes by virtue of their nodular architecture and compliment of histiocytes and giant cells can resemble L-TGCT. Para-articular deposits of monosodium urate (tophaceous gout) and calcium pyrophosphate dihydrate (tophaceous pesudogout) (19) may elicit a granulomatous response, in which case the granulomatous inflammation surrounds conspicuous deposits of proteinaceous debris harboring crystalline material. Tendinous xanthoma develops in tendons of patients with hyperlipoproteinemia. The predominance of lipid-laden, foamy histiocytes in the xanthoma and its characteristic location and clinical background allow proper distinction. The two most common necrobiotic processes occurring in this area, rheumatoid nodule formation and the deep form of granuloma annulare, can be differentiated from L-TGCT by the presence of granulomatous inflammation surrounding variably sized deposits of red to pale blue necrobiotic collagen.

The fibroma of tendon sheath shares many clinical, topographic, and macroscopic features with L-TGCT. At low magnification, both lesions are partitioned into lobules by cleft-like spaces, show varying degrees of fibrosis, and usually have an attachment to the tenosynovium. However, in contrast to the heterogeneous population of cells constituting L-TGCT, the cells of the fibroma of tendon sheath have a more uniform spindled and stellate appearance (Fig. 5). The cells of the fibroma of tendon sheath demonstrate more convincing expression of muscle-specific and smooth muscle actin than do cells of the tenosynovial giant cell tumor (16).

B. Diffuse Tenosynovial Giant Cell Tumor (Extra-Articular Pigmented Villonodular Tenosynovitis)

Jaffe et al. (5) first coined the term "pigmented villonodular synovitis" for the family of localized and diffuse tenosynovial and bursal-based giant cell tumors under discussion. In current practice, this appellation is typically reserved for the diffuse intra-articular form of the disease. This process is generally referred to as pigmented villonodular tenosynovitis (PVNS). In most cases of extra-articular diffuse giant cell tumor (D-TGCT), the lesion probably represents an extension of PVNS outside of the joint space. However, the literature contains examples of diffuse giant cell tumor with documented origin within bursae and tendon sheaths and lacking an intra-articular component (1,5).

1. Clinical Findings and Outcome

The clinical features and outcome of D-TGCT more closely parallel those of PVNS than L-TGCT. In comparison with L-TGCT, D-TGCT (and PVNS) occurs in a slightly younger population, with approximately 50% of patients diagnosed before age 40 years (1). The lesion involves females slightly more often than males (1). The para-articular soft tissue and intra-articular surface of the knee are the most common locations for D-TGCT and PVNS, respectively (1). The ankle, foot, and wrist are less commonly involved sites for D-TGCT, according to the records of the Armed Forces Institute of Pathology (AFIP) (1). Tumors have also

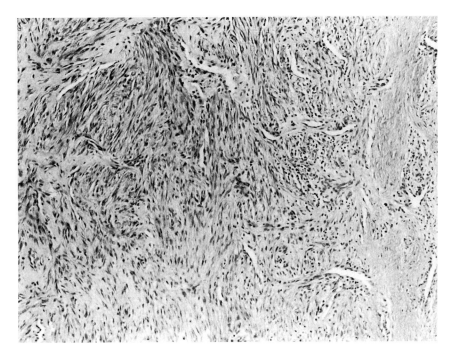

FIG. 5 The fibroma of tendon sheath shares a lobulated configuration and a well-circumscribed margin with the localized tenosynovial giant cell tumor. The fibroma of tendon sheath is characterized by a somewhat uniform population of predominantly spindled cells and an accompanying component of thin-walled, elongated capillary–sized vessels.

been reported in the hip, sacroiliac joint, vertebral column, and digits. Unlike the usual presentation for L-TGCT, D-TGCT (and PVNS) more commonly causes joint pain, functional impairment including limitation of motion of the joint, joint effusion, and hemarthrosis (1,13). The duration of symptoms range from months to decades.

The recurrence rate of D-TGCT is similar to that of PVNS. In the experience of AFIP (1), 40–50% of patients with D-TGCT develop local recurrence. The basic approach to treatment should be an attempt to remove as much of the tumor as possible while trying to maintain the function of the involved extremity (1).

2. Gross Findings

The bulky, sheet-like, and multinodular growth pattern of D-TGCT appreciated by both the surgeon at operation and the pathologist in the laboratory helps to distinguish it from the localized variant. Unfortunately, both tumors may show similar

gross features early in their evolution. D-TGCT has a firm consistency with a variegated tan–yellow to red–brown cut surface. In contrast to L-TGCT, the tumor
lacks a fibrous capsule and has more prominent cleft-like invaginations. The
shaggy, matted, villous projections so characteristic of PVNS are not generally
seen in the D-TGCT.

3. Microscopic Findings

The cellular makeup, character of the fibrous stroma, and formation of cleft-like
and rounded spaces differ little from those described for L-TGCT (see Figs. 2–4).
The tumor grows in an expansile manner and is not surrounded by a fibrous capsule. Capillary-sized vessels and elongated, branching cleft-like spaces are more
abundant, whereas multinucleation and xanthomatous change are less commonly
observed in D-TGCT than in the localized variant.

4. Differential Diagnosis

Reactive synovial hyperplasias associated with hemarthrosis, degenerative and
destructive joint diseases (osteoarthritis and rheumatoid arthritis), and failed orthopedic prosthetics ("detritic" synovitis) are processes that grossly and histologically imitate PVNS (Fig. 6A, B). These lesions exhibit an expansion of the synovium with villous formation. However, unlike PVNS, this synovial proliferation
is principally due to collagen deposition, an increase in the number of reactive vessels, and, in some instances, a more pronounced chronic inflammatory cell infiltrate. Although the number of synovial lining cells may be modestly increased in
these disorders, they do not form a tumoral mass as they do in the tenosynovial
giant cell tumor.

The failure of the pathologist or surgeon to identify a tenosynovial or bursal
origin for D-TGCT coupled with its expansile growth pattern may lead to a consideration of sarcoma. This macroscopic impression is further enhanced by the
monotonous population of somewhat primitive-appearing, mitotically active cells
and the lack of multinucleated giant cells, xanthoma cells, and fibrosis observed
microscopically early in the evolution of D-TGCT (1). Subtle histologic clues,
such as absence of cellular pleomorphism and atypical mitotic figures, presence of
cleft-like spaces, presence of an occasional multinucleated cell or cells containing
fat or hemosiderin, and presence of "peripheral maturation" (see above) at the periphery of the tumor, will help the pathologist arrive at the correct diagnosis.

C. Malignant Tenosynovial Giant Cell Tumor

The existence of a malignant form of tenosynovial giant cell tumor (M-TGCT)
has been the subject of controversy for a number of reasons. First, the nature of

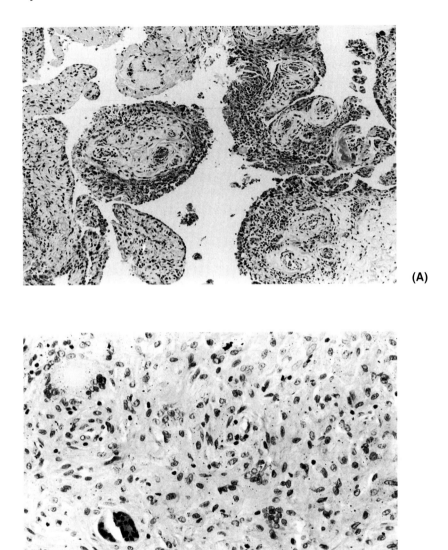

FIG. 6 Reactive intra-articular lesions that mimic the diffuse tenosynovial giant cell tumor (pigmented villonodular synovitis). (A) Hemarthrosis results in the formation of bulbous villi. However, these villi are composed primarily of collagen with only a thin layer of hemosiderin-laden mononuclear cells covering the surface. (B) "Detritic" synovitis due to a failed orthopedic prosthesis. The cellular element is composed chiefly of mononuclear cells and foreign-body giant cells containing intracellular deposits of finely granular foreign material.

the tenosynovial giant cell tumor is still a conundrum with some investigators favoring a reactive etiologic process. Second, early studies of tumors categorized as M-TGCT included unrelated neoplasms, such as giant cell malignant fibrous histiocytoma, clear cell sarcoma, and epithelioid sarcoma. Finally, histologic features of the TGCT do not always predict the pathobiological course of the lesion.

For the diagnosis of M-TGCT, Enzinger and Weiss from the AFIP (1) require that the malignant lesion either coexist with or present as a possible recurrence of a documented, conventional TGCT. Bertoni and associates (20) accepted the second criterion set forth by Enzinger and Weiss for their definition but broadened the definition to include any synovial-based sarcoma with overlapping histopathologic features of a conventional PVNS. Both of these investigative groups found that the true incidence of M-TGCT is exceedingly low.

1. Clinical Findings and Outcome

The location, age range, and clinical signs and symptoms of M-TGCT closely parallel those of D-TGCT. Females are affected more often than males (20). The mean age at the time of clinical recognition is about one or two decades later (sixth to seventh decade) than for D-TGCT. The majority of tumors occur in the knee, followed by ankle and foot (20). Commonly reported complaints include joint swelling, pain, and effusion.

The reported data on the behavior of these lesions is sparse but indicates that M-TGCT is a locally aggressive neoplasm with the potential for metastatic spread. Bertoni and associates (20) reported that 5 of 8 patients experienced at least one recurrence and 56% of patients developed metastatic disease. The lung was the most common metastatic site, and all patients with pulmonary metastasis died. Prompt wide (local) excision or amputation appears to be the therapy of choice.

2. Gross and Microscopic Findings

On gross examination, the neoplasm has a bulky, multinodular appearance. The tumors reported in the series by Bertoni and associates (20) had an intra-articular component, and all but one extended beyond the joint space into the surrounding skeletal muscle and fat.

According to Bertoni et al. (20), the cells of M-TGCT grow in infiltrating nodules and sheets and are accompanied by a sparse amount of stroma (Fig. 7). Necrosis is a conspicuous feature, and focal hemorrhage may also be present. In contrast to D-TGCT, M-TGCT has a more monotonous cytologic appearance as xanthoma cells and hemosiderin-laden cells are virtually absent. Osteoclast-like giant cells may be scattered about the tumor but typically are not as numerous as in D-TGCT. Instead, the principal neoplastic element is a round to oval cell possessing an enlarged, hyperchromatic nucleus with a prominent nucleolus and ex-

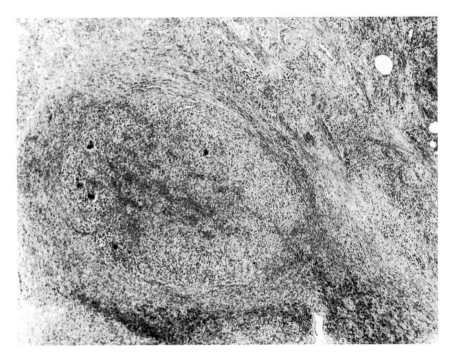

FIG. 7 Malignant tenosynovial giant cell tumor. At scanning magnification, the vaguely nodular growth pattern and presence of rare osteoclast-like giant cells are reminiscent of the benign tenosynovial giant cell tumor. However, the tumor is much more cellular and has a sparse stromal component. (Courtesy of Julie C. Fanburg-Smith, M.D., Armed Forces Institute of Pathology.)

hibiting a high nuclear/cytoplasmic ratio (Fig. 8). Mitotic activity is variable, but atypical mitotic figures can be observed. "Peripheral maturation" is absent in malignant lesions, and the cleft-like and rounded spaces are also markedly diminished in size and number.

3. Differential Diagnosis

Malignant fibrous histiocytoma (MFH), like M-TGCT, tends to arise in deep soft tissue, may have a nodular configuration, and microscopically may possess a component of osteoclast-like giant cells (giant cell variant of malignant fibrous histiocytoma) (Fig. 9). In contrast to M-TGCT, MFH rarely involves intra-articular surfaces. Furthermore, the cells of MFH are typically spindled, show a greater degree of pleomorphism, and are arranged in a storiform pattern or in short fascicular arrays.

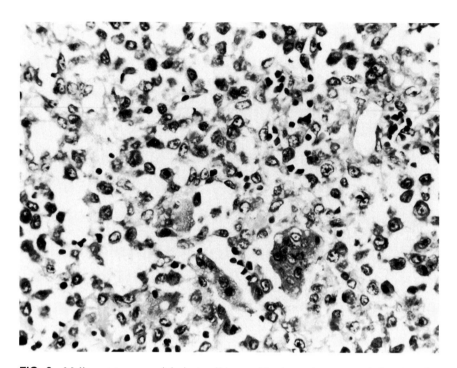

FIG. 8 Malignant tenosynovial giant cell tumor. The tumor is composed almost exclusively of round to oval cells with pleomorphic nuclei. The nuclear:cytoplasmic ratio of these cells is greater than that of the cells of conventional tenosynovial giant cell tumor. Note the virtual absence of stroma. (Courtesy of Julie C. Fanburg-Smith, M.D., Armed Forces Institute of Pathology.)

Epithelioid sarcoma tends to exhibit a nodular growth pattern within deep soft tissue as does the M-TGCT. Unlike the cells of M-TGCT, the spindled and epithelioid cells of the epithelioid sarcoma are closely associated with bundles of dense, eosinophilic collagen. The coexpression of cytokeratin and vimentin further distinguishes epithelioid sarcoma from M-TGCT.

The location close to bone and focal presence of hyalinized collagen reminiscent of osteoid in M-TGCT may elicit a diagnosis of osteosarcoma. The latter neoplasm exhibits clear-cut production of osteoid by malignant osteoblasts and often demonstrates areas of cartilagenous differentiation.

D. Inflammatory Myofibroblastic Tumor

Although sometimes interchanged with "inflammatory pseudotumor," the appellation "inflammatory myofibroblastic tumor" (IMT) is the currently favored term applied to a group of clinically diverse, histologically distinct, tumoral processes composed chiefly of myofibroblasts and fibroblasts (21). The prototype of IMT, "plasma cell granuloma" of the lung, was first described by Bahadori and Liebow (22) as a reactive proliferation of spindled fibroblasts and macrophages admixed with a rich plasma cell infiltrate in a predominantly sclerotic stroma. Since this initial series, tumors with histologic overlap with plasma cell granuloma but exhibiting a wider range of histomorphology have been reported in virtually every body site.

The true nature and, more importantly, the pathobiological potential of IMT is still uncertain and has generated intense debate. Although the majority of tumors seem to arise spontaneously, putative examples of IMT and reactive processes resembling IMT have been reported in association with prior trauma (23), resolving pneumonitis (24) or infection by bacterial (25), mycobacterial (26,27), and viral (28,29) organisms.

Studies have provided evidence that some examples of IMT may represent true neoplasms. Spencer first raised this possibility when he reported two cases of

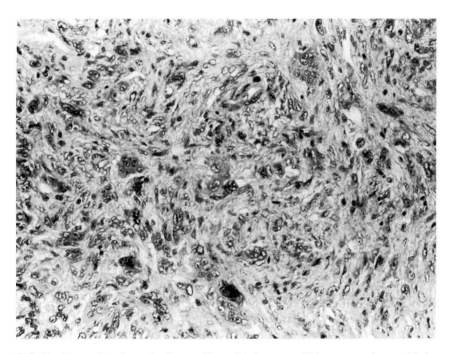

FIG. 9   Giant cell variant of malignant fibrous histiocytoma. This sarcoma shares with the malignant tenosynovial giant cell tumor a deep location and an osteoclast-like giant cell component. However, the former entity also possesses pleomorphic spindle and multinucleated cells that typically grow in a storiform pattern.

inflammatory pseudotumor of the lung ("plasma cell granuloma") with histologic features overlapping with malignant fibrous histiocytoma (30). In 1991, Meis and Enzinger (31) from the AFIP evaluated the clinicopathologic features of 38 tumors previously categorized as inflammatory pseudotumor. The majority arose as single or multiple masses within the mesentery and retroperitoneum of children and young adults. Ten patients experienced at least one recurrence (37%), three developed histologically confirmed metastatic disease (11%), and five died of their tumor (19%). Meis and Enzinger proposed that this subset of intra-abdominal tumors represented a low-grade sarcoma and introduced the term "inflammatory fibrosarcoma." In addition, reports of "metastasizing" IMTs without overt malignant features (32–36) and extrapulmonary IMTs that underwent sarcomatous histologic transformation on recurrence with (37) and without (38) documented metastatic spread have appeared in the literature. Cytogenetic studies demonstrating clonal cytogenetic abnormalities (39) and a flow cytometric study of pediatric IMTs showing aneuploidy (hyperdiploidy) (36) lend further support to the notion that some IMTs are neoplastic.

Other studies have offered an alternative view concerning the nature and pathobiological potential of these tumors. Coffin and colleagues (38) studying 84 patients with IMT noted, as did the AFIP, a young patient population, a predominance of intra-abdominal tumors, occasional multifocal presentation, and a significant recurrence rate. However, no tumor metastasized and four tumors regressed spontaneously. These investigators surmised that the increased morbidity and mortality exhibited by some of these lesions is due primarily to location of the tumor near vital structures and its potential for multifocality—features that make complete excision difficult.

Whether all of the tumoral processes designated under the rubric of IMT are truly etiologically related is doubtful as the clinical spectrum of IMT ranges from lesions acting like reactive processes to tumors exhibiting characteristics of true neoplasms. Current evidence supports the existence of a small subset of primarily intra-abdominal myofibroblastic tumors that demonstrate histologic features compatible with a sarcoma and have the potential to act aggressively.

1.   Clinical Findings and Outcome

The majority of IMTs arise in the lung. The remaining examples of IMT are found in a multitude of extrapulmonary sites, including head and neck (including oral cavity, upper respiratory tract, and thyroid); small and large bowel mesentery, omentum, and virtually all intra-abdominal viscera; mediastinum and heart; retroperitoneum; genitourinary tract (male genital tract, uterus, vagina, kidney, and urinary bladder); spleen and lymph nodes; breast; central and peripheral nervous system; skin, somatic soft tissue and bone (25,40,41). The tumors afflict patients over a wide age range, with the vast majority presenting in children and young adults. Overall, pulmonary tumors affect an older population than do extrapulmonary IMTs.

Incidental detection of an asymptomatic mass is the most common presenting manifestation of IMT. However, in approximately 15–30% of cases, the patient seeks medical attention because of constitutional symptoms, such as fever, night sweats, or unexplained weight loss (40). These symptoms are often accompanied by abnormal laboratory values, including a hypochromic microcytic iron deficiency anemia, elevated sedimentation rate, hypergammaglobulinemia, and thrombocytosis (40). In young children, parents may consult a physician because of persistent fever or impaired growth caused by an occult tumor.

The demographics and clinical symptomatology of IMT vary with its location. In general, extrapulmonary IMTs more frequently present with constitutional or site-specific complaints. The pulmonary IMT has a peak incidence in the third decade of life and is usually detected as an incidental chest x-ray finding. A prior respiratory infection is documented in between 5% (22) and 37% (30) of patients in large series. IMT of the bladder is more common in females and occurs over a wide age range, with most patients presenting in the third through fifth decades of life (42,43). IMT of the urinary bladder presents with hematuria and, occasionally, symptoms of acute cystitis (42,44). A recent history of a surgical procedure or trauma, although a characteristic clinical feature of the so-called postoperative spindle cell nodule of the urogenital tract, is not generally elicited with conventional forms of IMT (42,44). Intra-abdominal and retroperitoneal tumors have a peak incidence in the first two decades of life (31,38). Females are more commonly affected than males (31,38). The mesentery and omentum are the most common sites of origin reported in two large studies (31,38). Intra-abdominal tumors are associated with an increase in abdominal girth; vomiting, diarrhea, or ileus; jaundice and ascites; gastrointestinal obstruction or intussusception. Often the systemic manifestations of IMT vanish once the tumor is removed and reappear with recurrent disease (21,45).

On balance, the majority of IMTs, especially those arising in the lung, lower urogenital tract, and somatic soft tissue, are cured with complete excision. Approximately 25% of patients with extrapulmonary and less than 5% of patients with pulmonary IMTs experience local recurrence (38). Higher rates are reported for multinodular tumors and tumors located in close proximity to vital structures such as those involving the abdomen, retroperitoneum, mesentery, and upper airway (38). From a therapeutic standpoint, complete excision (without radical surgery, chemotherapy, or radiation), including all identifiable nodules, and close clinical follow-up is the recommended therapy for IMT (40).

2. Gross Findings

IMTs vary in size, texture, shape, and color. Extrapulmonary tumors, especially intra-abdominal, retroperitoneal, and mesenteric tumors, tend to be larger, are less well circumscribed, and are more often multinodular and/or multifocal than IMTs of the lung (38).

Intraparenchymal IMTs of the lung are typically round and well circumscribed, whereas endobronchial tumors tend to have a polypoid configuration. The tumors are mostly firm with a variegated cut surface. Fibrotic lesions have a white cut surface. The presence of xanthoma cells results in a yellow color, whereas red or brown foci represent hemorrhage. Abundant chronic inflammation imparts a tan lymphoid appearance. Calcification can be identified in 10–25% of cases (21).

IMT of the bladder presents as a nodular intramural mass that can protrude into the lumen in a polypoid fashion. The tumor may extend into the muscularis propria or even into the perivesicular connective tissue, raising concerns about a true sarcoma (46). Tumors with a fibrous composition have a firm consistency with a white cut surface, but most tumors have a more gelatinous or myxoid appearance.

IMTs of the mesentery, retroperitoneum, and mediastinum are mostly well-circumscribed, unencapsulated masses. Tumors composed of two or more separate or contiguous nodules are often encountered in abdominal and pelvic sites. Tumors arising in the mesentery can be attached to the wall of the large or small bowel. The cut surface of the IMT is firm, with a variably white fibrous and tan myxoid appearance. Occasionally, the cut surface reveals a central scar. Hemorrhage, microcyst formation, necrosis, and calcification are infrequently encountered.

3. Microscopic Findings

In their clinicopathologic study of IMT, Coffin and associates described three main histoarchitectural patterns of growth (38). No one pattern typically prevails in any given case but, more commonly, two or more patterns blend into one another, creating a multipatterned architecture.

The first pattern described resembles that of nodular fasciitis or granulation tissue with haphazardly dispersed spindle cells, strands of fine collagen, and numerous, capillary-sized vessels suspended in a variably inflamed, myxedematous stromal matrix. The main cellular element is spindle-shaped, possesses abundant pale eosinophilic cytoplasm, and has an oval or tapered nucleus with finely dispersed chromatin and a conspicuous nucleolus (Fig. 10). Some of these cells have abundant, fibrillar eosinophilic cytoplasm that may falsely suggest skeletal muscle differentiation. Histiocyte-like cells with rounded nuclei and foamy to granular eosinophilic cytoplasm represent another cellular element commonly identified. Cells with enlarged nuclei and prominent basophilic nucleoli, akin to the "ganglion-like" cells of proliferative fasciitis, can be found. The polymorphous

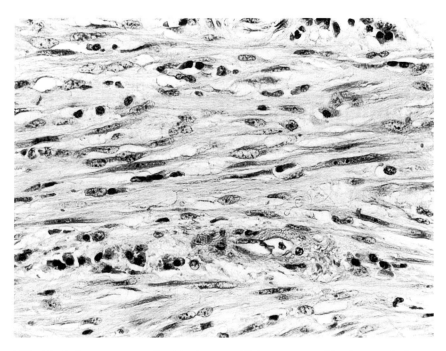

FIG. 10 Inflammatory myofibroblastic tumor. High-power magnification reveals the cytologic characteristics of myofibroblasts, which include a spindle shape, relatively abundant lightly eosinophilic cytoplasm, and a tapered nucleus. Note the interspersed plasma cells and lymphocytes.

inflammatory component consists of lymphocytes, plasma cells, neutrophils, and eosinophils.

A cellular myofibroblastic proliferation constitutes the second histologic pattern described in IMT. The proliferating, spindled myofibroblasts are arranged in a short interwoven fascicular or storiform pattern (Fig. 11). Broad, sweeping fascicles of cells are noted in a minority of cases. Even in the more cellular foci, the mitotic rate is low and abnormal figures are not identified. The stroma is variably collagenous. Lymphocytes, plasma cells, and lymphoid follicles are sprinkled throughout the process.

The third histomorphologic pattern has a scar-like quality and features thick bands of hypocellular, eosinophilic collagen (Fig. 12). Open, nonbranching capillaries and a paucicellular lymphoplasmacytic inflammatory component complete the histology. Dystrophic calcification and, less commonly, bone formation can be observed. These paucicellular, collagenous areas commonly alternate with the more cellular zones described above.

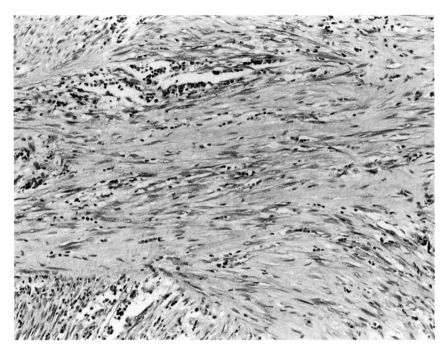

FIG. 11 Inflammatory myofibroblastic tumor. The tumor features a loosely organized fascicular growth pattern of spindle cells embedded in a collagenous stroma peppered with chronic inflammatory cells.

Several investigators have suggested that certain histomorphologic features should at least raise concern about the possibility of malignancy in IMT (31,47,48). Some authors further contend that only tumors harboring these histologic characteristics should be classified as examples of "inflammatory fibrosarcoma" (47,48). These features include cytologic atypia, manifested by a markedly enlarged nucleus exhibiting abnormally distributed chromatin and a prominent nucleolus, and the presence of hypercellular foci in which the cells adopt an elongated, fascicular growth pattern.

The immunohistochemical profile of IMT supports the basic myofibroblastic and fibroblastic nature of the process as the spindle cells convincingly express vimentin, muscle-specific and α-smooth muscle actin, and variably express desmin (40). Focal cytokeratin expression has been identified within spindle cells (31,38,42,44,49) and rarely in the large ganglion-like cells (31). The macrophage/histiocyte-related immunomarker, CD68 (KP1), highlights histiocytes within the lesions, but also variably stains spindle cells (31,38) and, occasionally, ganglion-

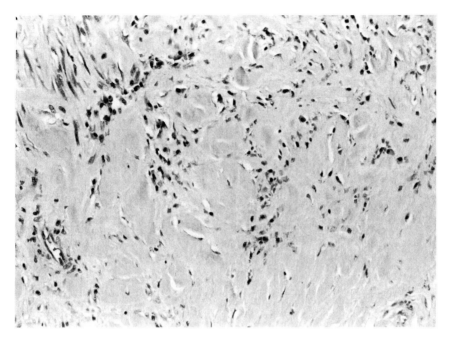

FIG. 12 Inflammatory myofibroblastic tumor. In this field, spindle cells (*upper left*) merge with a mildly inflamed, paucicellular, highly collagenous zone that is reminiscent of scar tissue.

like tumor cells (31). Focal CD30 (Ki-1) immunoreactivity within spindle tumor cells has been reported in IMT (38).

4. Differential Diagnosis

The differential diagnosis of IMT arising within the abdominal cavity, retroperitoneum, mediastinum, and pelvis includes benign processes, such as idiopathic inflammatory fibrosclerosing lesions and fibromatosis; sarcomas including MFH, leiomyosarcoma, rhabdomyosarcoma; and hematopoietic tumors such as follicular dendritic cell (FDC) tumor and lymphoma.

The family of primary idiopathic inflammatory fibrosclerosing lesions (idiopathic retroperitoneal fibrosis, idiopathic forms of sclerosing mediastinitis, and orbital pseudotumor) typically afflicts older individuals. As opposed to the circumscription of the IMT, these processes diffusely infiltrate adjacent soft tissues. Idiopathic retroperitoneal fibrosis takes the form of a sheet-like fibroplasia that centers around the distal aorta and characteristically results in ureteral obstruction, whereas sclerosing mediastinitis infiltrates around major mediastinal

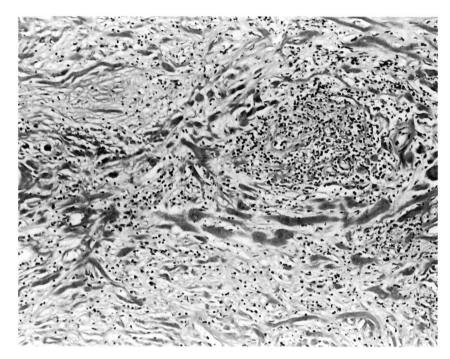

FIG. 13 Idiopathic inflammatory fibrosclerosing lesion. In contrast to the inflammatory myofibroblastic tumor, this process exhibits a more uniform histology characterized by densely sclerotic collagen and a conspicuous lymphoplasmacytic infiltrate with perivascular cuffing by lymphocytes (*upper right*).

vessels and bronchi (50). These lesions differ histologically from IMT by their overall lower cellularity and more uniform cytoarchitecture, greater degree of sclerosis, and frequent presence of a lymphocytic perivascular infiltrate (Fig. 13). Similar to IMT, retractile (sclerosing) mesenteritis generally presents as a well-circumscribed mass or as multiple nodules in the mesentery of the small and, less often, large bowel (51). The histomorphology of the lesion somewhat resembles that of idiopathic retroperitoneal fibrosis and sclerosing mediastinitis, but the process centers on lobules of degenerating mesenteric fat.

Intra-abdominal fibromatosis, like IMT, is often multifocal and grossly appears circumscribed (52). A subset of intra-abdominal fibromatoses arise in the setting of familial polyposis coli (Gardner's syndrome). On the microscopic level, intra-abdominal fibromatosis often demonstrates myxoid or keloidal-like foci that can mimic IMT, especially with small biopsies. However, in more typical areas, the bland spindle cell component of fibromatosis adopts an elongated fascicular growth pattern and characteristically infiltrates surrounding native soft tissue.

At variance with IMT, true sarcomas typically demonstrate obvious cellular pleomorphism, high mitotic activity, including the presence of atypical mitotic figures, and focal necrosis. However, some sarcomas have overlapping features with IMT. Inflammatory MFH can present with systemic symptoms, including fever and leukocytosis (53). Histologically, this MFH variant bears features of a reactive process, including the presence of an acute and chronic inflammatory infiltrate and a variable number of banal-appearing xanthoma cells. However, careful scrutiny will detect markedly atypical tumor cells scattered throughout the process and, on occasion, areas of more conventional MFH. Leiomyosarcoma can infrequently have a striking inflammatory component that masks the true nature of the neoplasm (54). Leiomyosarcoma is composed of intersecting fascicles of spindle cells with intensely eosinophilic, fibrillar cytoplasm, distinct cell borders, and a centrally located nucleus with blunt ends. The large, voluminous spindle cells occasionally identified in IMT could be misinterpreted as rhabdomyoblasts. Unlike the cells in IMT, rhabdomyoblasts typically exhibit more intense cytoplasmic eosinophilia and possess cross-striations. Moreover, rhabdomyoblasts strongly express desmin and MyoD1 (55).

FDC tumor is an indolent, low-grade neoplasm composed chiefly of follicular dendritic cells and is found primarily in lymph nodes (56) and, less often, in extranodal sites (57–60). FDC tumors occurring primarily in the liver and spleen have been reported to exhibit significant histologic overlap with IMT (28,29), including the presence of spindle cells admixed with a lymphoplasmacytic infiltrate. FDC tumor differs histologically from conventional IMT by exhibiting, at least focally, a syncytial growth pattern and greater degree of cytologic atypia (59). The inflammatory component of FDC tumor (excluding the "inflammatory" FDC tumors of the liver and spleen) consists of lymphocytes uniformly sprinkled throughout the process and typically lacks the intense plasmacytic infiltrate common to conventional IMT. The cells of FDC tumor variable express FDC markers, CD21 (IF8), and CD35 (Ber-Mac-DRC) (59). About 12% of reported FDC tumors are associated with Ebstein–Barr virus (59).

Non-Hodgkin's lymphoma and some forms of Hodgkin's lymphoma of the retroperitoneum and mediastinum can masquerade as a fibroinflammatory process due to the presence of a markedly fibrous stroma. Unlike the polymorphous inflammatory element of IMT, the neoplastic component of sclerosing non-Hodgkin's lymphomas is monotonous and cytologically malignant. Traversing bands of dense collagen are characteristic of nodular sclerosing Hodgkin's disease but are not observed in IMT. The large, atypical virocyte-like cells observed in some cases of IMT may resemble Reed–Sternberg cells of classical Hodgkin's disease, but the latter cells are immunoreactive for CD30 (Ki-1) in about 90% of cases and for CD15 (Leu-M1) in more than 80% of cases (61).

Lesions of the extra-abdominal soft tissues not already covered in the differential diagnosis of IMT include nodular and proliferative fasciitis, infectious processes, Rosai-Dorfman disease, and sarcomatoid carcinoma. One characteristic histologic pattern described in IMT overlaps with the histology of nodular and proliferative fasciitis. These latter lesions, in contrast to IMT, are usually small and reach their maximum size within months without causing systemic symptoms. Microscopically, the other characteristic patterns observed in IMT are at best minor components of nodular fasciitis.

A variety of infectious agents can elicit a histiocytic and spindle cell proliferation resulting in a tumefaction imitating IMT. This is particularly true with *Mycobacterium avium-intracellulare* infection in AIDS patients (27,62). Histochemical stains for mycobacterial organisms, especially Fite stain, or electron microscopic examination of tissue will expose the organisms. Pronounced tissue neutrophilia and/or the identification of more than an occasional microabscess should also suggest an infectious etiology.

Rosai-Dorfman disease of soft tissue (63) may histologically resemble IMT. The spindle cells composing the process differ from those of IMT by virtue of their more granular cytoplasm and, more importantly, by their ability to exhibit some degree of emperipolesis of inflammatory cells. Unlike IMT, the proliferating spindle and polygonal histiocytes comprising the lesion strongly express S-100 protein (63).

Spindle cell carcinoma (sarcomatoid carcinoma) arising from mucosal surfaces can prove difficult to distinguish from IMT, particularly if the spindle cell element is hypocellular, lacks significant pleomorphism and mitotic activity, and the epithelial component is not represented. Features that favor carcinoma are adjacent mucosal dysplasia and the finding of destructive invasion by a cellular infiltrate exhibiting cytologic atypia and atypical mitotic figures (64). Myogenic markers and cytokeratin can be expressed by spindle cells in both lesions, but diffuse cytokeratin immunoreactivity supports the diagnosis of spindle cell carcinoma.

E. Myxoid Lesions of Soft Tissue

Stromal deposition of mucin can be a focal or diffuse finding in any soft-tissue tumor. As the amount of stromal mucin increases, the lesional cells become splayed apart and the tumor tends to lose its characteristic architectural pattern of growth. Also, the vascular component becomes more easily visualized. The terms "myxoid" or "myxoid change" are used to reflect this alteration, but the tumor is still named according to its perceived histogenesis. True "myxomas," on the other hand, are benign tumors with copious amounts of stromal mucin that histologically resemble undifferentiated, embryonic connective tissue such as that composing the umbilical cord. By definition, its cells should not show evidence of a specific line of mesenchymal differentiation (65).

The lesional cells of the myxoma are small and mostly spindled in appearance. Some of the cells have a stellate or star-like morphology. Stout in his seminal paper on myxomas (65) stated that the stellate-shaped cell is the principal cell in myxoma and that the spindled element results from "pressure molding" of cells by densely concentrated collagen in areas containing less mucosubstance. Electron microscopic studies of soft-tissue myxomas have demonstrated a mixed population of cells, including fibroblast-like cells with well-developed, dilated, branching runs of rough endoplasmic reticulin; cells differentiating toward myofibroblasts; undifferentiated mesenchymal cells; and histiocytes (66,67).

The mucosubstance present in myxomas is predominantly the acidic nonsulfated mucopolysaccharide hyaluronic acid (68). This mucosubstance has a faint, pale blue appearance with standard hematoxylin and eosin stain. It is faintly periodic acid–Schiff (PAS)–positive, but stains intensely blue with Alcian blue at pH 2.5 and colloidal iron stain, and metachromatically with toluidine blue at pH 4.0. Pretreatment of the tissue with hyaluronidase abolishes the Alcian blue and colloidal iron stain by destroying hyaluronic acid. It has been shown experimentally that the hyaluronic acid inhibits the proper polymerization of precollagen fibers in the extracellular compartment (69).

In this chapter, only myxomas arising in the somatic soft tissue will be discussed. The most common of these lesions, the ganglion cyst, is encountered routinely in everyday practice. The characteristic location and gross and microscopic appearance of the ganglion and the digital mucous cyst, a closely related entity, allow for their immediate recognition. The prototype of soft-tissue myxomas, the intramuscular myxoma, is a rare tumor with a negligible recurrence rate that, by virtue of its deep location and sometimes large size, may be confused with other benign or malignant tumors with myxoid features. Unlike the intramuscular myxoma, which is surrounded by skeletal muscle and easily removed surgically, the "aggressive" angiomyxoma, superficial angiomyxoma (cutaneous angiomyxoma), and juxta-articular myxoma arise in more penetrable connective tissue, are less well circumscribed, and show higher rates of recurrence.

F. Ganglion Cysts and Digital Mucous Cysts

Ganglions are cystic lesions containing viscous, mucinous material that are found primarily in the hand and wrist in close proximity to joints and tenosynovial tissue. Ganglions have also been described in peripheral nerve (70) and in bone (69). Digital mucous cysts (DMCs) are located exclusively in the dermis of the distal finger or, less often, the distal toe.

The etiology of ganglion formation is still uncertain. A convincing relationship between trauma or repetitive joint motion and the development of the lesion has not been established. Theories advanced include herniation of synovium, formation of a tract from the joint space to the surrounding soft tissue, extravasation of synovial fluid from the joint space into the surrounding tissue, and excess production of synovial fluid by fibroblasts or metaplastic synovial cells (71).

1. Clinical Findings and Outcome

Ganglion cyst formation is a disease of young adults and affects females more commonly than males. The dorsal aspect of wrist represents the most common site for ganglion formation (70). Lesions also occur on the volar aspect of the wrist, hand, and fingers, dorsum of the foot and toes, and ankle (70). The ganglion usually presents as a nodule or swelling that seldom obtains a maximum single dimension greater than 3 cm and may even decrease in size with rest. Pain or minor discomfort is elicited in about 50% of patients (70). Carpal tunnel syndrome and nerve palsies have been associated with volar wrist ganglions (72).

DMC presents mainly in patients between 40 and 70 years of age and shows a female predominance (73). The dorsal aspect of the distal middle and index finger are the two most common locations for the lesion, followed by the distal aspect of the toes (73). The tumor presents as an asymptomatic, small nodule usually less than 2 cm in greatest dimension. Longitudinal grooving of the overlying nail and osteoarthritic changes of the distal interphalangeal joint are associated findings (73). The ability to transilluminate the lesion helps to differentiate the ganglion from a solid mass (73).

Approximately 50% of dorsal wrist ganglion disappear without treatment on long-term follow-up (72). DMC has also been reported to regress spontaneously. After surgical management, the recurrence rate for dorsal wrist ganglion and DMC ranges from 13% to 40% and 25% to 40%, respectively (72).

2. Gross and Microscopic Findings

Although the ganglion is frequently attached to the joint capsule or tendon sheath, most of the lesion is grossly identified within surrounding connective tissue. It appears as a rounded, cystic nodule lined by a fibrous wall of variable thickness. The lesion may be multiloculated. The surrounding connective tissue can have gelatinous foci suggestive of incipient ganglion formation.

Microscopically, the ganglion consists of an irregularly shaped cystic structure or cleft-like space devoid of a true cellular lining, but bordered by a dense collagenous wall (Fig. 14). The cavity contains a variable amount of mucin, histiocytes, or an occasional spindled or stellate-shaped fibroblast. Rarely, a modest proliferation of bland spindle cells without architectural complexity or increased vascularity is present. The surrounding connective tissue commonly exhibits focal myxoid change (Fig. 15).

DMC is histomorphologically similar to ganglion but arises directly under the skin of the distal digit. It appears first as a localized accumulation of hyaluronic acid–rich mucosubstance containing interspersed spindle and stellate-shaped cells and a scant number of delicate collagen fibers (Fig. 16). A cystic cavity or cleft-like space that is filled with mucosubstance and often lined by condensed dermal collagen eventually forms.

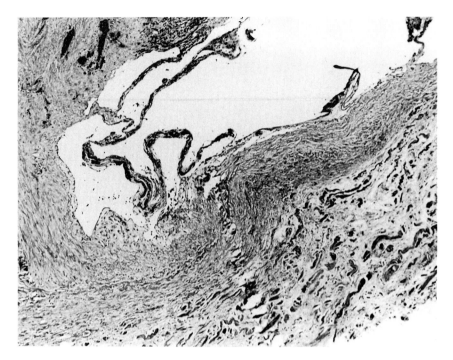

FIG. 14 Ganglion cyst. The lesion consists of an irregularly shaped cystic space with a dense collagenous wall but having no true cellular lining.

G. Intramuscular Myxoma

1. Clinical Findings and Outcome

The intramuscular myxoma (IM) affects individuals over an age range of 20–84 years but has a peak incidence in middle-aged adults (71). The majority of patients are female (71). The tumor develops in association with deep skeletal muscle. The thigh and pelvic girdle, shoulder, and upper arm represent the common sites of origin in decreasing order of frequency (75). The lesion usually presents as a slow-growing, painless mass, with fewer than 25% of tumors associated with discomfort or pain (75). The mass is movable when the affected muscle relaxes but becomes fixed when the muscle contracts (76). The duration of signs and symptoms prior to presentation varies from months to years.

The presence of multiple lesions is a rare phenomenon and is usually associated with a coexistent fibrous dysplasia of bone (77–79). In such cases, the manifestations of fibrous dysplasia typically appear first. In most cases reported in the literature, the fibrous dysplasia involves more than one bone (polyostotic) (78,79)

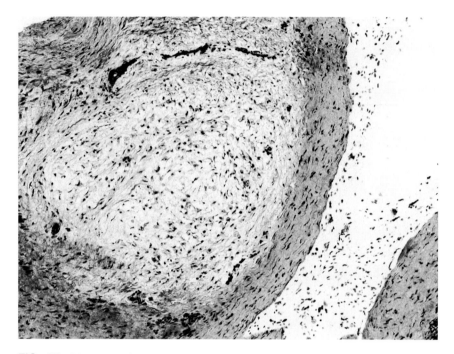

FIG. 15 The connective tissue adjacent to the ganglion cyst has undergone myxoid change.

and in some instances can be associated with Albright's syndrome (polyostotic fibrous dysplasia, café-au-lait spots on the skin, and endocrine abnormalities) (69,78). The IM typically arises in the same general vicinity as the bone(s) involved by fibrous dysplasia. The cause of this curious association is unknown, but Wirth (78) speculated that an inborn error of mesenchymal metabolism may be the etiologic factor.

IM is a wholly benign tumor that rarely recurs and is best managed with complete (local) excision.

2. Gross and Microscopic Findings

The tumors are located in skeletal muscle or attached to the muscular fascia. Most tumors range in size between 5 and 10 cm in greatest dimension (69). On gross inspection, the tumor has an oval or lobular shape and appears well circumscribed. The cut surface has a soft, mucoid consistency and a gray–white color. Thin, traversing fibrous trabeculae and small mucin-filled cysts are additional features identified on cut section. On close inspection, the process can be observed infiltrating into surrounding edematous skeletal muscle.

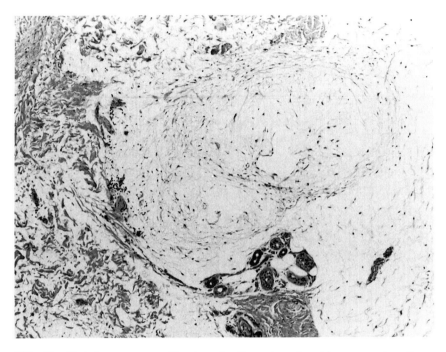

FIG. 16 Digital mucous cyst. The dermal collagen is replaced by myxomatous tissue with interspersed spindle cells. Cystification is observed near the center of the lesion.

On microscopic examination, IM is characterized by the presence of scattered, bland, spindled and stellate-shaped cells; a sparse number of small vessels; and numerous thin collagen fibers suspended in a richly myxoid stromal matrix (Fig. 17). The spindled and stellate-shaped cells have a small nucleus and a meager amount of pale, occasionally vacuolated, eosinophilic cytoplasm. The ill-defined cytoplasmic processes of the lesional cells are often continuous with delicate strands of collagen that run haphazardly throughout the tumor. The mitotic activity is virtually nonexistent. The hyaluronic acid–rich, mucinous stroma often contains small cystic spaces. Occasionally, residual atrophic skeletal muscle fibers, foamy histiocytes, and, rarely, mast cells are identified in the myxoid matrix. Simple, nonarborizing, capillary-sized vessels are scattered throughout the process. At the periphery of the lesion, skeletal muscle fibers adjacent to the tumor are atrophic and separated by edema fluid or infiltrating tumor. Fat cells are commonly interspersed in the skeletal muscle. Focally, collagen fibers condense to form an incomplete thin fibrous lining (Fig. 18).

Rarely, IM may have areas exhibiting increased cellularity, more abundant collagen, and an increase in the number of vessels, including vessels with thick walls. These "hypercellular and hypervascular myxomas" lack the mitotic activ-

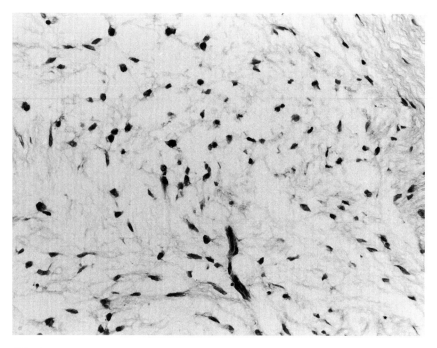

FIG. 17 Intramuscular myxoma. The tumor is composed of scattered spindle and stellate-shaped cells and nonbranched, capillary-sized vessels suspended in a richly myxomatous matrix containing wispy strands of collagen.

ity, cytologic atypia, branching vascular network, and necrosis characteristic of a sarcoma (80).

The immunohistochemical profile of lesional cells of IM includes strong expression of vimentin and weak, focal expression of actin, desmin, and CD34 (QBEND-10) (81).

H.   Juxta-Articular Myxoma

The juxta-articular myxoma (JAM) is a myxomatous process that arises in association with large joints. JAM and its variants have been reported in the literature under a variety of names, including juxta-articular or periarticular myxoma (82), parameniscal cyst (83), and cystic myxomatous tumors of the knee (84). As this tumor may exhibit large size, poor circumscription, and focal hypercellularity, recognition of JAM as a distinct benign entity is important with respect to proper treatment.

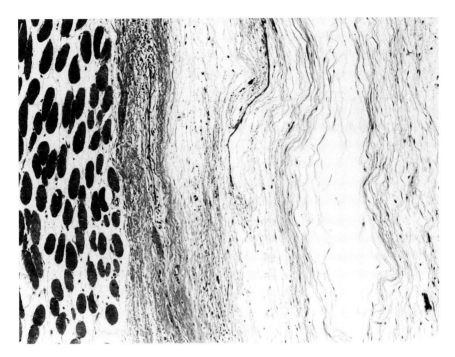

FIG. 18 At the periphery of the intramuscular myxoma, condensed collagen forms an incomplete wall around the tumor. The surrounding skeletal muscle is edematous.

1. Clinical Findings and Outcome

Although JAM affects patients over a wide age range (16–83 years), almost three-fourths of cases occur in men in the third to fifth decades of life (82). The vast majority of lesions develop around the lateral or medial aspect of the knee (82). Less commonly involved sites include shoulder, elbow, hip, and ankle (82).

JAM usually presents as a swelling or mass, with more than 50% of patients eliciting a history of pain or tenderness (82,84). Rarely, the patient complains of a "locking" or "snapping" sensation with mobilizing of the joint. A history of prior trauma is often elicited in these patients. Some patients exhibit radiographic manifestations of osteoarthritis. On rare occasion, the lesion is discovered incidentally during arthroplastic surgery for osteoarthritis (69,82).

Although JAM is a benign tumor with no potential for metastatic spread, it has a recurrence rate of 34%, with one half of these patients experiencing more than one recurrence (82). Complete conservative excision of the tumor accompanied by meniscectomy (if involved) with close clinical follow-up is considered the treatment of choice (82).

2. Gross and Microscopic Findings

JAM is centered primarily in the subcutaneous tissue but can extend to the over-lying dermis or the deep fibrous structures of the joint (82). JAM has been ob-served to abut the synovium or invade skeletal muscle (70,82). When the process involves the knee, the main tumor mass is not infrequently associated with smaller, ganglion-like structures within the lateral or medial semilunar cartilage (82–84).

The tumors range in size from lesions approximating the dimensions of a ganglion to masses over 10 cm in greatest dimension. The lesion appears as a lob-ulated, unilocular or multilocular cyst lined by a thin fibrous membrane. The tu-mor has a soft, jelly-like consistency. The cut surface is myxoid, gelatinous, or slimy in appearance and white to tan–yellow in color.

JAM is chiefly composed of bland-appearing, oval, spindle and stellate-shaped cells embedded in a relatively hypovascular, hyaluronic acid–rich mu-cinous stroma through which run numerous strands of delicate collagen (see Fig. 17). Cystic spaces of varying size and shape are identified in the vast major-ity of cases. JAM is often seen infiltrating and entrapping subcutaneous fat.

Focal increased cellularity or fibrosis, especially in recurrent lesions, is a feature peculiar to this myxoma variant. In the cellular foci, the spindle cells main-tain their benign cytologic appearance but proliferate in loosely organized fas-cicles or vaguely storiform arrays unaccompanied by increased mitotic activity. An increased number of capillary-sized vessels can also be identified within JAM, but an intricate, branching pattern of proliferating vessels, as seen in some sarco-mas, is not appreciated.

3. Differential Diagnosis

The ganglion cyst, IM, and JAM share histomorphologic features yet can be dis-tinguished from one another. Both ganglion and JAM exhibit cystic change and rarely a ganglion may show a modest cellular proliferation. However, the former entity occurs more commonly in females, is a smaller lesion, and arises chiefly in the joint capsule or tendinous tissue of the wrist. The ganglion cyst also contains lesser amounts of mucin than does IM or JAM.

IM differs from JAM by virtue of its deep location and association with the large muscle groups of the thigh, pelvic girdle, or shoulder. Microscopically, IM is better circumscribed than JAM and does not undergo as much cystification. Foci of increased cellularity or vascularity also occur less commonly in IM than in JAM.

A variety of myxoid-appearing, spindle cell lesions enter into the differen-tial diagnosis of IM and JAM. Nodular fasciitis arises primarily in the subcu-taneous tissue and rarely occurs in skeletal muscle. In contrast to IM and JAM, nodular fasciitis generally affects a younger population and achieves its maximum size in a few months. Although areas of nodular fasciitis with a loosely organized, granulation tissue-like appearance may suggest a myxoma, most examples of nodular fasciitis have more cellular areas composed of large, reactive-appearing spindle cells arranged in gently whorled fascicles and accompanied by elongated, thin-walled, nonarborizing vessels.

The solitary (localized) neurofibroma may be relatively hypocellular and exhibit marked myxoid change. Unlike the smoothly contoured nucleus of the fibroblast in the myxoma, the nucleus of the lesional cell in solitary neurofibroma exhibits greater contour irregularities. Another distinguishing feature when present is the close association of the cells of the neurofibroma with thick bundles of collagen. Small cells with an oval or fusiform morphology and a pattern of infiltrative growth into superficial soft tissue are two features shared by JAM and the diffuse form of neurofibroma. The cells of the latter entity adopt a more organized growth pattern with the occasional formation of neural palisades or Wagner-Meissner–like bodies. Immunohistochemical expression of S-100 protein and CD57 (Leu7) further serves to differentiate these entities from myxoma.

Deep forms of fibromatosis occasionally exhibit myxoid change with an associated loss of the characteristic fascicular growth pattern. In comparison with myxoma, deep fibromatosis is a more cellular process and its cells assume a more organized growth pattern. Infiltration of surrounding skeletal muscle is more pronounced in deep fibromatosis. Generally, a microscopic search will identify conventional areas of fibromatosis.

Some myxoid sarcomas, in particular low-grade myxoid malignant fibrous histiocytoma (myxofibrosarcoma), myxoid variant of dermatofibrosarcoma protuberans, and myxoid liposarcoma, may not exhibit overt pleomorphism. Careful scrutiny of the neoplasm will demonstrate, at least focally, requisite criteria for establishing a malignant diagnosis, including the presence of cytologic atypia (nuclear enlargement, hyperchromatism, and an abnormal chromatin distribution) and/or an occasional abnormal mitotic figure. Myxoid liposarcoma, like IM myxoma, is a large, deeply located, primarily myxoid neoplasm. The presence of lipoblasts and an arborizing, plexiform capillary network are the key histologic features of myxoid liposarcoma. Low-grade myxoid malignant fibrous histiocytoma (myxofibrosarcoma, grade 1) is distinguished from myxoma by the presence of cytologic atypia, multinucleated giant cells, and numerous branching capillaries and thicker walled, curvilinear vessels (Fig. 19A). The low-grade fibromyxoid sarcoma, as described by Evans (85,86), shares with IM myxoma a deep location, typically involving the musculature of the thigh and buttock; large size; and the presence of relatively hypocellular, myxoid foci. The overall cellularity, cytologic atypia, and vascularity of this sarcoma is greater than that of the myxoma (Fig. 19B).

I. Deep Angiomyxoma (Aggressive Angiomyxoma)

The aggressive angiomyxoma (AAM) is a well-vascularized, myxedematous spindle cell tumor that presents in the deep soft tissues of the pelvic and perineal

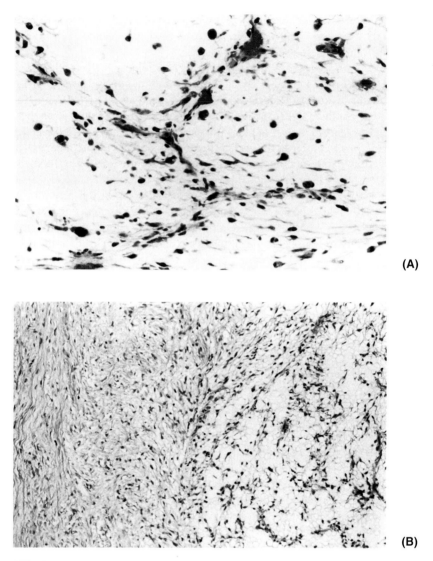

(A)

(B)

FIG. 19 Sarcomas that resemble benign soft-tissue myxomas. (A) Low-grade myxoid malignant fibrous histiocytoma (myxofibrosarcoma) possesses a more elaborate vascular network than benign myxoma, including branched and thick-walled, arcuate-shaped vessels. Note highly atypical cells scattered in the stroma. (B) Low-grade fibromyxoid sarcoma typically has contrasting myxoid and collagenous areas. Overall, the higher cellularity, more complex vascular growth pattern, and scattered atypical spindle cells distinguish this lesion from benign myxoma.

regions and has locally recurrent potential. This somewhat distinctive, site-specific tumor was first delineated by Steeper and Rosai in 1983 (87). Subsequent three largest studies of AAM (88–90) have reported nearly identical histologic findings and have confirmed the tumor's proclivity for local recurrence in both female and male patients.

In contradistinction to the controversy that surrounds the pathogenetic nature of some myxomatous lesions, most investigators agree that AAM is a true neoplasm composed of fibroblasts and cells showing variable smooth muscle differentiation. Minor cytogenetic aberrations involving the 12q14-15 region bolster support for the neoplastic nature of this tumor (91).

1. Clinical Findings and Outcome

AAM shows a striking female predominance, with a female-to-male ratio of about 6:1 (90). The age of patients at presentation ranges from the teens to 70 years, with a peak incidence in the fourth decade of life. In females, the vast majority of tumors present in the deep soft tissues of the vulvovaginal and pelvioperineal regions (87–90). Less common sites include the buttock, retroperitoneum, and inguinal region (87,90). The scrotum and spermatic cord, inguinal area (including presentation within hernia sacs), perianal area, and pelvioperineal region are primary sites for AAM in men (88,92,93).

The most common presenting signs and symptoms are pain or pressure in the vulvovaginal or pelvioperineal areas, dyspareunia, and increased frequency of urination. In males, AAM presents in a similar fashion to a hernia. The duration of clinical features before presentation varies from months to as long as 17 years (90).

AAM is benign but may locally infiltrate adjacent soft tissue, including fascia and muscle. Rare examples of AAM invading the gastrointestinal tract, bladder, and pubic bone have been detailed in the literature (94). The reported recurrence rate of AAM ranges from 36% to 72% (90). Late and multiple recurrences are not uncommon. The high recurrence rate experienced with AAM is thought to reflect inadequate initial resection of the tumor because it blends imperceptibly into surrounding tissue, making the interface between tumor and native tissue difficult to identify during surgery (95). The ability of CT, ultrasonography, and MRI to better access invasion of AAM into adjacent organs and soft tissue makes these radiologic techniques important in the planning of a surgical approach (94). The recommended treatment of AAM is to surgically excise as much of the tumor as technically possible.

2. Gross and Microscopic Findings

AAMs range in size from 3 cm to 60 cm, with the majority of lesions measuring at least 5 cm in greatest dimension (87,88,90). On gross examination, AAM is a large, lobulated mass that generally appears deceptively well circumscribed. The tumor is soft to rubbery in consistency. The cut surface has a glistening, gelatinous appearance and a gray–white to pink–tan color. Small cystic areas and foci of hemorrhage are occasionally observed.

Microscopically, AAM exhibits low to moderate cellularity and is composed of haphazardly arranged, short spindle and stellate-shaped cells set a myxoid-appearing, edematous stroma containing fine strands of collagen and a prominent component of variably sized vessels (Fig. 20). Multinucleated cells are infrequently observed. An increase in the cellularity is occasionally observed around vessels or at the periphery of the lesion where microscopic evidence of infiltration into surrounding tissue with entrapment of native fat, peripheral nerve, or muscle is common (Fig. 21). Mitotic activity is negligible.

The vascular element varies with respect to density and size of the vessels. Medium-sized to large vessels with a thickened wall composed of either condensed collagen fibers or smooth muscle are a consistent finding. Capillary-sized vessels with thin walls are found as scattered units or organized into tight congeries. Extravasation of red blood cells is commonly noted around these fragile capillary structures.

The stroma consists of a loose meshwork of delicate, wavy collagen fibers set in a myxedematous stromal matrix. Thin bundles or fascicles of mature smooth muscle can be identified in the stroma, generally running parallel to vessels or nerves (89,90,96). Microcysts occasionally form in the stroma. Histochemical stains demonstrate that the noncollagenous stroma consists of a small quantity of acidic mucopolysaccharide chiefly in the form of hyaluronic acid (90).

The immunohistochemical profile of the neoplastic cells indicates fibroblastic and variable smooth muscle differentiation. The cells strongly express vimentin and variably express muscle-specific and α-smooth muscle actin. Variable desmin immunoreactivity has been reported in the neoplastic cells (90,93,96). In one series, weak CD34 (QBEND-10) immunoreactivity was demonstrable in half of cases (90). The nuclei show strong expression of estrogen and progesterone receptor proteins (90).

3. Differential Diagnosis

The principal entities in the differential of AAM are angiomyofibroblastoma (AMF), superficial angiomyxoma (see below), myxoid smooth muscle tumor, lipomatous tumor with myxoid stroma, diffuse neurofibroma, and pelvic fibromatosis.

AMF is a neoplasm that arises principally in the vulvar region (97) and has a peak incidence in the fifth decade of life. In contrast to AAM, AMF is typically small, well circumscribed, and subcutaneous in location. Microscopically, the cells composing AMF differ from the short spindle and stellate-shaped cells of

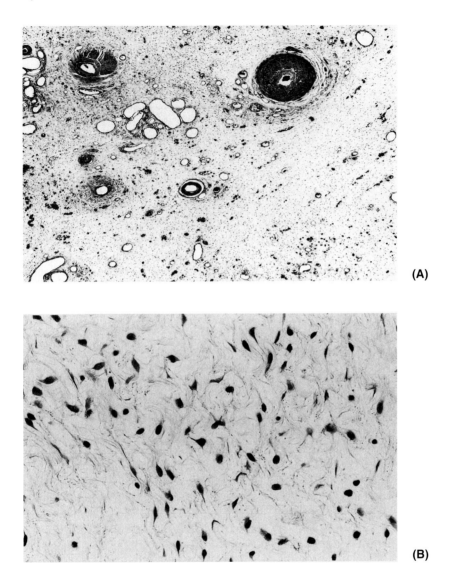

FIG. 20 Aggressive angiomyxoma. (A) Scanning magnification shows haphazardly arranged spindle cells within a loosely texture stroma containing both thick-walled and capillary-sized vessels. (B) The chief mesenchymal element is a cytologically bland cell with a spindle or stellate shape set in a myxedematous stromal matrix containing fine strands of collagen. (Courtesy of John F. Fetsch, M.D., Armed Forces Institute of Pathology.)

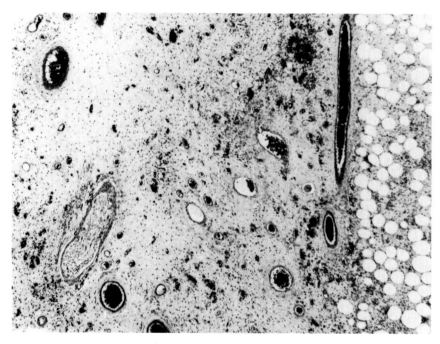

FIG. 21   At the periphery of the lesion, tumor is observed infiltrating around a peripheral nerve twig and invading surrounding native fat. (Courtesy of John F. Fetsch, M.D., Armed Forces Institute of Pathology.)

AAM by their plump, epithelioid appearance and their proclivity to concentrate around lesional vessels in a nested and cord-like arrangement (Fig. 22). The vessels of AMF are in greater number and more evenly distributed throughout the process than the vessels of AAM. Vessels with muscular walls and entrapped nerves are commonly identified in AAM but typically absent in AMF. As both neoplasms may express smooth muscle actin and desmin, immunohistochemistry is not particularly helpful in the differential diagnosis (90). AMF-like tumors have been described in the inguinoscrotal region of men (98). These tumors share some histomorphologic features with the female type of AMF. However, the cells of the AMF-like tumor do not concentrate around vessels as they do in the female AMF. A lesion nearly identical to some examples of the AMF-like tumor in males has been described in the vulvar region of females and designated "cellular angiofibroma" (99).

Smooth muscle tumors tend to lose their characteristic fascicular growth pattern when the stroma becomes edematous or myxoid, and thus may resemble

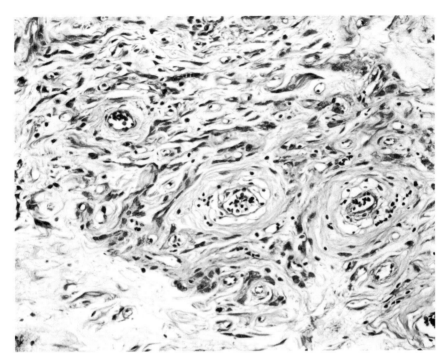

FIG. 22 Angiomyofibroblastoma. Unlike the cytologic features and growth pattern of the cells of aggressive angiomyoma, the angiomyofibroblastoma consists of epithelioid-appearing cells and spindle cells that grow in nested and cord-like arrangements around capillary-sized vessels. (From Laskin WB, Fetsch JF, Tavassoli FA. Hum Pathol 28:1046– 1055, 1997.)

AAM. The cells of a smooth muscle tumor are generally larger and possess more abundant eosinophilic cytoplasm than the cells of AAM (Fig. 23). Blunt-ended, centrally positioned nuclei and juxtanuclear vacuoles further characterize smooth muscle cells. The cells of the smooth muscle tumor typically retain, at least focally, a packeted or fascicular growth pattern.

Lipomatous lesions with myxoid stroma, especially on small biopsies, can imitate AAM. Myxolipomas do not possess the variety of vessels seen in AAM. Moreover, myxolipomas typically have areas of more conventional lipoma that will assist in its correct diagnosis. Myxoid variant of liposarcoma is composed of atypical short spindle and stellate-shaped cells along with immature lipoblasts set in an acidic mucopolysaccharide-rich stroma containing a well-developed plexiform capillary vascular network.

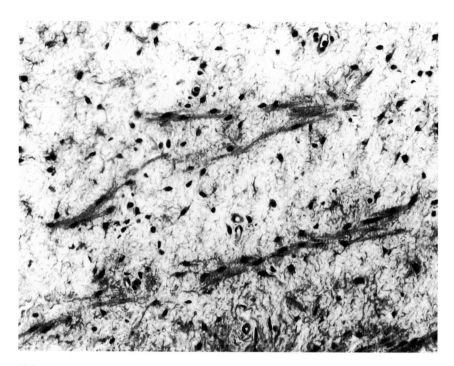

FIG. 23 Myxoid or edematous smooth muscle tumors. Although many of the cells have a short, spindled morphology similar to that of aggressive angiomyxoma, some cells possess more abundant cytoplasm and a more centrally placed nucleus. These larger cells are attempting to form loosely organized fascicles. (Courtesy of Armed Forces Institute of Pathology.)

The diffuse form of neurofibroma can be mistaken for AAM by virtue of its composition of oval and short spindle cells embedded in a loosely textured stroma. Neurofibroma is typically less vascular than AAM, and its cells exhibit a greater degree of alignment than those of AAM. Wagner-Meissner–like structures or neural palisades can be identified within neurofibroma. The immunoprofile of the lesional cells of neurofibroma include variable reactivity with neural markers S-100 protein and CD57 (Leu7).

Pelvic fibromatosis involves the iliac fossa and lower pelvic areas and may have myxoid-appearing areas. The cells in myxoid areas of fibromatosis display a greater degree of alignment than those of AAM. Compared to AAM, the fibromatosis is a less vascularized process. Generally, the myxoid foci of fibromatosis alternate with more characteristic areas of the tumor featuring cells arranged in long, infiltrating fascicles.

J. Superficial Angiomyxoma (Cutaneous Angiomyxoma)

Myxomas of the dermis and subcutaneous tissue are less well characterized than the more frequently encountered deep intramuscular myxomas and myxomas arising in the jaw bones and heart. In 1985, Carney et al. (100) described a complex of maladies (Carney's complex) in which myxomas, including cutaneous myxomas, were an integral part. In 1988, Allen et al. (101) delineated the clinicopathologic features of histologically similar-appearing myxoid lesions of the dermis and subcutaneous tissue that did not have an association with Carney's complex. After a critical review of the literature pertaining to the subject, Allen et al. (101) surmised that the lesions he described, many of the previously reported and variously named myxoid lesions of the dermis and subcutis, as well as the "cutaneous myxomas" of Carney's complex, were all closely related. He proposed the term "superficial angiomyxoma" (SAM) for both the syndromal and sporadic superficial myxomas. This term codifies these tumors under a simple descriptive heading and highlights two important distinguishing features of this variant of myxoma; its superficial location and salient histologic features.

1. Clinical Findings and Outcome

Allen et al. (101) described three clinical presentations of SAM. The most common presentation is that of a solitary lesion without stigmata of Carney's complex, followed by multiple lesions without features of Carney's complex; and lastly, lesions associated with the fully expressed Carney's complex.

SAM, not associated with Carney's complex, mostly presents as a painless, slow-growing, solitary skin nodule. In the series by Allen et al. (101), the incidence in males is slightly higher than that in females. The lesions are located primarily on the trunk and lower extremity, followed by the head and neck region and arm. SAMs have also been reported in the female and male genital regions (102).

Carney's complex (100,103,104) is a constellation of maladies, including pigmented skin lesions (lentigines and giant cell blue nevi), endocrine disorders (primary pigmented nodular adrenocortical disease, a variety of stromal tumors of the testis, and the growth hormone–producing pituitary adenoma), psammomatous melanocytic schwannoma, and myxomatous tumors (cardiac myxoma, myxoid fibroadenoma of the breast, myxoma of the external ear canal, and cutaneous myxoma). The disorder is familial and transmitted as an autosomal dominant trait. Females are affected slightly more often than males, and the initial lesions manifest at an early age (mean age of 18 years). The majority of afflicted patients do not manifest all of the lesions. However, as the cardiac myxoma and the psammomatous melanocytic schwannoma are the main causes of morbidity and mortality in this disorder (100,103), it is important to identify patients at risk for Carney's complex so that proper evaluation for these potentially lethal tumors can be performed.

SAMs associated with the Carney's complex are usually multiple and vary from small sessile papules to large pedunculated lesions. The eyelid represents the most common site at which lesions occur, but other sites, including head and neck, nipples of the breast, axilla, trunk, limbs, and perineum, may also be involved (100).

SAM is a totally benign lesion with no malignant potential. Local recurrence is not uncommon, however, and recurrence rates of 33% (102) and 38% (101) have been documented. Allen et al. (101) found a higher recurrence rate with SAMs containing epithelial components. Recurrences are generally single, and late recurrences have been reported on rare occasion (101,102).

2. Gross and Microscopic Findings

On gross examination, the lesion consists of soft, lobulated nodules. The tumor often elevates the overlying skin, imparting a polypoid or pedunculated configuration to the process. The tumors range in size from 0.5 to 9 cm, with the majority of lesions measuring between 1 and 5 cm (101). The cut surface is glistening, mucoid, or gelatinous in appearance and has a gray to white color. Incomplete collagenous bands traverse the cut surface, resulting in a nodular configuration.

Microscopically, the process typically involves both dermis and subcutaneous fat, but occasionally only one location is affected. The tumor consists of multiple, variably demarcated angiomyxoid nodules (Fig. 24A). The nodules are composed of a hypocellular to moderately cellular population of bland-appearing, short-spindled, stellate-shaped, and, occasionally, multinucleated cells scattered haphazardly throughout a highly myxoid stroma. Mitotic activity is negligible.

The stroma contains an overabundance of hyaluronic acid–rich mucosubstance that forms microcysts within the nodules and cleft-like spaces at the interface of the nodule with the surrounding native tissue (Fig. 24B). Thin, wavy collagen fibers course through the stroma. The vascular element consists of small to medium-sized, thin-walled, nonarborizing vessels. The vascular density of the nodules varies. Other features observed in SAM include some perivascular hyalinization, a "mixed" inflammatory infiltrate (including mast cells), fibrin and hemosiderin deposition, and interstitial hemorrhage.

Epithelial structures in the tumor nodules, including epidermal cysts with keratinous debris and linear strands of squamous cells emanating from the epidermal surface or from a cyst wall, have been identified in almost 30% of cases (101) and undoubtedly have contributed to the plethora of names assigned to SAM in the past.

In a large study of genital tract SAMs (102), the immunoprofile of the tumor was rather broad, with immunoreactivity reported for vimentin, CD34

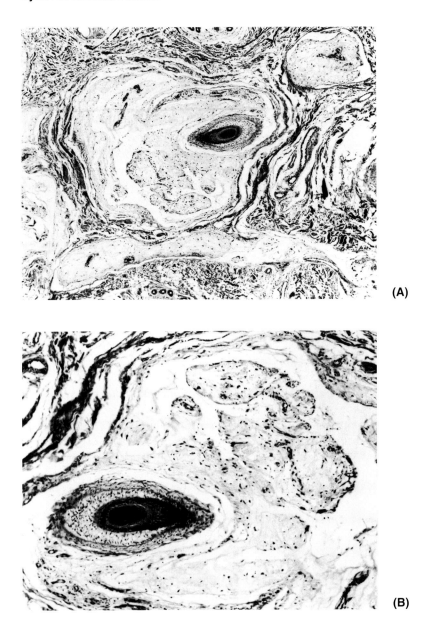

FIG. 24 (A) Superficial angiomyxoma (cutaneous myxoma). The lesion consists of multiple paucicellular, highly myxomatous nodules scattered throughout the dermis. (B) A myxomatous nodule of superficial angiomyxoma is composed of scattered bland-appearing mesenchymal cells and small to medium-sized vessels. Note characteristic cleft-like space separating the tumor nodule from the native dermal tissue (*upper right*).

(QBEND-10), muscle-specific and α-smooth muscle actins, and, to a lesser extent, factor XIIIa and S-100 protein.

3. Differential Diagnosis

Superficially located, myxoid mesenchymal processes enter into the differential of SAM and include cutaneous focal mucinosis and digital mucous cyst, neurothekeoma (nerve sheath myxoma), solitary (localized) and plexiform variants of neurofibroma, lipoma with myxoid stroma, myxoid variant of dermatofibrosarcoma protuberans (DFSP) and low-grade myxoid malignant fibrous histiocytoma (myxofibrosarcoma) and, in the lower genital tract, the vulvovaginal fibroepithelial (mesodermal stromal) polyp (FEP), aggressive angiomyxoma (AAM), and angiomyofibroblastoma (AMF).

Cutaneous focal mucinosis and digital mucous cyst are small, solitary lesions. The latter entity predilects to the dermis of the distal phalanx (see Fig. 16). Both lesions lack the prominent vasculature and cellularity of SAM.

The conventional form of neurothekeoma (nerve sheath myxoma) shares with SAM a superficial location, multinodularity, and an acidic mucopolysaccharide-rich stroma. In contrast to the random arrangement of cells in SAM, the lesional cells of neurothekeoma assume an "onion skin" or lamellar growth pattern in the nodule (Fig. 25). The nodules are often partially invested by dense collagen layer that may harbor EMA-immunoreactive perineurial-like cells. Its cells display a greater degree of S-100 protein expression than the cells of SAM.

Solitary (localized) and plexiform variants of neurofibroma share with SAM tumor nodules composed of spindle cells immersed in an acidic mucopolysaccharide-rich stromal matrix. The plexiform variant is typically a deep-seated lesion and is closely associated with neurofibromatosis type 1. In contrast to the cells of SAM, the cells composing the aforementioned neurofibroma variants have elongated serpentine nuclei and are often apposed to thick strands of collagen. The cells generally demonstrate a stronger expression of S-100 protein than the cells of SAM and can show CD57 (Leu-7) immunoreactivity.

FEP arises mainly in the vulvovaginal region. Similar to SAM, it is a superficial process composed of spindle, stellate-shaped, and multinucleated cells set in a myxedematous stroma. In contrast to SAM, the FEP presents chiefly in middle-aged women and during the reproductive age. At variance with the multinodular growth pattern of SAM, FEP is generally a solitary lesion. Some examples of FEP feature a significant component of bizarre-appearing, multinucleated giant cells and brisk mitotic activity. AAM is a deeply seated tumor composed of short spindle and stellate-shaped cells suspended in an edematous, myxoid-appearing stroma. In comparison with SAM, AAM is a much larger lesion, possesses less acidic mucopolysaccharide, and shows a wider morphologic array of vessels. AMF, although superficial, is better delineated than SAM and is composed of

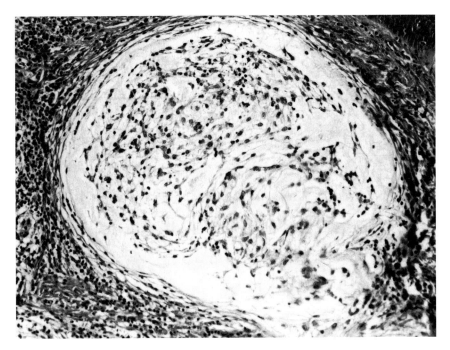

FIG. 25 Nerve sheath myxoma (neurothekeoma). In contrast to the haphazard arrangement of cells in the superficial angiomyxoma, the cells composing the nerve sheath myxoma are better oriented, frequently interconnect, and tend to grow in a lamellar or "onion skin" pattern.

spindle and epithelioid cells that condense around vessels in nested and cord-like arrangements. The tumor cells strongly express desmin in contrast to the cells of SAM.

Myxoid variant of DFSP forms large expansile nodules within the dermis and infiltrates the subcutaneous fat in a pericellular, honeycomb fashion. Its cells exhibit mild nuclear atypia and are better oriented than the cells of SAM. The sarcoma also features an arborizing, thin-walled vascular network. The cells of DFSP exhibit a greater degree of CD34 (QBEND-10) expression than the cells of SAM. Superficial, low-grade variant of myxoid malignant fibrous histiocytoma (myxofibrosarcoma) centers in the subcutaneous tissue and is rarely confined to the dermis. Although it may grow in a multinodular fashion, the myxoid malignant fibrous histiocytoma is more cellular than SAM and its cells exhibit at least focal cytologic atypia. An intricate vascular network of thick-walled, curvilinear vessels and branching, capillary-sized vessels is characteristic of this sarcoma (see Fig. 19A).

II. TUMORS OF UNCERTAIN HISTOGENESIS

Soft-tissue tumors are classified according to their presumed histogenesis, i.e., they are named for the normal adult soft tissue to which they have the most resemblance. This determination is accomplished primarily through critical histologic examination, with added support from immunohistochemical and electron microscopic studies. More recently, cytogenetics has found a useful niche in the classification of some soft-tissue lesions.

Although the majority of soft-tissue tumors can be codified in this way, there is a heterogeneous group of soft-tissue lesions that defy current attempts to establish a histogenesis. Tumors in this broad category that share clinical features, follow a similar pathobiological course, exhibit reproducible cytomorphologic features, and have a similar immunohistochemical profile seem to represent definable clinicopathologic entities. This chapter focuses on this interesting group of soft-tissue neoplasms.

A. Synovial Sarcoma

The synovial sarcoma is a well-recognized clinicopathologic entity and is the most commonly encountered tumor among the neoplasms of uncertain histogenesis. Over a 10-year period at AFIP, this neoplasm was the fourth most common sarcoma studied (105).

Morphologically, this sarcoma is composed of a spindle and an epithelial cell element. The best recognized variant consists of varying proportions of both components (biphasic synovial sarcoma). Tumors composed exclusively of spindle cells (monophasic fibrous type) are more commonly reported than the biphasic variant (106). The monophasic fibrous variant generally requires demonstration of cytokeratin or EMA expression for confirmation. The variant exhibiting only epithelial structures (monophasic epithelial type) is very uncommon and usually cannot be differentiated from carcinoma unless a spindle cell component is present.

The tumor originally derived its name from its rather close histomorphologic resemblance to normal and hyperplastic synovium. Yet several points seriously challenge a kinship between mature synovial tissue and the synovial sarcoma. First, synovial sarcoma only rarely arises from the intra-articular surface of joints and, in fact, can originate in tissue devoid of synovium. Second, normal and hyperplastic synovial tissue does not express cytokeratin or EMA, despite the characteristic expression of both proteins in the cells of synovial sarcoma. Third, the epithelial cells of synovial sarcoma ultrastructurally possess uniform microvilli and tight junctions, which are features not found in normal synovial cells (4). Lastly, while components of basal lamina are seen separating individual and groups of epithelioid cells from the spindle cells in synovial sarcoma by electron microscopic (107,108) and immunohistochemical (109) evaluation, synoviocytes lack basal lamina (3).

Currently, most investigators favor that both components of the synovial sarcoma are derived from a primitive mesenchymal cell that has the capacity to undergo epithelial differentiation. Demonstration of a conversion of cells and their associated matrix proteins from a spindled mesenchymal to an epithelial phenotype supports this hypothesis (109) and has prompted some observers to consider the synovial sarcoma as a "carcinoma" or "carcinosarcoma" of connective tissue (108,110). No specific etiologic factor, including prior trauma, has been definitely linked to the development of synovial sarcoma.

1. Clinical Findings and Outcome

In the vast experience of the AFIP (105), most patients with synovial sarcoma range in age from 15 to 40 years, with 90% of patients presenting before age 50. Older individuals and children under the age of 10 years are less commonly affected. The sarcoma occurs more commonly in men.

The overwhelming majority of tumors present in the deep, para-articular soft tissue of the extremities, with the area around the knee and distal thigh representing the most commonly involved site (105), followed by the deep soft tissues of the lower leg, foot, shoulder, and upper extremity. Intra-articular synovial sarcomas represent fewer than 5% of all reported cases and occur mostly in the knee (111). Tumors located in the head and neck region usually arise in the paravertebral soft tissue and present as parapharyngeal or retropharangeal masses (105). Less commonly involved head and neck sites include the hypopharynx, tonsillar fossa, orofacial region, and soft tissues of the neck. A small number of cases of synovial sarcoma have been documented in the lung, mediastinum, and pleura (112–114), anterior abdominal wall (115), heart (116), and vulva (117).

The sarcoma usually presents as a slow-growing mass or a swelling within deep soft tissue. It is associated with tenderness or pain in about half of cases (105). Rarely, the patient may present with symptoms of pain but no palpable mass. Numbness or paresthesias can result from nerve involvement by the tumor. Radiographs often demonstrate spotty calcifications within the mass.

Synovial sarcoma is a fully malignant neoplasm with recurrent and metastatic potential. Extremely high recurrence rates approaching 80% have been reported with inadequate initial surgery and no radiotherapy (105). The performance of a more extensive excision with or without the addition of radiation therapy has resulted in recurrence rates ranging from 18% (118) to as low as 0% (119). As with most sarcomas, recurrences generally manifest within 2 years of initial surgery, but longer intervals before recurrence have been documented. Most recurrences are single, but multiple recurrences are not rare.

Metastatic lesions develop in 50–70% of patients in most series (119). As with other forms of sarcoma, synovial sarcoma metastasizes most often to the lung, followed by lymph nodes, then bone marrow (105). Late lung metastases are not uncommon and adversely influence long-term survival.

The reported 5-year survival for synovial sarcoma ranges from 25% (120) to 82% (121), with most recent studies claiming a 5-year survival rate of about 50%. The 10-year survival for this sarcoma ranges from 34% (119) to as low as 11.2% (120), primarily due to the presence of late metastases. Parameters associated with a better survival include heavy calcification or ossification within the tumor (121), small size (less than 5 cm) (122), location of the tumor in the distal extremity (122), and young age at presentation (122). Features noted to adversely affect prognosis include high mitotic activity (greater than 15 mitoses per 10 high-power fields) (123), high nuclear grade and presence of cells with "rhabdoid" morphology (124), poor differentiation (see below) (125), vascular invasion (105), extensive necrosis (126), and aneuploid cell population detected by flow cytometry (127). Although previous studies suggested a slightly more favorable prognosis for patients with biphasic tumors (123,128,129), more recent studies have failed to demonstrate a significant survival difference (118,124,126,127).

Cytogenetic studies have provided an important diagnostic and, perhaps, prognostic marker for synovial sarcoma. A characteristic fusion gene (*SYT-SSX*) resulting from the translocation of the *SYT* gene on chromosome 18 to one of two loci on chromosome Xp11 (130,131) has been identified in more than 90% of all synovial sarcomas, regardless of type (132). In the experience of one group (132), all biphasic tumors (and some monophasic tumors) harbored the *SYT-SSX1* transcript, whereas the *SYT-SSX2*-bearing tumors were all monophasic variants. Moreover, the latter subset demonstrated a significantly better metastasis-free survival.

2. Gross Findings

The size of the tumor varies according to its location and ranges from small lesions about 1 cm in greatest dimension to large bulky masses. In the AFIP series of 345 cases (105), most tumors excised ranged in size from 3 to 5 cm in greatest dimension. The neoplasm tends to exhibit a lobulated contour with smooth margins and is commonly surrounded by a fibrous pseudocapsule. Fast-growing tumors have less well-circumscribed margins and may present as infiltrative, multinodular masses. The tumors may be soft or firm (depending on the relative cellularity and collagen content). The cut surface is generally gray–white to yellow. Cyst formation is not uncommon and in some cases can be pronounced. Gritty foci of calcification may be identified. In fast-growing tumors, red–brown hemorrhagic foci and yellow necrotic areas can be identified.

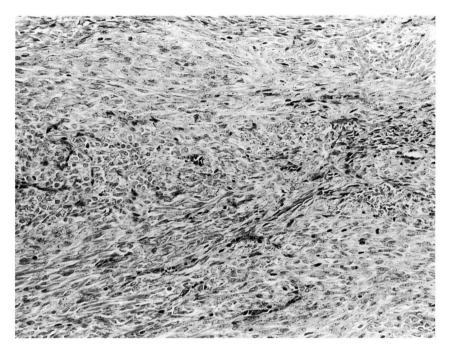

FIG. 26 Synovial sarcoma, monophasic, fibrous type. Spindled neoplastic cells are arranged in a short, fascicular growth pattern.

3.   Microscopic Findings

The two main histologic subtypes of synovial sarcoma, the biphasic and the monophasic fibrous variants, share a common spindle cell element. The spindle cells are arranged in short, cellular, intersecting fascicles or in broad sheets (Fig. 26). On occasion, the cells exhibit palisading of their nuclei or form vague pseudorosettes. Microscopically, they have a short spindled configuration with a small amount of pale cytoplasm and ill-defined cell borders. The cells possess rather uniform-appearing, oval, hyperchromatic nuclei with small, distinct nucleoli (Fig. 27). Cellular zones with a meager amount of stroma alternate with less cellular areas rich in stromal matrix. In these latter foci, thick bands of dense collagen prevail and can have a hyalinized placque-like (Fig. 28) or osteoid-like (pseudo-osteoid) appearance. Calcium deposits and bone appear within this hyalinized collagen and, in some cases, are found in abundance (121). Cartilage is a rare finding. Less often, a hyaluronic acid–rich myxoid stroma predominates, in which case the embedded spindle cells tend to adopt a laciform pattern of growth (133). Although

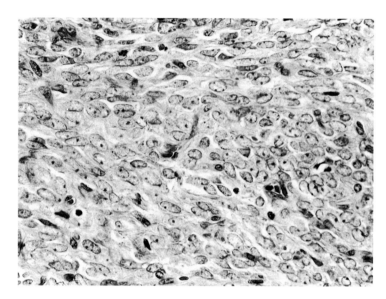

FIG. 27 Spindle cell component of the monophasic synovial sarcoma generally has a uniform cytologic appearance. The neoplastic cells have ill-defined cytoplasmic borders and overlapping, oval-shaped, hyperchromatic nuclei with small, conspicuous nucleoli.

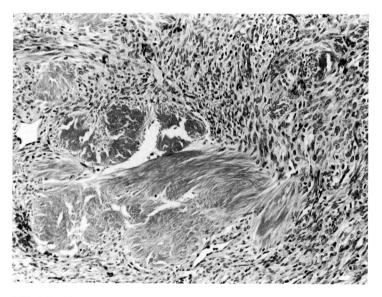

FIG. 28 Placque-like deposits of hyalinized collagen within a monophasic fibrous synovial sarcoma. Deposits of stromal matrix are commonly identified in synovial sarcoma.

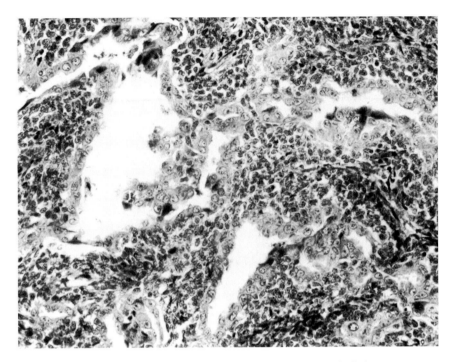

FIG. 29 Synovial sarcoma, biphasic type. Intermingled with the spindled component are irregularly shaped glandular structures lined by cuboidal cells with pale cytoplasm and rounded nuclei.

the degree of vascularity varies in synovial sarcoma, a well-developed hemangio-pericytoma-like network of thin-walled vessels is often identified in areas of the tumor. Foci of hemorrhage or hemosiderin deposition are not uncommonly observed. Mast cells are commonly sprinkled throughout the stroma, but other inflammatory elements are sparse.

The epithelial cells of the biphasic variant are arranged in nests, solid cords, or trabeculae; line rounded and elongated gland-like and cystic spaces; or mount small papillary structures (Fig. 29). The epithelial cell has a cuboidal to columnar shape with pale cytoplasm and a vesicular nucleus. Eosinophilic secretions are found within pseudoglandular lumina and, rarely, within the cytoplasm of the epithelial cells. This product has histochemical staining characteristics of epithelial mucin. The epithelial cell component can undergo squamous metaplasia replete with keratin pearls and keratohyaline granules. The interface between the juxtaposed spindled and epithelial components is generally sharp. However, in spindled areas, small aggregates of cells with oval contours, relatively more abundant cytoplasm, and better defined cell borders blend with the spindled element

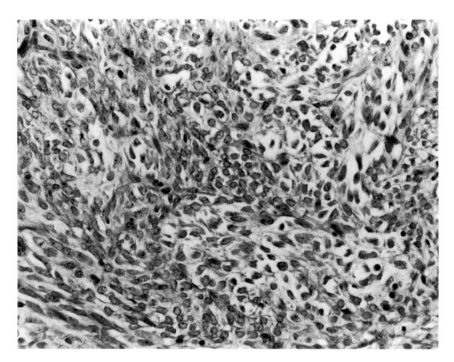

FIG. 30 Ill-defined clusters of cells with cleared cytoplasm, better defined cell borders, and rounded nuclei are identified within a spindle cell area of the synovial sarcoma. This finding signifies spindle cells transitioning to an epithelial morphology.

and appear to represent cells transitioning to an epithelial morphology (Fig. 30). In these foci, reticulin stain highlights this early epithelial differentiation by surrounding clusters of these plump, ovoid cells. Mitotic activity is found in both components of the conventional synovial sarcoma and typically is less than 2 mitoses per 10 high-power fields.

The monophasic epithelial synovial sarcoma is a poorly recognized variant given its close histologic resemblance to carcinoma. It is composed almost exclusively of epithelial cells forming solid nests or gland-like structures. The diagnosis is virtually impossible if only the epithelial component is identified. However, in the experience of the AFIP (105), tumors with this overwhelming epithelial component typically have microscopic foci of conventional spindle cell sarcoma (and, by definition, should be classified as biphasic).

Poorly differentiated synovial sarcoma is a fourth subtype of synovial sarcoma that may present in a pure form or as a component of a conventional synovial sarcoma. This variant composes about 20% of cases of synovial sarcoma according to the records of the AFIP (105). Such neoplasms not only are difficult to classify as synovial sarcomas but also appear to act more aggressively than conventional forms. Three histologic variants of poorly differentiated synovial sarcoma are recognized (134). One variant consists of cellular fascicles of cytologically high-grade-appearing spindle cells resembling the growth pattern of a fibrosarcoma or a malignant peripheral nerve sheath tumor. The cells exhibit brisk mitotic activity and areas of necrosis. The second subtype is composed of epithelioid-appearing cells that exhibit high-grade cytologic characteristics, including the presence of cells with a "rhabdoid" morphology, and high mitotic activity (Fig. 31A). The third variant is composed of small, rounded cells with high nuclear/cytoplasmic ratios reminiscent of a Ewing's sarcoma/primitive neuroectodermal tumor (Fig. 31B).

Immunohistochemically, the spindle cell component, in addition to the epithelial cell element, expresses cytokeratin and EMA. EMA and cytokeratin expression can be spotty in the spindled component or completely absent, particularly in poorly differentiated foci. Overall, EMA appears to be a more sensitive immunomarker than cytokeratin for synovial sarcoma, especially with the poorly differentiated variants (135). Cytokeratins 8 and 18 are commonly expressed as in other sarcomas, but cytokeratins 7 and 19 (136) and high molecular weight keratin (135) have been touted as being more specific for synovial sarcoma. Vimentin is strongly expressed in the spindle cells but is usually absent in the epithelial cell component. Variable S-100 protein as well as CD57 (Leu-7) immunoreactivity has been identified in conventional synovial sarcoma (137). The epithelial cells and, rarely, the spindle cells can express carcinoembryonic antigen (138). Strong expression of the proto-oncogene bcl-2 was observed in the spindled component of all synovial sarcomas tested in one study (139). In addition, focal immunoreactivity for the *MIC2* oncogene product (Ewing's sarcoma marker) using the HBA71 antibody has been reported (140).

4. Differential Diagnosis

Deep-seated spindle cell neoplasms and tumors having a biphasic appearance enter into the differential diagnosis of the synovial sarcoma and include fibrosarcoma, malignant peripheral nerve sheath tumor (malignant schwannoma), leiomyosarcoma, and mesothelioma.

Although a fascicular pattern of growth is common to both fibrosarcoma and the spindled areas of synovial sarcoma, the cells of fibrosarcoma are generally more pleomorphic, exhibit higher mitotic activity, and are typically arranged in longer fascicles. The presence of mast cells, stromal calcification, and bone formation are features more commonly observed in synovial sarcoma. In contrast to the spindled element of synovial sarcoma, the cells of conventional fibrosarcoma do not express cytokeratin or EMA. Sclerosing epithelioid fibrosarcoma (141) shares with synovial sarcoma the presence of epithelioid cells, foci of bone

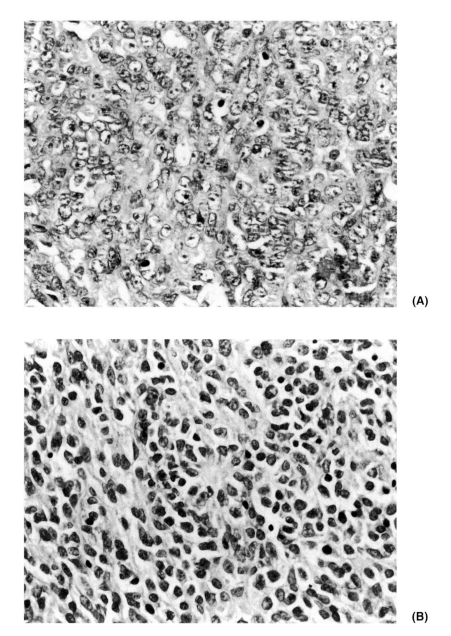

FIG. 31 Poorly differentiated variants of synovial sarcoma. (A) The cells within this focus have high nuclear/cytoplasmic ratios and large, pleomorphic nuclei with prominent nucleoli. (B) Small neoplastic cells with little cytoplasm are reminiscent of the cells composing a primitive neuroectodermal tumor. Note the formation of a pseudorosette (near center).

formation or calcification, and immunoreactivity for EMA, cytokeratin, and S-100 protein. In contrast to synovial sarcoma, the sclerosing epithelioid fibrosarcoma is relatively hypocellular and extremely hyalinized. The epithelioid cells are arranged in cords and small nests simulating the appearance of infiltrating carcinoma. The focal EMA and cytokeratin immunoreactivity has not been described in the more conventional fibrosarcomatous areas of the tumor that are present in the majority of cases. Malignant peripheral nerve sheath tumor (malignant schwannoma) is usually located close to a large peripheral nerve and/or associated with neurofibromatosis type 1. The high-grade histology, occasional presence of nuclear palisading and subendothelial cellular proliferation, and the presence of cells with bent and buckled nuclei are features more in keeping with a malignant peripheral nerve sheath tumor. Some poorly differentiated synovial sarcomas can closely resemble malignant peripheral nerve sheath tumor, but the former typically demonstrate areas of conventional synovial sarcoma. As both the malignant peripheral nerve sheath tumor and synovial sarcoma lesions can express S-100 protein and CD57 (Leu-7), only convincing cytokeratin immunoreactivity (particularly with antibodies directed against cytokeratins 7 or 19 or high molecular weight keratin) within the spindled component will help distinguish these two lesions. The rare glandular malignant peripheral nerve sheath tumor histologically imitates biphasic synovial sarcoma. In contrast to the epithelial component of the biphasic synovial sarcoma, the epithelial component of this malignant peripheral nerve sheath tumor shows neuroendocrine differentiation (with immunohistochemical stains) and intestinal differentiation (by the presence of goblet cells) (142).

Leiomyosarcoma can arise in the deep soft tissue of the extremities. Although a fascicular growth pattern of spindle cells is shared by both leiomyosarcoma and synovial sarcoma, the fascicles of the former entity tend to intersect at more acute angles. In contrast to the spindle cells of synovial sarcoma, the cells of leiomyosarcoma possess intensely eosinophilic cytoplasm and have distinct cell borders. Delicate fuscinophilic longitudinal fibers can be demonstrated in the smooth muscle cells with the trichrome histochemical stain. The nuclei of the leiomyosarcoma are blunt-ended and often possess characteristic paranuclear vacuoles. Immunohistochemically, the absence of cytokeratin and bcl-2 expression and presence of desmin immunoreactivity in leiomyosarcoma help to differentiate these two sarcomas.

Biphasic mesothelioma of the pleura can be difficult to distinguish microscopically from primary pleural synovial sarcoma. The former neoplasm afflicts an older population and is strongly associated with asbestos exposure. The mucin associated with epithelial cells in synovial sarcoma has staining properties similar to those of epithelial mucin, whereas the intracellular mucin in mesothelioma shows the staining profile of hyaluronic acid. Expression of S-100 protein (114) and bcl-2 (143) (in spindle cells) and BerEP4 (114) (in epithelial cells) is reported to favor the diagnosis of synovial sarcoma over a mesothelioma. Ultrastructurally, the cells of synovial sarcoma lack the long, slender microvilli and perinuclear concentration of tonofilaments characteristic of mesothelioma.

B. Epithelioid Sarcoma

Tumors with the appearance of epithelioid sarcoma were first described by Laskowski in 1961 (144). However, it was not until 1970 when Enzinger (145) reported the clinicopathologic features of 62 cases and coined the term "epithelioid sarcoma" (ES) that the neoplasm became recognized as a distinct entity separate from synovial sarcoma and clear cell sarcoma.

ES represents the most common primary sarcoma of the hand and wrist (146). Unfortunately, the clinical and histologic features of ES can mimic those of a nonneoplastic process, so that the sarcoma may be misdiagnosed for a considerable period of time until recurrence or metastasis reveals its true neoplastic nature.

The histogenesis of ES is still an enigma. Electron microscopic analysis of ES reveals a spectrum of ultrastructural differentiation ranging from epithelial-appearing cells with intercellular junctions and surface microvilli to near-totally undifferentiated, fibroblast-like cells with a paucity of organelles (147). Recent cytogenetic evaluation of ES has disclosed loss of heterozygosity of chromosome 22q in 60% of informative cases (148). As this chromosomal region carries the tumor suppressor gene implicated in neurofibromatosis type 2, this finding suggests that the suppressor gene may be involved in the pathogenesis of ES.

1. Clinical Findings and Outcome

ES has been reported in almost all age groups but is more prevalent in patients between 10 and 39 years of age (149). It tends to involve males more frequently than females, especially when the tumor presents in the second through fifth decade of life (150). The flexor surface of the hand, fingers, and forearm represent the most commonly involved sites, followed by knee and lower leg, proximal lower and upper extremity, ankle, and feet and toes (146). The trunk and head and neck regions are the least commonly involved sites. The penis and vulva are also reported sites of primary disease (146). A history of prior trauma is elicited in about 20% (149) to 25% (150) of cases.

ES arising in the dermis most often presents as a slow-growing, painless, usually solitary nodule or plaque. ES situated in the subcutaneous or fascial tissue frequently presents as a fixed, relatively hard nodule. Tumors occurring in the hand (151) and penis (152) can mimic the clinical manifestations of superficial fibromatosis. Dermal and subcutaneous lesions characteristically develop a cleft of overlying skin, which eventually ulcerates (153). These seemingly innocuous clinical presentations not uncommonly lead the clinician to an erroneous diagnosis of a benign lesion. As the neoplasm spreads proximally up the extremity producing numerous cutaneous nodules and ulcerative lesions, a dramatic clinical picture unveils.

ES propagates along fascial planes, tendon sheaths, and aponeuroses. The tumor frequently recurs after inadequate excision and eventually metastasizes via the lymphatics to locoregional lymph nodes and, later, through the bloodstream. In a study of 202 patients with follow-up over 10 years from the AFIP (149), more than 77% of patients developed at least one recurrence. More recent series document recurrence rates ranging from 69% (154) to 34% (155). Multiple recurrences are characteristic. Recurrences generally manifest within a year after diagnosis, but late recurrences are also not unusual.

Metastases were reported in 45% of patients followed over 10 years in the AFIP study (149). Lung and regional lymph nodes are the most common metastatic sites, followed by skin, soft tissue, and central nervous system (146). Lymph node metastases develop in about 45% of cases (149,150,154). The scalp is a commonly reported site of skin and soft-tissue metastasis (146). Although local recurrence generally precedes systemic spread, a visceral metastasis occasionally presents as the first form of recurrent disease (149).

Although the reported 5-year survival for ES is at least 60% in most studies (150,154–157), the overall survival of patients with ES is probably quite low. Parameters that impact adversely on survival include large size (particularly tumors 5 cm or larger) (149), vascular invasion (149), and lymph node metastasis (150), and the presence of necrosis (149). Proximal location (149), deep location (149), male sex (156), older age (149), high mitotic activity (149), and presence of pulmonary metastasis (154) have also been reported to correlate with decreased survival. Although local recurrence has been reported to adversely affect prognosis lin some studies (150,156), others have found that recurrence is a function of the adequacy of initial surgery and is unrelated to survival or development of distant metastases (157).

Radical local excision or amputation is the recommended therapy. Adjuvant radiotherapy helps to provide local control. Since lymph node involvement is more common in ES than in other types of sarcoma (149), regional lymph node dissection should be attempted.

2. Gross Findings

Tumors in the distal aspect of the extremity are situated in the superficial soft tissue (dermis and/or subcutaneous tissue) and appear as small (generally less than 5 cm), nonencapsulated nodules with a firm to hard consistency. The lesions may appear well circumscribed or invade surrounding tissue in a fashion similar to that of squamous cell carcinoma. The cut surface of the tumor is gray–white to tan, with centrally located yellow to brown foci of necrosis and/or hemorrhage.

Tumors arising in the more proximal locations tend to be large, deeply situated masses (deep fascia or tendons) with a multinodular growth pattern and an ill-defined, infiltrating margin. The nodules grow along fascial planes, surround nerves and vessels, or diffusely invade tendons and muscle.

3. Microscopic Findings

At low-power magnification, ES is characterized by a predominantly nodular growth pattern of epithelioid and plump spindle cells (Fig. 32). The center of the nodule commonly undergoes degenerative change characterized by necrosis, hemorrhage, cystification, focal calcification, or replacement of tumor cells by a myxohyaline stroma. At the periphery of the nodules, the epithelioid cells occasionally grow in a cord-like fashion and the spindle cells form vague fascicles as these elements mingle with dense, eosinophilic collagen. The nodules have a tendency to coalesce. When the tumor spreads along fascial planes and aponeurotic connective tissue, the confluent nodules align themselves along the length of the tissue plane, resulting in an undulating band of tumor cells surrounding hypocellular or necrotic zones (garland-like configuration).

The neoplastic cells have an epithelioid or plump spindle cell morphology and usually exhibit a mild to moderate degree of pleomorphism (Fig. 33). No sharp demarcation between the two cells types is appreciated. Instead, the epithelioid cells, concentrated more toward the center of the nodule, blend imperceptibly with the spindled element. The cells possess eosinophilic cytoplasm with fairly well-defined cell borders. Clear cell change and the presence of intracytoplasmic lipid vacuoles (probably a degenerative change) are occasionally observed. The nucleus has a round to slightly irregular, ovoid contour with irregularly distributed, vesicular chromatin and a conspicuous nucleolus. Multinucleated cells can be identified as a minor component in some cases. The mitotic rate in ES varies but usually is less than 10 mitoses per 10 high-power fields.

Cells with an eccentrically positioned nucleus, prominent nucleolus, and a pale eosinophilic intracytoplasm inclusion ("rhabdoid" cell morphology) may be interspersed in the tumor cell population or, in some cases, represent a significant component of the tumor. The "proximal type" of ES (158), which arises primarily in axial sites as a large, generally deeply seated mass, is composed of pleomorphic epithelioid cells, including a significant rhabdoid component (Fig. 34). This variant has histologic overlap with both the "extrarenal malignant rhabdoid tumor" and carcinoma. Rarely, ES consists predominantly of bland-appearing spindle cells arranged in a storiform or fascicular growth pattern with interspersed epithelioid and rhabdoid cells ("fibroma-like" variant) (159).

The stroma of ES is generally composed of dense, eosinophilic collagen that can have a hyalinized appearance. Focal myxoid change is infrequently encountered. Osseous metaplasia is reported in up to 20% of cases, whereas cartilaginous metaplasia is exceedingly rare (146). A chronic inflammatory infiltrate commonly accompanies the process and on occasion can be quite striking. Small amounts of hemosiderin may be identified in the tumor.

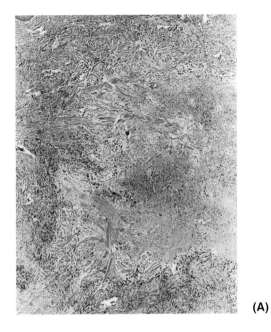

(A)

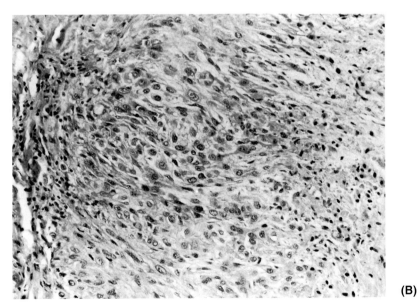

(B)

FIG. 32 Epithelioid sarcoma. (A) Scanning view of an ill-defined nodule of tumor cells surrounding a central area of necrosis within the dermis. Epidermal surface is on top. (B) Portion of the nodule showing epithelioid and spindled tumor cells merging with the central area of necrosis (*right*).

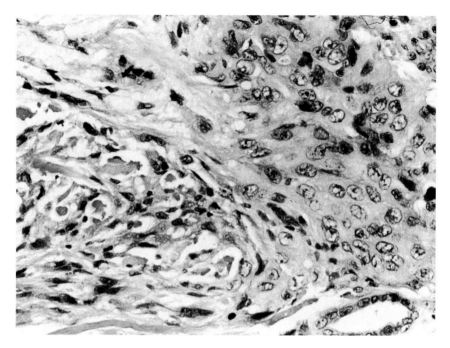

FIG. 33 Epithelioid sarcoma is composed of epithelioid-appearing cells with eosinophilic cytoplasm and moderately atypical nuclei with a vesicular chromatin pattern and
spindled tumor cells with elongated nuclei.

The characteristic immunoprofile of ES is the coexpression of keratin and
vimentin. Cytokeratin is expressed in more than 75% of cases (149). Its expression is somewhat variable in a given tumor but generally is more pronounced in
the epithelioid cell component. EMA is expressed in more than 50% of tumors
(160,161) and its pattern of reactivity also demonstrates variability in the same lesion. CD34 (QBEND-10) is reportedly expressed in about 50% of tumors tested
(162). Carcinoembryonic antigen (CEA) (149) immunoreactivity can be focally
identified in ES. Desmin expression has been observed mainly in the rhabdoid cell
component of the proximal type of ES (158).

4. Differential Diagnosis

Reactive processes and neoplasms displaying a nodular arrangement of epithelioid-appearing cells constitute entities that require separation from ES.
Necrobiotic granulomas (NGs), including granuloma annulare and rheumatoid nodule, are reactive lesions that may histologically resemble ES. In contrast

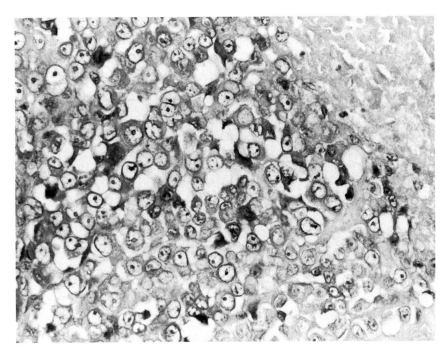

FIG. 34 "Proximal-type" epithelioid sarcoma. Epithelioid cells with abundant eosino-philic cytoplasm and large nuclei possessing prominent nucleoli. Some cells have "rhab-doid" features.

to ES, NG exhibits less cellular atypia and lower mitotic activity. The inflam-matory infiltrate of the latter is generally heavier than that of ES. Langhans giant cells may be present in NG but are not a component of ES. While the cells of NG express histiocyte/monocyte-related immunomarkers, they do not show keratin, EMA, or convincing CD34 (QBEND-10) immunoreactivity.

The presence of eosinophilic, epithelioid cells attached to and ulcerating the skin may evoke the diagnosis of squamous cell carcinoma. In addition, the proxi-mal type of ES, with its deeply located nodules of large, eosinophilic, epithelioid-appearing cells, may masquerade as a squamous cell carcinoma. As most cases of squamous carcinoma arise in actinically damaged skin, the absence of atypical squamous epithelium in the adjacent nonulcerated epidermis is a feature against squamous carcinoma. Unlike the cells of squamous carcinoma, the cells of ES lack intercellular bridges and do not exhibit keratinization. The cells of squamous car-cinoma also do not express CD34 (QBEND-10) (162).

Malignant melanoma, especially a tumor devoid of pigment (amelanotic melanoma), may be mistaken for ES. The cytoplasm of melanoma cells has a more "dusty," amphophilic appearance than that of ES cells. Importantly, melanoma cells express S-100 protein and HMB-45, but not EMA or keratin.

Vascular tumors with epithelioid endothelial cells, including epithelioid hemangioendothelioma (EHE) and epithelioid angiosarcoma, may resemble ES histologically. In contrast to the cells of ES, the cells of EHE have pale cytoplasm and typically exhibit intracytoplasmic lumina containing red blood cells or their debris. They are arranged in small nests or thin trabeculae and attempt to form primitive vascular lumina. Large nodules with central necrosis are not indicative of EHE. The epithelioid variant of angiosarcoma is the most common morphologic expression of high-grade angiosarcoma involving the soft tissues (163). The epithelioid appearance of the cells and formation of solid nests without discernible vascular differentiation mimic the histopathologic features of ES, particularly, the proximal type of ES. However, careful search will typically uncover vascular channels lined by the neoplastic cells or the presence of intracellular vacuoles containing red blood cells or their debris. The cells of both vascular neoplasms express CD34 and can focally express keratin and EMA (164,165). However, in contrast to ES, they also express factor VIII–related antigen and CD31.

C. Alveolar Soft-Part Sarcoma

In 1952, Christopherson (166) delineated the clinical and pathologic features of a morphologically distinct soft-tissue entity in his seminal paper "Alveolar Soft-Part Sarcomas: Structurally Characteristic Tumors of Uncertain Histogenesis." The continued relevance of this title, almost five decades later, stands in testament to the frustration experienced by investigators who have attempted to uncover the etiogenesis of this rare sarcoma. Despite the fact that the alveolar soft-part sarcoma (ASPS) accounts for less than 1.0% of all soft-tissue sarcomas (146), the literature is replete with studies attempting to ascertain its histogenesis. Early studies claimed that ASPS is a variant of paraganglioma or granular cell tumor, a neoplasm exhibiting skeletal muscle differentiation, or a neoplasm capable of producing renin.

Presently, the most intriguing theory is that the ASPS is derived from skeletal muscle. This hypothesis gained initial support when investigators claimed that the intracytoplasmic, membrane-bound crystals in ASPS ultrastructurally resembled the crystalline structures detected in nemaline myopathy and within tumor cells of adult rhabdomyoma (167). Furthermore, a few studies have identified myogenic proteins, including the highly sensitive and specific skeletal muscle marker MyoD1, within cells of ASPS on frozen tissue (168). However, this evidence for skeletal muscle differentiation has been recently contested because specific ultrastructural features of muscle differentiation have not been identified within ASPS and researchers have not been able to demonstrate nuclear expression of MyoD1 or myogenin—two key proteins in skeletal muscle differentiation—using immunohistochemistry (169), Western blot analysis (169), and molecular techniques (170).

1. Clinical Findings and Outcome

According to the files of the AFIP, ASPS principally affects adolescents and young adults in the 15- to 35-year-old range (146). However, the neoplasm can afflict children and older adults. Females are involved slightly more often than males.

The tumor arises primarily in the deep soft tissues of the lower extremity, with the anterior thigh and buttock representing the two most frequently involved sites (171), followed by the chest and abdominal wall. Unusual locations include retroperitoneum (171), mediastinum (172), and female genital tract (173). In children, ASPS predilects to the head and neck region, especially the periorbital soft tissue and tongue (146). ASPS clinically presents as a slow-growing, painless mass that may be apparent for months to years before the patient seeks medical attention. Unfortunately, sometimes metastatic disease to the lung or brain heralds the presence of an occult sarcoma.

ASPS has a poor long-term survival. In a clinicopathologic study covering more than 60 years, Lieberman et al. (171) documented a 5-year survival for patients presenting without metastatic disease of 60%; a 10-year survival of 38%; and a 20-year survival of only 15%. Death usually results from metastases to vital organs. The principal metastatic sites are lung, followed by brain and bone. The majority of metastases occur early, with approximately one-fourth to one-third of patients presenting with metastatic disease at time of diagnosis (146,171,174). The likelihood of metastatic spread of the sarcoma at the time of diagnosis increased with age at initial presentation in one study (171). Local recurrence of tumor has been reported in about 20% of patients in one study (174) and tended to occur in patients who had inadequate initial surgery. Children with ASPS have a better prognosis than adults. Compared with adult tumors, ASPS in children tends to be detected earlier when the sarcoma is smaller and less invasive (175,176).

Because ASPS grows slowly even at metastatic sites, surgery combined with radiotherapy and/or chemotherapy is the recommended treatment (146).

2. Gross Findings

ASPS varies in size from lesions less than 5 cm in greatest dimension to bulky masses over 20 cm. The tumor is generally well circumscribed and may be partially surrounded by a fibrous pseudocapsule. Large, tortuous vessels can be identified in the surrounding normal tissue. The tumor has a firm but friable consistency. The cut surface has an overall gray color with areas of hemorrhage and necrosis resulting in red-tan and yellow-white foci, respectively. Thin fibrous septa may be observed coursing through the mass.

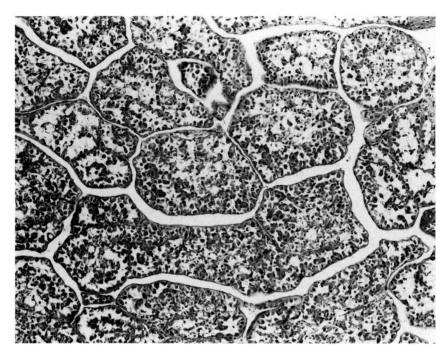

FIG. 35 Alveolar soft-part sarcoma. Epithelioid tumor cells are arranged in well-delineated nests separated by thin-walled, sinusoidal vascular channels.

3. Microscopic Findings

At low-power magnification, ASPS displays a distinctive nested or organoid arrangement of large, polygonal cells with eosinophilic cytoplasm (Fig. 35). The nests are separated from one another by thin-walled, sinusoidal vascular channels. Protrusion of nests of tumor into these vessels as well as frank vascular invasion are common findings in ASPS. Loss of cellular cohesion results in intact and degenerated cells floating in the center of the nest and imparts a "pseudoalveolar" appearance to the otherwise ball-like arrangement of cells (Fig. 36). ASPS can be composed of small, compact nests of cells without discernible intervening vascular structures (Fig. 37). This architectural pattern is more commonly seen in children (146).

The tumor cells have a uniform, oval to polygonal shape with distinct cell borders and an ample amount of finely granular, eosinophilic cytoplasm (Fig. 36). Cytoplasmic vacuolization is observed in some instances and probably represents a degenerative phenomenon. The cells possess one or two, eccentrically positioned, uniformly round to reniform-shaped nuclei with vesicular chromatin and prominent nucleoli. Mitotic activity is characteristically low. PAS stain detects

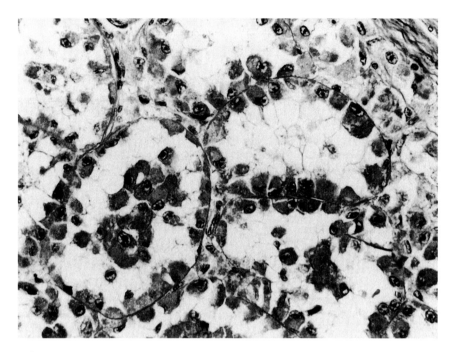

FIG. 36   The neoplastic cells of alveolar soft-part sarcoma exhibit very little cytologic variability. They have abundant, finely granular, eosinophilic cytoplasm and a large, oval-shaped nucleus with vesicular chromatin and prominent nucleoli. Loss of cellular cohesion results in intact and degenerated cells floating in the center of the nest (pseudoalveolar pattern).

intracytoplasmic glycogen and highlights elongated and rhomboid-shaped crystalline structures commonly disposed in sheaf-like aggregates in the cytoplasm (146).

Unusual histomorphologic variants include a pleomorphic form of ASPS characterized by loss of the nest-like growth, cellular pleomorphism, and high mitotic activity (177). Examples of ASPS featuring a spindle cell component (178) and psammomatous calcifications (179) have been documented in the literature.

The immunohistochemical profile of ASPS is broad and somewhat nonspecific. Most patients with ASPS exhibit some degree of vimentin, desmin, and muscle-specific actin expression (146). S-100 protein immunoreactivity has been observed in some cases (171,175,178,180).

4. Differential Diagnosis

Tumors exhibiting an alveolar or nested arrangement of relatively large, epithelioid-appearing cells enter into the differential diagnosis of the ASPS and include

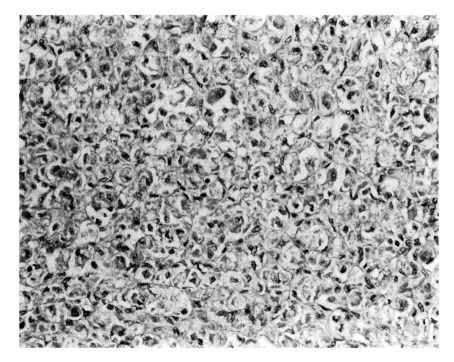

FIG. 37 Alveolar soft-part sarcoma consisting of small, compact nests of cells without a conspicuous sinusoidal vascular component. This variant is more commonly observed in children.

paraganglioma, adult form of rhabdomyoma, granular cell tumor (GCT), rhabdo-myosarcoma, and metastatic renal cell carcinoma.

The paraganglioma is not known to arise in the soft tissue of the extrem-ity. Compared with ASPS, the alveolar nests of paraganglioma tend to be smaller and the cells do not typically exhibit as much cellular dyscohesion (Fig. 38). Al-though both tumors exhibit S-100 protein immunoreactivity, only the sustentacu-lar cells surrounding nests of tumor cells in paraganglioma express this protein. Furthermore, tumor cells of paraganglioma are known to express synaptophysin, chromogranin, and neurofilament protein.

Adult rhabdomyoma arises primarily in deep soft tissue of the head and neck region. In contrast to the loosely cohesive pattern of growth exhibited by cells of ASPS, the large, polygonal-shaped cells of adult rhabdomyoma form tightly packed nodules. Phosphotungstic acid–hematoxylin (PTAH) highlights the cross-striations and characteristic crystalline material in the cells of the rhabdomyoma. Furthermore, cells of rhabdomyoma show strong immunoexpression of myogenic proteins, including desmin and myoglobin.

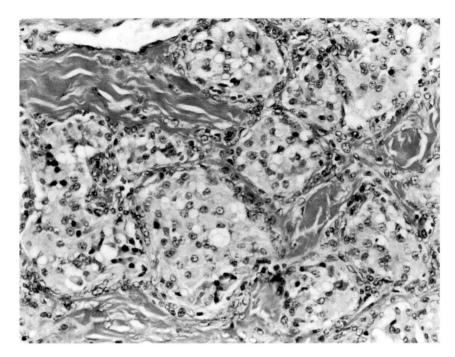

FIG. 38 The paraganglioma consists of cells with ill-defined cytoplasmic borders arranged in small, cohesive nests surrounded by a collagenous stroma.

Although GCT is rarely encountered in the deep soft tissue, its composition of intensely granular cells is a feature shared with ASPS. GCT does not demonstrate the uniform nested pattern of growth characteristic of ASPS but infiltrates surrounding tissue as irregularly shaped nests and trabeculae. The cells of classical GCT display more intensely granular cytoplasm and possess smaller nuclei with less prominent nucleoli than cells of ASPS. In contrast to ASPS, the cells of GCT show strong and diffuse S-100 protein immunoreactivity as well as CD57 (Leu-7) immunoreactivity.

Rhabdomyosarcoma is a disease of infants and children and less frequently affects young adults. Some examples of embryonal rhabdomyosarcoma are composed of rather well-differentiated rhabdomyoblasts with voluminous eosinophilic cytoplasm that can mimic the cells of ASPS. Similar to ASPS, the cells of the alveolar variant of rhabdomyosarcoma undergo loss of cohesion resulting in a "pseudoalveolar" architecture. Unlike ASPS, both forms of rhabdomyosarcoma are more infiltrative and composed of a more pleomorphic population of cells that exhibit high mitotic activity. The distinctive thin-walled vascular channels present in ASPS are not found in rhabdomyosarcoma. Immunohistochemically, rhabdomyosarcoma generally shows a greater degree of myogenic protein expression than ASPS.

Metastatic renal cell carcinoma features a prominent thin-walled vascular network and can exhibit an alveolar arrangement of cells with granular, eosinophilic cytoplasm. Renal cell carcinoma occurs in an older population than ASPS and is rare before age 40 years. Renal cell carcinoma usually expresses the epithelial immunomarkers cytokeratin and EMA.

D. Ossifying Fibromyxoid Tumor of Soft Parts

In 1989, Enzinger and colleagues from the AFIP (181) detailed the clinicopathologic features of 59 examples of a previously undescribed soft-tissue tumor that they termed "ossifying fibromyxoid tumor of soft parts" (OFT), based chiefly on the tumor's histomorphologic attributes.

Since this initial report, other examples of OFT have been reported in the literature as case reports and small series. Many studies have concentrated on the immunohistochemical profile or ultrastructural features of the tumor in an attempt to clarify its histogenesis. The imunoexpression of neural markers, including S-100 protein (181–184) in the majority of these tumors, and the presence of discontinuous runs of thick basal lamina and interdigitating cytoplasmic processes on ultrastructural examination (181–183) support the view that the OFT is closely related to elements of the peripheral nerve sheath.

1. Clinical Findings and Outcome

OFT occurs over a wide age range (14–79 years) but shows a peak incidence in the fifth decade of life (181). Men were affected more often than women. The tumor clinically presents as a slow-growing, asymptomatic nodule or mass in the subcutaneous tissue or, less often, skeletal muscle. Multiple lesions have been documented at presentation (182,185) and are usually grouped in the same general area. The shoulder, upper arm, buttock, and thigh are the preferentially involved sites of origin (181). The tumor arises less frequently in the head and neck region and trunk. The duration of preoperative disease varied from less than 1 year to over 20 years in one study (181).

Although a relatively new entity with only short-term follow-up, the OFT, as classically defined, appears to possess a low-grade malignant potential. In the AFIP series (181), the local recurrence rate was 27%, with multiple recurrences documented in three patients. One patient with three recurrences developed a presumed metastasis to the opposite thigh 20 years after initial excision. The authors observed that tumors that acted more aggressively were larger, more deeply seated, and exhibited a higher mitotic count than nonrecurrent lesions.

One group of investigators defined a subset of "atypical and malignant" OFTs characterized by tumors exhibiting increased cellularity and mitotic activity(186). Two of the six patients in this study developed recurrent disease and one experienced a pulmonary metastasis. Two additional OFTs cited in the literature with worrisome histologic features pursued an aggressive clinical course (184,187).

Surgery is presently the mainstay of therapy for OFT. A complete local excision is recommended for small lesions, whereas a wide local excision is reserved for large, deep tumors featuring aggressive histologic characteristics (hypercellularity accompanied by high mitotic activity), and for recurrent lesions (181).

2. Gross Findings

The tumors vary in size from about 1 cm to as large as 17 cm (181). The OFT appears as either a well-circumscribed, single round to oval nodule or as a multinodular or lobulated mass. The tumor is surrounded by a thick fibrous pseudocapsule. Most lesions have a firm to hard, cartilage-like consistency. The tumor may feel gritty on sectioning due to its variably calcified or ossified pseudocapsule. The cut surface of the lesion usually has a glistening appearance and a white–tan color with occasional foci of hemorrhage.

3. Microscopic Findings

At low-power magnification, OFT is composed of uniform-appearing, small round to polygonal-shaped cells embedded in a myxohyaline to collagenous stromal matrix (Fig. 39). The cells are arranged in lobules that vary in size and cellularity, and are partially separated by fibrous bands. The tumor is surrounded by an incomplete fibrous pseudocapsule composed of dense fibrous and hyalinized connective tissue (Fig. 40). Nests of tumor may be seen infiltrating through rents in this fibrous shell. More than 80% of tumors (181,183) have varying amounts of calcified lamellar (sometimes replete with marrow spaces) or woven bone within the pseudocapsule. Spicules of bone can be observed extending into the substance of the tumor along the fibrous tracts (Fig. 39).

The neoplastic element of the OFT is a relatively small cell with lightly eosinophilic to clear cytoplasm and a cytologically bland-appearing, round to spindle-shaped nucleus containing a small nucleolus (Fig. 41). The occasional presence of a clear space around the cell mimics the appearance of chondrocytic differentiation. The cells assume a variety of patterns within the tumor nests and lobules. They may be evenly dispersed without a distinct growth pattern (Fig. 41). In zones with an abundant myxocollagenous stromal matrix, the cells interconnect to form anastomosing, thin, cord-like or laciform arrangements (Fig. 42). A vaguely fascicular growth pattern of spindle cells occurs in the more collagenous areas of the tumor. Polygonal-shaped cells with distinct cell borders may aggregate around vessels in a manner reminiscent of a glomus tumor. In conventional examples, the mitotic activity is low, averaging less than 2 mitotic figures per 10 high-power fields.

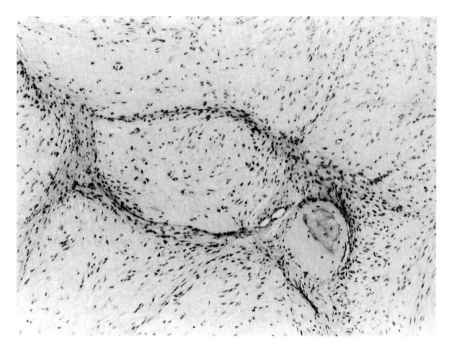

FIG. 39 Ossifying fibromyxoid tumor of soft parts. At low power, bland-appearing spindle cells embedded in a myxohyalin stroma are separated into lobules by the fibrous bands. Note spicule of bone in one of the fibrous partitions (*lower right*).

The stroma of OFT varies in amount and composition. The stromal mucin is chiefly composed of hyaluronic acid. Only minuscule amounts of sulfated mucopolysaccharide are detectable with aldehyde fuchsin stain at pH 1.0 or 1.7 (181). Microcysts are occasionally identified in these mucin-rich areas. Collagen deposition varies from delicate fibers in the myxoid zones to thick bands of hyalinized collagen that occasionally contain spicules of bone or osteoid. Mature cartilage is infrequently identified in OFT. A rich network of thin-walled vessels, often showing perivascular fibrosis, is a consistent finding.

OFTs with aggressive histopathologic features have been described. At variance with classical OFTs, tumors reported in the literature as "atypical" or "malignant" OFTs (186) show increased cellularity and are composed of a slightly more pleomorphic cell population exhibiting nuclear hyperchromatism and increased mitotic activity (greater than 2 mitoses per 10 high-power fields). Kilpatrick et al. (186) commented on the relative lack of a bony shell around the tumors in their study and the prominence of osteoid and bone in the substance of the tumor. Williams et al. (184) reported a malignant OFT that featured necrosis and complete absence of bone formation.

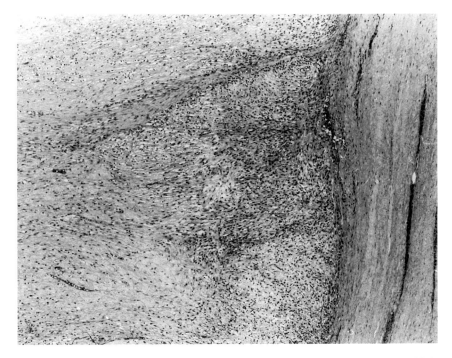

FIG. 40   The ossifying fibromyxoid tumor of soft parts is generally surrounded by a thick, collagenous pseudocapsule.

The immunohistochemical profile of conventional OFT includes immunoreactivity for neural and myogenic markers. Along with strong and diffuse expression of vimentin, approximately 75% of tumors tested variably express S-100 protein and over half express CD57 (Leu-7) (182–184). In one study (183), 70% of tumors expressed desmin. Limited expression of neuron-specific enolase (NSE) (184), glial fibrillary acidic protein (182–184), α-smooth muscle actin (183,184) and muscle-specific actin (184) has also been documented.

4. Differential Diagnosis

The lobular configuration of OFT, coupled with its multipatterned microscopic appearance, bone formation, and immunohistochemical profile, elicits a wide range of histogenetically diverse neoplasms in its differential diagnosis.

OFT can be misdiagnosed as a variant of a cartilaginous tumor, such as myxoid chondrosarcoma, chondroblastoma, or chondromyxofibroma, by virtue of the focal presence of pericellular haloes, myxocollagenous matrix, and S-100 protein expression. Unlike OFT, the stromal mucin of cartilaginous tumors is predominantly a sulfated mucopolysaccharide. The cells of extraskeletal myxoid chondro-

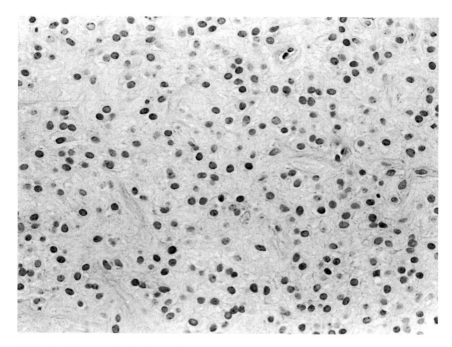

FIG. 41 Tumor cells haphazardly arranged in a myxohyaline stromal matrix possess pale cytoplasm and uniform, oval to round nuclei with evenly dispersed, finely granular chromatin.

sarcoma and chondroblastoma differ from the cells of OFT by their deeply eosinophilic cytoplasm and intracytoplasmic deposition of glycogen (as demonstrated with PAS stain) (see Fig. 45B). Cytologic atypia is more pronounced in myxoid chondrosarcoma and chondromyxofibroma than in OFT. Linear deposition of calcium in the pericellular interstitium and the presence of osteoclast-like giant cells are characteristic of chondroblastoma and chondromyxofibroma, but not of OFT.

Benign peripheral nerve sheath tumors, especially schwannoma and the nerve sheath myxoma (neurothekeoma), are included in the differential diagnosis of OFT. In contrast to the small, uniform cells of OFT, the schwannoma is composed of larger cells with elongated, serpentine nuclei. The OFT does not exhibit the alternating pattern of cellular Antoni A and hypocellular Antoni B areas characteristic of schwannoma. Moreover, no case of OFT has been documented to arise directly from a peripheral nerve. Nerve sheath myxoma (neurothekeoma) has in common with OFT a lobulated architecture and a cord-like growth pattern of short spindle cells suspended in a myxoid stroma (see Fig. 25). Unlike OFT, the nodules composing neurothekeoma are often surrounded by a dense collagenous

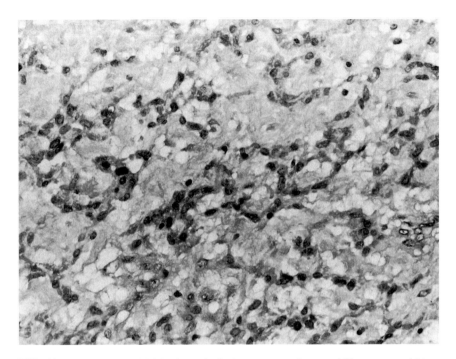

FIG. 42 Tumor cells with bland cytologic features grow in a cord-like pattern within a myxocollagenous stromal matrix.

collar that is devoid of metaplastic bone but may contain perineurial fibroblasts that express EMA. Although the cells of both neoplasms express S-100 protein, conventional nerve sheath myxoma does not express myogenic markers.

Clear cell sarcoma has in common with OFT a nest-like arrangement of pale spindle cells that express S-100 protein. Unlike OFT, clear cell sarcoma is not encapsulated and has little interstitial matrix between cells. The lesional cell of clear cell sarcoma differs from the cell composing OFT by virtue of its larger, more vesicular nucleus, more prominent nucleolus, and greater quantity of intracytoplasmic glycogen. Small numbers of multinucleated giant cells often accompany the spindled element in clear cell sarcoma. In contrast to OFT, clear cell sarcoma demonstrates evidence of melanin production and is HMB-45-immunoreactive in the majority of cases.

Epithelioid smooth muscle tumors and glomus tumors share with OFT a component of polygonal-shaped cells with eosinophilic cytoplasm set in a myxocollagenous stroma. Epithelioid smooth muscle tumors are rare in the soft tissues of the extremities. Moreover, the neoplastic cell is larger and generally has more intensely eosinophilic cytoplasm than the cell composing OFT. Although areas of

OFT may resemble glomus tumor, the other morphologic patterns present in OFT are not identified in the latter. In contrast to OFT, the epithelioid smooth muscle tumor and glomus tumor do not show strong S-100 protein immunoreactivity and commonly exhibit a greater degree of muscle-specific and α-smooth muscle actin immunoexpression.

OFTs must be distinguished from "mixed" tumors of salivary gland (pleomorphic adenoma), skin (chondroid syringoma), and soft-tissue origin, as well as tumors composed primarily of myoepithelial cells. In contrast to OFT, the matrix of "mixed" tumor is composed of a chondroid-appearing mucin rich in sulfated mucopolysaccharides. The presence of epithelial differentiation in the form of ductal structures, squamous islands, and epithelial cysts in pleomorphic adenoma and chondroid syringoma excludes OFT as a diagnostic consideration. Myoepitheliomas, on the other hand, are composed of cellular fascicles of spindle cells, or epithelioid-appearing and plasmacytoid cells set in a variably myxoid stroma. The immunoprofile of OFT and the "mixed" tumors are very similar, except for the cytokeratin expression in the epithelial structures of the "mixed" tumor and within the neoplastic cells of the myoepithelioma.

The proposed examples of OFTs with atypical microscopic features must be differentiated from conventional extraskeletal osteosarcoma and malignant peripheral nerve sheath tumor (malignant schwannoma). Extraskeletal osteosarcoma characteristically features lace-like osteoid, which is produced by markedly atypical neoplastic cells. This contrasts the mature-appearing bone found in the substance of some "atypical" or "malignant" OFTs and the lower grade cytologic atypia displayed by its cells. Malignant peripheral nerve sheath tumors on occasion produce mature bone or cartilage. Most malignant peripheral nerve sheath tumors are composed of cells with hyperchromatic, cytologically atypical nuclei arrayed in elongated, cellular fascicles. While approximately 50% of patients with a malignant peripheral nerve sheath tumor have neurofibromatosis type 1, to date no patients with OFT have been found to have this disorder. In further distinction from the above-discussed sarcomas, the "atypical" or "malignant" OFTs show, at least focally, cytomorphologic features more closely resembling classical OFTs and do not exhibit the full constellation of malignant features attending these high-grade sarcomas.

E. Parachordoma

The parachordoma is an extremely rare soft-tissue neoplasm with histomorphologic features that overlap with classical chordoma and, to some extent, with extraskeletal myxoid chondrosarcoma and "mixed" tumor of skin and soft tissue. Dabska (188) is credited with fully characterizing the clinicopathologic features of this unusual neoplasm in a study of 10 cases, which included five examples reported earlier by Laskowski as "chordoma periphericum." She concluded that parachordoma is histologically similar to chordoma, arises in the deep soft tissue of the extremities, and follows a benign clinical course if adequately excised.

Since Dabska's seminal study, only scattered reports of parachordoma or "chordoma periphericum" have appeared in the literature. Recent investigations have focused on the ultrastructural characteristics and immunoprofile of the parachordoma in an attempt to help differentiate it from tumors with similar histology and to establish its histogenesis. In general, electron microscopic and immunohistochemical studies have shown that the cells of parachordoma possess features resembling those of chordoma (189–191).

Several histogenetic origins have been proposed for the parachordoma, but none are universally accepted. Laskowski considered a specialized synovial cell with the capability of undergoing chondroid differentiation as the progenitor cell of parachordoma (188). Another group of investigators proposed that the tumor arises from the ectopic notochord cells displaced by migration of developing structures (191).

At present, the term "parachordoma" denotes a benign soft-tissue neoplasm with histomorphologic, immunohistochemical, and ultrastructural features comparable to chordoma, but taking origin in extra-axial sites.

1. Clinical Findings and Outcome

Parachordoma arises mainly in tenosynovial and aponeurotic tissue, or on the surface of bone in close relation to the periosteum (188). One tumor in subcutaneous tissue has been reported (192).

The tumor presents as a slow-growing mass in adolescents and adults (188). There is no established sex predilection. Most patients claim that the tumor was present for years before they sought medical attention. Although the majority of lesions are painless, Dabska (188) reported that the two patients with subperiosteal tumor complained of pain at the time of presentation.

Parachordoma is a benign neoplasm that can recur with inadequate excision, but to date no metastasis has been reported. In Dabska's study of 10 cases (188), 3 of the 8 patients with 5 or more years of follow-up developed recurrence, but all were cured with local reexcision. Complete local excision is the current recommended treatment.

2. Gross Findings

The tumor is described as an ovoid, lobulated, well-circumscribed mass that is sometimes surrounded by a thin fibrous pseudocapsule. In the series by Dabska (188), the tumors ranged in size from 2.5 cm to 8 cm in greatest dimension, with the majority measuring 5 cm or less. The mass generally has a firm to hard consistency. The cut surface has a pink–gray to white color and is frequently traversed by fibrous bands. Gelatinous-appearing areas and variably sized cysts containing mucoid material can often be identified.

3. Microscopic Findings

At low-power magnification, the neoplasm is characterized by epithelioid-appearing cells arranged in small nests, cord-like arrays, and pseudoglandular structures in a myxohyaline stroma (Fig. 43). Irregular bands of fibrous tissue traverse the tumor, imparting a lobular architecture.

The main neoplastic element possesses abundant clear to pale eosinophilic cytoplasm, which is variably vacuolated (Fig. 44). The cytoplasm may be extremely vacuolated similar to the "physalipherous" cell of classical chordoma. Myxoid material can be identified in the intracytoplasmic vacuoles (with Alcian blue stain). PAS stain demonstrates the presence of intracytoplasmic glycogen. The nuclei range in morphology from a large structure with bland, vesicular chromatin and a prominent nucleolus to a small, pyknotic form. Multinucleation is occasionally observed. Mitotic activity is minimal, and lymphatic or vascular invasion is not observed. Some tumors have a minor component of short, spindle-shaped cells with scant cytoplasm and elongated, hyperchromatic nuclei arranged in cords within a fibrous matrix.

The stromal matrix of the lobules varies from a purely myxoid to a more chondroid or hyaline-like composition. Most investigators claim that the stromal mucin has staining characteristics of a nonsulfated acidic mucopolysaccharide (69,192).

Immunohistochemical analysis of parachordoma demonstrates immunoexpression of vimentin, S-100 protein, and EMA in most tumors tested (190,192–196). Some investigators have reported cytokeratin immunoexpression in parachordoma (191–194,196). However, in a recent study of four cases, all tumors exhibited CAM5.2 (cytokeratin 8 and 18) immunoreactivity, but not AE1 or CK19 expression (192).

4. Differential Diagnosis

Convention chordoma and extraskeletal myxoid chondrosarcoma represent two relatively common soft-tissue neoplasms that demonstrate histomorphologic overlap with parachordoma. Their separation from the latter neoplasm is clinically important as both of these sarcomas have the potential to act in a malignant fashion.

Although chordoma shares histomorphologic, immunohistochemical, and ultrastructural features with parachordoma, it differs substantially in its site of origin and clinical features. Chordomas develop exclusively in the axial skeleton, with the majority of neoplasms occurring in the sacrococcygeal region, followed by the spheno-occipital area of the cranium. In contradistinction to the relatively

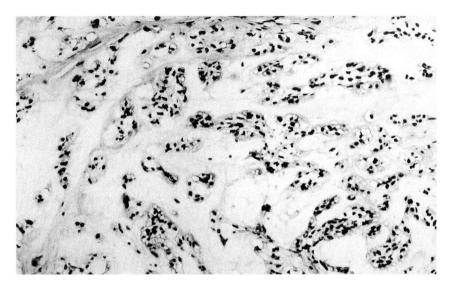

FIG. 43 Parachordoma. Epithelioid-appearing neoplastic cells are arranged in nests and elongated cord-like structures within a myxohyaline stroma. (From Fisher C, Miettinen M. Ann Diagn Pathol 1:3–10, 1997.)

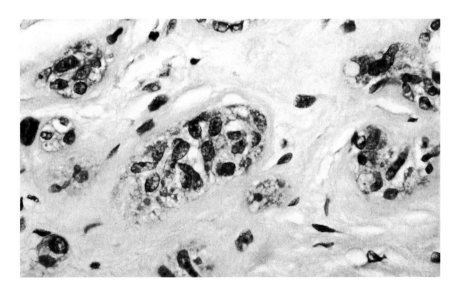

FIG. 44 The tumor cells have clear to pale eosinophilic cytoplasm and variably sized nuclei (From Fisher C, Miettinen M. Ann Diagn Pathol 1:3–10, 1997.)

asymptomatic clinical presentation exhibited by most parachordomas, the chordoma almost always produces symptoms related to its location in the axial skeleton. The radiograph of the latter neoplasm characteristically shows destruction of the involved bone and soft-tissue spread of tumor. Histologically, the cells of chordoma generally grow in a more cord-like fashion and do not exhibit the nested and gland-like growth patterns seen in parachordoma (Fig. 45A).

Extraskeletal myxoid chondrosarcoma bears resemblance to parachordoma due to its lobular architecture and mucopolysaccharide-rich stroma. However, this sarcoma generally arises in deep skeletal muscle. The cells of the myxoid chondrosarcoma are smaller and contain more intensely eosinophilic, less vacuolated cytoplasm than the cells of parachordoma (Fig. 45B). Moreover, they have a tendency to grow in anastomosing thin trabecula, unlike the cells within parachordoma. Although the cells of both neoplasms express S-100 protein, the cells of the myxoid chondrosarcoma rarely express cytokeratin or EMA. Ultrastructurally, the cells of myxoid chondrosarcoma possess microtubular aggregates within dilated rough endoplasmic reticulum and lack features of epithelial differentiation (192).

Most examples of the "mixed" tumor of the soft tissues arise in the skin (chondroid syringoma), but rare cases have been reported in deep subcutaneous and subfascial sites (197). Tumors with a preponderance of myoepithelial cells may show histologic features reminiscent of parachordoma, including lobular arrays of rounded myoepithelial cells arranged in nests or cords within a chondromyxoid matrix. The presence of any epithelial differentiation, such as the formation of ductal structures or epithelial-lined cysts, favors a mixed tumor. As both myoepithelial cells and the cells of parachordoma express S-100 protein, cytokeratin, and EMA, other discriminating immunomarkers for myoepithelial differentiation, such as α-smooth muscle actin, glial fibrillary acidic protein, or calponin, as well as evaluation of ultrastructure, may be helpful in differentiating these lesions.

Chondroid lipoma is a rare form of lipomatous tumor with chondroid features that exhibits histomorphologic and immunohistochemical overlap with parachordoma (198,199). Similar to parachordoma, this tumor frequently arises in deep soft tissue, is well circumscribed, and is composed of epithelioid-appearing cells with eosinophilic and vacuolated cytoplasm arranged in nests, strands, and sheets in a myxohyaline stroma. The neoplastic cells of both entities express S-100 protein and cytokeratin. Chondroid lipoma differs from parachordoma by demonstrating unequivocal lipomatous differentiation, no EMA immunoreactivity, and only focal CAM5.2 (cytokeratin 8 and 18) immunoreactivity.

F. Extrarenal Rhabdoid Tumor of Soft Tissue

The malignant rhabdoid tumor was initially characterized as a highly aggressive renal neoplasm affecting children younger than 2 years (200). The tumor derives

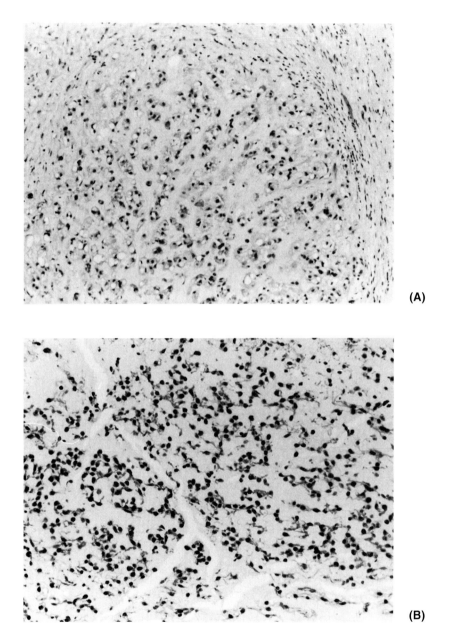

(A)

(B)

FIG. 45 Common soft-tissue neoplasms that may be confused with parachordoma. (A) In contrast to the nested arrangement of cells in parachordoma, the cells of the chordoma generally proliferate in a cord-like or trabecular pattern. (B) The cells of extraskeletal myxoid chondrosarcoma are smaller and more eosinophilic than the cells of parachordoma and grow in thin anastomosing cords.

its name from the early observation that the cells composing this unique renal tumor cytologically resembled those of rhabdomyosarcoma but lacked ultrastructural evidence of skeletal muscle differentiation (201). However, concerns were soon raised that malignant rhabdoid tumor may not represent a specific clinico-pathologic entity as reports of neoplasms exhibiting the characteristic cytomor-phologic features of malignant renal rhabdoid tumor, but having a wider topo-graphic distribution and age range, as well as showing a more variable clinical course, emerged in the literature. Presently, many investigators consider malig-nant rhabdoid tumor to be not a specific entity but rather a distinctive morphotype that is shared by neoplasms of diverse histogenesis as they progress to a more aggressive pathobiological state.

Despite the continuing controversy that surrounds the specificity of the rhabdoid phenotype, there appears to be a narrow subset of childhood soft-tissue tumors with rhabdoid features that display sufficient clinicopathological overlap with the malignant renal rhabdoid tumor to be considered as much of a distinct clinicopathologic entity as the latter neoplasm. Monosomy or deletion of chromo-some band 22q11.2 in a group of congenital malignant extrarenal rhabdoid tumors and in some examples of malignant rhabdoid tumor of kidney, brain, liver, and retroperitoneum (202) further suggest that there exists a select group of malignant rhabdoid tumors that are interrelated. It is the extrarenal rhabdoid tumors of soft tissue (ERTs) that share features with malignant renal rhabdoid tumor that will be discussed below.

1. Clinical Findings and Outcome

The vast majority of ERTs occurs in infants and young children, although the dis-ease may rarely affect adolescents and adults. ERTs have been described in the soft tissues of the head and neck, paravertebral region, shoulder, trunk, extremities, mediastinum, and retroperitoneum (146,202,203). ERTs also have been reported in the central nervous system, liver, thymus, prostate, and skin (146,202,203). The clinical course of the ERT is marked by early dissemination and death. This is par-ticularly true for tumors presenting at birth or within the first year of life (202). Survival rates of 27% (203) and 36% (204) have been documented in two large se-ries of ERT with median follow-up intervals of 6 and 19 months, respectively.

2. Gross and Microscopic Findings

Nearly all of the tumors arising in the soft tissues of the neck, thorax, and extrem-ities are deep, intramuscular lesions (203). The masses are partially pseudoencap-sulated and have a soft to firm consistency. Their cut surface is gray–tan to white with foci of necrosis.

Microscopically, the hallmark cytologic features of the rhabdoid cell are (a) a round to polygonal shape and amphophilic to lightly basophilic cytoplasm that commonly has a weakly PAS-positive, paranuclear globoid inclusion with a

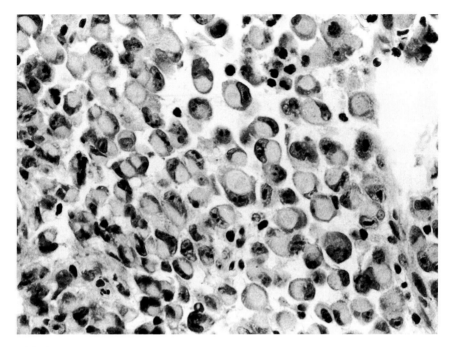

FIG. 46 Extrarenal malignant rhabdoid tumor. The tumor is characterized by a population of dyscohesive cells with pale paranuclear cytoplasmic inclusions and eccentrically positioned, large, vesicular nuclei containing prominent nucleoli.

pale eosinophilic, "glassy" appearance, and (b) a large, eccentrically positioned nucleus with a round to reniform configuration and prominent nucleoli (Fig. 46).

The cells are generally noncohesive but may focally grow in a trabecular pattern or adhere to vessel walls or fibrous septa. Mitotic figures are easily observed, but atypical mitotic figures are uncommon. The cells form bulky, ill-defined sheets or large irregular nests. The stromal matrix is usually edematous but may be myxoid. Lymphatic and blood vessel invasion is frequently identified.

ERT shows rather consistent immunoexpression of vimentin, and the majority of tumors display keratin and EMA expression (202–204). In one study (204), more than 50% of tumors tested expressed the Ewing marker (CD99), synaptophysin, Leu-7 (CD57), and NSE. Focal immunoreactivity has been reported for desmin (202,203) and muscle-specific actin (202–204).

3. Differential Diagnosis

As a number of neoplasms, including carcinomas, melanomas, and soft-tissue sarcomas, may have foci exhibiting the cytomorphologic features of a malignant rhabdoid tumor, a carefully taken history to exclude other malignancies, a thorough histopathologic examination of the entire specimen, a complete immuno-profile, and even an ultrastructural analysis should be performed before the diagnosis of ERT is rendered. Poorly differentiated foci of synovial sarcoma, malignant epithelioid schwannoma, extraskeletal myxoid chondrosarcoma, mesothelioma, and the intra-abdominal desmoplastic small round cell tumor are some of the soft-tissue sarcomas that can demonstrate rhabdoid features. However, rhabdomyosarcoma and the epithelioid sarcoma are the two neoplasms that bear the closest histologic resemblance to ERT.

Rhabdomyosarcoma, like ERT, arises principally in the deep soft tissues and mostly affects children. The embryonal variant may harbor polygonal-shaped rhabdomyoblasts that mimic the cells of ERT. The dyshesive growth pattern of round rhabdomyoblasts in the alveolar variant somewhat resembles the growth pattern of ERT. At variance with the cells composing ERT, rhabdomyoblasts demonstrate cross-striations on light microscopic and convincingly express desmin and MyoD1, but not keratin or EMA. Electron microscopic examination demonstrates ultrastructural differences between the two sarcomas. Rhabdomyoblasts possess thin actin filaments (6–8 nm) in association with thick myosin filaments (12–15 nm). The finding of myosin filaments intimately associated with rows of ribosomes represents the minimal criterion for the diagnosis of skeletal muscle differentiation. In contrast, the ERT shows no definitive evidence of differentiation but features characteristic paranuclear whorled aggregates of intermediate filaments (which correspond to the eosinophilic cytoplasmic inclusions observed with light microscopy), scattered organelles, and primitive to moderately developed desmosomes (203).

Epithelioid sarcoma can have cells with rhabdoid features. In contrast to ERT, epithelioid sarcoma affects mostly adolescents and young adults and predilects to the hand and forearm area. The tumoral cells of epithelioid sarcoma form cohesive nodules that frequently coalesce and exhibit central necrosis. The "proximal type" of epithelioid sarcoma is composed of large epithelioid cells, including a significant component of rhabdoid-appearing cells arranged in large, bulky nodules. In some instances, the number of rhabdoid-appearing cells in this variant of epithelioid sarcoma may make separation from ERT almost impossible. Although coexpression of vimentin and keratin is a feature shared by both epithelioid sarcoma and ERT, the former neoplasm demonstrates CD34 immunoreactivity in 50% of cases (162).

G. Pleomorphic Hyalinizing Angiectatic Tumor

The pleomorphic hyalinizing angiectatic tumor (PHAT), described in 1996 (205). represents a recent addition to the list of soft-tissue tumors of uncertain histogenesis. This extremely rare neoplasm exhibits histologic features that overlap with both "ancient" schwannoma and pleomorphic sarcoma. Some investigators have even speculated that some examples of PHAT may be related to a variant of hemangioma that features bizarre stromal cells ("symplastic" hemangioma) (206). Nevertheless, PHAT shows no immunohistochemical or electron microscopic features characteristic of a specific line of mesenchymal differentiation (205). Moreover, unlike schwannoma and high-grade-appearing sarcomas, PHAT appears to act in a low-grade malignant fashion with the potential for local recurrence but not for metastatic spread.

1. Clinical Findings and Outcome

PHAT occurs in adults ranging in age from 32 to 83 years (205). The chief complaint is the presence of a slow-growing mass. Eleven of the 14 tumors reported in the series by Smith et al. (205) arose in subcutaneous tissue, whereas the remaining three tumors were intramuscular. The lower extremity is the most common site of origin of PHAT. In the series by Smith et al. (205), 4 of 8 patients with follow-up data experienced a recurrence, and 1 patient suffered multiple recurrences over a 25-year period. No patient was reported to have had metastatic spread of the tumor.

2. Gross Findings

PHAT is described as a lobulated tumor ranging in size from more than 2 cm to 8 cm in greatest dimension (205). The tumors are not encapsulated, and the majority exhibit an infiltrative border. The cut surface of the neoplasm is white–tan and shows areas of hemorrhage.

3. Microscopic Findings

A low-power magnification, PHAT features clusters of dilated, irregularly contoured blood vessels and an accompanying relatively cellular population of pleomorphic, plump spindle and multinucleated cells proliferating haphazardly in a variably collagenous stroma (Figs. 47 and 48). In less vascularized examples, a fascicular growth pattern can be observed. The tumors usually have an infiltrative border (Fig. 47B).

The ectatic vessels in the tumor show marked fibrinoid change, perivascular hyaline fibrosis, and occasionally contain intraluminal fibrin and thrombi (Fig. 47). Hemosiderin deposition is noted in the tumor cells adjacent to the ectatic vessels. The stroma is composed of loosely textured collagen, but small quantities of mucin can be observed in some cases. Mast cells are commonly identified, and a few tumors contain collections of lymphocytes.

The tumor cells possess hyperchromatic, pleomorphic nuclei (Fig. 48). Intranuclear pseudoinclusions are frequently identified. Despite the marked degree of cytologic atypia exhibited by the tumor cells, mitotic acitivy is scarce.

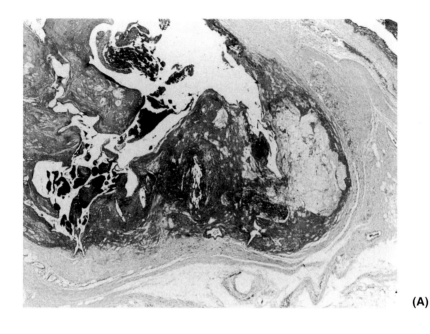

(A)

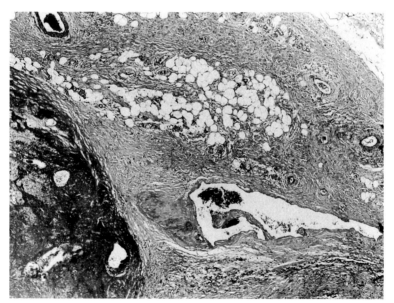

(B)

FIG. 47 Pleomorphic hyalinizing angiectatic tumor of soft parts. (A) At scanning magnification, the most striking feature of this tumor is the presence of large, ectatic blood vessels containing intraluminal fibrin and thrombus. (B) The process commonly infiltrates surrounding native tissue.

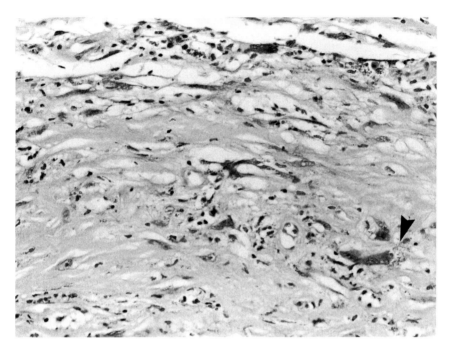

FIG. 48   The tumor cells surrounding the angiectatic vessels are spindled or polygonal in shape and can exhibit marked nuclear pleomorphism. Note hemosiderin deposition associated with lesional cell (*arrowhead*).

Smith et al. (205) reported that the tumor cells lack S-100 protein, EMA, CD31, and desmin expression. CD34 immunoreactivity was demonstrated in 6 of the 12 tumors tested. Furthermore, immunoelectron microscopy revealed large numbers of cytoplasmic vimentin filaments within the tumor cells.

4.   Differential Diagnosis

Dilated vessels with hyalinized walls and pleomorphic spindle cells with intranuclear pseudoinclusions are microscopic features shared by PHAT and "ancient" schwannoma (neurilemmoma). Unlike PHAT, the neurilemmoma is generally encapsulated and noninvasive. Its cells are arranged in sharply demarcated Antoni A and Antoni B zones and they strongly express S-100 protein in contrast to the spindle cell element of PHAT.

The marked pleomorphism exhibited by cells of PHAT may lead to the consideration of a high-grade sarcoma, like MFH. Microscopically, the striking cytologic atypia exhibited by high-grade MFH is accompanied by high mitotic activity, which is absent in PHAT. Intranuclear pseudoinclusions and CD34 expression identified in the tumor cells of PHAT are rarely observed in MFH. Moreover, the ectatic vessels with perivascular hyaline and intraluminal fibrin and thrombus formation characteristically present in PHAT differ significantly from the thick-walled, branching, curvilinear vessels of MFH.

REFERENCES

1. Enzinger FM, Weiss SW. Benign tumors and tumorlike lesions of synovial tissue. In: FM Enzinger, SW Weiss, eds. Soft Tissue Tumors, 3rd ed. St. Louis: Mosby, 1995, pp. 735–755.
2. Hough AJ. Joints. In: I Damjanov, J Linder, eds. Anderson's Pathology, 10th ed. St. Louis: Mosby, 1996, pp. 2612–2652.
3. Barland P, Novikoff AB, Hamerman D. Electron microscopy of the human synovial membrane. J Cell Biol 14:207–220, 1962.
4. Schmidt D, Mackay B. Ultrastructure of human tendon sheath and synovium. Implications for tumor histogenesis. Ultrastruct Pathol 3:269–283, 1982.
5. Jaffe HL, Lichtenstein L, Sutro CJ. Pigmented villonodular synovitis, bursitis and tenosynovitis. A discussion of the synovial and bursal equivalents of the tenosynovial lesion commonly denoted as xanthoma, xanthogranuloma, giant cell tumor or myeloplaxoma of the tendon sheath, with some consideration of this tendon sheath lesion itself. Arch Pathol 31:731–765, 1941.
6. Ushijima M, Hashimoto H, Tsuneyoshi M, Enjoji M. Giant cell tumor of the tendon sheath (nodular tenosynovitis). A study of 207 cases to compare the large joint group with the common digit group. Cancer 57:875–884, 1986.
7. Young JM, Hudacek AG. Experimental production of pigmented villonodular synovitis in dogs. Am J Pathol 30:799–810, 1954.
8. Hoaglund FT. Experimental hemarthrosis: the response of canine knees to injections of autologous blood. J Bone Joint Surg 49:285–298, 1967.
9. El-Naggar AK, Abdul-Karim FW. Tenosynovial giant cell tumors and other lesions traditionally considered to be reactive: further evidence for neoplastic etiology. Adv Anat Pathol 2:329–331, 1995.
10. Vogrincic GS, O'Connell JX, Gilks CB. Giant cell tumor of tendon sheath is a polyclonal cellular proliferation. Hum Pathol 28:815–819, 1997.
11. Biddulph SL. Synovial lesions. In: GP Bogumill, EJ Fleegler, eds. Tumors of the Hand and Upper Limb. Edinburgh: Churchill Livingstone, 1993, pp. 183–191.
12. Rao AS, Vigorita VJ. Pigmented villonodular synovitis (giant-cell tumor of the tendon sheath and synovial membrane). J Bone Joint Surg A 66:76–94, 1984.
13. Jones FE, Soule EH, Coventry MB. Fibrous histiocytoma of synovium (giant cell tumor of tendon sheath, pigmented nodular synovitis). J Bone Joint Surg A 51:76–86, 1969.
14. Fletcher AG, Horn RC. Giant cell tumors of tendon sheath origin. Ann Surg 133:374–385, 1951.
15. Wright CJE. Benign giant cell synovioma. An investigation of 85 cases. Br J Surg 38:257–271, 1951.

16. Maluf HM, DeYoung BR, Swanson PE, Wick MR. Fibroma and giant cell tumor of tendon sheath: a comparative histological and immunohistological study. Mod Pathol 8:155–159, 1995.

17. O'Connell JX, Fanburg JC, Rosenberg AE. Giant cell tumor of tendon sheath and pigmented villonodular synovitis: immunophenotype suggests a synovial cell origin. Hum Pathol 26:771–775, 1995.

18. Silverman JS, Knapik M. Correspond re: H. Maluf, B.R. DeYoung, P.E. Swanson, M.R. Wick. Fibroma and giant cell tumor of tendon sheath: a comparative histological and immunohistological study. Mod Pathol (letter) 9:82–84, 1996.

19. Ishida T, Dorfman HD, Bullough PG. Tophaceous pseudogout (tumoral calcium pyrophosphate dihydrate crystal deposition disease). Hum Pathol 26:587–593, 1995.

20. Bertoni F, Unni KK, Beabout JW, Sim FH. Malignant giant cell tumor of the tendon sheaths and joints (malignant pigmented villonodular synovitis). Am J Surg Pathol 21:153–163, 1997.

21. Pettinato G, Manivel JC, DeRosa N, Dehner LP. Inflammatory myofibroblastic tumor (plasma cell granuloma): clinicopathologic study of 20 cases with immunohistochemical and ultrastructural observations. Am J Clin Pathol 94:538–546, 1990.

22. Bahadori M, Liebow AA. Plasma cell granulomas of the lung. Cancer 31:191–208, 1973.

23. Proppe KH, Scully RE, Rosai J. Postoperative spindle cell nodules of genitourinary tract resembling sarcomas: a report of eight cases. Am J Surg Pathol 8:101–108, 1984.

24. Matsubara O, Tan-Liu NS, Kenney RM, Mark EJ. Inflammatory pseudotumors of the lung: progression from organizing pneumonia to fibrous histiocytoma or to plasma cell granuloma in 32 cases. Hum Pathol 19:807–814, 1988.

25. Chan JKC. Inflammatory pseudotumor: A family of lesions of diverse nature and etiologies. Adv Anat Pathol 3:156–171, 1996.

26. Wade HW. The histoid variety of lepromatous leprosy. Int Lepr 31:129–142, 1963.

27. Brandwein M, Choi H-SH, Stauchen J, Stoler M, Jagirdar J. Spindle cell reaction to nontuberculous mycobacteriosis in AIDS mimicking a spindle cell neoplasm: evidence for dual histiocytic and fibroblast-like characteristics of spindle cells. Virchows Arch A 416:281–286, 1990.

28. Arber DA, Kamel OW, Van de Rijn M, Daivs RE, Medeiros LJ, Jaffe ES, Weiss LM. Frequent presence of the Epstein-Barr virus in inflammatory pseudotumor. Hum Pathol 26:1093–1098, 1995.

29. Selves J, Meggetto F, Brousset P, Voigt J-J, Pradere B, Grasset D, Icart J, Mariame B, Knecht H, Delsol G. Inflammatory pseudotumor of the liver: evidence for follicular dendritic reticulum cell proliferation associated with clonal Epstein-Barr virus. Am J Surg Pathol 20:747–753, 1996.

30. Spencer H. The pulmonary plasma cell/histiocytoma complex. Histopathology 8:903–916, 1984.

31. Meis JM, Enzinger FM. Inflammatory fibrosarcoma of the mesentery and retroperitoneum: a tumor closely simulating inflammatory pseudotumor. Am J Surg Pathol 15:1146–1156, 1991.

32. Maier HC, Sommers SC. Recurrent and metastatic pulmonary fibrous histiocytoma/plasma cell granuloma in a child. Cancer 60:1073–1076, 1987.

33. Malhotra V, Tatke M, Malik R, Gondal R, Beohar PC, Kumar S, Puri V. An unusual
     case of plasma cell granuloma involving lung and brain. Ind J Cancer 28:223–227,
     1991.
34. Chan YF, White J, Brash H. Metachronous pulmonary and cerebral inflammatory
     pseudotumors in a child. Pediatr Pathol 14:805–815, 1994.
35. Myint MA, Medeiros LF, Sulaiman RA, Aswad BI, Glantz L. Inflammatory pseudo-
     tumor of the ileum: a report of a multifocal, transmural lesion with regional lymph
     node involvement. Arch Pathol Lab Med 118:1138–1142, 1994.
36. Biselli R, Ferlini C, Fattorossi A, Boldrini R, Bosman C. Inflammatory myofibro-
     blastic tumor (inflammatory pseudotumor): DNA flow cytometric analysis of nine pe-
     diatric cases. Cancer 77:778–784, 1996.
37. Donner LR, Trompler RA, White RR. Progression of inflammatory myofibroblastic
     tumor (inflammatory pseudotumor) of soft tissue into sarcoma after several recur-
     rences. Hum Pathol 27:1095–1098, 1996.
38. Coffin CM, Watterson J, Priest JR, Dehner LP. Extrapulmonary inflammatory myo-
     fibroblastic tumor (inflammatory pseudotumor). A clinicopathologic and immuno-
     histochemical study of 84 cases. Am J Surg Pathol 19:859–872, 1995.
39. Su LD, Atayde-Perez A, Sheldon S, Fletcher JA, Weiss SW. Inflammatory myofibro-
     blastic tumor: cytogenetic evidence supporting clonal origin. Mod Pathol 11:364–
     368, 1998.
40. Coffin CM, Humphrey PA, Dehner LP. Extrapulmonary inflammatory myofibro-
     blastic tumor: a clinical and pathological survey. Semin Diagn Pathol 15:85–101,
     1998.
41. Sciot R, Dal Cin P, Fletcher CDM, Hernandez JM, Garcia JL, Samson I, Ramos L,
     Brys P, Van Damme B, Van den Berghe H. Inflammatory myofibroblastic tumor of
     bone: report of two cases with evidence of clonal chromosomal changes. Am J Surg
     Pathol 21:1166–1172, 1997.
42. Jones EC, Clement PB, Young RH. Inflammatory pseudotumor of the urinary blad-
     der. A clinicopathological, immunohistochemical, ultrastructural, and flow cytomet-
     ric study of 13 cases. Am J Surg Pathol 17:264–274, 1993.
43. Ro JY, El-Naggar AK, Amin MB, Sahin AA, Ordonez NG, Ayala AG. Pseudosarco-
     matous fibromyxoid tumor of the urinary bladder and prostate: immunohistochemi-
     cal, ultrastructural, and DNA flow cytometric analyses of nine cases. Hum Pathol 24:
     1203–1210, 1993.
44. Hojo H, Newton WA, Hamoudi AB, Qualman SJ, Wakasa H, Suzuki S, Jaynes F.
     Pseudosarcomatous myofibroblastic tumor of the urinary bladder in children: a study
     of 11 cases with review of the literature. An intergroup rhabdomyosarcoma study. Am
     J Surg Pathol 19:1224–1236, 1995.
45. Tang TT, Segura AD, Oechler HW, Harb JM, Adair SE, Gregg DC, Camitta BM,
     Franciosi RA. Inflammatory myofibrohistiocytic proliferation simulating sarcoma in
     children. Cancer 65:1626–1634, 1990.
46. Weidner N. Inflammatory (myofibroblastic) pseudotumor of the bladder: a review and
     differential diagnosis. Adv Anat Pathol 2:362–375, 1995.
47. Hollowood K, Fletcher CDM. Soft tissue sarcomas that mimic benign lesions. Semin
     Diagn Pathol 12:87–97, 1995.
48. Batsakis JG, El-Naggar AK, Luna MA, Goepfert H. "Inflammatory pseudotumor":
     What is it? How does it behave? Ann Otol Rhinol Laryngol 104:329–331, 1995.

49. Albores-Saavedra J, Manivel JC, Essenfeld H, Dehner LP, Drut R, Gould E, Rosai J. Pseudosarcomatous myofibroblastic proliferations in the urinary bladder of children. Cancer 66:1234–1241, 1990.

50. Mitchinson MJ. The pathology of idiopathic retroperitoneal fibrosis. J Clin Pathol 23: 681–689, 1970.

51. Kelly JK, Hwang W S. Idiopathic retractile (sclerosing) mesenteritis and its differential diagnosis. Am J Surg Pathol 13:513–521, 1989.

52. Burke AP, Sobin LH, Shekitka KM, Federspiel BH, Helwig EB. Intra-abdominal fibromatosis. A pathologic analysis of 130 tumors with comparison of clinical subgroups. Am J Surg Pathol 14:335–341, 1990.

53. Kyriakos M, Kempson RL. Inflammatory fibrous histiocytoma: an aggressive and lethal lesion. Cancer 37:1584–1606, 1976.

54. Merchant W, Calonje E, Fletcher CDM. Inflammatory leiomyosarcoma: a morphological subgroup within the heterogeneous family of so-called inflammmatory malignant fibrous histiocytoma. Histopathology 27:525–532, 1995.

55. Dias P, Parham DM, Shapiro DN, Webber BL, Houghton PJ. Myogenic regulatory protein (MyoD1) expression in childhood solid tumors: diagnostic utility in rhabdomyosarcoma. Am J Pathol 137:1283–1291, 1990.

56. Monda L, Warnke R, Rosai J. A primary lymph node malignancy with features suggestive of dendritic reticulum cell differentiation: a report of 4 cases. Am J Pathol 122:562–572, 1986.

57. Perez-Ordonez B, Erlandson RA, Rosai J. Follicular dendritic cell tumor: report of 13 additional cases of a distinctive entity. Am J Surg Pathol 20:944–955, 1996.

58. Chan JKC, Fletcher CDM, Nayler SJ, Cooper K. Follicular dendritic cell sarcoma: clinicopathologic analysis of 17 cases suggesting a malignant potential higher than currently recognized. Cancer 79:294–313, 1997.

59. Chan JKC. Proliferative lesions of follicular dendritic cells: an overview, including a detailed account of follicular dendritic cell sarcoma, a neoplasm with many faces and uncommon etiologic associations. Adv Anat Pathol 4:387–411, 1997.

60. Shek TWH, Ho FCS, Ng IOL, Chan ACL, Ma L, Srivastava G. Follicular dendritic cell tumor of the liver. Evidence for an Epstein-Barr virus–related clonal proliferation of follicular dendritic cells. Am J Surg Pathol 20:313–324, 1996.

61. Classic Hodgkin's Disease. In: RA Warnke, LM Weiss, JKC Chan, ML Cleary, RF Dorfman, eds. Atlas of Tumor Pathology. Tumors of the Lymph Nodes and Spleen. Washington, DC: Armed Forces Institute of Pathology, 1994, pp. 277–304.

62. Wood, C, Nickoloff BJ, Todes-Taylor NR. Pseudotumor resulting from atypical mycobacterial infection: A "histoid" variety of Mycobacteria avium-intracellulare complex infection. Am J Clin Pathol 83:524–527, 1985.

63. Montgomery EA, Meis JM, Frizzera G. Rosai-Dorfman disease of soft tissue. Am J Surg Pathol 16:122–129, 1992.

64. Wenig BM, Devaney K, Bisceglia M. Inflammatory myofibroblastic tumor of the larynx. A clinicopathologic study of eight cases simulating a malignant spindle cell neoplasm. Cancer 76:2217–2229, 1995.

65. Stout AP. Myxoma: the tumor of primitive mesenchyme. Ann Surg 127:706–719, 1948.

66. Miettinen M, Hockerstedt K, Reitamo J, Totterman S. Intramuscular myxoma: a clinicopathological study of twenty-three cases. Am J Clin Pathol 84:265–272, 1985.

67. Hashimoto H, Tsuneyoshi M, Daimaru Y, Enjoji M, Shinohara N. Intramuscular myxoma. A clinicopathologic, immunohistochemical, and electron microscopic study. Cancer 58:740–747, 1986.

68. Kindblom L-G, Angervall L. Histochemical characterization of mucosubstances in bone and soft tissue tumors. Cancer 36:985–994, 1975.

69. Enzinger FM, Weiss SW. Benign soft tissue tumors of uncertain type. In: FM Enzinger, SW Weiss, eds. Soft Tissue Tumors, 3rd ed. St. Louis: Mosby, 1996, pp. 1039–1066.

70. Enzinger FM, Weiss SW. Benign tumors of peripheral nerves. In: FM Enzinger, SW Weiss, eds. Soft Tissue Tumors, 3rd ed. St. Louis: Mosby, 1996, pp. 821–888.

71. Allen PW. Myxoid tumors of soft tissues. Pathol Ann 15(Pt 1):133–192, 1980.

72. Hooper G. Cystic swellings. In: GP Bogumill, EJ Fleegler, eds. Tumors of the Hand and Upper Limb. Edinburgh: Churchill Livingstone, 1993, pp. 172–182.

73. Sonnex TS. Digital myxoid cysts: a review. Cutis 37:89–94, 1986.

74. Kleinert HE, Kutz JE, Fishmen JH, McCraw LH. Etiology and treatment of the so-called mucous cyst of the finger. J Bone Joint Surg A 54:1455–1458, 1972.

75. Enzinger FM. Intramuscular myxoma. A review and follow-up study of 34 cases. Am J Clin Pathol 43:104–113, 1965.

76. Kindblom L-G, Stener B, Angervall L. Intramuscular myxoma. Cancer 34:1737–1744, 1974.

77. Mazabraud A, Semat P, Roze R. A propos de l'association de fibromyxomes des tissus mous a la dyplasie fibreuse des os. Presse Med 75:2223–2228, 1967.

78. Wirth WA, Leavitt D, Enzinger FM. Multiple intramuscular myxomas: another extraskeletal manifestation of fibrous dysplasia. Cancer 27:1167–1173, 1971.

79. Ireland DCR, Soule EH, Ivins JC. Myxoma of somatic soft tissues. A report of 58 patients, 3 with multiple tumors and fibrous dysplasia of bone. Mayo Clin Proc 48:401–410, 1973.

80. Nielsen GP, O'Connell JX, Rosenberg AE. Intramuscular myxoma. A clinicopathologic study of 51 cases with emphasis on hypercellular and hypervascular variants. Am J Surg Pathol 22:1222–1227, 1998.

81. Remstein ED, Goldstein NS, Nascimento AG. Soft tissue myxoma: a histologic and immunohistochemical analysis of 40 cases. Am J Clin Pathol 105:495 (abs.), 1996.

82. Meis JM, Enzinger FM. Juxta-articular myxoma: a clinical and pathologic study of 65 cases. Hum Pathol 23:639–646, 1992.

83. Bennett GE, Shaw MB. Cysts of the semilunar cartilages. Arch Surg 33:92–105, 1936.

84. Ghormley RK, Dockerty MB. Cystic myxomatous tumors about the knee: their relation to cysts of the menisci. J Bone Joint Surg 25:306–318, 1943.

85. Evans HL. Low-grade fibromyxoid sarcoma. A report of two metastasizing neoplasms having a deceptively benign appearance. Am J Clin Pathol 88:615–619, 1987.

86. Evans HL. Low-grade fibromyxoid sarcoma. A report of 12 cases. Am J Surg Pathol 17:595–600, 1993.

87. Steeper TA, Rosai J. Aggressive angiomyxoma of the female pelvis and perineum: report of nine cases of a distinctive type of gynecologic soft-tissue neoplasm. Am J Surg Pathol 7:463–475, 1983.

88. Begin LR, Clement PB, Kirk ME, Jothy S, McCaughey WTE, Ferenczy A. Aggressive angiomyxoma of pelvic soft parts: a clinicopathologic study of nine cases. Hum Pathol 16:621–628, 1985.

89. Skalova A, Michal M, Husek K, Zamecnik M, Leivo I. Aggressive angiomyxoma of the pelvioperineal region: immunohistological and ultrastructural study of seven cases. Am J Dermatopathol 15:446 451, 1993.

90. Fetsch JF, Laskin WB, Lefkowitz M, Kindblom L-G, Meis-Kindblom J. Aggressive angiomyxoma. A clinicopathologic study of 29 female patients. Cancer 78:79–90, 1996.

91. Kazmierczak B, Wanschura S, Meyer-Bolte K, Caselitz J, Meister P, Bartnitzke S, Van de Ven W, Bullerdiek J. Cytogenic and molecular analysis of an aggressive angiomyxoma. Am J Pathol 147:580–585, 1995.

92. Tsang WYW, Chan JKC, Lee KC, Fisher C, Fletcher CDM. Aggressive angiomyxoma. A report of four cases occurring in men. Am J Surg Pathol 16:1059–1065, 1992.

93. Clatch RJ, Drake WK, Gonzalez JG. Aggressive angiomyxoma in men. A report of two cases associated with inguinal hernias. Arch Pathol Lab Med 117:911–913, 1993.

94. Smith HO, Worrell RV, Smith AY, Dorin MH, Rosenberg RD, Bartow SA. Aggressive angiomyxoma of the female pelvis and perineum: review of the literature. Gynecol Oncol 42:79–85, 1991.

95. Hilgers RD, Pai R, Bartow SA, Aisenbrey G, Bowling MC. Aggressive angiomyxoma of the vulva. Obstet Gynecol 68:60S–62S, 1986.

96. Granter SR, Nucci MR, Fletcher CDM. Aggressive angiomyxoma: reappraisal of its relationship to angiomyofibroblastoma in a series of 16 cases. Histopathology 30:3–10, 1997.

97. Fletcher CDM, Tsang WYW, Fisher C, Lee KC, Chan JKC. Angiomyofibroblastoma of the vulva. A benign neoplasm distinct from aggressive angiomyxoma. Am J Surg Pathol 16:373–382, 1992.

98. Laskin WB, Fetsch JF, Mostofi FK. Angiomyofibroblastomalike tumor of the male genital tract. Analysis of 11 cases with comparison to female angiomyofibroblastoma and spindle cell lipoma. Am J Surg Pathol 22:6–16, 1998.

99. Nucci MR, Granter SR, Fletcher CDM. Cellular angiofibroma: a benign neoplasm distinct from angiomyofibroblastoma and spindle cell lipoma. Am J Surg Pathol 21:636–644, 1997.

100. Carney JA, Gordon H, Carpenter PC, Shenoy BV, Go VLW. The complex of myxomas, spotty pigmentation, and endocrine overactivity. Medicine 64:270–283, 1985.

101. Allen PW, Dymock RB, MacCormac LB. Superficial angiomyxomas with and without epithelial components: report of 30 tumors in 28 patients. Am J Surg Pathol 12:519–530, 1988.

102. Fetsch JF, Laskin WB, Tavassoli FA. Superficial angiomyxoma (cutaneous myxoma). A clinicopathologic study of 17 cases arising in the genital region. Int J Gynecol Pathol 16:325–334, 1997.

103. Carney JA. Psammomatous melanotic schwannoma: a distinctive, heritable tumor with special associations, including cardiac myxoma and the Cushing syndrome. Am J Surg Pathol 14:206–222, 1990.

104. Ferreiro JA, Carney JA. Myxomas of the external ear and their significance. Am J Surg Pathol 18:274–280, 1994.
105. Enzinger FM, Weiss SW. Synovial sarcoma. In: FM Enzinger, SW Weiss, eds. Soft Tissue Tumors, 3rd ed. St. Louis: Mosby, 1995, pp. 757–786.
106. Folpe AL, Schmidt RA, Chapman D, Gown AM. Poorly differentiated synovial sarcoma. Immunohistochemical distinction from primitive neuroectodermal tumors and high-grade malignant peripheral nerve sheath tumors. Am J Surg Pathol 22: 673–682, 1998.
107. Fisher C. Synovial sarcoma: ultrastructural and immunohistochemical features of epithelial differentiation in monophasic and biphasic tumors. Hum Pathol 17:996–1008, 1986.
108. Dardick I, Ramjohn S, Thomas MJ, Jeans D, Hammar SP. Synovial sarcoma. Interrelationship of the biphasic and monophasic subtypes. Res Pract 187:871–885, 1991.
109. Guardino M, Christensen L. Immunohistochemical analysis of extracellular matrix components in synovial sarcoma. J Pathol 172:279–286, 1994.
110. Miettinen M, Virtanen I. Synovial sarcoma—a misnomer. Am J Pathol 117:18–25, 1984.
111. Fetsch JF, Meis JM. Intra-articular synovial sarcoma. Mod Pathol 5:6(abs.), 1992.
112. Zeren H, Moran C, Suster S, Fishback NF, Koss MN. Primary pulmonary sarcomas with features of monophasic synovial sarcoma: a clinicopathological, immunohistochemical, and ultrastructural study of 25 cases. Hum Pathol 26:474–480, 1995.
113. Witkin GB, Miettinen M, Rosai J. A biphasic tumor of the mediastinum with features of synovial sarcoma. A report of four cases. Am J Surg Pathol 13:490–499, 1989.
114. Gaertner E, Zeren EH, Fleming MV, Colby TW, Travis WD. Biphasic synovial sarcomas arising in the pleural cavity. A clinicopathologic study of five cases. Am J Surg Pathol 20:36–45, 1996.
115. Fetsch JF, Meis JM. Synovial sarcoma of the abdominal wall. Cancer 72:469–477, 1993.
116. Burke A, Virmani R. Primary cardiac sarcomas. In: A Burke, R Virmani, eds. Tumors of the Heart and Great Vessels. Washington, DC: Armed Forces Institute of Pathology, 1995, pp. 127–170.
117. Nielsen GP, Shaw PA, Rosenberg AE, Dickersin GR, Young RH, Scully RE. Synovial sarcoma of the vulva: a report of two cases. Mod Pathol 9:970–974, 1996.
118. Brodsky JT, Burt ME, Hajdu SI, Casper ES, Brennan MF. Tendosynovial sarcoma. Clinicopathologic features, treatment, and prognosis. Cancer 70:484–489, 1992.
119. Singer S, Baldini EH, Demetri GD, Fletcher JA, Corson JM. Synovial sarcoma: prognostic significance of tumor size, margin of resection, and mitotic activity for survival. J Clin Oncol 14:1201–1208, 1996.
120. Cadman N, Soule E, Kelly P. Synovial sarcoma: an analysis of 134 tumors. Cancer 18:613–627, 1965.
121. Varela-Duran J, Enzinger FM. Calcifying synovial sarcoma. Cancer 50:345–352, 1982.
122. Soule EH. Synovial sarcoma. Am J Surg Pathol 10 (Suppl 1):78–82, 1986.
123. Cagle LA, Mirra JM, Storm FK, Roe DJ, Eilber FR. Histologic features relating to prognosis in synovial sarcoma. Cancer 59:1810–1814, 1987.

124. Oda Y, Hashimoto H, Tsuneyoshi M, Takeshita S. Survival in synovial sarcoma. A multivariate study of prognostic factors with special emphasis on the comparison between early death and long-term survival. Am J Surg Pathol 17:35–44, 1993.

125. Bergh P, Meis-Kindblom JM, Gherlinzoni F, Berlin O, Bacchini P, Bertoni F, Gunterberg B, Kindblom L-G. Synovial sarcoma: identification of low and high risk groups. Cancer 85:2596–2607, 1999.

126. Rooser B, Willen H, Hugoson A, Rydholm A. Prognostic factors in synovial sarcoma. Cancer 63:2182–2185, 1989.

127. El-Naggar AL, Ayala AG, Abdul-Karim FW, McLemore D, Ballance WW, Garnsey L, Ro JY, Batsakis JG. Synovial sarcoma. A DNA flow cytometric study. Cancer 65:2295–2300, 1990.

128. Krall RA, Kostianovsky M, Patchefsky AS. Synovial sarcoma: A clinical, pathological, and ultrastructural study of 26 cases supporting the recognition of a monophasic variant. Am J Surg Pathol 5:137–151, 1981.

129. Zito R. Synovial sarcoma: an Australian series of 48 cases. Pathology 16:45–52, 1984.

130. Crew AJ, Clark J, Fisher C, Gill S, Grimer R, Chand A, Shipley J, Gusterson BA, Cooper CS. Fusion of SYT to two genes, SSX1 and SSX2, encoding proteins with homology to the Kruppel-associated box in human synovial sarcoma. EMBO J 14:2333–2340, 1995.

131. de Leeuw B, Suijkerbuijk RF, Olde Weghuis D, Meloni AM, Stenman G, Kindblom LG, Balemans M, van den Berg E, Sandberg AA et al. Distinct Xp11.2 breakpoints in synovial sarcoma revealed by metaphase and interphase FISH: relationship to histologic subtypes. Cancer Genet Cytogenet 73:89–94, 1994.

132. Kawai A, Woodruff J, Healey JH, Brennan MF, Antonescu CR, Ladanyi M. SYT-SSX gene fusion as a determinant of morphology and prognosis in synovial sarcoma. N Engl J Med 338:153–160, 1998.

133. Krane JF, Bertoni F, Fletcher CD. Myxoid synovial sarcoma: an underappreciated monphologic subset. Mod Pathol 12:456–462, 1999.

134. Meis-Kindblom JM, Stenman G, Kindblom L-G. Differential diagnosis of small round cell tumors. Semin Diagn Pathol 13:213–241, 1996.

135. Folpe AL, Schmidt RA, Chapman D, Gown AM. Poorly differentiated synovial sarcoma. Immunohistochemical distinction from primitive neuroectodermal tumors and high-grade malignant peripheral nerve sheath tumors. Am J Surg Pathol 22: 673–682, 1998.

136. Miettinen M. Keratin subsets in spindle cell sarcomas: keratins are widespread but synovial sarcoma contains a distinctive keratin polypeptide pattern and desmoplakins. Am J Pathol 138:505–513, 1991.

137. Ordonez NG, Mahfouz SM, Mackay B. Synovial sarcoma: an immunohistochemical and ultrastructural study. Hum Pathol 21:733–749, 1990.

138. Corson JM, Weiss LM, Banks-Schlegel SP, Pinkus GS. Keratin proteins and carcinoembryonic antigen in synovial sarcomas: an immunohistochemical study of 24 cases. Hum Pathol 15:615–621, 1984.

139. Hirakawa N, Naka T, Yamamoto I, Fukuda T, Tsuneyoshi M. Overexpression of bcl-2 protein in synovial sarcoma: a comparative study of other soft tissue spindle cell sarcomas and an additional analysis by fluorescence in-situ hybridization. Hum Pathol 27:1060–1065, 1996.

140. DeiTos AP, Wadden C, Calonje E, Sciot R, Pauwels P, Knight JC, Dal Cin P, Fletcher CDM. Immunohistochemical demonstration of glycoprotein p30/32MIC2 (CD99) in synovial sarcoma: a potential cause of diagnostic confusion. Appl Immunohistochem 3:168–173, 1995.

141. Meis-Kindblom JM, Kindblom L-G, Enzinger FM. Sclerosing epithelioid fibrosarcoma. A variant of fibrosarcoma simulating carcinoma. Am J Surg Pathol 19:979–993, 1995.

142. Christensen WN, Strong EW, Bains MS, Woodruff JW. Neuroendocrine differentiation in the glandular peripheral nerve sheath tumor: pathologic distinction from the biphasic synovial sarcoma with glands. Am J Surg Pathol 12:417–426, 1988.

143. Nicholson AG, Goldstraw P, Fisher C. Synovial sarcoma of the pleura and its differentiation from other primary pleural tumours: a clinicopathological and immunohistochemical review of three cases. Histopathology 33:508–513, 1998.

144. Laskowski J. Sarcoma aponeuroticum. Nowotwory 11:61–67, 1961.

145. Enzinger FM. Epithelioid sarcoma. A sarcoma simulating a granuloma or a carcinoma. Cancer 26:1029–1041, 1970.

146. Enzinger FM, Weiss SW. Malignant soft tissue tumors of uncertain type. In: FM Enzinger, SW Weiss, eds. Soft Tissue Tumors, 3rd. ed. St. Louis: Mosby, 1995, pp. 1067–1093.

147. Fisher C. Epithelioid sarcoma: the spectrum of ultrastructural differentiation in seven immunohistochemically defined cases. Hum Pathol 19:265–275, 1988.

148. Quezado MM, Middleton LP, Bryant B, Lane K, Weiss SW, Merino MJ. Allelic loss on chromosome 22Q in epithelioid sarcomas. Hum Pathol 29:604–608, 1998.

149. Chase DR, Enzinger FM. Epithelioid sarcoma. Diagnosis, prognostic indicators, and treatment. Am J Surg Pathol 9:241–263, 1985.

150. Prat J, Woodruff JM, Marcove RC. Epithelioid sarcoma. An analysis of 22 cases indicating the prognostic significance of vascular invasion and regional lymph node metastasis. Cancer 41:1472–1487, 1978.

151. Erdmann MW, Quaba AA, Sommerlad BC. Epithelioid sarcoma masquerading as Dupuytren's disease. Br J Plast Surg 48:39–42, 1995.

152. Moore SW, Wheeler JE, Hefter LG. Epithelioid sarcoma masquerading as Peyronie's disease. Cancer 35:1706–1710, 1975.

153. Dabska M, Koszarowski T. Clinical and pathologic study of aponeurotic (epithelioid) sarcoma. Pathol Annu 17:129–153, 1982.

154. Ross HM, Lewis JJ, Woodruff JM, Brennan MF. Epithelioid sarcoma: clinical behavior and prognostic factors of survival. Ann Surg Oncol 4:491–495, 1997.

155. Halling AC, Wollan PC, Pritchard DJ, Vlasak R, Nascimento AG. Epithelioid sarcoma: a clinicopathologic review of 55 cases. Mayo Clin Proc 71:636–642, 1996.

156. Bos GD, Pritchard DJ, Reiman HM, Dobyns JH, Ilstrup DM, Landon GC. Epithelioid sarcoma. An analysis of fifty-one cases. J Bone Joint Surg A 70:862–870, 1988.

157. Evans HL, Baer SC. Epithelioid sarcoma: a clinicopathologic and prognostic study of 26 cases. Semin Diagn Pathol 10:286–291, 1993.

158. Guillou L, Wadden C, Coindre J-M, Krausz T, Fletcher CDM. "Proximal-type" epithelioid sarcoma, a distinctive aggressive neoplasm showing rhabdoid features. Clinicopathologic, immunohistochemical, and ultrastructural study of a series. Am J Surg Pathol 21:130–146, 1997.

159. Mirra JM, Kessler S, Bhuta S, Eckardt J. The fibroma-like variant of epithelioid sarcoma. A fibrohistiocytic/myoid cell lesion often confused with benign and malignant spindle cell tumors. Cancer 69:1382–1395, 1992.

160. Wick MR, Manivel JC. Epithelioid sarcoma and isolated necrobiotic granuloma: a comparative immunochemical study. J Cutan Pathol 13:253–260, 1986.

161. Daimura Y, Hashimoto H, Tsuneyoshi M, Enjoji M. Epithelial profile of epithelioid sarcoma: an immunohistochemical analysis of eight cases. Cancer 59:134–141, 1987.

162. Arber DA, Kandalaft PL, Mehta P, Battifora H. Vimentin-negative epithelioid sarcoma: the value of an immunohistochemical panel that includes CD34. Am J Surg Pathol 17:302–307, 1993.

163. Meis-Kindblom JM, Kindblom L-G. Angiosarcoma of soft tissue. A study of 80 cases. Am J Surg Pathol 22:683–697, 1998.

164. Ohsawa M, Naka N, Tomita Y, Kawamori D, Kanno H, Aozasa K. Use of immunohistochemical procedures in diagnosing angiosarcoma. Evaluation of 98 cases. Cancer 75:2867–2874, 1995.

165. Mentzel T, Beham A, Calonje E, Katenkamp D, Fletcher CDM. Epithelioid hemangioendothelioma of skin and soft tissues: clinicopathologic and immunohistochemical study of 30 cases. Am J Surg Pathol 21:363–374, 1997.

166. Christopherson WM, Foote FW, Stewart FW. Alveolar soft-part sarcomas: structurally characteristic tumors of uncertain histogenesis. Cancer 5:100–111, 1952.

167. Fisher ER, Reidbord H. Electron microscopic evidence suggesting myogenous derivation of the so-called alveolar soft part sarcoma. Cancer 27:150–159, 1971.

168. Rosai J, Dias P, Parham DM, Shapiro DN, Houghton P. MyoD1 protein expression in alveolar soft part sarcoma as confirmatory evidence of its skeletal muscle nature. Am J Surg Pathol 15:974–981, 1991.

169. Wang NP, Bacchi CE, Jiang JJ, McNutt MA, Gown AM. Does alveolar soft-part sarcoma exhibit skeletal muscle differentiation? An immunocytochemical and biochemical study of myogenic regulatory protein expression. Mod Pathol 9:496–506, 1996.

170. Cullinane C, Thorner PS, Greenberg ML, Kwan Y, Kumar M, Squire J. Molecular genetic, cytogenetic, and immunohistochemical characterization of alveolar soft-part sarcoma. Implications for cell of origin. Cancer 70:2444–2450, 1992.

171. Lieberman PH, Brennan MF, Kimmel M, Erlandson RA, Garin-Chesa P, Flehinger BY. Alveolar soft-part sarcoma. A clinico-pathologic study of half a century. Cancer 63:1–13, 1989.

172. Flieder DB, Moran CA, Suster S. Primary alveolar soft-part sarcoma of the mediastinum: a clinicopathological and immunohistochemical study of two cases. Histopathology 31:469–473, 1997.

173. Nielsen GP, Oliva E, Young RH, Rosenberg AE, Dickersin GR, Scully RE. Alveolar soft-part sarcoma of the female genital tract: a report of nine cases and review of the literature. Int J Gynecol Pathol 14:283–292, 1995.

174. Auerbach HE, Brooks JJ. Alveolar soft part sarcoma. A clinicopathologic and immunohistochemical study. Cancer 60:66–73, 1987.

175. Matsuno Y, Mukai K, Itabashi M, Yamauchi Y, Hirota T, Nakajima T, Shimosato Y. Alveolar soft part sarcoma. A clinicopathologic and immunohistochemical study of 12 cases. Acta Pathologica Japonica 40:199–205, 1990.

176. Pappo AS, Parham DM, Cain A, Luo X, Bowman LC, Furman WL, Rao BN, Pratt CB. Alveolar soft part sarcoma in children and adolescents: clinical features and outcome of 11 patients. Med Pediatr Oncol 26:81–84, 1996.
177. Evans HL. Alveolar soft-part sarcoma. A study of 13 typical examples and one with a histologically atypical component. Cancer 55:912–917, 1985.
178. Jong R, Kandel R, Fornasier V, Bell R, Bedard Y. Alveolar soft part sarcoma: review of nine cases including two cases with unusual histology. Histopathology 32:63–68, 1998.
179. Persson S, Willems JS, Kindblom LG, Angervall L. Alveolar soft part sarcoma. An immunohistochemical, cytologic and electron-microscopic study and a quantitative DNA analysis. Virchows Arch A 412:499–513, 1988.
180. Miettinen M, Ekfors T. Alveolar soft part sarcoma. Immunohistochemical evidence for muscle cell differentiation. Am J Clin Pathol 93:32–38, 1990.
181. Enzinger FM, Weiss SW, Liang CY. Ossifying fibromyxoid tumor of soft parts. A clinicopathologic analysis of 59 cases. Am J Surg Pathol 13:817–827, 1989.
182. Miettinen M. Ossifying fibromyxoid tumor of soft parts. Additional observations of a distinctive soft tissue tumor. Am J Clin Pathol 95:142–149, 1991.
183. Schofield JB, Krausz T, Stamp GWH, Fletcher CDM, Fisher C. Ossifying fibromyxoid tumour of soft parts: immunohistochemical and ultrastructural analysis. Histopathology 22:101–112, 1993.
184. Williams SB, Ellis GL, Meis JM, Heffner DK. Ossifying fibromyxoid tumour (of soft parts) of the head and neck: a clinicopathological and immunohistochemical study of nine cases. J Laryngol Otol 107:75–80, 1993.
185. Yoshida H, Minamizaki T, Yumoto T, Furuse K, Nakadera T. Ossifying fibromyxoid tumor of soft parts. Acta Pathol Jpn 41:480–486, 1991.
186. Kilpatrick SE, Ward WG, Mozes M, Miettinen M, Fukunaga M, Fletcher CDM. Atypical and malignant variants of ossifying fibromyxoid tumor. Clinicopathologic analysis of six cases. Am J Surg Pathol 19:1039–1046, 1995.
187. Schaffler G, Raith J, Ranner G, Weybora W, Jeserschek R. Radiographic appearance of an ossifying fibromyxoid tumor of soft parts. Skel Radiol 26:615–618, 1997.
188. Dabska M. Parachordoma. A new clinicopathologic entity. Cancer 40:1586–1592, 1977.
189. Povysil C, Matejovsky Z. A comparative ultrastructural study of chondrosarcoma, chordoid sarcoma, chordoma and chordoma periphericum. Pathol Res Pract 179:546–559, 1985.
190. Ishida T, Oda H, Oka T, Imamura T, Machinami R. Parachordoma: an ultrastructural and immunohistochemical study. Virchows Arch A 422:239–245, 1993.
191. Shin HJC, Mackay B, Ichinose H, Ayala AG, Romsdahl MM. Parachordoma. Ultrastruct Pathol 18:249–256, 1994.
192. Fisher C, Miettinen M. Parachordoma: A clinicopathologic and immunohistochemical study of four cases of an unusual soft tissue neoplasm. Ann Diagn Pathol 1:3–10, 1997.
193. Hirokawa M, Manabe T, Sugihara K. Parachordoma of the buttock: An immunohistochemical case study and review. Jpn J Clin Oncol 24:336–339, 1994.
194. Sangueza OP, White CR. Parachordoma. Am J Dermatopathol 16:185–188, 1994.

195. Niezabitowski A, Limon J, Wasilewska A, Rys J, Lackowska B, Nedoszytko B. Parachordoma—a clinicopathologic, immunohistochemical, electron microscopic, flow cytometric, and cytogenetic study. Gen Diagn Pathol 141:49–55, 1995.

196. Karabela-Bouropoulou V, Skourtas C, Liapi-Avgeri G, Mahaira H. Parachordoma. A case report of a very rare soft tissue tumor. Pathol Res Pract 192:972–978, 1996.

197. Kilpatrick SE, Hitchcock MG, Kraus MD, Calonje E, Fletcher CDM. Mixed tumors and myoepitheliomas of soft tissue: a clinicopathologic study of 19 cases with a unifying concept. Am J Surg Pathol 21:13–22, 1997.

198. Meis JM, Enzinger FM. Chondroid lipoma. A unique tumor simulating liposarcoma and myxoid chondrosarcoma. A brief report of two cases with ultrastructural analysis. Am J Surg Pathol 17:1103–1112, 1993.

199. Kindblom L-G, Meis-Kindblom JM. Chondroid lipoma: an ultrastructural and immunohistochemical analysis with further observations regarding its differentiation. Hum Pathol 26:706–715, 1995.

200. Beckwith JB, Palmer NF. Histopathology and prognosis of Wilms' tumor: results from the First National Wilms' Tumor Study. Cancer 41:1937–1948, 1978.

201. Haas JE, Palmer NF, Weinberg AG, Beckwith JB. Ultrastructure of malignant rhabdoid tumor of the kidney: a distinctive renal tumor of children. Hum Pathol 12:646–657, 1981.

202. White FV, Dehner LP, Belchis DA, Conard K, Davis MM, Stocker JT, Zuppan CW, Biegel JA, Perlman EJ. Congenital disseminated malignant rhabdoid tumor. A distinct clinicopathologic entity demonstrating abnormalities of chromosome 22q11. Am J Surg Pathol 23:249–256, 1999.

203. Kodet R, Newton WA, Sachs N, Hamoudi AB, Raney RB, Asmar L, Gehan EA. Rhabdoid tumors of soft tissues: a clinicopathologic study of 26 cases enrolled on the intergroup rhabdomyosarcoma study. Hum Pathol 22:674–684, 1991.

204. Fanburg-Smith JC, Hengge M, Hengge UR, Smith JSC, Miettinen M. Extrarenal rhabdoid tumors of soft tissue: A clinicopathologic and immunohistochemical study of 18 cases. Ann Diagn Pathol 2:351–362, 1998.

205. Smith MEF, Fisher C, Weiss SW. Pleomorphic hyalinizing angiectatic tumor of soft parts. A low-grade neoplasm resembling neurilemoma. Am J Surg Pathol 20:21–29, 1996.

206. Mentzel T, Fletcher CDM. Recent advances in soft tissue tumor diagnosis. Am J Clin Pathol 110:660–670, 1998.

15
Pediatric Small-Cell Tumors of Soft Tissue

David M. Parham
University of Arkansas for Medical Sciences and
Arkansas Children's Hospital Research Institute
Little Rock, Arkansas

I. INTRODUCTION

Small-cell tumors of childhood are a clinically distinct category of tumors sharing a number of important characteristics that set them apart from other soft-tissue neoplasms. These highly malignant cancers share a common cardinal feature of histologically and biologically recapitulating the primitive, multipotential nature of embryonal tissue; hence, they are often referred to as "embryonal" neoplasms. In fact, these tumors are not uncommonly found in neonates and abortuses (1,2). Because embryonal tissues exhibit little to no terminal differentiation, this cardinal property of small-cell tumors can lead to considerable diagnostic difficulty resolvable only by ancillary techniques, such as electron microscopy, immunohistochemical staining, and cytogenetics/molecular genetics (3).

   Small-cell neoplasms can arise in and recapitulate the embryogenesis of virtually every organ, a phenomenon best theorized by Sir Rupert Willis. In his classic text, *The Borderland of Embryology and Pathology* (4), Willis described embryonic tumors as arising during embryonic, fetal, or early postnatal development from an immature organ rudiment (Table 1) and recognized their fundamental differences from cancers of mature adult tissues. Although the latter concept is correct, the former one is overstated in that small-cell neoplasms may arise in adult tissues that undergo regressive transformation as a result of genetic perturbations, so that "embryonal neoplasms" uncommonly occur in adults (2,5). Diagnostic

TABLE 1A Embryonic Tumors Discussed by Willis (4)

Organ	Derivative tumor
Sympathetic neuron	Neuroblastoma
CNS neuron	Medulloblastoma/neuroepithelioma
Eye	Retinoblastoma
Kidney	Nephroblastoma (Wilms tumor)
Liver	Hepatoblastoma
Soft tissue/skeletal muscle	Rhabdomyosarcoma

TABLE 1B Other Embryonic Tumors

Organ	Derivative tumor
Lung	Pleuropulmonary blastoma
Salivary gland	Sialoblastoma/salivary gland anlage tumor
Pancreas	Pancreatoblastoma
Germ cells	Germinoma/embryonal carcinoma
Placenta	Choriocarcinoma
Yolk sac	Yolk sac tumor
Mesothelium	Desmoplastic small-cell tumor?
Parasympathetic neuron	Ewing sarcoma/peripheral neuroectodermal tumor
Fat	Lipoblastoma

confusion is compounded in adults, who are more commonly susceptible to a wide variety of small-cell carcinomas.

Of the small-cell tumors, sarcomas comprise a relatively common and clinically important category of pediatric and adolescent cancers, surpassed in frequency in the United States only by leukemia/lymphoma, brain tumors, and neuroblastomas (6). By far the most common lesion of this class is the rhabdomyosarcoma; however, others, such as peripheral neuroectodermal tumor and desmoplastic small-cell tumor, are not as uncommon as one might expect (7). Separation of these morphologically overlapping tumors is critical to proper therapy and prognosis as well as to assignment to various multi-institutional protocols (8). During the past several decades, many strides have been made in the successful management of these highly malignant lesions, but adequate diagnosis is key to this process.

A major factor that directly affects the outcome of sarcoma patients is early tumor recognition, as lower stage patients have better survival and require less morbid treatment. Unfortunately, failure to consider these tumors in the clinical differential diagnosis of various masses has led to many instances of delayed treatment. A similar failure may occur at the histologic level if biopsies contain inadequate or crushed material or if the pathologist fails to consider these often treacherous lesions as possible diagnoses. Thus, a primary rule is to always consider the possibility of sarcoma in pediatric masses, particularly if the patient fails early conservative therapy. Also, pathologists must be willing to obtain additional studies or seek more experienced consultation if clinical suspicion is high.

II. RHABDOMYOSARCOMA

A. Classification

Rhabdomyosarcoma constitutes the largest subgroup of pediatric soft-tissue sarcomas, comprising from 80% to 90% of reported cases in this category (9). Although the name implies that these tumors arise from striated muscle, in fact a large number of them arise from areas devoid of this tissue, such as the urinary bladder, prostate, common bile duct, and vagina. Thus, the term actually reflects the tendency of the tumors to *form* skeletal myoblasts rather than *originate* from the musculoskeletal system.

The larger category of rhabdomyosarcoma is composed of a series of subcategories defined by histologic features. This heterogeneity was recognized in the 1950s by several groups, who subclassified rhabdomyosarcoma into embryonal, alveolar, botryoid, and pleomorphic subtypes (10). The histologic category of the tumor was soon found to correspond to clinical groupings, as discussed below, and more recently it has become apparent that they correlate with genetic features, as will also be discussed. The implication is that the generic diagnosis "rhabdomyosarcoma" encompasses a group of biologically dissimilar entities, all of which have a tendency to recapitulate the myogenesis pathway of embryonic tissues.

In more recent years, particularly the 1980s, it became apparent that there were imperfections in the rhabdomyosarcoma classification scheme. Several independent groups of investigators noted that the alveolar category could be expanded to encompass cytologically similar but histologically dissimilar tumors (11). Similarly, it was found that the embryonal category could be further subdivided into more differentiated spindle cell lesions dissimilar from typical embryonal lesions (12,13) and might encompass lesions without overt myogenesis (14). Concurrently, the development of biological means of confirmation gave credence to some of these observations (15), and the existence of a large multi-institutional database and slide depository, the Intergroup Rhabdomyosarcoma Study, lent a means of testing and verification (16,17). As a result, a modern international classification of rhabdomyosarcomas has been formulated and is in current use by the Intergroup Rhabdomyosarcoma Study Group (IRSG) (Table 2). The following discussion will offer further elucidation.

TABLE 2   International Classification of Pediatric Rhabdomyosarcoma (17)[a]

Embryonal rhabdomyosarcoma [includes embryonal sarcoma (14)]
Alveolar rhabdomyosarcoma (includes solid variants)
Botryoid rhabdomyosarcoma
Spindle cell rhabdomyosarcoma
Rhabdomyosarcoma, not otherwise classified
Undifferentiated sarcoma
Sarcoma, not classifiable

[a]Pleomorphic rhabdomyosarcoma, though the most common form of adult rhabdomyosarcoma, is vanishingly rare in children and is not included in this pediatric classification.

B. Clinical Features

Because rhabdomyosarcomas may arise virtually anywhere within the body, their presenting clinical features are protean. For more detailed information, the reader is referred to the excellent review by Ruymann (18). However, unlike some soft-tissue lesions, clinical manifestations are generally related to mass effect, and systemic symptoms are rare. One reported systemic effect has been hypercalcemia caused by tumor secretion of a parathormone-like substance (19).

Clinical symptomatology may be related to the affected organ system. Orbital soft tissue is a relatively common site of origin and presents as proptosis and diplopia. Parameningeal tumors often cause neurologic defects related to pressure on the spinal cord. Urinary tract tumors arising within the bladder or prostate typically present as urinary retention. Cervicovaginal tumors cause vaginal bleeding, and large extruding masses may be evident. Painless growing masses are typical of extremity tumors. Biliary tumors lead to jaundice, and nasal/paranasal lesions may cause obstructive symptoms. The rare cardiac lesions are associated with valvular dysfunction and filling defects, causing congestive heart failure and fetal demise (1).

Of particular note is that occasional extremely aggressive lesions may present with widespread bone marrow metastases lacking an apparent primary source (20). These are generally alveolar rhabdomyosarcomas that create diagnostic confusion with hematologic malignancies (21). The dilemma may be compounded by the rare ability of these tumors to express B-cell markers (22).

In predicting clinical behavior and prognosis, stage, histology, and site of origin are the most important considerations. Stage can be expressed either as a surgicopathologic grouping (Table 3) or clinical stage (Table 4). Grouping (Table 3) has been the traditional method of separating patients into treatment groups and is based on combined surgical, pathologic, and radiologic determination of residual tumor burden following surgery. However, outcome variables re-

TABLE 3   Rhabdomyosarcoma Surgicopathologic Grouping (148)

Group 1
- Localized tumors, completely excised
  A. Confined to the organ or muscle of origin
  B. Infiltration outside organ or muscle; regional lymph nodes not involved

Group 2
- Tumors with compromised or regional resection, including:
  A. Tumors grossly excised but with microscopic residual (i.e., positive microscopic margins)
  B. Regional disease, completely excised, but with regional lymph node involvement or extension to an adjacent organ
  C. Regional disease with involved lymph nodes, macroscopically resected but with microscopic residual

Group 3
- Tumors with incomplete resection or biopsy and gross residual disease

Group 4
- Tumors with distant metastases at presentation

lated to tumor site and degree of invasiveness has led to a rhabdomyosarcoma-specific staging system (Table 4). This system is based on behavioral aspects of this neoplasm that give superior predictions for planning multiagent therapy and surgical approach.

Histology repeatedly has also been shown to be predictive of rhabdomyosarcoma therapy response and clinical outcome (17,23), independent of clinical grouping. To some degree this observation reflects the tendency of certain histologies to occur in particular sites and ages. As examples, rhabdomyosarcomas are most common in head and neck and genitourinary lesions arising in young children, whereas alveolar rhabdomyosarcomas are most common in extremity and parameningeal lesions arising in adolescents and young adults. Nevertheless, even within a given site of origin, histology has significant prognostic significance (13,24).

Over the past century, the prognosis for embryonal rhabdomyosarcomas has changed remarkably. This trend is illustrated dramatically by comparing outcomes for the large consecutive trials directed by the IRSG (25), which has been a leader in the search for more effective means of surgery, diagnosis, radiotherapy, and chemotherapy. This multi-institutional group was founded in 1972 by combining sarcoma sections of the Pediatric Oncology Group and the Children's Cancer Study Group in an effort to standardize therapy and diagnosis and to accumulate a sufficient number of patients for timely statistical analysis of prospective

TABLE 4A Rhabdomyosarcoma TNM Pretreatment Staging System (148)

Stage	Sites	T	Tumor size	N	M
I	Orbit	T1 or T2	a or b	N0 or N1 or Nx	M0
	Head and neck (excluding parameningeal)				
	GU–nonbladder/nonprostate				
II	Bladder/prostate	T1 or T2	a	N0 or Nx	M0
	Extremity				
	Head and neck parameningeal				
	Other (including trunk, retroperitoneum, etc.)				
III	Bladder/prostate	T1 or T2	a	N1	M0
	Extremity		b	N0 or N1 or Nx	
	Head and neck parameningeal				
	Other (including trunk, retroperitoneum, etc.)				
IV	All	T1 or T2	a or b	N0 or N1	M1

GU, genitourinary; for definitions of T, N, and M, see text.

TABLE 4B Definitions of T, N, and M Classifications

Classification	Description
Tumor	
T1	Confined to anatomical site of origin
A	<5 cm in diameter
B	≥5 cm in diameter
T2	Extended into or fixed in surrounding tissue
A	<5 cm in diameter
B	≥5 cm in diameter
Regional lymph nodes	
N0	Regional lymph nodes not clinically involved
N1	Regional lymph nodes clinically involved
Nx	Clinical status of regional lymph nodes unknown
Metastasis	
M0	No distant metastasis
M1	Metastasis present

trials. Since that time, outcome for group 3 embryonal rhabdomyosarcoma treated with IRSG therapy improved from an overall 5-year survival rate of 50% (8) to a progression-free 5-year survival rate of 65% (26), in papers published in 1988 and 1995, respectively. Additional data from IRS-IV promises even more remarkable gains.

Unfortunately, the gains made in successfully treating embryonal rhabdomyosarcoma have not been matched by similar success with alveolar rhabdomyosarcoma, although the more aggressive therapy used with the latter tumors on IRS-III appear to ameliorate some of the differences in outcome (26). Newer agents are needed for these aggressive lesions, which paradoxically appear to show good initial response in some studies (24), only to recur with untamable ferocity and relentlessness.

Conversely, the substantial improvements in outcome seen with embryonal rhabdomyosarcoma have lead to cautious attempts to limit therapy, which can have considerable morbidity. For example, successfully treated patients with paratesticular rhabdomyosarcomas have suffered abdominal adhesions, lymphedema, and sterility (27), and bladder tumor patients treated by exenteration are at risk for the infections and other complications attendant on ileal diversion (28). Surgical questions have thus focused on limited bladder excision and lymph node staging. Similarly, chemotherapeutic agents effective with rhabdomyosarcoma are also associated with neuropathy, deafness, Fanconi's syndrome, pancytopenia, and second malignancies (29), so that limiting therapy without decreasing effectiveness again becomes a desirable goal.

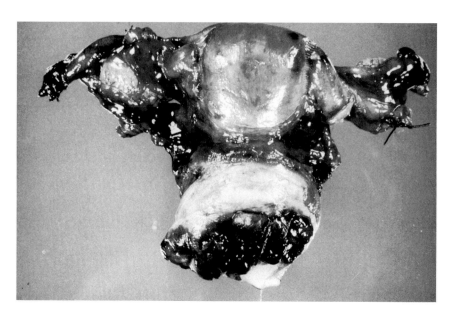

FIG. 1 Botryoid rhabdomyosarcoma of the upper vagina. A hemorrhagic, grape-like, polypoid mass protrudes from the vagina os of this resected uterus and fallopian tubes.

C. Gross Appearance

Rhabdomyosarcomas, like most small-cell neoplasms, are generally fleshy, nondescript, pale gray–yellow masses punctuated by areas of necrosis and hemorrhage. They insidiously invade adjacent tissues, so that microscopic areas of marginal involvement may be apparent even with grossly resected lesions. It thus generally behooves the surgeon to perform a standard cancer operation with wide margins if possible and to remove previous biopsy tracks. However, in areas such as the orbit, total exenteration is impractical, mutilating, and unnecessary, so that therapy must be tailored to fit the clinical and anatomical circumstances.

Of particular note is the gross appearance of the botryoid variant of rhabdomyosarcoma, so named for its resemblance to a cluster of grapes (Fig. 1). This tumor arises exclusively along mucosa-lined surfaces, such as the bladder or vagina, and externally situated examples may arise from the conjunctiva. Because of its distinctive topography, botryoid rhabdomyosarcoma produces remarkable images with computed tomography (CT). Whether these lesions represent embryonal rhabdomyosarcoma with mucosal involvement or constitute a separate entity has been debated, but there are no genetic data to date that indicate a difference. Nevertheless, botryoid rhabdomyosarcoma has a statistically proven superior prognosis (30), although it is difficult to completely discount the effects of site in the ex-

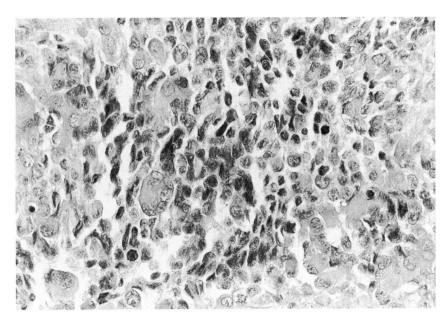

FIG. 2 Rhabdomyosarcoma. In this photomicrograph, numerous rhabdomyoblasts are present. They are recognized by their content of abundant cytoplasm with eccentric nuclei. Multinucleated forms can be seen.

cellent outcome. Of interest is that myogenous Wilms' tumor also produces this botryoid morphology when it involves the renal pelvis (31).

D. Microscopic Appearance

The primary distinguishing characteristic of rhabdomyosarcoma is its capacity for myogenesis at the microscopic level. This proclivity to manufacture muscle is manifested as a defining cell, the rhabdomyoblast. Rhabdomyoblasts are characterized by the progressive acquisition of a brightly pink cytoplasm that reflects their content of myofilament proteins (Fig. 2). This process is typically exhibited in a heterogeneous fashion indicative of variable levels of myofilament expression among tumor cells. At the more differentiated end of the spectrum, rhabdomyoblasts acquire microscopically visible cytoplasmic cross striations that result from the submicroscopic alignment of myofilaments in register. At the less differentiated (and unfortunately more common) end of the spectrum, the cells show minimal if any cytoplasmic pinkness, so that ancillary methods of demonstrating myogenesis are often necessary for diagnostic confirmation. This difficulty may be compounded in small samples.

As with many high-grade cancers, the tumor cells of rhabdomyosarcoma acquire unusual and peculiar shapes that render them a caricature of their derivative normal tissues. Rhabdomyoblasts thus occur in a variety of odd forms, such as tadpole cells, racquet cells, strap cells, spider cells, and multinucleated giant cells. The multinucleated giant cells may contain nuclei arranged in a tandem fashion, reflecting the normal embryonic formation of multinucleated myofibers. Cytoplasmic glycogen is often abundant and may be manifested as clear cytoplasm rather than pink (32). This feature has been used diagnostically with the periodic acid–Schiff (PAS) stain, which imbues glycogenated cells with a bright mauve color that is removed with diastase digestion. In contradistinction, morphologically similar neoplasms, such as lymphomas and neuroblastomas, generally do not contain glycogen, though exceptions do occur (33).

After finding clear evidence of myogenesis, diagnosis of rhabdomyosarcoma then becomes a matter of histologic subclassification, which is critical to both therapy and prognosis. Table 2 lists the classification scheme in current use by the IRSG. Most crucial to therapy is proper recognition of the alveolar subtype. Although prognostically diverse, the other histologies are currently lumped together for treatment purposes.

The most common subtype of rhabdomyosarcoma is embryonal rhabdomyosarcoma. This lesion is named for its remarkable resemblance to developing muscle in embryos and fetuses. Just as embryonal skeletal musculature appears to condense out of a primordial soup of gelatinous matrix and primitive mesenchyme, so embryonal rhabdomyosarcoma is typified by alternating areas of cellular condensation and laxity, with cells floating in a sea of primitive mucoid ground substance (Fig. 3A). Analogous to the variable appearance of the developing musculoskeletal system, these tumors may exhibit a heterogeneous degree of differentiation, matrix, and cellularity from case to case or even within individual tumors. Under the influence of differentiation agents, such as oncolytic drugs, x-irradiation, cyclic AMP, or *cis*-retinoic acid, the cells may terminally differentiate into mature myoblasts that histologically resemble normal muscle cells (34). This phenomenon can lead to diagnostic dilemmas during microscopic examination of posttreatment excisions or biopsies, as tumor cells may not be separable from entrapped normal muscle (Fig. 3B). Although some data indicate that these terminally differentiated cells are essentially benign (35), further experience is needed to verify that reentry into the cell cycle and malignant behavior does not occur. This may be a particular issue when planning postexcision therapy and follow-up of patients with microscopically positive margins consisting only of differentiated tumor cells.

Mention must be made of embryonal sarcoma, a category of soft-tissue sacoma described by the Societé Internationale d'Oncologie Pédiatrique (SIOP) (14,36). This particular species of pediatric sarcoma (not related to embryonal sar-

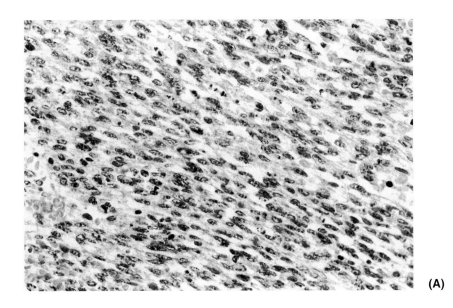

(A)

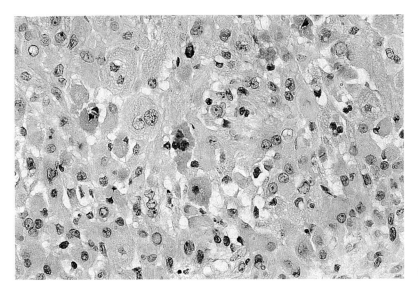

(B)

FIG. 3 Embryonal rhabdomyosarcoma. (A) At biopsy, this tumor contains primitive spindle cells arrayed with varying degrees of condensation, reminiscent of developing skeletal muscle. (B) This tumor, which was excised following combination chemotherapy, shows differentiation of myoblasts into more mature myotubes and myofibers. There is abundant fibrillar cytoplasm.

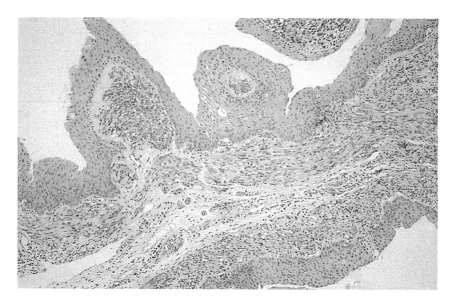

FIG. 4 Botryoid rhabdomyosarcoma. A condensation of tumor cells, or cambium layer, abuts the squamous epithelial lining of this tumor.

coma of the liver) is characterized histologically by a resemblance to embryonal rhabdomyosarcoma but lacks definite histologic evidence of myogenesis. Theoretically, it represents the most primitive end of the mesenchymal spectrum of embryonal rhabdomyosarcoma, and muscle proteins may be demonstrable by immunohistochemical means. It has thus been included in the embryonal rhabdomyosarcoma category in the International Classification. Of note is that it appears to have a better prognosis than typical embryonal rhabdomyosarcoma (36).

A more responsive variant of rhabdomyosarcoma is the botryoid tumor. Just as it displays a typical gross appearance that resembles a cluster of grapes, so botryoid rhabdomyosarcoma should exhibit a key histologic feature, the cambium layer (Fig. 4). A cambium layer comprises a subepithelial condensation of tumor cells, so named for its resemblance to the more rapidly growing woody layer of a tree subjacent to its bark. In the current International Classification (17), this feature is necessary for diagnosis, although mucosal erosion overlying the tumor can obscure its recognition. Happily, only focal epithelial condensation is sufficient. As stated above, patients with botryoid rhabdomyosarcoma enjoy a better clinical outlook than those with other subtypes (30).

Spindle cell rhabdomyosarcoma is another subtype that is associated with a superior clinical behavior among tumors of this class. However, spindle cell variants arise almost exclusively in the paratesticular region, a site with independently

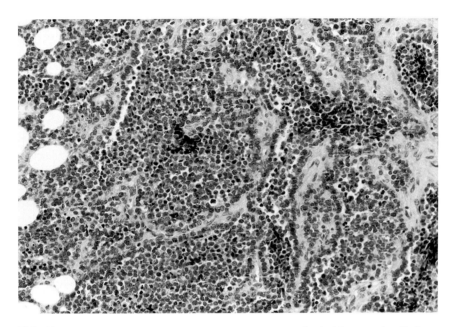

FIG. 5 Alveolar rhabdomyosarcoma. Dense aggregates of primitive round cells form nests subtended by fibrous septa, from which the cells hang in a picket fence pattern.

better prognosis, so that an argument might again be made that this observation is site-dependent. Nevertheless, within the total group of paratesticular rhabdomyosarcomas, spindle cell tumors show a less aggressive clinical behavior (12,13). Grossly, spindle cell rhabdomyosarcomas have a fibrous, whorled appearance more akin to fibrosarcoma than to embryonal tumor, and that analogy is also true microscopically. These tumors are more differentiated than the usual rhabdomyosarcoma and exhibit a heavy content of muscle proteins by immunohistochemistry (12). They histologically mimic other spindle cell sarcomas, as storiform areas may resemble fibrous histiocytoma and wavy neuroid foci may mimic nerve sheath tumors. Scattered individual round cells with larger, atypical nuclei or multinucleated giant cells with bright pink cytoplasm often punctuate these wavy and whorled bundles of spindle cells. The molecular basis for this particular variant of rhabdomyosarcoma is uncertain at present, but its clinical, morphologic, and immunohistochemical distinctiveness cannot be denied.

Contrasting with the relative benignity and cellular differentiation of spindle cell rhabdomyosarcoma is the alveolar rhabdomyosarcoma, which is accorded special treatment status and research priority because of its aggressive, inexorable behavior. Microscopically, alveolar rhabdomyosarcomas are highly cellular, aggressive-appearing lesions that typically form nests separated by a prominent framework of fibrovascular septa (Fig. 5). From this fibrous buttress hang rows of tumor cells that are suspended in a "picket fence" arrangement, with loss of tumor cell cohesion in the periphery of the alveolar nests and increased cohesion in their central portions. The majority of tumor cells are usually poorly differentiated with little cytoplasm, but scattered multinucleated tumor giant cells are common.

Although recognition of this nested pattern with fibrous septa has been the diagnostic sine qua non of alveolar rhabdomyosarcoma for decades, it has become apparent that these foci may be missing in small biopsies and even absent in some cases. Otherwise these "solid variants" show the crowded, highly cellular, undifferentiated round cell cytohistologic features of typical alveolar tumors. This concept has been met with some degree of skepticism, but the fact remains that solid alveolar rhabdomyosarcomas have biological features and clinical behavior identical to those of typical alveolar rhabdomyosarcomas (11,15). They are thus included in this diagnostic category in the current International Classification (Table 2).

Pleomorphic rhabdomyosarcoma is the most common variant in adults, but it is so rare in children that it is not included in the current classification scheme. Childhood examples usually include at least a focal embryonal component (30). These tumors have gone in and out of fashion like hemlines, with some disputing their existence (37). Because biological markers confirm their myogenesis (38), they are currently in vogue. The controversy centers on their similarity to malignant fibrous histiocytoma, another hotly disputed concept (39). Regardless of nosology, pleomorphic rhabdomyosarcomas have a distinctive whorled appearance accented by large plump spindle cells with eosinophilic cytoplasm, and a myogenous phenotype can be demonstrated by immunohistochemical and electron microscopic examination (37,38). Cytoplasmic cross-striations are occasionally present. In contrast to juvenile rhabdomyosarcomas, which are composed of small cells, these lesions contain large cells akin to other adult spindle cell sarcomas.

An overlapping concept between pleomorphic rhabdomyosarcoma and juvenile rhabdomyosarcoma is anaplastic rhabdomyosarcoma. Anaplasia may occur focally or diffusely in rhabdomyosarcoma and is defined by the present of enlarged cells with hyperchromatic, angry-appearing nuclei and often bizarre, multipolar mitoses (Fig. 6). These cytologic changes are sometimes seen in other pediatric tumors, such as Wilms' tumor (40) and neuroblastoma (41), and they may occur in any variety of rhabdomyosarcoma. When anaplasia occurs diffusely, it portends a poor prognosis, whereas focal anaplasia has less significance (42). At present, anaplastic rhabdomyosarcoma is not listed in the International Classification and does not determine therapy, but its occurrence is being following in present in IRSG pathology reviews for possible future action. Biologically, anaplasia likely signifies a malignant progression similar to that seen in Wilms' tumor (43).

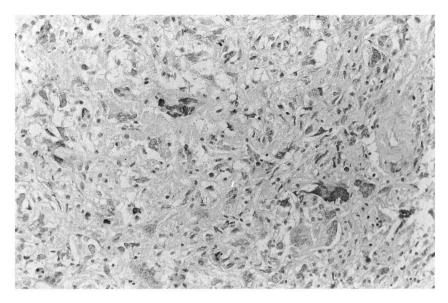

FIG. 6 Anaplastic rhabdomyosarcoma. This rhabdomyosarcoma contains scattered large cells with distorted, markedly hyperchromatic nuclei.

Mention must be made of other diagnostic categories used by the International Classification, i.e., rhabdomyosarcoma, not otherwise specified; sarcoma, not otherwise specified; and undifferentiated sarcoma. Rhabdomyosarcoma, not otherwise specified, refers to those biopsies that contain rhabdomyoblasts but that have limited material, thus precluding further characterization. Similarly, sarcoma, not otherwise specified, refers to lesions that contain limited material without definitive rhabdomyoblasts but with cells resembling rhabdomyosarcoma. Both of these categories generally represent rhabdomyosarcomas, but with biopsies with scant material or abundant artifact or cellular degeneration; the patients from these groups are placed on study but without further pathologic categorization. On the other hand, undifferentiated sarcomas generally contain adequate material, but they consist of primitive cells that lack sufficient morphologic or biological differentiation for further categorization. These lesions cannot be proven at present to be rhabdomyosarcomas and probably represent a mixed bag of high-grade pediatric sarcomas. Regardless of nosology, in IRS-I and II they composed a group with poor clinical outcome similar to alveolar rhabdomyosarcoma (44).

The IRSG now recognizes a group of rare and unusual lesions that express features of both muscle cells and nerve cells, i.e., ectomesenchymomas. At one end of the spectrum, these comprise spindle cell or embryonal rhabdomyosarcomas containing scattered mature ganglion cells. Conversely, primitive lesions with peripheral primitive neuroectodermal tumor–like areas may coexist with primitive rhabdomyosarcoma, either alveolar or embryonal. Their behavior generally correlates with the histologic pattern of rhabdomyosarcoma (45). Immunohistochemistry and electron microscopy may be used to confirm the coexistence of two cell types, and molecular biological studies have intriguingly demonstrated features of either alveolar rhabdomyosarcoma, peripheral primitive neuroectodermal tumor (PNET) (see below), or both (46,47). One hypothetical reason for the development of these tumors is that neuroectoderm forms muscle and other mesenchymal tissues in the head (48); another is that transcription factors responsible for the formation of muscle and nerve have similar molecular structures and substrates, and neoplastic transformation might be associated with aberrant gene activation independent of cell lineage (49).

E. Ancillary Studies

Because of their often primitive nature, rhabdomyosarcomas can easily be mistaken for a variety of other small-cell neoplasms. In previous decades, diagnosis was resolved by prolonged and often futile searches for cross-striations. Happily, in the current era there are a number of ancillary techniques that may be used to demonstrate myogenesis; the liberality with which these are applied generally depends on the experience of the surgical pathologist, as these tumors are unusual in general practice. Unfortunately, caveats exist for any given technique.

1.   Electron Microscopy

Electron microscopy was perhaps the earliest technique to be used for ancillary diagnosis of rhabdomyosarcoma, as bundles of "thick" (15-nm) myosin and "thin" (6-nm) actin filaments in hexagonal arrays could be found in cells lacking microscopic cross-striations (Fig. 7). However, as the histologic diagnostic criteria for rhabdomyoblasts loosened, so did the utility of electron microscopy, for cells that are well-differentiated ultrastructurally are usually recognizable microscopically. Earlier ultrastructural stages of myogenesis were then defined, and the sine qua non has become complexes of thick (myosin) filaments associated with free ribosomes (50). Even earlier mesenchymal stages have been described (51), but there is potential overlap with other primitive sarcomas using these criteria. Nevertheless, experienced electron microscopists can attain diagnostic sensitivity and specificity that rivals other techniques (52).

2.   Immunohistochemistry

Special stains have long been used to augment the diagnosis of rhabdomyosarcoma; these stains include the PAS reaction to demonstrate glycogen and the phosphotungstic acid-hematoxylin (PTAH) to demonstrate cross-striations. With

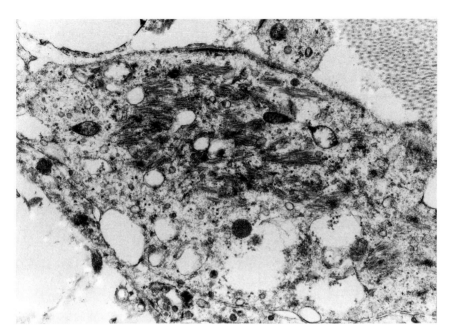

FIG. 7 Electron micrograph of rhabdomyosarcoma cell. The cell contains disorganized cytoplasmic bundles of thick and thin filaments.

the advent of immunohistochemistry came a new concept: the demonstration of muscle-specific proteins by use of antibodies that were then tagged using fluorescent or enzymatic dyes. Using this methodology, unique muscle proteins, such as myoglobin, titin, dystrophin, desmin, and creatine kinase M, can be visualized (Fig. 8), and muscle cells are replete with a host of energy transfer and filamentous proteins designed for contraction and locomotion. Similar to creatine kinase, muscle-specific isoenzymes of various filamentous proteins, such as actin and myosin, broaden the diagnostic armamentarium. More recently, a family of muscle protein transcription promoters has been discovered that includes MyoD and myogenin; these act by binding to DNA and initiating the molecular events leading to the formation of the aforementioned muscle-specific proteins. In this manner, it is possible to visualize proteins like MyoD (Fig. 9), which are formed early in the myogenesis pathway, and proteins like myogenin, which are created later (34).

The major problem with this scenario of diagnostic "magic bullets" has been their ability to repeatedly find their target (i.e., sensitivity) and not hit others (i.e., specificity). Some proteins, like myoglobin, are found primarily in differentiated cells and so are of little utility in primitive tumors. Others, like muscle-

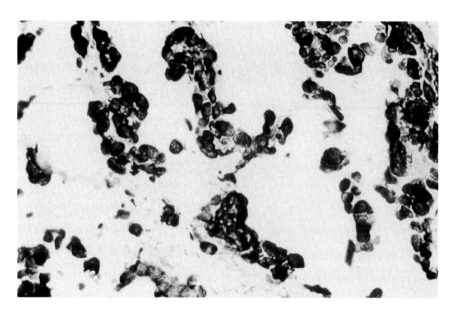

FIG. 8 Desmin immunostain of rhabdomyosarcoma. The product of the immunostaining reaction forms a dark precipitate that deeply colors the cytoplasm of the tumor cells and indicates the presence of abundant desmin protein.

specific actin, are actually shared by all muscle cells, including smooth and cardiac muscle and myogenic hybrids like myofibroblasts and myoepithelial cells. Nonspecific cytoplasmic staining and decreased sensitivity result from use of paraffin-embedded tissues rather than frozen materials for MyoD staining (53). Unexpected desmin staining rarely may be seen with primitive neural tumors (54), and newer methods to improve its detection have decreased its specificity (55). Yet in spite of these caveats, immunohistochemical evaluation is currently the most popular approach to verification of rhabdomyosarcoma diagnosis, and it generally works well and requires a comparative minimum of technical and professional time if automated immunostaining is employed.

3. Cytogenetics/Molecular Genetics

The newest additions to the diagnostic array for rhabdomyosarcoma are the complementary tools of cytogenetics and molecular genetics. Molecular genetics using the polymerase chain reaction (PCR) has an incredible amount of sensitivity and specificity, with a turnaround time comparable to that of histologic methods. Cytogenetics still requires several days to weeks for tumor cells to grow in vitro, and it is often unsuccessful if insufficient tumor tissue is submitted, if bacterial

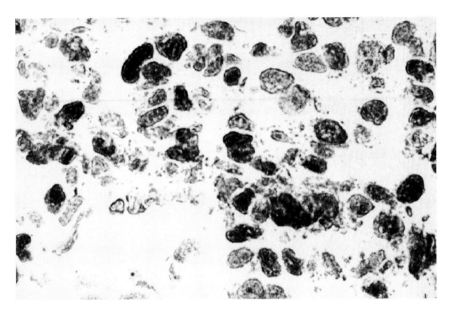

FIG. 9   MyoD immunostain of rhabdomyosarcoma. In this immunostain, the reaction product is localized to the tumor cell nuclei, whose dark color indicates the presence of MyoD protein.

contamination occurs, or if normal tissue is submitted instead or overgrows the neoplastic component. However, it is much less susceptible to contamination by other specimens than PCR methods, which require a high degree of fastidiousness and vigilance.

The value of either technique to rhabdomyosarcoma diagnosis is limited to alveolar rhabdomyosarcoma, which displays a characteristic fusion between the *PAX3* gene on chromosome 2 and the *FKHR* gene of chromosome 13, visualized by standard karyotyping as the t(2;13)(q35;q14) (Fig. 10). This translocation fuses two DNA-binding transcription factors and appears to cause the abnormal cell proliferation (56). Another *PAX* gene, *PAX7*, located on chromosome 1, may also fuse with the *FKHR* gene and produce alveolar rhabdomyosarcomas containing a similar aberrant fusion gene, the t(1;13)(p36;q14) (Fig. 11). Although similar in molecular composition and in tumorigenesis, the two translocations are dissimilar in affected patient age, stage, location, and metastatic pattern, with t(1;13)(p36;q14) lesions representing less aggressive tumors and occurring in younger children (57).

In order to demonstrate these genes using molecular genetics, the standard approach has been to utilize reverse transcriptase (RT), an enzyme discovered in

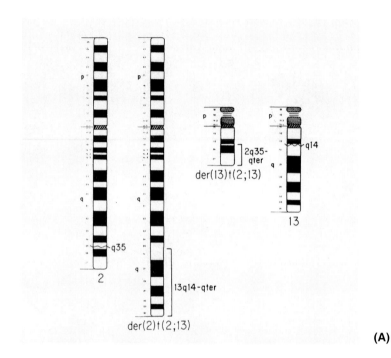

(A)

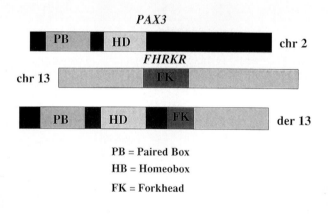

PAX3

| PB | HD | | chr 2 |

FHRKR

chr 13 | | FK | |

| PB | HD | FK | | der 13 |

PB = Paired Box
HB = Homeobox
FK = Forkhead

(B)

FIG. 10 Alveolar rhabdomyosarcoma translocation, the t(2;13)(q14;q35). (A) In this illustration, the normal chromosomes 2 and 13 are on the far left and right, respectively. With the reciprocal translocation, portions of the long arms of the two chromosomes are juxtaposed, creating two derivative chromosomes as illustrated by the two central ones in the figure. (B) A model of the translocation shows that the *PAX3* gene on chromosome 2 (*top*) is fused with the *FHRKR* gene on chromosome 13 (*middle*) to produce a derivative fusion gene (*bottom*). This unites the paired box, homeobox, and forkhead domains into one gene.

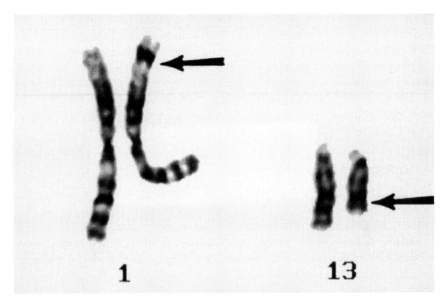

FIG. 11 Alveolar rhabdomyosarcoma. In this tumor, a portion of the long arm chromosome 13 is inserted into the short arm of chromosome 1 (*arrows*), producing a fusion of the 1p36 and 13q14 regions similar to that produced by the t(1;13)(p36;q14). (Courtesy of Dr. Jeff Sawyer, Department of Pathology, University of Arkansas for Medical Sciences, and the Cytogenetics Laboratory, Arkansas Children's Hospital.)

retroviruses, to convert single-stranded mRNA to double-stranded DNA. Oligonucleotide primers attaching to opposite ends of the fusion gene are then used to generate multiple copies of this cDNA, using a thermocycler and PCR. This process greatly increases the DNA available for standard hybridization using a signal-tagged probe, which then is detected autoradiographically or enzymatically in a predictable electrophoretic pattern. The primers and probes may be composed of consensus sequences allowing detection of both fusions in one step (58), and primers and probes to other tumor-specific fusions (see below) can be added to the mixture as a single test for multiple tumors (or multiplex test) (59). Although RT-PCR is a very specific test, about 15–20% of alveolar rhabdomyosarcomas diagnosed by standard histologic testing are negative for unknown reasons (60).

Currently, there is no genetic test for embryonal rhabdomyosarcoma, as no specific gene or mutation has been found to date. Mutations of the short arm of chromosome 11 have been demonstrated (61), but these genetic lesions are shared by other pediatric tumors, including Wilms' tumor, hepatoblastoma, and adrenal cortical carcinoma (62), and thus are not specific to embryonal rhabdomyosarcoma. Recent studies have demonstrated that embryonal rhabdomyosarcomas show epigenetic alterations distinct from those of alveolar rhabdomyosarcoma and similar to those of fetal muscle (63); verification of these results is needed before their acceptance as standard diagnostic tests. Similarly, myogenin immunostaining shows a distinct difference in embryonal as compared to alveolar rhabdomyosarcoma, using a small series of cases (64). These phenomena could be related to aberrant biological consequences of the *PAX;FKHR* fusion, as the *PAX* gene normally functions to initiate MyoD synthesis during embryogenesis (65), and MyoD in turn initiates myogenin synthesis (66).

F. Differential Diagnosis

Differential diagnosis of rhabdomyosarcoma hinges around two unrelated phenomena: their primitive, undifferentiated nature and their tendency to form muscle. As a result, the differential list must include not only the host of small round blue cell tumors but also the vast number of nonrhabdomyosarcomatous lesions capable of forming skeletal muscle (or in the case of the rhabdoid tumor, appearing to form muscle). A partial list of the former is given in Table 5 and a summary of the latter in Table 6. Note that there is some degree of overlap, which should not be unexpected. Other considerations for pleomorphic rhabdomyosarcoma are the pleomorphic spindle cell tumors covered in other chapters of this text.

The most important step in differential diagnosis is to obtain a well-stained, well-sectioned slice of viable, pristine tumor tissue. Most mistakes are made at this simple step, using inadequate material for definitive characterization. If this is suitably accomplished, then it becomes a matter of what ancillary tissue is available for further analysis using the techniques listed above. Electron microscopy requires optimally fixed tissue, preferably in cooled, fresh glutaraldehyde, for best visualization, necessitating consideration soon after specimen receipt in the pathology laboratory or frozen-section room. These tissues are often degenerate, and

TABLE 5   Differential Diagnosis of Rhabdomyosarcoma—Small Round Blue Cell Tumors

Ewing sarcoma	Embryonal sarcoma of liver
Primitive peripheral neuroectodermal tumor	Pleuropulmonary blastoma
Neuroblastoma	Malignant melanoma
Pigmented neuroectodermal tumor	Desmoplastic small round cell tumor
Esthesioneuroblastoma	Synovial sarcoma
Lymphoblastic lymphoma	Malignant peripheral nerve sheath tumor
Small noncleaved cell lymphoma	Germ cell tumors
Wilms' tumor	Histiocytoses

TABLE 6   Differential Diagnosis of Rhabdomyosarcoma—
Myogenous/Pseudomyogenous Tumors

Rhabdomyoma
Nerve sheath tumors, benign and malignant (Triton tumor)
Rhabdoid tumor
Inflammatory myofibroblastic tumor
Eosinophilic cystitis
Various carcinomas with heterologous muscle
Various sarcomas with heterologous muscle
Sex cord tumors with heterologous muscle
Germ cell tumors
Embryonal sarcoma of liver
Pleuropulmonary blastoma
Ectomesenchymoma (primitive neuroectodermal tumor plus rhabdomyosarcoma)
Malignant mesenchymoma (fibrosarcoma/malignant fibrous histiocytoma plus rhabdo-
    myosarcoma and/or other heterologous elements)

glutaraldehyde penetrates slowly, so the submitted tissue should be paper thin and fresh. Immunohistochemistry is less dependent on specimen preparation, but optimal fixation is still required. The use of newer retrieval techniques has optimized some staining, but unexpected patterns of reactivity may result (55). Finally, cytogenetic analysis has an absolute requirement for fresh, preferably sterile tissue; molecular techniques work best with fresh tissue that is snap-frozen soon after biopsy.

The aforesaid preparations made, differential diagnosis essentially becomes a matter of careful observation of cytohistologic detail to detect rhabdomyoblasts and to rule out other patterns, with confirmation of myogenous differentiation if needed by electron microscopic and/or immunohistochemical examination. If alveolar rhabdomyosarcoma is a consideration, confirmation may be obtained by cytogenetic or molecular genetic examination as above.

III.   EWING FAMILY OF TUMORS (EWING/PNETS)

A.   Classification and History

It is only within the past couple of decades that we have realized that two histologically disparate neoplasms, Ewing's sarcoma and peripheral primitive neuroectodermal tumor (PNET; also referred to as peripheral neuroepithelioma), are biologically related. Interestingly, both entities were described within 4 years of each other, by New York pathologists who published their findings in a state medical journal (67,68). James Ewing, later to found Memorial Hospital for the Treatment of Cancer and Allied Diseases in New York City (now Memorial Sloan-Kettering Cancer Center), described a peculiar undifferentiated round cell tumor of bone in adolescents, and Arthur Purdy Stout of Columbia University published a case report of a primitive rosette–forming neoplasm of the ulnar nerve of a young adult. In spite of vehement skepticism by Sir Rupert Willis (69), Ewing's sarcoma became a standard diagnosis by the 1950s and was accepted as an entity of unknown origin by prominent bone pathologists, such as Jaffe and Lichtenstein (70). On the other hand, PNET underwent diagnostic atrophy and was only noted in sporadic case reports or small series until the mid-1970s. At that point, Askin and colleagues published a paper describing a peculiar small-cell tumor of the chest wall in adolescents (71), later to become known as the Askin tumor. Thanks to cytogenetic, ultrastructural, and biological studies, the commonality of these three lesions—Ewing's sarcoma, PNET, and Askin's tumor, became unveiled, so that today they are referred to as the PNET or Ewing family of tumors (72). Soft-tissue examples of these lesions have also become commonly recognized, so that now, instead of thinking of them as rare, we consider them to be the second most common pediatric soft-tissue sarcoma, following rhabdomyosarcoma (7,73). For a more detailed accounting of this historical saga, the reader is referred to excellent review articles by Dehner and Yunis (69,74).

Classification of Ewing family tumors has also incurred its share of controversy. When the PNET of bone was first described, there was evidence that these lesions were more aggressive than standard Ewing's sarcomas (75), although atypical features in Ewing's sarcoma had not been found to have prognostic significance in a larger series (76). Later studies yielded evidence that the presence of the neural features seen with PNET (discussed below) were indeed of serious import (77). This prompted Schmidt and colleagues to publish an article reporting that the presence of rosettes or immunopositivity for two or more neural markers was sufficient evidence that PNET was the diagnosis and aggressive clinical behavior would ensue (78). However, more recent studies have not confirmed the prognostic significance of Ewing family subclassification (79,80). Nevertheless, standardization of future analyses would dictate utilization of a classification system similar to that shown in Table 7.

B. Clinical Features

Ewing family tumors are primarily lesions of bone; only a relatively small percentage arises in soft tissue. Among the latter, the chest wall, paravertebral region, pelvis, and proximal extremities are favored sites (81). Typically, these tumors arise in adolescents and young adults, although small children may be affected (82,83). Often they arise from peripheral nerve, inviting confusion with malignant peripheral nerve sheath tumor (84). Among organ systems, the kidneys are more commonly affected than is appreciated (85) and are probably the most common

TABLE 7 Histologic Classification of Ewing Family Tumors

Diagnosis	Histology	Immunohistochemistry	Electron microscopy
Ewing's sarcoma	Rosettes absent, no atypia [a]	CD99 and/or vimentin pos. only	Pools of glycogen only, no neuro-secretory granules
Atypical Ewing's sarcoma	Rosettes absent, atypia present	Above plus only one neural marker	Pools of glycogen with only rare neurosecretory granules, or vague neural features
Primitive neuroectodermal tumor	Rosettes present	Two or more neural markers	Neurosecretory granules and neural features easily identified

[a] For definition of atypia, see text.

site of origin among solid organs (86). Because these latter tumors more typically arise in older children and adults, they may be mistaken for adult Wilms' tumors. Finally, parameningeal and dural examples have been reported (87–89), further muddying the semantic distinction between these lesions and the similarly named but biologically distinct PNETs of the central nervous system.

Ewing family tumors are aggressive lesions that are best considered systemic rather than localized phenomena, and therapy should be planned accordingly. Nevertheless, size and stage of the tumor are important predictors of outcome (81,90,91). Furthermore, site of origin is important, as pelvic primaries are relatively aggressive, and renal primaries would appear to be so as well (85). Systemic symptoms, such as fever and elevated erythrocyte sedimentation rate, may occur and invite confusion with infections. As with all sarcomas, metastases at presentation are an ominous sight. With Ewing family lesions these typically occur in the lungs, in contradistinction to the histologically similar neuroblastoma (81). Soft-tissue examples have histologically been clinically aggressive with poor outcome (81), although when previously treated on IRSG protocols they attained a survival rate similar to that of embryonal rhabdomyosarcoma (92). Because of their biological relatedness, soft-tissue lesions in this group currently are treated in a manner similar to that of bony lesions in the Intergroup Ewing's Sarcoma Study. Recent advances in chemotherapy, such as the addition of ifosfamide to the therapeutic regimen, have been accompanied by marked improvements in outcome (93,94).

C. Gross Appearance

Ewing family tumors are typically fleshy yellow–tan lesions that may contain degenerate areas of necrosis and hemorrhage. By gross examination they possess no distinguishing characteristics that would separate them from other high-grade sarcomas, except that occasional examples arise from peripheral nerves. Chest wall examples may or may not arise from rib; by definition, the so-called Askin tumor does not (71). This distinction must be made radiographically, as soft-tissue lesions are capable of invading bone, and bony lesions typically have an associated soft-tissue mass. After therapy, the Ewing tumors often regress, leaving a fibrous scar that may contain microscopic nests of residual viable tumor. This tumor regression may be associated with serous atrophy and edema of the adjacent fibrofatty tissue (95,96). Postchemotherapy tumor regression is associated with a good prognosis (97,98).

D. Microscopic Appearance

As stated above, the classification of Ewing family tumors is defined by their histologic and ultrastructural appearance and immunostaining properties. This di-

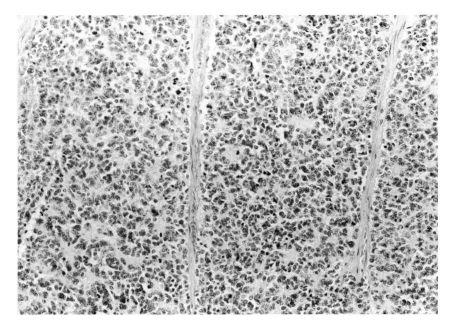

FIG. 12   Peripheral primitive neuroectodermal tumor (PNET). This tumor contains numerous Homer Wright rosettes, with wreaths of nuclei arrayed around wispy neurofibrillary cores.

versity is related primarily to their capacity for neuroectodermal differentiation, expressed histologically as Homer Wright rosettes (Fig. 12). These microscopic structures comprise wreaths of dark, oval nuclei that circumscribe wispy, lightly pink, neurofibrillary cores. By electron microscopy, these neurofibrillary cores correspond to elongated, dendritic tumor cell processes that intertwine in a fashion similar to that of a skein of yarn. The presence of well-defined rosettes de facto suffices to categorize a lesion histologically as PNET.

On the other end of the differentiation spectrum lies typical Ewing's sarcoma, which by its primitive nature is the penultimate small round blue cell tumor. These are composed of highly compressed cellular masses that usually occur in diffuse sheets (Fig. 13). The tumor cell nuclei typically possess round, even contours and smooth chromatin with inconspicuous nuclei, being similar to but larger than lymphoid cells. One prominent distinction is their cytoplasm, which is often clear or bubbly due to an abundance of glycogen demonstrable by PAS stains. At first glance, this cytoplasmic vacuolization may resemble the neurofibrillary material found in rosettes, but neural similarities are otherwise lacking. Another prominent feature is the presence of interspersed amorphous clusters of cells with

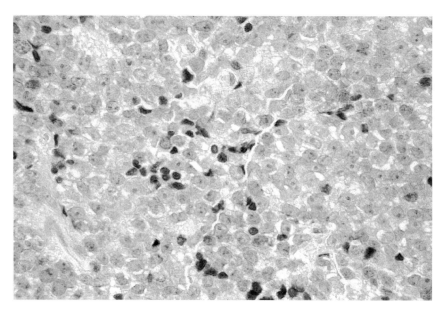

FIG. 13 Ewing's sarcoma. This tumor contains monotonous sheets of undifferentiated tumor cells with round nuclei, minimal bubbly cytoplasm, and scattered "dark" cells.

more condensed nuclei and lightly eosinophilic cytoplasm; this creates a pattern of alternating "light" cells and "dark" cells. Although these are rapidly growing lesions, the mitotic index is often paradoxically low in typical Ewing's tumors.

In some Ewing's tumors, the above typical features are distorted, so that cells are larger and display more uneven contours, irregular chromatin, and an increased mitotic index. These tumors are referred to as "atypical Ewing's sarcomas" or "large-cell Ewing's sarcomas," and they were recognized among soft-tissue examples in the early IRSG studies (99). However, PNET-defining rosettes should be absent, although admittedly some irregular small aggregates of cells may have abortive rosette-like features. Nevertheless, one should not be able to see a discrete neurofibrillary core or a well-defined circular nuclear wreath. Not surprisingly, some observers have noted that atypical Ewing's sarcomas comprise a "missing link" between typical Ewing's sarcomas and PNETs, as they often express a solitary neural marker, such as neuron-specific enolase, or show rudimentary neuronal features by ultrastructural examination (see below) (100,101). Regardless of nosology, prevailing opinion dictates that the presence of atypia does not confer prognostic significance (76).

Like the neural crest that they recapitulate, PNETs are capable of more than simple neural differentiation. Schwann cell, glial, ependymal, and epithelial differentiation have been described (102), and, as noted above, ectomesenchymomatous differentiation into skeletal muscle and other soft tissues is theoretically possible. I have personally seen examples with neuroendocrine differentiation, and hormonal secretion of polypeptides such as glucagon or cholecystekinin may occur (103). This panoply of cellular multipotentiality leads to diagnostic and nosologic confusion, and questions regarding treatment implications for nonneuronal differentiation have not been completely answered. However, ectomesenchymomatous tumors appear to respond similarly to rhabdomyosarcoma and are currently included on IRSG protocols (45).

E. Ancillary Findings

1. Electron Microscopy

Due to the above-mentioned capacity of PNETs for multipotential differentiation, electron microscopy can be fruitfully used to resolve questions posed by unexpected immunostaining results or unusual histologies (101). However, with more primitive Ewing-like tumors, evidence for differentiation may be sparse and require careful searching. One prominent feature is the formation of elongated, tenuous cytoplasmic processes, but one must be careful not to confuse short extensions with other structures, such as filopodia. The best evidence is the presence of 80- to 100-nm neurosecretory granules (Fig. 14) and/or parallel stacks of 25-nm microtubules within the processes. Better differentiated examples may contain synaptic junctions and secretory vesicles within neurofibrillary cores. However, one must beware of overinterpretation of neurosecretory granules, which are easily confused with primary lysosomes, and isolated microtubules, which are a nonspecific finding typical of mitotically active cells. As with rhabdomyosarcomas, in spite of these caveats experienced electron microscopists can attain a degree of diagnostic accuracy that rivals that of other commonly used tests (104).

True to their more primitive nature, typical Ewing's sarcomas are ultrastructurally characterized by the prominence of their round, bland nuclei and the blandness of their elementary cytoplasm, distinguished mainly by its abundant pools of glycogen. This latter feature may be partially dissolved in processing, leaving large irregular cytoplasmic spaces lacking a membranous border. The "dark cells" noted by light microscopic examination typically display more condensed chromatin and busier cytoplasm that contains increased numbers of mitochondria or lysosomes, suggesting that these are effete cells entering the throes of apoptosis. Atypical Ewing's tumors may contain these features as well as primitive neural features without the well-defined differentiation of PNET (101,105). Rare tumors may have primitive mesenchymal features suggestive of sarcomatous differentiation; these have been termed "primitive sarcomas of bone" (101).

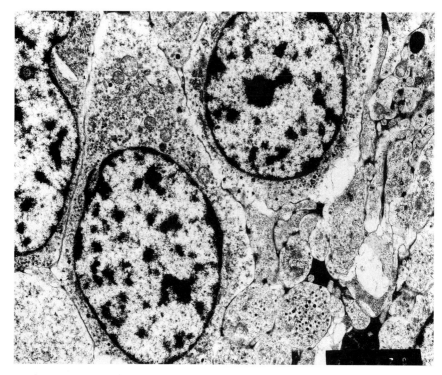

FIG. 14 Electron micrograph of peripheral primitive neuroectodermal tumor. There are aggregates of short cytoplasmic processes containing small dark neurosecretory granules.

2. Immunohistochemistry

Similar to muscle cells, neurons possess a complex machinery of cell-specific proteins, in this case dedicated to electrical excitation and signal transmission. As such, a wide variety of markers can be utilized to demonstrate the neurility of tumors. Commonly used neural markers include synaptophysin and chromogranin, proteins unique to the neurosecretory granule/synaptic vesicle apparatus, and neuron-specific enolase, an isoenzyme of the anaerobic glycolytic enzyme that catalyzes degradation of 2,3-diphosphoglycerate into phosphoenolpyruvate. Other examples include CD57 (also known as Leu-7), a membrane protein shared by natural killer lymphocytes and neuroendocrine cells, and S-100, a nuclear protein linked to cell cycle proteins. Each of these markers has inherent problems; for example, the more sensitive synaptophysin requires optimal fixation, whereas the more stable chromogranin unfortunately is rarely seen in PNET, perhaps because of the relative rarity of neurosecretory granules. Nonspecificity is a problem with the other markers. Ironically, neuron-specific enolase is perhaps the least specific of all, but it is very sensitive and often is expressed by atypical Ewing's tumors (100). CD57 (or Leu-7), an isoform of the neural cell adhesion molecule, is expressed not only by some lymphocytes but also by epithelial tumors (106). S-100 is a poorly characterized protein named for its solubility when bovine brain is exposed to a 100% solution of ammonium sulfate. It is present in a host of cell types, including cartilage, fat, and Schwann cells, so that its presence in PNET may indicate differentiation into the latter elements. Because of the risk of diagnostic misadventure, these markers are thus best applied in conjunction with staining for other cell types, such as myogenous and lymphoid ones.

A more recently characterized marker that has found great popularity in Ewing tumor diagnosis is CD99, formerly known as MIC2 antigen. This marker is expressed in more than 95% of Ewing/PNET cases and shows a distinctive diffuse membranous pattern of immunoreactivity (107). However, being derived from a lymphoblastic cell line (108), it suffers from similar reactivity in lymphoblastic tumors (109). Rhabdomyosarcomas occasionally may also yield positive immunostaining, although generally in a focal cytoplasmic or nuclear pattern of reactivity (107,110). More recent results indicate that other sarcomas, such as synovial sarcomas, may be positive (107). Thus, as with the other markers, CD99 stains are best interpreted in the context of a diagnostic panel of immunostains that includes lymphoid, neural, and muscle antigens.

3. Cytogenetics/Molecular Genetics

Like alveolar rhabdomyosarcoma, the Ewing family of tumors is genetically characterized by a gene fusion, in this case between the *FLI1* gene on chromosome 11 and the *EWS* gene on chromosome 22. Karyotypically this is expressed by the reciprocal translocation, t(11;22)(q24;q12). Unlike alveolar rhabdomyosarcoma, which has a single reproducible fusion point, a variety of combinatorial fusions may occur (111), all of which fuse the two translated protein molecules. In this chimeric protein, a DNA transcription factor (EWS) is joined to an RNA-binding factor (FLI1), causing abnormal DNA regulation and leading to tumorigenesis (112). The length of the resultant protein, which varies with the fusion combination, may have prognostic significance (113). It is of note that the *FLI1* gene is an oncogene whose murine counterpart causes erythroleukemia (114).

As is frequently the case with nature's intrigues, the *EWS* story has become more complicated with each passing investigation. For one thing, *FLI1* is a member of the *ETS* family of genes, and although it is by far the most commonly affected, a variety of other *ETS* genes may fuse with *EWS* to produce morphologically identical tumors. To date, Ewing's tumor associated fusions of the chromosome 22q breakpoint with genes on chromosomes 21 (*ERG*), 7, and 17 have been described (115–117), and undoubtedly more are yet to come. Another intriguing phenomenon is that fusions of non-*ETS* genes with *EWS*, such as with the *WT1* gene or the *ATF-1* (118) genes on chromosomes 11 and 12, respectively, produce dissimilar tumors, in these instances the desmoplastic small-cell tumor (see below) and the clear cell tumor of soft parts (see Chapter 14). Extraskeletal myxoid chondrosarcoma is also characterized by an *EWS* gene type of fusion (119). Thus, the *EWS* gene is a promiscuous locus whose dalliances beget a variety of tumorigenetic offspring with dissimilar histologies.

In spite of their various convolutions, the genetic aberrations of the Ewing family tumors can be profitably utilized for ancillary diagnosis. Standard karyotyping will reveal the t(11;22)(q24;q12), and the resultant mRNA can be probed using RT-PCR (60). However, additional testing is required to more completely screen for the host of fusions possible with the *EWS* gene. Another caveat is that apparent cases of rhabdomyosarcoma bearing this genetic brand have been described (47), and desmoplastic small-cell tumors may also display it rather than their more characteristic *WT1;EWS* fusion (120). These rare exceptions raise currently unanswered issues regarding use of histology versus molecular testing for treatment decisions. For the present and until gene-specific treatment is available, the wiser source is probably to defer to histology rather than genetics in unquestionable cases.

F. Differential Diagnosis

Diagnosis of Ewing family tumors has undergone much change since the beginning of my career, when it was largely a diagnosis of exclusion based on presence of typical clinical findings and absence of histologic characteristics of other tumors. Happily, with the advent of the genetic and immunochemical tools currently available, it is now routinely possible to make an unabashedly firm pathologic diagnosis. This transformation has led to recognition, as stated above, that these soft-tissue tumors are relatively common neoplasms, not the fuel for isolated case reports as in the past. However, the sine qua non remains the availability of adequate optimally prepared tissue for microscopic and genetic examination, which is a not uncommon problem with the fragile cells that constitute these lesions. I have often observed biopsies containing only blue smudges of crushed nuclei that cannot even be distinguished from normal lymphocytes. I would therefore offer the following advice: Exercise the utmost care when obtaining and handling these brittle tumors, and be prepared to liberally rebiopsy a patient if unsatisfactory material is obtained on the initial attempt.

Given the availability of pristine tissue, differential diagnosis includes the list of small-cell neoplasms found in Table 5. A common mimic is the solid variant of alveolar rhabdomyosarcoma, which may lack the fibrous septa of its typical form. A converse consideration is that fibrovascular strands may traverse atypical Ewing's tumors and PNETs, yielding a resemblance to typical alveolar rhabdomyosarcoma. These two tumor entities occur in identical locations and affect identical age groups of patients, with the caveat that Ewing's tumors are exceedingly rare in black children. Lymphoma would appear to be less of a problem, given its usual presentation in lymph nodes, but soft-tissue examples are well known (121). Diagnosis of this latter tumor is made particularly treacherous because of its reactivity with CD99 and frequent nonreactivity with CD45, the common lymphocyte antigen. Attention to cytologic detail is thus important, as is use of a panel that includes neural, muscle, and lymphoid antigens.

The diagnostician is also advised that unexpected results, such as desmin positivity, may occasionally occur with PNET (54), so that cases with incongruous staining patterns may require additional studies, such as electron microscopy and/or genetics/cytogenetics, for verification. As above, these latter techniques require optimal tissue preparation and submission while fresh sterile tumor is available, even if the tests are ultimately not performed. Therefore, at Arkansas Children's Hospital, we immerse small portions of fresh tumor tissue in glutaraldehyde, freeze a healthy portion in liquid nitrogen, and submit a 1-g sterile portion to cytogenetics when ample biopsy samples of suspected cases are received.

IV. NEUROBLASTIC TUMORS

A. Classification

Neuroblastic tumors are frequently confused with PNETs, as witnessed by a series of exchanges in one pathology journal after the publication of an article on "adult neuroblastoma" (102,122). In fact, they are distinctly dissimilar lesions, affecting different age groups, metastasizing to different locations, presenting in different foci, having different differentiation potentials and biological features, and, most importantly, requiring different therapy and staging. Happily, their distinction is generally easily accomplished, as noted below. The key biological difference is that neuroblastomas are adrenergic tumors, as reflected by their predilection for the adrenal glands and sympathetic ganglia, whereas PNETs are cholinergic tumors (123).

Neuroblastic tumors are generally classified by their differentiation capacity, which reflects an active proclivity to produce mature ganglia and Schwann cells. This tendency reaches its apogee in the benign member of the group, ganglioneuroma, which is solely composed of nonmetastasizing mature elements and is most frequently encountered in the posterior mediastina of young children. Its more virulent and primal cousin, neuroblastoma, resides most frequently in the adrenal gland and is one of the most common congenital neoplasms, often differentiating into mature tissues in prenatal and early life. However, unresolved neuroblastomas constitute one of the most common malignant groups in children, following leukemias and brain tumors. In between neuroblastoma and ganglioneuroma lies the ganglioneuroblastoma, a partially differentiated lesion that nevertheless has full metastatic potential because of its content of malignant neuroblasts. Neuroblastic tumors may also commence from immature teratomas, and they have similar clinical and biological features to de novo tumors when arising in this milieu (124).

B. Clinical Features

Clinically, neuroblastic tumors produce not only mass effects but also a host of systemic symptoms engendered from their capacity for neurohormonal production and autoantibody stimulation (125). Besides the typical abdominal mass produced from adrenal neuroblastomas, examples of clinical lesions include Horner's syndrome caused by mediastinal pressure, myoclonus caused by production of a motor endplate–related autoantibody, and watery diarrhea secondary to secretion of vasoactive intestinal polypeptide.

Neuroblastomas are potentially aggressive lesions whose clinical behavior depends on genetic, histologic, and staging factors. Genetic and histologic factors will be discussed below. Of primary importance to staging is examination of the bone marrow, which is a common site of metastatic disease. The staging system in current use by the Pediatric Oncology Group is given in Table 8. Of note in this system is that multifocal primary tumors (e.g., bilateral adrenal primary tumors) should be staged according to the greatest extent of disease. The midline is defined as the vertebral column; tumors arising unilaterally and extending past the midline must cross into the opposite side of the vertebral column. Finally, note that metastatic disease may be present in stage 4S tumors, which paradoxically have a good

TABLE 8 International Neuroblastoma Staging System (INSS) (149)

Stage 1—Localized tumor with complete gross excision, with or without microscopic residual disease; representative ipsilateral lymph nodes negative for tumor microscopically. (Nodes attached to and removed with the primary tumor may be positive.)

Stage 2A—Localized tumor with incomplete gross resection; representative ipsilateral nonadherent lymph nodes negative for tumor microscopically.

Stage 2B—Localized tumor with or without complete gross excision, with ipsilateral nonadherent lymph nodes positive for tumor; enlarged contralateral lymph nodes must be negative microscopically.

Stage 3—Unresectable unilateral tumor infiltrating across the midline, with or without regional lymph node involvement; or localized unilateral tumor with contralateral regional lymph node involvement; or midline tumor with bilateral extension by infiltration (unresectable) or by lymph node involvement.

Stage 4—Any primary tumor with dissemination to distant lymph nodes, bone, bone marrow, liver, skin, and/or other organs (except as defined for stage 4S).

Stage 4S—Localized primary tumor (as defined for stage 1, 2A, or 2B) with dissemination limited to skin, liver, and/or bone marrow (limited to infants less than 1 year of age).

outcome. Marrow involvement at stage 4S nevertheless should be minimal, with fewer than 10% of total nucleated cells being malignant. The unexpectedly excellent behavior of stage 4S neuroblastomas has been confirmed by a number of investigators and has led to speculation concerning their biology (126,127).

C. Gross Findings

Neuroblastomas are typically fleshy masses discolored by abundant purple to plum-colored hemorrhage (Fig. 15). As such they produce raised purplish masses when metastasizing to skin and subcutaneous soft tissues; as a result, affected infants have been termed "blueberry-muffin babies." Adrenal masses usually compress the normal gland into a thin cap that partially rims the fibrous capsule. Paravertebral tumors invade through the neural foramina in a dumbbell fashion that is apparent on nuclear magnetic resonance images. Paravertebral lesions may also completely swallow adjacent lymph nodes, but this finding does not have the significance of separate metastases. Chalky foci of calcification are typically present.

On the opposite side of the coin, ganglioneuromas form firm yellow–tan masses with a whorled, fibroma-like cut surface (Fig. 16). These lesions may appear locally invasive, but they are terminally differentiated lesions by definition

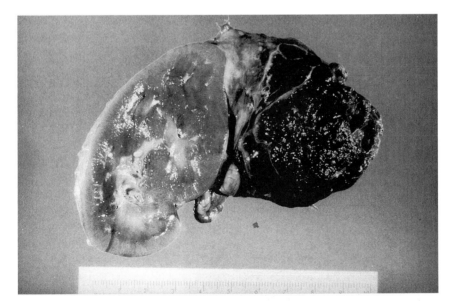

FIG. 15 Neuroblastoma. The adrenal gland is replaced by a large, fleshy, hemorrhagic mass on the right. The tumor is sharply delimited from the adjacent kidney on the left.

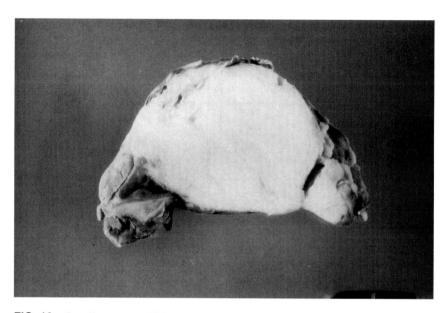

FIG. 16 Ganglioneuroma. This mass has a whorled, fibrous cut surface, without hemorrhage.

and usually don't grow if incompletely excised (128). Ganglioneuroblastomas in the composite form comprise firm yellow–tan ganglioneuromatous masses, but containing nodular foci of fleshy, hemorrhagic tissue constituting their neuroblastomatous elements (Fig. 17). Otherwise the gross appearance of ganglioneuroblastomas reflects their relative proportions of mature schwannian and immature neuroblastic tissues.

D. Microscopic Features

Histologically, neuroblastic tumors compose a maturationally heterogeneous group, ranging from primitive neuroblastoma to terminally differentiated ganglioneuroma. The key histologic element of neuroblastoma is the production of neuropil, a wispy, light pink, fibrillar material, by otherwise undifferentiated-appearing neuroblasts; these cells are characterized otherwise by their granular, "salt and pepper" chromatin. This material corresponds ultrastructurally to the formation of elongated dendritic processes that interdigitate in a manner reminiscent of normal nervous system development. Undifferentiated tumors with minimal amounts of neuropil do occur, but this material generally is not difficult to find. Rosettes similar to those described above for PNET are commonly seen and have cores filled with neuropil (Fig. 18). As noted grossly, abundant hemorrhage is typically present, so that fibrosis and hemosiderin deposition are common con-

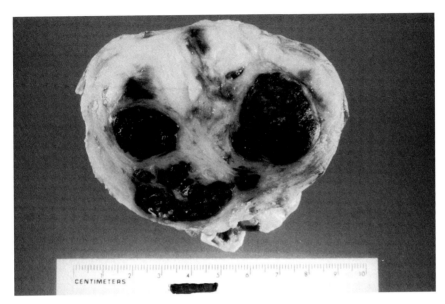

FIG. 17 Composite ganglioneuroblastoma. This mass is composed of pale, whorled, fibrous tumor (ganglioneuroma) punctuated by dark hemorrhagic nodules of neuroblastoma.

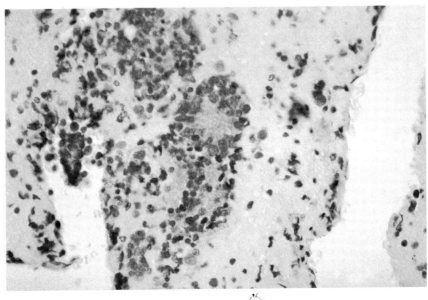

FIG. 18 Neuroblastoma. This fine-needle aspirate contains an easily recognizable Homer Wright rosette.

comitant features. Clusters of lymphocytes also appear and relate to the immunologic stimulation produced by this tumor. Another reactive but diagnostically significant feature is the presence of islands of dystrophic calcification, which often grow to sufficient size to be detectable radiographically and grossly.

Early cytologic differentiation into ganglionic cells is evidenced in neuroblasts that contain nuclei with prominent nucleoli and acquire an eccentric triangular rim of cytoplasm. In ganglioneuroblastomas, which can be graded by their degree of differentiation (125), progressive acquisition of neural features results in mature ganglion cells with pale nuclei, prominent nucleoli, and abundant cytoplasm with Nissl substance (Fig. 19). Mature neuronal cells tend to be diffusely dispersed among the less differentiated elements, except in the more compartmentalized composite ganglioneuroblastoma. Schwann cell and satellite cell elements also progressively differentiate out of this primordial neural stew, and melanocytic differentiation may rarely be seen.

In the terminally differentiated ganglioneuromas, scattered isolated nests of mature ganglion cells actually become subsumed by the Schwann cell element, which lends to these tumors their fibrous gross appearance. Ganglioneuromas also typically contain the scattered clusters of mature lymphocytes seen in more primitive lesions, so that caution is advised in interpreting fine-needle aspirations to

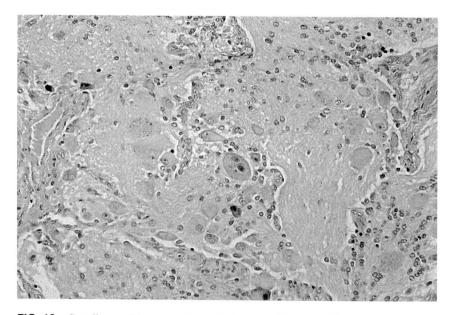

FIG. 19 Ganglioneuroblastoma (differentiating neuroblastoma). The tumor comprises a mixture of undifferentiated cells and mature ganglion cells embedded in a prominent fibrillary stroma. Note the mature binucleated ganglion cell in the center of the photograph.

avoid overdiagnosis of benign small-cell elements. Ganglioneuromatous areas frequently occur in posttreatment excisions of primary and metastatic lesions and represent therapy-induced maturation analogous to that frequently seen with congenital neuroblastomas. In the occasional lucky patient, this maturation into a benign differentiated tumor occurs spontaneously; its relationship to immunologic phenomena has been the subject of biological and therapeutic investigation (128,129).

Histologic examination is important in neuroblastoma not only for diagnosis but also for grading, which has distinct prognostic significance. The currently used grading system is that of Shimada (130), as outlined in Table 9. Note that besides maturation, age of the patient and amount of mitosis/apoptosis are important in dividing patients into prognosis groups. The latter feature requires counting mitotic figures and karyolytic bodies among 5000 tumor cells, an onerous chore that may be made more palatable to the busy surgical pathologist by estimation of the total number of tumor cells per microscopic field. In spite of this statistically treacherous maneuver, Shimada grading is a predictably reproducible, prognostically significant, and commonly accepted practice.

E. Ancillary Findings

1. Electron Microscopy

Ultrastructural examination has been used in the past to diagnose neuroblastomas, which typically show some degree of differentiation at the submicroscopic level, even in its absence at the microscopic level. Thus, one generally finds

TABLE 9 Neuroblastoma Grading System of Shimada (130)

Good prognostic lesions
Stroma-rich (Schwann cell–rich) tumors with intermixed differentiating neuroblastic
  elements
Stroma-poor (Schwann cell–poor) tumors in patients younger than 1.5 years with MKI[a]
  < 200
Stroma-poor tumors in patients 1.5–5 years of age, with ganglionic differentiation and
  MKI > 100.

Poor prognostic lesions
Stroma-rich nodular tumors (nodular ganglioneuroblastomas; see text description)
Stroma-poor tumors in patients younger than 1.5 years, with MKI > 200
Stroma-poor tumors in patients 1.5–5 years of age, with MKI > 100
Stroma-poor tumors of all types in patients older than 5 years

[a]MKI, mitotic karyorrhectic index (determining by counting the number of mitoses and karyolytic bodies among 5000 tumor cells).

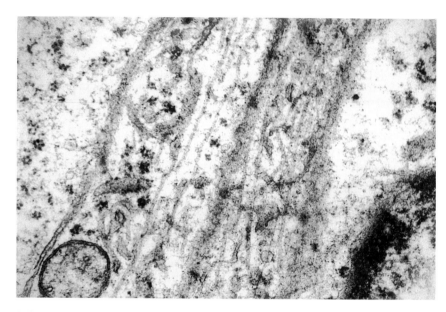

FIG. 20   Electron micrograph of neuroblastoma. In this high-power magnification, parallel strands of microtubules are seen within tapered cytoplasmic processes.

well-developed, intertwining, nontapering processes containing fairly numerous, uniform, 80- to 100-nm neurosecretory granules and parallel arrays of 25-nm microtubules (Fig. 20). Overlap with well-differentiated examples of PNET is theoretically possible, but seasoned electron microscopists note that the latter tumors typically contain more pleomorphic neurosecretory granules, more tapering processes, and a relative dearth of microtubules (52). Another feature more typical of PNET is cytoplasmic glycogen, but rare examples of neuroblastoma containing this element have been reported (33).

2.   Immunohistochemistry

In general, the markers used for immunohistochemical diagnosis of neuroblastoma have been those noted above in the description of Ewing's tumor immunohistochemistry. Two important exceptions should be noted: chromogranin is more likely to be positive with neuroblastoma, and to my knowledge a case of CD99-positive neuroblastoma has yet to be reported. This latter feature makes CD99 staining a robust tool in the diagnostic distinction between PNET and neuroblastoma (131). Newer markers, such as NB84 (132) and NCAM (133), have been described for neuroblastoma, but their diagnostic utility has not been fully confirmed.

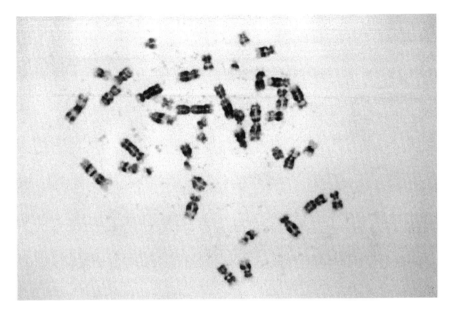

FIG. 21 Neuroblastoma metaphase spread. Besides the darker normal chromosomes, note the numerous, lightly staining doublets. These are double-minute chromosomes that contain markedly amplified segments of the N-*myc* gene.

3. Cytogenetics/Molecular Genetics

Cytogenetics also shows a distinct difference between neuroblastoma and PNET. Whereas *EWS;ETS* fusions are characteristic of the latter lesion (see above), neuroblastomas are distinguished by frequent deletions in chromosome 1p, common but deadly amplifications of the N-*myc* oncogene, and resultant double-minute chromosomes (Fig. 21) and homogeneous staining regions that contain the amplified oncogene segments. This N-*myc* amplification phenomenon results in a dramatic increase in the number of DNA segments transcribing this gene and causes unrestrained growth in vitro and aggressive clinical behavior in vivo. Fluorescence in situ hybridization (FISH), in which fluorescein-tagged segments of N-*myc* DNA are hybridized to cytologic preparations of neuroblastoma cells, can be used to directly visualize and count the number of copies per tumor cell nucleus. This technique has become the standard method of genetic testing for N-*myc* amplification and is being routinely performed in all new cases.

Another prognostic genetic feature of neuroblastoma is ploidy, an estimate of the amount of DNA per tumor cell. This test is routinely performed by flow cytometry or image cytometry. Ironically, aneuploidy, or an abnormal amount of DNA, is associated with good prognosis in neuroblastomas, whereas this feature is usually a bad omen in adult tumors. The combination of stage, Shimada grade, N-*myc* copy number, and ploidy yields an often interrelated but sometimes independent system of prognostication that has become standard practice in assignment of neuroblastoma patients to treatment strata (134).

Newer prognostic indicators for neuroblastoma include Ha-*ras* and *trk A* gene expression. Tanaka et al. (135) found that favorable outcome of neuroblastoma was associated with high expression of these genes, whereas unfavorable outcomes were distinguished by low expression. Also, localized low-stage tumors tended to be associated with high gene expression.

F. Differential Diagnosis

Diagnosis of neuroblastoma is based on the recognition of the neural elements that constitute it, and in general this neurility is present in sufficient quantities for ready identification. As a result, cytologic preparations and bone marrow aspirates are often used for primary diagnosis. However, occasional examples show minimal or no differentiation at the light microscopic level, necessitating use of the ancillary techniques described above. Essential elements to consider are the clinical settings and radiographic images, as calcified adrenal masses in infants and very young children are also uniformly neuroblastomas. Another important feature is urinary catecholamine secretion, whose measurement should be considered prior to excision of these lesions to avoid postexcisional declines to nondiagnostic levels. Neuroblastic tumors are also morphologically similar to PNETs, but there are great treatment differences, so that it behooves the pathologist to perform ancillary studies as described above if distinction is an issue. Usually this is a problem with paravertebral, thoracic, and pelvic tumors, as both entities may occur in these locations.

Other entities that may be considered include Wilms' tumors, as distinction between Wilms' tumors with adrenal extension and neuroblastomas with renal extension or origin can be an issue both radiographically and clinically. Happily, distinction can usually be made because of the neurogenic tendencies of the former and the nephroblastic proclivity of the latter. However, Wilms' tumors may contain neural elements, so that some degree of caution is advised in questionable cases. Another overlapping element is anaplasia, which may occur in both tumors.

Finally, another lesion to be aware of is the pigmented neuroectodermal tumor (or retinal anlage tumor). This tumor is a neuroblastic lesion, unrelated to typical neuroblastoma and usually occurring in the head and neck region of young children. Because neuroblastoma may occur in the neck, there is potential clinical overlap, but the pigmented neuroectodermal lesion generally does not metastasize and thus deserves an entirely different therapeutic approach. Distinction between the two entities is made by the presence of nests of melanocytic cells laden with dark brown melanin pigment, which is the key diagnostic feature of pigmented neuroectodermal tumor.

Another neuroblastic look-alike is the esthesioneuroblastoma, a primitive neural tumor arising from the neuroepithelium of the olfactory placode. This tumor is an invasive, aggressive neoplasm that erodes into the cribriform plate and thus into the base of the brain, and it deserves aggressive combined therapy. Some geneticists have observed the *EWS;FLI1* fusion of PNET in these tumors (136), linking it to the Ewing family, but others have not (137). Distinctive features are the presence of epithelial markers expected of its neuroepithelial origin and the absence of CD99 expression, which would suggest nonrelatedness to PNET (138).

V. DESMOPLASTIC SMALL-CELL TUMOR

A. Clinical Features

Desmoplastic small-cell tumor is descriptively named malignancy that primarily affects adolescents and young adults and arises in the peritoneal cavity and retroperitoneum. Although initially considered to arise exclusively from these sites, recent reports have expanded its sites of origin to the head and thorax (139,140). Scrotal tumors have also been described, but these likely arise from the peritoneal extension into this region via the tunica vaginalis.

Desmoplastic small-cell tumor is an aggressive, highly malignant neoplasm. Its unrestrained behavior, with peritoneal seeding, abdominal adhesion, and omental cake formation, is reminiscent of mesothelioma and ovarian surface carcinomas, and some have considered it a primitive variety of the former tumor. Treatment attempts have been largely unsuccessful with incompletely excised lesions, and it is hoped that future protocols will be more successful in eradicating this pernicious neoplasm.

B. Gross Features

In its typical intra-abdominal location, desmoplastic small-cell tumor occurs as a sclerotic, locally invasive mass that may arise anywhere from the surface of the ovary (141) to the pancreas. As noted above, there is often evidence of peritoneal spread, so that the surgeon should carefully examine the mesothelial surfaces.

C. Microscopic Features

Desmoplastic small-cell tumor has only recently been added to our diagnostic lexicon (142). Its descriptive sobriquet encompasses its usual histology, comprising

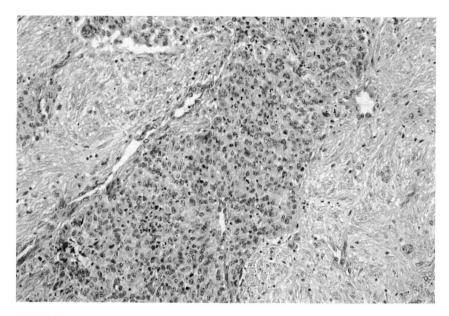

FIG. 22 Desmoplastic small-cell tumor. In this photomicrograph, a central cellular strand of primitive small cells is surrounded by dense fibrous tissue.

nests of primitive small cells encircled by a mass of dense fibrotic tissue (Fig. 22). The small-cell foci may contain vague rosettes or epithelioid features, and often cells have a rhabdoid appearance, raising a consideration of alveolar rhabdomyosarcoma because of their abundant pinkish cytoplasm that contains hyaline inclusions.

D. Ancillary Techniques

1. Electron Microscopy and Immunohistochemistry

As might be anticipated from the above histologic description, desmoplastic small-cell tumors exhibit a vague mixture of primitive neural and epithelial features by electron microscopy, i.e., scattered neurosecretory granules and microvillous surfaces. Mostly the cells are primitive and seemingly undifferentiated, in stark contrast to the panoply of markers they exhibit by immunohistochemistry. It is thus the multipotentiality of desmoplastic small-cell tumor that characterizes it phenotypically. One should thus observe varying levels of positivity for desmin, vimentin, epithelial membrane antigen, cytokeratin, neuron-specific enolase,

S-100 protein, synaptophysin, and CD57 (143,144). It is apparent that desmoplastic small-cell tumors are a hybrid of mesenchymal, epithelial, and neural cells.

2. Cytogenetics/Molecular Genetics

As might be expected from a hybrid lesion, desmoplastic small-ccll tumor is genetically characterized by a fusion of the *WT1* gene on chromosome 11 and the *EWS* gene on chromosome 22, karyotypically expressed by a reciprocal translocation, the t(11;22)(p13;q12). It is important to note that although similar chromosomes are involved, the breakpoint on chromosome 11 is totally different from that of the Ewing family of tumors but rather is mutated in some Wilms' tumors. As with Ewing's tumors and alveolar rhabdomyosarcomas, RT-PCR or FISH can be profitably used for ancillary diagnosis by demonstration of this chimeric gene. One caveat is that occasional desmoplastic small-cell tumors may contain the *EWS;FLI1* fusion typical of Ewing's tumors rather than the *EWS;WT1* fusion (120), so that histopathologic correlation is advisable.

A noteworthy feature of the *WT1* gene involvement in desmoplastic small-cell tumor is that this gene is important not only to normal kidney development but also mesothelial development. Strong expression of *WT1* by splanchnic mesoderm occurs during embryogenesis. Hypothetically, this may link the desmoplastic small-cell tumor with its predilection for mesothelial tissues in both origin and spread. Another link is that some tumors previously diagnosed as adult Wilms' tumors or extrarenal Wilms' tumors could represent examples of this lesion.

E. Differential Diagnosis

Besides consideration of Wilms' tumors in the differential diagnosis, thought should be given to Ewing family tumors, which as noted may have a nested alveolar-like pattern, and alveolar rhabdomyosarcoma, in which this pattern is typical. The key distinguishing features are the typical clinical presentation, the polyphenotypia with combined expression of epithelial, neural, and mesenchymal markers, and the *EWS;WT1* genetic marker, which is demonstrable by the t(11;22)(p13;q12) with standard karyotyping.

VI. OTHER TUMORS THAT MAY PRESENT AS SMALL-CELL SARCOMAS

The following brief dissertation will touch on the variety of other neoplasms that may present as small-cell sarcomas. For more detailed discussions, please consult the appropriate chapters in this text. It should be apparent to the reader that the differential diagnosis of small-cell tumors encompasses a wide range of pathologic entities. This dilemma is usually solved by careful histologic examination and correlation with clinical, radiographic, clinical laboratory, immunohistochemical, ultrastructural, cytogenetic, and genetic findings. Thus, it is no wonder that pathologists often become equivocating and demanding when dealing with these lesions, particularly since the tumors are often highly malignant and require toxic therapies. Experience levels, clinical settings, and availability of tests vary from institution to institution, so that a variety of ancillary test algorithms may be used for any given case. It is also a truism that even in experienced hands, a small percentage of cases remain a nosologic mystery and so continue to deserve the title of "undifferentiated small-cell malignancy." However, these can still be entered on protocols such as those of the IRSG, which accepts undifferentiated sarcomas (see above).

The most critical neoplasms to exclude when diagnosing a small-cell malignancy are the hematologic cancers, as both lymphomas and leukemias may present as soft-tissue masses (121,145). This requires close attention to cytologic details, which may be more apparent on touch preps than on histologic sections. One should also avoid the occasional overlap in phenotypic marker expression that may occur, as lymphoblastic lesions commonly express the CD99 "Ewing" marker (109), and rhabdomyosarcoma rarely expresses B-cell markers (22). Finally, an unfortunate observation that I have rarely made is the possible confusion of Langerhans cell histiocytosis with rhabdomyosarcoma.

Another group of neoplasms to consider when dealing with small-cell sarcomas is those that usually have a spindle cell predominance. Monophasic synovial sarcoma and malignant peripheral nerve sheath tumor are foremost in this category. Monophasic synovial sarcoma lacks the distinctive epithelial component that facilitates diagnosis of its biphasic counterpart, and it occurs in locations, clinical settings, and ages typical of the other tumors discussed above. Furthermore, synovial sarcomas may invade a variety of structures, such as nerve or bone, and its cytologic features may overlap with PNET or atypical Ewing's tumor; furthermore, it can express S-100 protein. However, diagnosis is usually resolvable by the cytokeratin and epithelial membrane antigen positivity, the typical genetic fusion, *SSX;SYT*, expressed karyotypically as t(X;18)(p11;q11), and the finding of microcalcifications (see Chapter 14).

Malignant peripheral nerve sheath tumors in children often contain small-cell foci (84), inviting confusion with PNET (Fig. 23). In rare instances, neuroepithelial canals as seen with medulloepithelioma, a rare brain tumor, may occur. Another potentially confusing aspect of peripheral nerve sheath tumors is their potential for rhabdomyoblastic differentiation. This form of nerve sheath tumor is known as Triton tumor because its origin was once thought to be analogous to the capacity for limb regeneration seen in Triton salamanders. Confusion with rhab-

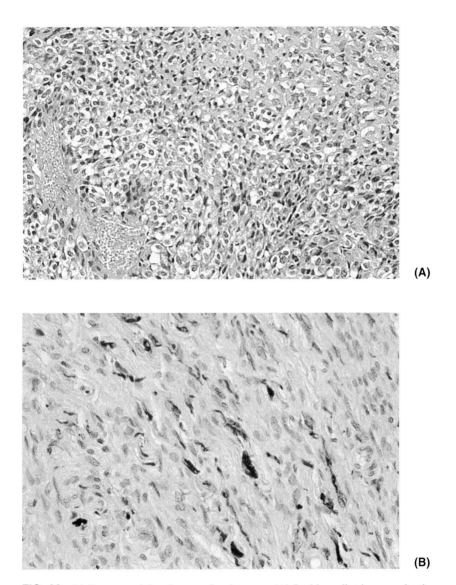

(A)

(B)

FIG. 23 Malignant peripheral nerve sheath tumor. (A) In this pediatric example, there are prominent aggregates of primitive Ewing's sarcoma–like cells. (B) Other areas of this tumor are composed of more typical, wavy, spindle cells. In this immunostain, the darkly staining nuclei indicate the presence of S-100 protein, a marker of Schwann cell differentiation.

domyosarcoma is possible if the nerve sheath component is not recognized. For additional discussion of peripheral nerve sheath tumors, see Chapter 9.

A number of organ-specific blastomas, or tumors that recapitulate organogenesis, consist largely of a small-cell complement. These are listed in Table 1. These lesions generally only arise within their derivative organs, although extrarenal Wilms' tumors exist (146). The differential diagnosis is made more difficult by the fact that small-cell sarcomas may occur in the same organs as blastomas; for example, PNET may occur in the kidney and desmoplastic small-cell tumor in the pancreas. Careful microscopic examination of the tumor should reveal the embryonal histology seen in these blastomatous neoplasms, as Wilms' tumor is recognized by its tubulogenesis and glomerulogenesis. Problems may arise, even with Wilms' tumors, when a sarcomatous element resembling rhabdomyosarcoma overgrows the other elements, if the blastoma is completely undifferentiated, or if sampling error clouds the picture. For further discussion of these various tumors, the reader is advised to consult more detailed texts (147).

Germ cell tumors arise in a variety of locations, including the retroperitoneum, and thus should also be considered in the differential diagnosis of small-cell tumors. In particular, germinomas (dysgerminomas, seminomas) are composed of primitive cells with monotonous round nuclei and glycogenated cytoplasm. Immunohistochemical stains for placental alkaline phosphatase can help in identifying these lesions, which usually contain a mononuclear inflammatory cell component that may form granulomas. Often germ cell tumors show partial differentiation into other forms, so that careful examination may reveal additional foci of teratoma, embryonal carcinoma, yolk sac carcinoma, or choriocarcinoma. It is always advisable to save a preoperative blood sample from suspected germ cell tumor patients, as α-fetoprotein or human chorionic gonadotropin levels are useful in both diagnosing and monitoring these lesions. Metabolism of these compounds occurs after surgery, and the resultant drop in postoperative blood levels renders them unreliable.

A final category of small-cell tumors, probably the most common group overall, is small-cell carcinomas, which are very rare in children but unfortunately common in adults. These are epithelial lesions that generally arise from mucosal surfaces such as the bronchus or urothelium, so that clinical distinction is usually possible. Overlap occurs with neuroendocrine lesions such as carcinoids, but small-cell carcinomas do not occur in soft tissues. On the other hand, small-cell sarcomas may occur in solid organs, so they are worth diagnostic consideration, particularly if rosettes or rhabdomyoblasts are identified. Definitive diagnosis may require immunohistochemistry for cytokeratin as well as the neural and muscle markers described above, and electron microscopy can also be used to identify epithelial features, such as tonofilaments and desmosomes. Of note is the occasional finding of neuroendocrine and rhabdomyosarcomatous differentiation in adult carcinomas.

REFERENCES

1. Issacs H. Tumors of the Fetus and Newborn. Philadelphia: WB Saunders, 1997.
2. Hentrich M, Hartenstein R. Wilms' tumor in adults. Onkologie 18:310–315, 1995.
3. Triche TJ. Neuroblastoma and other childhood neural tumors: a review. Pediatr Pathol 10:175–193, 1990.
4. Willis RA. The Borderland of Embryology and Pathology. London: Butterworths, 1962, pp. 422–466.
5. Moody AM, Norman AR, Tait D. Paediatric tumours in the adult population—the experience of the Royal Marsden Hospital 1974–1990. Med Pediatr Oncol 26:153–159, 1996.
6. Ross JA, Severson RK, Pollock BH, Robison LL. Childhood cancer in the United States. A geographical analysis of cases from the Pediatric Cooperative Clinical Trials groups. Cancer 77:201–207, 1996.
7. Coffin CM, Dehner LP. Peripheral neurogenic tumors of the soft tissues in children and adolescents: a clinicopathologic study of 139 cases. Pediatr Pathol 9:387–407, 1989.
8. Maurer HM, Beltangady M, Gehan EA, Crist W, Hammond D, Hays DM, Heyn R, Lawrence W, Newton W, Ortega J, Ragab AH, Raney RB, Ruymann FB, Soule E, Tefft M, Webber B, Wharam M, Vietti TJ. The Intergroup Rhabdomyosarcoma Study—I: a final report. Cancer 61:209–220, 1988.
9. Schmidt D, Harms D. The applicability of immunohistochemistry in the diagnosis and differential diagnosis of malignant soft tissue tumors. A reevaluation based on the material of the Kiel Pediatric Tumor Registry. Klin Padiatr 202:224–229, 1990.
10. Horn RC, Enterline HT. Rhabdomyosarcoma: a clinicopathologic study of 39 cases. Cancer 11:181–199, 1958.
11. Tsokos M, Webber B, Parham D, Wesley R, Miser A, Miser JS, Etcubanas E, Kinsella T, Grayson J, Galtstein E, Pizzo PA, Triche TJ. Rhabdomyosarcoma: a new classification scheme related to prognosis. Arch Pathol Lab Med 116:847–855, 1992.
12. Cavazzana AO, Schmidt D, Ninfo V, Harms D, Tollot M, Carli M, Treuner J, Betto R, Salviati G. Spindle cell rhabdomyosarcoma: a prognostically favorable variant of rhabdomyosarcoma. Am J Surg Pathol 16:229–235, 1992.
13. Leuschner I, Newton WA Jr, Schmidt D, Sachs N, Asmar L, Hamoudi A, Harms D, Maurer HM. Spindle cell variants of embryonal rhabdomyosarcoma in the paratesticular region: a report of the intergroup rhabdomyosarcoma study. Am J Surg Pathol 17:221–230, 1993.
14. Caillaud JM, Gérard-Marchant R, Marsden HB, van Unnik AJM, Rodary C, Rey A, Flamant F. Histopathologic classification of childhood rhabdomyosarcoma: a report from the International Society of Pediatric Oncology Pathology Panel. Med Pediatr Oncol 17:391–400, 1989.
15. Parham DM, Shapiro DN, Downing JR, Webber BL, Douglass EC. Solid alveolar rhabdomyosarcomas with the t(2;13). Report of two cases with diagnostic implications. Am J Surg Pathol 18:474–478, 1994.
16. Asmar L, Gehan EA, Newton WA, Webber BL, Marsden HB, van Unnik AJM, Hamoudi AB, Shimada H, Tsokos M, Harms D, Ninfo V, Schmidt D, Cavazzana A, Gonzalez-Crussi F, Parham DM, Reiman HM, Beltangady MS, Sachs N, Triche TJ,

Maurer HM. Agreement among and within groups of pathologists in the classification of rhabdomyosarcoma and related childhood sarcomas: report of an international study of four pathology classifications. Cancer 74:2579–2588, 1994.

17. Newton WA Jr, Gehan EA, Webber BL, Marsden HB, van Unnik AJM, Hamoudi AB, Tsokos M, Shimada H, Harms D, Schmidt D, Ninfo V, Cavazzana A, Gonzales-Crussi F, Parham DM, Reiman HM, Asmar L, Beltangady MS, Sachs N, Triche TJ, Maurer HM. Classification of rhabdomyosarcoma and related sarcomas: pathologic aspects and proposal for a new classification—an Intergroup Rhabdomyosarcoma Study. Cancer 76:1073–1085, 1995.

18. Ruymann FB. Rhabdomyosarcoma in children and adolescents: a review. Hematol Oncol Clin North Am 1:621–654, 1987.

19. Choi YS, Lundy RO. Rhabdomyosarcoma and hypercalcemia. Arch Intern Med 149:1189–1189, 1989.

20. Etcubanas E, Peiper S, Stass S, Green A. Rhabdomyosarcoma, presenting as disseminated malignancy from an unknown primary site: a retrospective study of ten pediatric cases. Med Pediatr Oncol 17:39–44, 1989.

21. Kahn DG. Rhabdomyosarcoma mimicking acute leukemia in an adult: report of a case with histologic, flow cytometric, cytogenetic, immunohistochemical, and ultrastructural studies. Arch Pathol Lab Med 122:375–378, 1998.

22. Pinto A, Tallini G, Novak RW, Bowen T, Parham DM. Undifferentiated rhabdomyosarcoma with lymphoid phenotype expression. Med Pediatr Oncol 28:165–170, 1997.

23. Crist WM, Garnsey L, Beltangady MS, Gehan E, Ruymann F, Webber B, Hays DM, Wharam M, Maurer HM. Prognosis in children with rhabdomyosarcoma: a report of the Intergroup Rhabdomyosarcoma Studies I and II. J Clin Oncol 8:443–452, 1990.

24. Koscielniak E, Rodary C, Flamant F, Carli M, Treuner J, Pinkerton CR, Grotto P. Metastatic rhabdomyosarcoma and histologically similar tumors in childhood: a retrospective European multi-center analysis. Med Pediatr Oncol 20:209–214, 1992.

25. Maurer HM, Gehan EA, Beltangady M, Crist W, Dickman PS, Donaldson SS, Fryer C, Hammond D, Hays DM, Herrmann J, Heyn R, Jones PM, Lawrence W, Newton W, Ortega J, Ragab AH, Raney RB, Ruymann FB, Soule E, Tefft M, Webber B, Weiner E, Wharam M, Vietti TJ. The Intergroup Rhabdomyosarcoma Study–II. Cancer 71:1904–1922, 1993.

26. Crist W, Gehan EA, Ragab AH, Dickman PS, Donaldson SS, Fryer C, Hammond D, Hays DM, Herrmann J, Heyn R. The Third Intergroup Rhabdomyosarcoma Study. J Clin Oncol 13:610–630, 1995.

27. Heyn R, Raney RB Jr, Hays DM, Tefft M, Gehan E, Webber B, Maurer HM. Late effects of therapy in patients with paratesticular rhabdomyosarcoma. Intergroup Rhabdomyosarcoma Study Committee. J Clin Oncol 10:614–623, 1992.

28. Lobe TE, Wiener E, Andrassy RJ, Bagwell CE, Hays D, Crist WM, Webber B, Breneman JC, Reed MM, Tefft MC, Heyn R. The argument for conservative, delayed surgery in the management of prostatic rhabdomyosarcoma. J Pediatr Surg 31:1084–1087, 1996.

29. Heyn R, Haeberlen V, Newton WA, Ragab AH, Raney RB, Tefft M, Wharam M, Ensign LG, Maurer HM. Second malignant neoplasms in children treated for rhabdo-

myosarcoma. Intergroup Rhabdomyosarcoma Study Committee [see comments]. J Clin Oncol 11:262–270, 1993.

30. Newton WA Jr, Soule EH, Hamoudi AB, Reiman HM, Shimada H, Beltangady M, Maurer H. Histopathology of childhood sarcomas, Intergroup Rhabdomyosarcoma Studies I and II: clinicopathologic correlation. J Clin Oncol 6:67–75, 1988.

31. Weinberg AG, Currarino G, Hurt GE Jr. Botryoid Wilms' tumor of the renal pelvis. Arch Pathol Lab Med 108:147–148, 1984.

32. Boman F, Champigneulle J, Schmitt C, Beurey P, Floquet J, Boccon G. Clear cell rhabdomyosarcoma. Pediatr Pathol Lab Med 16:951–959, 1996.

33. Triche TJ, Ross WE. Glycogen-containing neuroblastoma with clinical and histopathologic features of Ewing's sarcoma. Cancer 41:1425–1432, 1978.

34. Parham DM. The molecular biology of childhood rhabdomyosarcoma. Semin Diagn Pathol 11:39–46, 1994.

35. Heyn R, Newton WA, Raney RB, Hamoudi A, Bagwell C, Vietti T, Wharam M, Gehan E, Maurer HM. Preservation of the bladder in patients with rhabdomyosarcoma. J Clin Oncol 15:69–75, 1997.

36. Wijnaendts LCD, van der Linden JC, van Unnik AJM, Delemarre JFM, Voute PA, Meijer CJLM. Histologic classification of childhood rhabdomyosarcomas: relationship with clinical parameters and prognosis. Hum Pathol 25:900–907, 1994.

37. Gaffney EF, Dervan PA, Fletcher CDM. Pleomorphic rhabdomyosarcoma in adulthood: Analysis of 11 cases with definition of diagnostic criteria. Am J Surg Pathol 17:601–609, 1993.

38. Wesche WA, Fletcher CDM, Dias P, Houghton PJ, Parham DM. Immunohistochemistry of MyoD1 in adult pleomorphic soft tissue sarcomas. Am J Surg Pathol 19:261–269, 1995.

39. Fletcher CDM. Pleomorphic malignant fibrous histiocytoma: fact or fiction? A critical reappraisal based on 159 tumors diagnosed as pleomorphic sarcoma. Am J Surg Pathol 16:213–228, 1992.

40. Faria P, Beckwith JB, Mishra K, Zuppan C, Weeks DA, Breslow N, Green DM. Focal versus diffuse anaplasia in wilms tumor—New definitions with prognostic significance: a report from the National Wilms Tumor Study Group. Am J Surg Pathol 20:909–920, 1996.

41. Joshi VV, Silverman JF, Altshuler G, Cantor AB, Larkin EW, Neill JSA, Norris HT, Shuster JJ, Tate Holbrook C, Hayes FA, Smith EI, Castleberry RP. Systematization of primary histopathologic and fine-needle aspiration cytologic features and description of unusual histopathologic features of neuroblastic tumors: A report from the Pediatric Oncology Group. Hum Pathol 24:493–504, 1993.

42. Kodet R, Newton WA Jr, Hamoudi AB, Asmar L, Jacobs DL, Maurer HM. Childhood rhabdomyosarcoma with anaplastic (pleomorphic) features: a report of the Intergroup Rhabdomyosarcoma Study. Am J Surg Pathol 17:443–453, 1993.

43. Douglass EC, Look AT, Webber B, Parham D, Wilimas JA, Green AA, Roberson PK. Hyperdiploidy and chromosomal rearrangements define the anaplastic variant of Wilms' tumor. J Clin Oncol 4:975–981, 1986.

44. Pawel BR, Hamoudi AB, Asmar L, Newton WAJ, Ruymann FB, Qualman SJ, Webber BL, Maurer HM. Undifferentiated sarcomas of children: pathology and clinical

behavior—an intergroup Rhabdomyosarcoma study. Med Pediatr Oncol 29:170–180, 1997.

45. Boue D, Parham D, Webber B, Maurer H, Qualman S. Clinicopathologic study of pediatric ectomesenchymoma from IRS III and IV. Mod Pathol 10:2P, 1997 (abstr).

46. Sorensen PH, Shimada H, Liu XF, Lim JF, Thomas G, Triche TJ. Biphenotypic sarcomas with myogenic and neural differentiation express the Ewing's sarcoma EWS/FLI1 fusion gene. Cancer Res 55:1385–1392, 1995.

47. Thorner P, Squire J, Chilton-MacNeill S, Marrano P, Bayani J, Malkin D, Greenberg M, Lorenzana A, Zielenska M. Is the EWS/FLI-1 fusion transcript specific for Ewing sarcoma and peripheral primitive neuroectodermal tumor? A report of four cases showing this transcript in a wider range of tumor types. Am J Pathol 148:1125–1138, 1996.

48. Le Douarin NM, Ziller C. Plasticity in neural crest cell differentiation. Curr Opin Cell Biol 5:1036–1043, 1993.

49. Weintraub H. The MyoD family and myogenesis: Redundancy, networks, and thresholds. Cell 75:1241–1244, 1993.

50. Erlandson RA. The ultrastructural distinction between rhabdomyosarcoma and other undifferentiated "sarcomas." Ultrastruct Pathol 11:83–101, 1987.

51. Dickman PS, Triche TJ. Extraosseous Ewing's sarcoma versus primitive rhabdomyosarcoma: diagnostic criteria and clinical correlation. Hum Pathol 17:881–893, 1986.

52. Mierau GW, Berry PJ, Malott RL, Weeks DA. Appraisal of the comparative utility of immunohistochemistry and electron microscopy in the diagnosis of childhood round cell tumors. Ultrastruct Pathol 20:507–517, 1996.

53. Wang NP, Marx J, McNutt MA, Rutledge JC, Gown AM. Expression of myogenic regulatory proteins (myogenin and MyoD1) in small blue round cell tumors of childhood. Am J Pathol 147:1799–1810, 1995.

54. Parham DM, Dias P, Kelly DR, Rutledge JC, Houghton P. Desmin positivity in primitive neuroectodermal tumors of childhood. Am J Surg Pathol 16:483–492, 1992.

55. Folpe AL, Patterson K, Gown AM. Antibodies to desmin identify the blastemal component of nephroblastoma. Mod Pathol 10:895–900, 1997.

56. Shapiro DN, Sublett JE, Li B, Downing JR, Naeve CW. Fusion of *PAX3* to a member of the forkhead family of transcription factors in human alveolar rhabdomyosarcoma. Cancer Res 53:5108–5112, 1993.

57. Kelly KM, Womer RB, Sorensen PH, Xiong QB, Barr FG. Common and variant gene fusions predict distinct clinical phenotypes in rhabdomyosarcoma. J Clin Oncol 15:1831–1836, 1997.

58. Barr FG, Xiong QB, Kelly K. A consensus polymerase chain reaction-oligonucleotide hybridization approach for the detection of chromosomal translocations in pediatric bone and soft tissue sarcomas. Am J Clin Pathol 104:627–633, 1995.

59. Downing JR, Head D, Parham DM, Shapiro DN. A multiplex RT-PCR assay for the diagnosis of alveolar rhabdomyosarcoma and Ewing's sarcoma. Mod Pathol 7:146A, 1994 (abstr).

60. Barr FG, Chatten J, D'Cruz CM, Wilson AE, Nauta LE, Nycum LM, Biegel JA, Womer RB. Molecular assays for chromosomal translocations in the diagnosis of pediatric soft tissue sarcomas. JAMA 273:553–557, 1995.

61. Scrable H, Witte D, Shimada H, Seemayer T, Wang-Wuu S, Soukup S, Koufos A, Houghton P, Lampkin B, Cavenee W. Molecular differential pathology in rhabdomyosarcoma. Genes Chrom Cancer 1:23–35, 1989.

62. Koufos A, Hansen MF, Copeland NG, Jenkins NA, Lampkin BC, Cavenee WK. Loss of heterozygosity in three embryonal tumours suggests a common pathogenetic mechanism. Nature 316:330–334, 1985.

63. Chen B, Dias P, Jenkins JJ, Savell VH, Parham DM. Methylation alterations of the MyoD1 upstream region are predictive of subclassification of human rhabdomyosarcomas. Am J Pathol 152:1071–1079, 1998.

64. Palmer H, Parham D, Chen B, Dilday B, Houghton P, Dias P. Strong immunohistochemical expression of myoglobin correlates with alveolar histology in rhabdomyosarcoma. Mod Pathol 11:14A, 1998 (abstr).

65. Rawls A, Olson EN. MyoD meets its maker. Cell 89:5–8, 1997.

66. Rudnicki MA, Schnegelsberg PNJ, Stead RH, Braun T, Arnold H-H, Jaenisch R. MyoD or Myf-5 is required for the formation of skeletal muscle. Cell 75:1351–1359, 1993.

67. Ewing J. Diffuse endothelioma of bone. Proc NY Pathol Soc 21:17–24, 1921.

68. Stout AP. A tumor of the ulnar nerve. Proc NY Pathol Soc 18:2–2, 1918.

69. Dehner LP. Primitive neuroectodermal tumor and Ewing's sarcoma. Am J Surg Pathol 17:1–13, 1993.

70. Lichtenstein L: Bone Tumors. 5th ed. St. Louis: C.V. Mosby, 1977, pp. 267–287.

71. Askin FB, Rosai J, Sibley RK, Dehner LP, McAlister WH. Malignant small cell tumor of the thoracopulmonary region in childhood: a distinctive clinicopathologic entity of uncertain histogenesis. Cancer 43:2438–2451, 1979.

72. Delattre O, Zucman J, Melot T, Garau XS, Zucker J-M, Lenoir GM, Ambros PF, Sheer D, Turc-Carel C, Triche TJ, Aurias A, Thomas G. The Ewing family of tumors—a subgroup of small-round-cell tumors defined by specific chimeric transcripts. N Engl J Med 331:294–299, 1994.

73. Harms D, Schmidt D. Rare tumors in childhood: pathologic aspects. Experience of the Kiel Pediatric Tumor Registry. Med Pediatr Oncol 21:239–248, 1993.

74. Yunis EJ. Ewing's sarcoma and related small round cell neoplasms in children. Am J Surg Pathol 10(Supp.1):54–62, 1986.

75. Jaffe R, Santamaria M, Yunis EJ, Tannery NH, Agostini RM, Medina J, Goodman M. The neuroectodermal tumor of bone. Am J Surg Pathol 8:885–898, 1984.

76. Nascimento AG, Unni KK, Pritchard DJ, Cooper KL, Dahlin DC. A clinicopathologic study of 20 cases of large-cell (atypical) Ewing's sarcoma of bone. Am J Surg Pathol 4:29–36, 1980.

77. Hartman KR, Triche TJ, Kinsella TJ, Miser JS. Prognostic value of histopathology in Ewing's sarcoma: long-term follow-up of distal extremity primary tumors. Cancer 67:163–171, 1991.

78. Schmidt D, Herrmann C, Jurgens H, Harms D. Malignant peripheral neuroectodermal tumor and its necessary distinction from Ewing's sarcoma. A report from the Kiel Pediatric Tumor Registry. Cancer 68:2251–2259, 1991.

79. Terrier P, Henry-Amar M, Triche TJ, Horowitz ME, Terrier-Lacombe MJ, Miser JS, Kinsella TJ, Contesso G, Llombart-Bosch A. Is neuro-ectodermal differentiation of

Ewing's sarcoma of bone associated with an unfavourable prognosis? Eur J Cancer 31A:307–314, 1995.

80. Hijazi Y, Worthy E, Steinberg S, Horowitz M, Tsokos M. Ewing's sarcoma (ES) vs. primitive neuroectodermal tumor (PNET)—does histology play a role in prognosis? Mod Pathol 6:126A, 1993 (abstr).

81. Marina NM, Etcubanas E, Parham DM, Bowman LC, Green A. Peripheral primitive neuroectodermal tumor (peripheral neuroepithelioma) in children: a review of the St. Jude experience and controversies in diagnosis and management. Cancer 64: 1952–1960, 1989.

82. Pratt CB, Meyer WH, Marina N, Pappo A, Luo X, Kun L. Ewing sarcoma under the age of 12 years. Proc Annu Meet Am Soc Clin Oncol 12:A1431, 1994 (abstr).

83. Maygarden SJ, Askin FB, Siegal GP, Gilula LA, Schoppe J, Foulkes M, Kissane JM, Nesbit M. Ewing sarcoma of bone in infants and toddlers: a clinicopathologic report from the Intergroup Ewing's Study. Cancer 71:2109–2118, 1993.

84. Meis JM, Enzinger FM, Martz KL, Neal JA. Malignant peripheral nerve sheath tumors (malignant schwannomas) in children. Am J Surg Pathol 16:694–707, 1992.

85. Rodriguez-Galindo C, Marina NM, Fletcher BD, Parham DM, Bodner SM, Meyer WH. Is primitive neuroectodermal tumor of the kidney a distinct entity? Cancer 79:2243–2250, 1997.

86. Marley EF, Liapis H, Humphrey PA, Nadler RB, Siegel CL, Zhu X, Brandt JM, Dehner LP. Primitive neuroectodermal tumor of the kidney—another enigma: a pathologic, immunohistochemical, and molecular diagnostic study. Am J Surg Pathol 21:354–359, 1997.

87. Lazzara EW, Ragland RL, Smith TW, Knorr JR, Weiner MA, Kamath SV, Law KY. Basimeningeal/spinal axis primitive neuroectodermal tumor without intraaxial lesion: radiological features. J Neuroimag 8:49–54, 1998.

88. Hisaoka M, Hashimoto H, Murao T. Peripheral primitive neuroectodermal tumour with ganglioneuroma-like areas arising in the cauda equina. Virchows Arch 431: 365–369, 1997.

89. Akai T, Iizuka H, Kadoya S, Nojima T, Kohno M. Primitive neuroectodermal tumor in the spinal epidural space—case report. Neurol Med Chir 38:508–511, 1998.

90. Donaldson SS. The value of adjuvant chemotherapy in the management of sarcomas in children. Cancer 55:2184–2197, 1985.

91. Meyer WH, Kun L, Marina N, Roberson P, Parham D, Rao B, Fletcher B, Pratt CB. Ifosfamide plus etoposide in newly diagnosed Ewing's sarcoma of bone. J Clin Oncol 10:1737–1742, 1992.

92. Raney RB, Asmar L, Newton WAJ, Bagwell C, Breneman JC, Crist W, Gehan EA, Webber B, Wharam M, Wiener ES, Anderson JR, Maurer HM. Ewing's sarcoma of soft tissues in childhood: a report from the Intergroup Rhabdomyosarcoma Study, 1972 to 1991. J Clin Oncol 15:574–582, 1997.

93. Wexler LH, Delaney TF, Tsokos M, Avila N, Steinberg SM, Weaver-McClure L, Jacobson J, Jarosinski P, Hijazi YM, Balis FM, Horowitz ME. Ifosfamide and etoposide plus vincristine, doxorubicin, and cyclophosphamide for newly diagnosed Ewing's sarcoma family of tumors. Cancer 78:901–911, 1996.

94. Gururangan S, Marina NM, Luo X, Parham DM, Tzen C-Y, Greenwald CA, Rao BN, Kun LE, Meyer WH. Treatment of children with peripheral neuroectodermal tumor or extraosseous Ewing's tumor with Ewing's directed therapy. J Pediatr Hematol Oncol 20:55–61, 1998.

95. Lemmi MA, Fletcher BD, Marina NM, Slade W, Parham DM, Jenkins JJ, Meyer WH. Use of MR imaging to assess results of chemotherapy for Ewing sarcoma. AJR Am J Roentgenol 155:343–346, 1990.

96. MacVicar AD, Olliff JF, Pringle J, Pinkerton CR, Husband JE. Ewing sarcoma: MR imaging of chemotherapy-induced changes with histologic correlation. Radiology 184:859–864, 1992.

97. Oberlin O, Patte C, Demeocq R, Lacombe MJ, Brunat-Mentigny M, Demaille M-C, Tron P, Bui BN, Lemerle J. The response to initial chemotherapy as a prognostic factor in localized Ewing's sarcoma. Eur J Cancer Clin Oncol 21:463–467, 1985.

98. Picci P, Bohling T, Bacci G, Ferrari S, Sangiorgi L, Mercuri M, Ruggieri P, Manfrini M, Ferraro A, Casadei R, Benassi MS, Mancini AF, Rosito P, Cazzola A, Barbieri E, Tienghi A, Brach dP, Comandone A, Bacchini P, Bertoni F. Chemotherapy-induced tumor necrosis as a prognostic factor in localized Ewing's sarcoma of the extremities. J Clin Oncol 15:1553–1559, 1997.

99. Soule EH, Newton W Jr, Moon TE, Tefft M. Extraskeletal Ewing's sarcoma: a preliminary review of 26 cases encountered in the Intergroup Rhabdomyosarcoma Study. Cancer 42:259–264, 1978.

100. Pinto A, Grant LH, Hayes FA, Schell MJ, Parham DM. Immunohistochemical expression of neuron-specific enolase and Leu 7 in Ewing's sarcoma of bone. Cancer 64:1266–1273, 1989.

101. Tsokos M. Peripheral primitive neuroectodermal tumors: diagnosis, classification, and prognosis. In: AJ Garvin, TJ O'Leary, J Bernstein, HS Rosenberg, eds. Pediatric Molecular Pathology: Quantitation and Applications. Perspectives in Pediatric Pathology, Vol. 16. Basel: Karger, 1992, pp. 27–98.

102. Dehner LP. Whence the primitive neuroectodermal tumor. Arch Pathol Lab Med 114:16–17, 1990.

103. Schneider BS, Helson L, Monahan JW, Friedman JM. Expression of cholecystokinin gene by cultured human primitive neuroepithelioma cell lines. J Clin Endocrinol Metab 69:411–419, 1989.

104. Mierau GW, Berry PJ, Orsini EN. Small round cell neoplasms: can electron microscopy and immunohistochemical studies accurately classify them. Ultrastruct Pathol 9:99–111, 1985.

105. Mierau GW. Extraskeletal Ewing's sarcoma (peripheral neuroepithelioma). Ultrastruct Pathol 9:91–98, 1985.

106. Ghali VS, Jimenez EJS, Garcia RL. Distribution of Leu-7 antigen (HNK-1) in thyroid tumors: its usefulness as a diagnostic marker for follicular and papillary carcinomas. Hum Pathol 23:21–25, 1992.

107. Stevenson AJ, Chatten J, Bertoni F, Miettinen M. CD99 (p30/32^{MIC2}) neuroectodermal/Ewing's sarcoma antigen as an immunohistochemical marker: review of more than 600 tumors and the literature experience. Appl Immunohistochem 2:231–240, 1994.

108. Ramani P, Rampling D, Link M. Immunocytochemical study of 12E7 in small round-cell tumours of childhood: an assessment of its sensitivity and specificity. Histopathology 23:557–561, 1993.

109. Riopel M, Dickman PS, Link MP, Perlman EJ. MIC2 analysis in pediatric lymphomas and leukemias. Hum Pathol 25:396–399, 1994.

110. Qualman SJ, Coffin CM, Newton WA, Hojo H, Triche TJ, Parham DM, Crist WM. Intergroup Rhabdomyosarcoma Study: update for pathologists. Pediatr Dev Pathol 1:463–474, 1998.

111. Zucman J, Melot T, Desmaze C, Ghysdael J, Plougastel B, Peter M, Zucker JM, Triche TJ, Sheer D, Turc-Carel C, Ambros P, Combaret V, Lenoir G, Aurias A, Thomas G, Delattre O. Combinatorial generation of variable fusion proteins in the Ewing family of tumours. EMBO J 12:4481–4487, 1993.

112. Delattre O, Zucman J, Plougastel B, Desmaze C, Melot T, Peter M, Kovar H, Joubert I, de Jong P, Rouleau G, Aurias A, Thomas G. Gene fusion with an ETS DNA-binding domain caused by chromosome translocation in human tumours. Nature 359:162–165, 1992.

113. de Alava E, Kawai A, Healey JH, Fligman I, Meyers PA, Huvos AG, Gerald WL, Jhanwar SC, Argani P, Antonescu CR, Pardo-Mindan FJ, Ginsberg J, Womer R, Lawlor ER, Wunder J, Andrulis I, Sorensen PH, Barr FG, Ladanyi M. EWS-FLI1 fusion transcript structure is an independent determinant of prognosis in Ewing's sarcoma. J Clin Oncol 16:1248–1255, 1998.

114. Ben-David Y, Giddens EB, Letwin K, Bernstein A. Erythroleukemia induction by Friend murine leukemia virus: insertional activation of a new member of the ets gene family, Fli-1, closely linked to c-ets-1. Genes Dev 5:908–918, 1991.

115. Peter M, Courturier J, Pacquement H, Michon J, Thomas G, Magdelenat H, Delattre O. A new member of the ETS family fused to EWS in Ewing tumors. Oncogene 14:1159–1164, 1997.

116. Urano F, Umezawa A, Yabe H, Hong W, Yoshida K, Fujinaga K, Hata J. Molecular analysis of Ewing's sarcoma: another fusion gene, EWS-E1AF, available for diagnosis. Jap J Cancer Res 89:703–711, 1998.

117. Jeon IS, Davis JN, Braun BS, Sublett JE, Roussel MF, Denny CT, Shapiro DN. A variant Ewing's sarcoma translocation (7;22) fuses the EWS gene to the ETS gene ETV1. Oncogene 10:1229–1234, 1995.

118. Zucman J, Delattre O, Desmaze C, Epstein A, Stenman G, Speleman F, Fletcher CDM, Aurias A, Thomas G. EWS and ATF-1 gene fusion induced by t(12;22) translocation in malignant melanoma of soft parts. Nature Genet 4:341–345, 1993.

119. Brody RI, Ueda T, Hamelin A, Jhanwar SC, Bridge JA, Healey JH, Huvos AG, Gerald WL, Ladanyi M. Molecular analysis of the fusion of EWS to an orphan nuclear receptor gene in extraskeletal myxoid chondrosarcoma. Am J Pathol 150:1049–1058, 1997.

120. Katz RL, Quezado M, Senderowicz AM, Villalba L, Laskin WB, Tsokos M. An intra-abdominal small round cell neoplasm with features of primitive neuroectodermal and desmoplastic round cell tumor and a EWS/FLI-1 fusion transcript. Hum Pathol 28:502–509, 1997.

121. Lanham GR, Weiss SW, Enzinger FM. Malignant lymphoma. A study of 75 cases presenting in soft tissue. Am J Surg Pathol 13:1–10, 1989.

122. Dehner LP. Peripheral and central primitive neuroectodermal tumors. A nosologic concept seeking a consensus. Arch Pathol Lab Med 110:997–1005, 1986.

123. Thiele CJ, McKeon C, Triche TJ, Ross RA, Reynolds CP, Israel MA. Differential protooncogene expression characterizes histopathologically indistinguishable tumors of the peripheral nervous system. J Clin Invest 80:804–811, 1987.

124. Lo R, Perlman E, Hawkins AL, Hayashi R, Wechsler DS, Look AT, Griffin CA. Cytogenetic abnormalities in two cases of neuroblastoma. Cancer Genet Cytogenet 74:30–34, 1994.

125. Kelly DR, Joshi VV. Neuroblastoma and related tumors. In: DM Parham, ed. Pediatric Neoplasia: Morphology and Biology. Philadelphia: Lippincott-Raven, 1996, pp. 105–152.

126. Hann H-W, Evans AE, Cohen IJ, Leitmeyer JE. Biologic differences between neuroblastoma stages IV-S and IV: measurement of serum ferritin and E-rosette inhibition in 30 children. N Engl J Med 305:425–429, 1981.

127. Tonini GP. Neuroblastoma: a multiple biological disease. Eur J Cancer A 29:802–804, 1993.

128. Hayes FA, Green AA, Rao BN. Clinical manifestations of ganglioneuroma. Cancer 63:1211–1214, 1989.

129. Bolande RP. A natural immune system in pregnancy serum lethal to human neuroblastoma cells: A possible mechanism of spontaneous regression. Perspect Pediatr Pathol 16:120–133, 1992.

130. Shimada H, Chatten J, Newton WA Jr, Sachs N, Hamoudi AB, Chiba T, Marsden HB, Misugi K. Histopathologic prognostic factors in neuroblastic tumors: definition of subtypes of ganglioneuroblastoma and an age-linked classification of neuroblastomas. J Natl Cancer Inst 73:405–416, 1984.

131. Pappo AS, Douglass EC, Meyer WH, Marina N, Parham DM. Use of HBA71 and anti-b2-microglobulin to distinguish peripheral neuroepithelioma from neuroblastoma. Hum Pathol 24:880–885, 1993.

132. Miettinen M, Chatten J, Paetau A, Stevenson A. Monoclonal antibody NB84 in the differential diagnosis of neuroblastoma and other small round cell tumors. Am J Surg Pathol 22:327–332, 1998.

133. Garin-Chesa P, Fellinger EJ, Huvos AG, Beresford HR, Melamed MR, Triche TJ, Rettig WJ. Immunohistochemical analysis of neural cell adhesion molecules: differential expression in small round cell tumors of childhood and adolescence. Am J Pathol 139:275–286, 1991.

134. Brodeur GM, Moley JF. Biology of tumors of the peripheral nervous system. Cancer Metast Rev 10:321–333, 1991.

135. Tanaka T, Sugimoto T, Sawada T. Prognostic discrimination among neuroblastomas according to Ha-ras/trk A gene expression: a comparison of the profiles of neuroblastomas detected clinically and those detected through mass screening. Cancer 83:1626–1633, 1998.

136. Sorensen PH, Wu JK, Berean KW, Lim JF, Donn W, Frierson HF, Reynolds CP, Lopez-Terrada D, Triche TJ. Olfactory neuroblastoma is a peripheral primitive neuroectodermal tumor related to Ewing sarcoma. Proc Natl Acad Sci USA 93:1038–1043, 1996.

137. Argani P, Perez-Ordonez B, Xiao H, Caruana SM, Huvos AG, Ladanyi M. Olfactory

neuroblastoma is not related to the Ewing family of tumors: absence of EWS/FLI1 gene fusion and MIC2 expression. Am J Surg Pathol 22:391–398, 1998.

138. Parham DM. Ewing's sarcoma, peripheral neuroepithelioma, and related tumors. In: DM Parham, ed. Pediatric Neoplasia: Morphology and Biology. Philadelphia: Lippincott-Raven, 1996, pp. 65–85.

139. Bian Y, Jordan AG, Rupp M, Cohn H, McLaughlin CJ, Miettinen M. Effusion cytology of desmoplastic small round cell tumor of the pleura: A case report. Acta Cytol 37:77–82, 1993.

140. Tison V, Cerasoli S, Morigi F, Ladanyi M, Gerald WL, Rosai J. Intracranial desmoplastic small-cell tumor. Report of a case. Am J Surg Pathol 20:112–117, 1996.

141. Young RH, Eichhorn JH, Dickersin GR, Scully RE. Ovarian involvement by the intra-abdominal desmoplastic small round cell tumor with divergent differentiation: a report of three cases. Hum Pathol 23:454–464, 1992.

142. Gerald WL, Miller HK, Battifora H, Miettinen M, Silva EG, Rosai J. Intra-abdominal desmoplastic small round-cell tumor: report of 19 cases of a distinctive type of high-grade polyphenotypic malignancy affecting young individuals. Am J Surg Pathol 15:499–513, 1991.

143. Layfield LJ, Lenarsky C. Desmoplastic small cell tumors of the peritoneum co-expressing mesenchymal and epithelial markers. Am J Clin Pathol 96:536–543, 1991.

144. Ordóñez NG, El-Naggar AK, Ro JY, Silva EG, Mackay B. Intra-abdominal desmoplastic small cell tumor: a light microscopic, immunocytochemical, ultrastructural, and flow cytometric study. Hum Pathol 24:850–865, 1993.

145. Behm FG. Malignancies of the bone marrow. In: DM Parham, ed. Pediatric Neoplasia: Morphology and Biology. Philadelphia: Lippincott-Raven, 1996, pp. 449–504.

146. Fernandes ET, Kumar M, Douglass EC, Wilimas J, Parham DM, Rao BN. Extrarenal Wilms' tumor. J Pediatr Surg 24:483–485, 1989.

147. Parham DM. Pediatric Neoplasia: Morphology and Biology. Philadelphia: Lippincott-Raven, 1996.

148. Lawrence W, Gehan EA, Hays DM, Beltangady M, Maurer HM. Prognostic significance of staging factors of the UICC staging system in childhood rhabdomyosarcoma: a report from the Intergroup Rhabdomyosarcoma Study (IRS-II). J Clin Oncol 5:46–54, 1987.

149. Kushner BH, Cheung NKV, LaQuaglia MP, Ambros PF, Ambros IM, Bonilla MA, Ladanyi M, Gerald WL. International Neuroblastoma Staging System stage 1 neuroblastoma: a prospective study and literature review. J Clin Oncol 14:2174–2180, 1996.

16

Surgical Management of Soft-Tissue Sarcoma

Alan D. Aaron
Georgetown University Hospital
Washington, DC, and
National Institutes of Health
Bethesda, Maryland

Brian Shannon and Christopher A. Attinger
Georgetown University Hospital
Washington, DC

I. INTRODUCTION

Surgical resection is the mainstay of treatment for soft-tissue sarcomas. Surgical excision is divided into one of four categories depending on the extent of resection (1,2). These include intracapsular excision, marginal excision, wide resection, and radical resection (Fig. 1). Intracapsular excision refers to a surgical procedure that involves incising the tumor capsule and removing the central neoplastic contents while leaving the capsule in situ. With this type of limited excision, neoplastic tissue is often left behind as tumor cells are contained within the capsule. Marginal excision refers to the removal of the tumor by separating or shelling out the tumor at the normal tissue–tumor capsule interface. Often the pseudocapsule of compressed normal tissue surrounding the tumor capsule is left behind. Marginal excision is considered adequate surgical treatment for a number of benign neoplasms but is considered inadequate for malignant tumors because cells that have migrated into the surrounding pseudocapsule tissue are left behind. Wide resec-

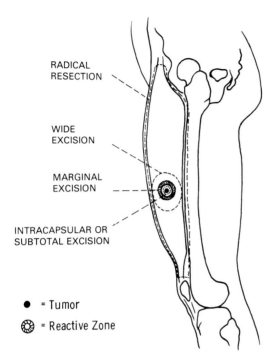

RADICAL
RESECTION

WIDE
EXCISION

MARGINAL
EXCISION

INTRACAPSULAR OR
SUBTOTAL EXCISION

● = Tumor

⊛ = Reactive Zone

FIG. 1 Diagrammatic representation of types of tumor resection based on a soft-tissue sarcoma located in the anterior compartment of the thigh. The small solid black circle represents the sarcoma. The cross-hatched region represents the surrounding reactive zone. The dotted lines represent levels of resection. Intracapsular resection enters the tumor capsule. Marginal resection is carried through the reactive zone. Wide resection goes through the normal tissue surrounding the reactive zone. Radical resection involves removal of the entire compartment. (From Enneking WF. Musculoskeletal tumor surgery, Vol. 1. New York: Churchill Livingtone, 1983, pp. 1–60.)

tion refers to the removal of a cuff of normal tissue in conjunction with the tumor, tumor capsule, and pseudocapsule. This is also considered an en bloc resection, as the tumor capsule is not violated during this procedure. Wide resection is the recommended surgical procedure for soft-tissue sarcomas. Radical resection denotes the removal of the tumor, pseudocapsule, and the entire surrounding anatomical compartment (3). By definition, an intracapsular and oftentimes a marginal resection results in the discovery of positive margins containing neoplastic tissue. Amputation is a surgical procedure and does not reflect the type or adequacy of resection (Fig. 2). For example, a soft-tissue sarcoma of the quadriceps muscle would require removal of the entire quadriceps muscle to be considered a radical resection. Using the above surgical categorization criteria, an above-the-knee amputa-

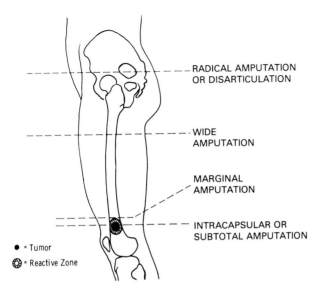

FIG. 2 Diagrammatic representation of tumor resection type when amputation is employed for a distal femoral sarcoma. It is notable that an above-knee amputation is considered a wide resection, not a radical resection, using this method of classifying tumor resection level. (From Enneking WF. Musculoskeletal tumor surgery, Vol. 1. New York: Churchill Livingtone, 1983, pp. 1–60.)

tion would be considered a wide resection. A hip disarticulation would be necessary to achieve a radical resection if amputation was employed.

II. LIPOMAS

The majority of benign soft-tissue tumors can be treated surgically with either intralesional or marginal resection. A notable exception to this is extra-abdominal desmoids, which require a wide resection when surgically feasible. Lipomas are the most common benign neoplasm and can arise in any fat-containing region. The majority of lipomas are asymptomatic and contained within the superficial subcutaneous fat. Deep-seated or intramuscular lipomas, though less common, can be painful. While their presence alone does not result in pain, compression of surrounding tissue or neurovascular structures may result in discomfort. The recurrence rate for lipomas has been reported to be as high as 5%. However, this figure is derived from historical series, which may have included patients with unrecognized atypical lipomas or low-grade liposarcomas (4).

III. HEMANGIOMAS

Hemangiomas are the most common tumor of infancy and childhood, with the majority being cutaneous in location. Intramuscular hemangiomas, though less common, are the most common benign tumor of skeletal muscle (5). Pain and swelling coupled with joint contractures and continued tumor growth are often presenting complaints. As the majority of lesions do not proliferate beyond childhood, treatment is generally reserved for those few lesions that continue to grow or cause local symptoms (6). Surgical excision is difficult, as hemangiomas often infiltrate the surrounding musculature. This requires surgical removal of a significant portion of adjacent muscle to achieve local control, which can result in predictable and potentially unacceptable functional impairment.

IV. BENIGN TUMORS OF PERIPHERAL NERVES

Benign nerve sheath tumors can be divided into two main categories: schwannomas (neurilemmomas) and neurofibromas. Benign schwannomas are solitary neoplasms that often present in the head, neck, and flexor surfaces of the extremities. Generally painless, large schwannomas that involve sensory nerves can cause local paresthesias, often manifesting with a positive Tinel's sign on physical examination. As these neoplasms emanate from the surrounding Schwann cells of the nerve, marginal excision is adequate. Sacrifice of the adjacent nerve is not necessary (7). Neurofibromas may be solitary or multiple, with the multiple variety being a component of neurofibromatosis type 1 (Von Recklinghausen's disease). As these neoplasms directly involve the nerve, surgical removal often requires removal of the nerve, with predictable loss of function.

V. EXTRA-ABDOMINAL DESMOIDS

Extra-abdominal desmoid tumors, commonly known as aggressive fibromatosis, are rare, with an incidence of between 2–4% (8–11). Although most studies have reported an equal incidence between men and women, two large series demonstrated a strong (2:1) predilection of these tumors for women (12,13). When controlled for gender, women were found to demonstrate a higher incidence during their fertile years. In addition, extra-abdominal desmoid tumors in premenopausal female patients had 4 times the rate of growth of tumors in their male counterparts (13). Extra-abdominal desmoids are characteristically nonmetastasizing but locally aggressive soft-tissue tumors, which invade adjacent normal structures (14). Local growth and tissue invasion may result in pain, deformity, organ dysfunction, and, occasionally, death in up to 8% of cases (15). Mortality is often related to direct erosion of the tumor into the trachea or the chest wall. As extra-abdominal desmoids are not malignant, local control is the most significant complication that surgeons confront. As with soft-tissue sarcomas, local recurrence can approach 90% in patients undergoing an intralesional or marginal resection (12). This is in comparison with a 48% recurrence rate in patients treated with a wide resection. As with soft-tissue sarcomas, a histologically clear margin of resection is an important predictor of successful local surgical control. In several studies, patients with close or contaminated surgical margins demonstrated higher rates of local recurrence (16–19). Because of the relatively poor local control rates with surgery alone, radiation therapy has been utilized in a number of studies.

Sherman et al. reported local recurrence in 1 of 9 patients who had negative surgical margins when treated with combined adjuvant radiation therapy (20). In a more recent review of 14 patients, 78% (11 patients) demonstrated a local control rate with adjuvant radiation therapy for positive, questionable, or reactive margins (21). Other studies have reported good results even in the event of positive or reactive margins. In a study by Miralbell et al., local control was achieved in 81% (17 of 21 patients) with histologically positive margins (19). In a recent review of 44 patients undergoing either surgery alone (34 patients) or surgery combined with radiation therapy (10 patients), the results of local control were evaluated. Local control was achieved in 22 of 34 patients (65%) treated with surgery alone, whereas 8 of 10 treated with combined surgery and radiation therapy were well controlled (22). In a recent series consisting of 107 patients with aggressive fibromatosis, patients were evaluated regarding treatment with either surgery alone (51 patients), radiation alone (15 patients), and surgery combined with radiation (41 patients) (23). Control rates among surgery, radiation therapy, and combined-modality groups were 69%, 93%, and 72%, respectively. Patients treated with surgery alone had control rates of 50% for gross residual disease, 56% for microscopically positive margins, and 77% for negative margins. Radiation and surgery resulted in rates of 59% for gross residual disease, 78% for microscopically positive margins, and 100% for negative margins. As expected, recurrent tumors demonstrated a higher risk of local recurrence regardless of the modality employed. Predictors of failure included patients under the age of 18, recurrent disease, positive surgical margins, and treatment with surgery alone. Recommended dosing of radiation therapy was 50–60 Gy for residual microscopic and 60–65 Gy for gross disease. Age of onset may impact the results of treatment. Higher recurrence rates have been reported in children in a study by Lopez et al., with children having an increased risk of recurrence (88%) as compared with adults (38%) (24).

Radiation therapy without surgical resection has been utilized in a small number of patients with acceptable results (25). Of 10 patients treated with radiation alone, 8 either achieved a complete response or stabilization of their disease.

In a study by Catton et al., better results using radiation alone (75%) versus combined therapy (54%) were reported (26). In another study by Kamath et al., 100% control rates were reported with radiation alone (27). Data from M.D. Anderson demonstrated a relatively high rate of local control (71.4%) with radiation therapy (20). The observation that patients with aggressive fibromatosis appear to have a greater risk of local recurrence following combined surgery and radiation therapy rather then radiation alone seems counterintuitive. Fibromatosis has been felt by some authors to be a reactive type of tumor as it has been described in previous surgical scars or burns (12,28–30). Surgery may actually play a role in stimulating growth of these tumors by either direct tumor extension or stimulation of neighboring pleuripotential cells to grow rapidly (31). Because abdominal wall desmoids appear to have a predilection for women during or following pregnancy, a hormonal or traumatic etiologic process is suspected as contributing to desmoid growth.

The theory that desmoids are hormone-responsive is supported by clinical regression of these tumors following menopause and the onset of menstruation (10,32). In addition, estrogen receptor status has been studied in these tumors, with estimates of 25–67% of desmoids binding estrogen and approximately 79% binding tamoxifen (33,34). For this reason, medical management has been undertaken to control growth of both abdominal and extra-abdominal lesions. Clinical responses have been reported following chemotherapy with cytotoxic agents, hormone antagonists such as tamoxifen, and nonsteroidal anti-inflammatory agents (35,36). More recent studies have promoted the use of combined therapy utilizing both antiestrogens and nonsteroidal anti-inflammatory treatment (37). In a study of 10 patients with large inoperable desmoid tumors in various body locations, 40% were found to respond to testolactone treatment. In a separate group of seven patients, nonsteroidal anti-inflammatory drugs were utilized concurrently with or after testolactone or tamoxifen with five major regressions, one partial regression, and one failure to respond reported. However, because of low patient numbers, variation between regimens, and the possibility of spontaneous regression, these modalities are still considered experimental.

The surgical resection of extra-abdominal desmoids is still considered to be the mainstay of treatment. However, radiation therapy should be strongly considered as an adjuvant modality in the management of these tumors. As with soft-tissue sarcomas, nonmutilating surgical resection should be entertained with radiation therapy being administered in large tumors regardless of negative margins. The use of antiestrogen therapy is considered to be experimental at this time; however, it is clear that a hormonal connection exists between these tumors and their growth characteristics. It is hoped that further research into nonsurgical modalities will yield a more functional and possibly reliable method for managing these nonmalignant neoplasms.

VI. SURGICAL MANAGEMENT
OF SOFT-TISSUE SARCOMAS

Once an appropriate biopsy specimen confirms the diagnosis of a primary soft-tissue sarcoma and staging is completed, surgical resection is the treatment of choice. Historically surgery has been the mainstay of treatment for localized soft-tissue sarcomas. Intralesional excision was initially employed, with high rates of recurrence being reported (38). Wide resection resulted in a decrease in local recurrence to approximately 60%. In a large series of 653 patients treated with soft-tissue sarcomas from 1935 to 1959 at Memorial Hospital, there was a 29% recurrence rate (39). Anatomical location was a key component of surgical failure, with radical resection or amputation reducing the recurrence rate to less than 20% (38,40,41). Unfortunately, to achieve local control of greater than 80%, the need for amputation approached 50% (3,40). Though local control was greater than 10% in patients undergoing amputation, distant metastasis developed in over one third of patients. Shiu et al. reported a 41% survival rate at 10 years, with distant metastases being the cause of death in 90% of patients who died of their disease (38). Because of these issues, radiation has been recommended by several authors to improve local control while reducing the need for radical resection or amputation (42–44). Rosenberg et al. reported a statistically equivalent risk of local recurrence and overall patient survival when comparing amputation and more conservative surgery combined with radiation therapy (45).

Wide surgical resection combined with radiation therapy is considered the treatment of choice in the management of high-grade soft-tissue sarcomas (46). Acceptable local control rates can be achieved while preventing amputation and maximizing function. However, radiation therapy should not be used to augment an inadequate surgical resection with contaminated margins (46). Though soft-tissue sarcomas often are located adjacent to neurovascular structures, direct invasion or encasement of these structures is uncommon. The neurovascular bundle can be dissected free of the sarcoma and retained in the majority of cases, thereby avoiding the need for amputation. Though these margins may be close, the use of either preoperative or postoperative radiation therapy avails the surgeon of the ability to retain these structures. In those cases where arterial or venous structures must be sacrificed, prosthetic or autogenous vein grafts may be used to reconstruct the vessel (47). Sacrifice of a major nerve does not preclude limb sparing, if the expected functional loss will permit ambulation at a level that is superior to a comparable amputation. Resection of the sciatic nerve, once thought to be an indication for amputation, results in functionally acceptable deficits in ambulation treatable with both bracing and supportive aids (walker, canes, etc.) (48). Amputation should be strongly considered in patients with sarcomas not amenable to limb sparing or when a marginally functional or painful extremity is the expected outcome (49). This includes patients with multiple skip lesions that make an en bloc resection impossible. Amputation often needs to be considered in the case of recurrent soft-tissue sarcomas (49). Complications of a previous biopsy, such as a deep infection, poor placement of a biopsy incision, or massive contamination, can make limb sparing impossible. The negative impact on local disease control is a major concern in the event of a poorly performed biopsy. In a study by Mankin et al., complications resulting in a less than optimal outcome were significant and included errors in diagnosis (17.8%), poorly performed biopsy (19.3%), nonrepresentative sample (3.4%), and amputation (3.0%) (50).

It is clear that the risk of local recurrence is closely tied to the adequacy of the surgical margin. Though "surgical margin" is a term that is familiar to most pratitioners, little is known about the interaction between sarcomas and the surrounding normal tissues (Fig. 3) (51). In a study of multiple samples of the tumor border in 36 musculoskeletal tumors, even highly malignant tumors did not demonstrate a reactive zone. Enneking et al. reported high recurrence rates for low-grade sarcoma (90%) in patients undergoing marginal resection as opposed to wide resection (10%) (1,52). Similar results are reflected in a series of 89 patients, who had been referred without biopsy with soft-tissue sarcomas. In an effort to avoid contamination of soft-tissue margins and to preserve muscle compartments, Stener advocated surgical resection without performing a biopsy (53,54). With more than 80% of the sarcomas being high grade and larger than 5 cm, patients underwent wide resection resulting in 13 amputations and 37 limb-sparing operations without biopsy prior to resection. One recurrence was reported. Of 16 patients undergoing wide resection after fine-needle aspiration, 3 demonstrated recurrence, and 6 of 22 patients had local recurrence if open biopsy was performed prior to resection. Of note, radiotherapy was not employed in this study (55). It is clear that the quality of the margin is at least as important as the physical distance. Some authors have suggested a new classification of surgical margins, with 5 cm outside the reactive zone being considered adequate (56). Unfortunately, application of this definition of an adequate surgical margin would result in a high rate of amputations, as most sarcomas of the upper extremity and a large number located in the thigh have difficulty achieving both a 5-cm margin and a limb-sparing procedure (57). Because of these issues, Rydholm and Rooser proposed a slight modification of the Enneking system (58). They proposed that margins be divided into subcutaneous and fascial margins as well as areolar–muscle margins. Areolar–muscle margins took into account the violation of facial margins while preserving at least a muscle margin. The local recurrence rate for the wide subcutaneous and facial margins in 72 high-grade sarcomas without adjuvant therapy was less than 10%. Karakousis reported similar results, with a 10% local recurrence rate for primary soft-tissue sarcomas in the extremities without radiation therapy, after wide resection (59). A local recurrence occurred in 30% after a wide areolar muscle margin.

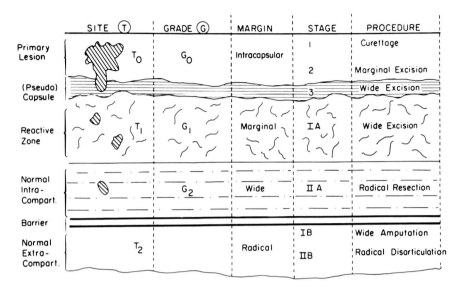

SITE Ⓣ	GRADE Ⓖ	MARGIN	STAGE	PROCEDURE

FIG. 3   On the left side of the chart are shown the tissue planes and lesions in progressive stages. In the second column, site is shown progressing from an intracapsular lesion to penetration of the capsule, satellites in the reactive zone, and skips in the normal intracompartmental tissue. In the third column, the grades advance from a benign intracapsular lesion to an aggressive extracapsular lesion without satellites, a low-grade malignant lesion with satellites, to a high-grade malignant lesion with both satellites and skips. In the fourth column, the various margins produced by dissection intracapsularly, through reactive tissue, through intracompartmental normal tissue, and through extracompartmental normal tissue are shown in relation to both site and grade. The fifth column shows the stages in relation to site, grade, and margin. Stage 1 and 2 are intracapsular, benign lesions: stage 3 lesions, though still benign, penetrate the capsule; stage IA lesions have satellites in the reactive zone within the compartment; and stage IIA lesions have both satellites and skips within the compartment. Extracompartmental low- and high-grade lesions are found beyond the normal compartmental barriers. In the last column, the recommended levels of surgical resection to achieve control of each lesion type based on site, grade, margin, and stage are provided. (From Enneking WF. Musculoskeletal tumor surgery, Vol. 1. New York: Churchill Livingstone, 1983, pp. 1–60.)

Marginal resection results in a predictably high recurrence rate of 60% for high-grade sarcomas and 30% for low-grade sarcomas without adjuvant therapy. Though it is clear that a positive margin demonstrates tumor cells at the surgical margin, defining a negative margin is more difficult. In a large series of 1000 patients from Memorial Hospital, a positive surgical margin was defined as "tumor present to be within less than one half of a $10\times$ microscopic field (1 mm) from the inked margin" (60). In another report from the same center, the pathologic margin was defined as positive when tumor was identified at the margin of resection (61). In a recent study of 95 preoperatively irradiated soft-tissue sarcomas of the extremities, the authors considered a surgical margin as positive if tumor cells were present at the tumor edge (62). In this study, 6 of 71 patients with negative margins had a local recurrence, as compared with 8 of 24 patients with positive margins.

Occasionally, patients undergo a marginal resection either because anatomic constraints prevent complete resection or more commonly a presumably benign neoplasm is later proven to be a sarcoma. In patients with incomplete or positive surgical margins, repeat resection should be undertaken whenever possible. In a study of 65 patients who had initially undergone inadequate surgical resection of a primary sarcoma and were subsequently found to have microscopically positive histologic margins without gross disease, patients were evaluated for histologic evidence of residual disease at repeat resection (63). Following a second resection, residual sarcoma was identified in 23 (35%) of the 65 patients. The margins of the second resection were positive in 9 (39%) of the 23 patients who had residual sarcoma. Five (22%) of the 23 patients had a local recurrence. Four of these 5 patients were found to have positive margins at repeat resection. This rate of recurrence was significantly higher than the 16 of 227 patients (7%) reported for patients undergoing wide resection with negative margins. In a follow-up study, which included 239 patients with soft-tissue sarcomas of the extremity treated with limb salvage surgery, patients were evaluated for risk of local recurrence (64). Using a univariate analysis, only status of the surgical margin and prior surgery were significant for local recurrence. In another study of 90 patients undergoing second resection of an initially inadequate first resection, the incidence of residual tumor was reported. Forty-four patients (48.9%) had identifiable macroscopic residual disease in the reoperative specimen (65). Goodlad et al. reported on 95 patients with a primary soft-tissue sarcoma excised inadequately elsewhere. Following a second resection, 56 of the 95 patients (59%) were found to have undergone an incomplete initial excision (66). In a large series of 189 patients, 67 were found to have incomplete resections, with residual tumor being found in 30 specimens (45%) (67).

A larger problem is when patients present with local recurrence following initial surgical resection. Once felt to be a clear indication for amputation, further studies have supported wide resection of recurrent sarcomas. In a study of 93 patients treated for local recurrence, 59 patients initially presented with extremity tumors (68). Of the 93 sarcomas, 65 (70%) of patients presented with a first recurrence, 15 (16%) with a second, 7 with a third (8%), and 6 with a fourth or more (6%). Of the 59 patients with extremity sarcomas, amputation was required in only 6 patients (10%). At 66 months, further local recurrence was noted in 27% of patients. The estimated 5-year survival rate was 100% for patients with grade 1 tumors, 77% for grade 2, and 45% for grade 3 tumors. Size also impacted patient outcome, as patients with small tumors ($<$5 cm) had a better outcome (78%) then patients with larger tumors ($>$5 cm) (57%). The overall 5-year survival rate was 65%. In a study by Ueda et al., the significance of local recurrence on patient survival was evaluated in 173 patients (69). The overall survival rates were 75.2% and 68.0% for 5 and 10 years, respectively. Inadequate surgical excision resulted in a higher rate of local recurrence (28.3%), as compared with patients undergoing initial definitive surgery (9.0%). Significant prognostic factors for local recurrence included histologic grade, tumor size, tumor depth, and surgical margin. Local recurrence after definitive surgery did not affect patient survival. Effect of local recurrence on patient survival is still debatable. In a study of 175 patients, local recurrence was reported in 74 patients. Of these patients, 55 developed metastasis after diagnosis, with 23 (42%) having previously experienced a local recurrence (70). Overall 5-year survival for the group was 72%. Factors associated with local recurrence included a wide surgical excision margin and the use of adjuvant radiotherapy. It is unlikely that radiation contributed to patient death but rather that larger, more aggressive sarcomas required the use of adjuvant radiotherapy and that these sarcomas by themselves were at higher risk for distal failure.

In an extensive review of 1041 patients with extremity soft-tissue sarcomas, patients presenting with local recurrence were at much higher risk for subsequent local failure (71). A patient with a lesion greater than 5 cm had about a 40% greater chance of local recurrence as compared with patients whose lesion was smaller than 5 cm. Studies have confirmed that disease-free survival and overall survival for patients do not differ between patients undergoing either amputation or limb sparing (71). Though local recurrence was higher in patients undergoing limb-sparing surgery and adjuvant radiation (25%), this was not statistically significant and did not result in reduced patient survival. These results were confirmed by Pisters et al., with overall survival not being affected even in those patients with local recurrence (72). More important risk factors included presence of high-grade sarcomas and large lesions. Even with an anticipated higher local recurrence rate in patients with positive surgical margins, overall patient survival has not been affected. In a study of 271 low-grade sarcomas, 56 (21%) were found to have a positive surgical margin (61). This subsequently translated into local recurrence in 14 (25%) patients. This is in comparison with 191 (70%) patients with negative surgical margins following surgical resection and local recurrence in 22 (11%) patients. This increased local recurrence rate did not translate to a higher risk of disease-specific death. Management of local recurrence includes either repeat surgical resection alone or surgery with reirradiation. In a small series, 25 patients with locally recurrent soft-tissue sarcoma following an initial wide resection and irradiation were assessed with regard to local control and overall survival (73). Nine patients were excluded either because they were not candidates for limb sparing requiring amputation (7 patients) or because they were offered palliative treatment secondary to systemic metastases (2 patients). Eleven patients underwent reresection without irradiation. Five patients received surgery combined with irradiation. Added to this group were seven patients who relapsed following re-resection. These patients were treated with repeat surgery and irradiation. The local control rate for patients undergoing surgery alone was 39% (4 of 11 patients), whereas patients undergoing combined surgery and irradiation was 100% (10 of 10 patients). Complications in the combined-therapy group included wound healing problems in six (60%) patients, with three patients recovering fully. Though the study population is small and heterogeneous with respect to tumor grade, the results suggest that even local recurrence can be treated with combined therapy when possible.

VII. COMPLICATIONS OF SURGERY

The impact of adjuvant treatment on wound healing in patients undergoing surgical resection is a major concern. One study reported a 34.4% incidence of soft-tissue complications following resection of extremity sarcomas (74). Though only 10% of patients required rehospitalization for management of complications, a delay of adjuvant treatment was seen in most patients. Severe complications resulted in delays of as long as 210 days. In the series by Lindberg et al., a 6.5% incidence of significant complications in 200 extremity soft-tissue sarcomas treated with postoperative radiation therapy was reported (75). One amputation was necessary 42 months after completion of radiation therapy. Two fractures were seen late following irradiation and were treated successfully. Bujko et al. reported an overall wound complication rate of 37% in 202 patients with soft-tissue sarcoma treated with preoperative irradiation (76). Secondary surgery was required in 33 patients (16%), including six amputations. Complication rates may vary depending on timing of radiation therapy. In a series of patients treated with brachytherapy a complication rate of 44% was reported when the catheters were loaded before the fifth postoperative day. Delaying the loading of the catheters after the fifth postoperative day reduced the complication rate to 14% (77). The use of vascularized tissue transfer in irradiated wounds can decrease wound complications (78,79). In a study of 180 patients undergoing limb salvage surgery for soft-tissue sarcoma, 137 patients (16%) treated with primary wound closure sustained complications (80). In a univariate analysis, the cross-sectional area of tumor resection, the use of preoperative irradiation, the width of the skin excision, a history of smoking, and a history of diabetes and/or vascular disease were factors associated with wound failure. Twenty-four patients, 18 empirically, underwent vascularized free-tissue transfer because of concerns regarding potential wound complications. There were 2 major wound complications in this group (11%), as compared with 56 patients who underwent primary closure with 16 major complications (30%) being reported.

　　Wound healing complications following musculoskeletal sarcoma resections are well documented, with ranges of 5–35% being reported. The incidence of flap necrosis ranges from 15% to 40%, and infection rates as high as 10–15% are reported (81–83). Wound healing complications have been associated with several variables, including chemotherapy, radiation therapy, endoprosthetic or allograft implant use, extensiveness of operative procedure, nutritional status, and allogeneic blood transfusions. Serum albumin levels of less than 35 g/L and a total lymphocyte count of less than 1.5×10^9/L have been equated with the failure of patients to heal lower extremity amputations (84,85). Albumin levels less than 28 g/L may indicate a need for active nutritional support preoperatively (86). A 10% incidence of severe (<30 g/L) hypoalbuminemia was found among 129 consecutive adult orthopedic patients awaiting elective or trauma surgery (87). In the study by Peat et al., 14% of the 35 patients tested prior to sarcoma resection were found to have low albumin levels, with several of these patients developing wound healing problems (80). In the same study, preoperative radiation therapy was associated with a higher wound complication rate, with 15 of 23 patients suffering from eventual wound complications (80). In a study of 87 patients who underwent wide resection for musculoskeletal sarcomas, 21 (25.3%) demonstrated wound healing complications (88). Types of complications included wound dehiscence (10 patients), hematoma or seroma (3 patients), and infection (9 patients). In this study, all patients were adequately nourished, with mean albumin levels greater than 3.5 g/dL. Statistical analysis determined that preoperative chemotherapy, depressed preoperative hematocrit, and allogeneic blood transfusion were significant factors adversely affecting wound healing.

VIII. SOFT-TISSUE RECONSTRUCTION

The utilization of microvascular flaps in surgical reconstructions has greatly expanded the indications for wide resection in the treatment of soft-tissue sarcomas (89). Large soft-tissue defects or delicate neurovascular structures that otherwise might be exposed following surgical resection can be covered with muscle flaps that expedite healing and provide increased radiation durability when utilizing postoperative irradiation. In the case of preoperative irradiation, free-tissue transfer often provides improved vascularized tissue to relatively hypoxic regions. This can greatly improve local wound healing in these patients. In patients undergoing large-bone resection in conjunction with soft-tissue resection, microvascular tissue transfer provides improved coverage for allograft or prosthetic reconstructions. The disadvantages of free-tissue transfer include increased operating time, absence of recipient vessels (especially in the limbs), possible loss of the flap due to microvascular failure, and the need for specialized nursing staff. Reece et al. reported on a prospective evaluation of the use of free-tissue transfer in managing soft-tissue defects created following wide surgical resection (90). Nineteen patients were divided into two groups according to those undergoing immediate versus delayed reconstruction. Eleven patients had free-tissue transfer performed

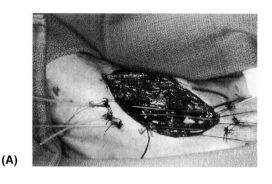

(A)

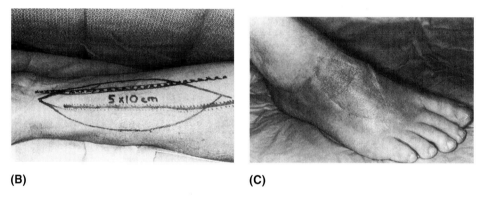

(B)   (C)

FIG. 4 (A) Photograph of the dorsum of the foot following wide resection of a high-grade cutaneous epithelial sarcoma. The dorsal long toe extensors have been resected to achieve clear surgical margins, followed by placement of brachytherapy catheters for anticipated postoperative radiation therapy. (B) Photograph of the volar forearm demonstrating the planned free-tissue transfer. This flap included vascularized tissue (radial artery and vein), tendon (palmaris longus tendon), and nerve (lateral antebrachial cutaneous nerve). (C) Photograph of the dorsum of the foot 1 year following sarcoma resection and reconstruction. The flap is sensate and well healed, with toe extensor function being restored by the palmaris longus tendon transfer. The patient is disease-free without local recurrence 5 years after surgery.

during the same operative procedure as the wide resection (immediate). The remaining eight patients presented with soft-tissue defects resulting from complications of the initial resection (delayed) that required soft-tissue coverage. Wide surgical margins were achieved in all patients. Preoperative irradiation was delivered with a mean dose of 53 Gy in 74% of patients. As with most series, the thigh was the most common location, followed by the calf and the knee (45,91,92). The postirradiation defects measured 40–575 cm^2. Complications occurred in 47% of patients, with no perioperative mortalities. Free-tissue transfer was successful in 95% of patients, with the only graft failure resulting from venous outflow obstruction. One amputation occurred secondarily to a pathologic femur fracture, with amputations not being a result of complications of free-tissue transfer. Heiner et al. reported on 10 patients who successfully underwent immediate free-tissue reconstruction for extremity sarcomas (93). Two patients experienced delayed flap complications secondary to radiation therapy with subsequent skin slough. In a large series of 26 patients who underwent flap reconstruction for treatment of malignant tumors of the knee or of tissue adjacent to the knee, the success of microvascular tissue transfer was greater than 90%. Though functional evaluation was considered good for the group as a whole, 5 patients (20%) underwent amputation for associated complications of local recurrence, flap necrosis, or secondary infection (94). In a recent study of 82 patients, primary closure with vascularized tissue transfer, as opposed to direct closure, led to fewer complications (19–51%) (78). Fewer secondary procedures for wound closure (10% vs. 35%), shorter average hospitalization (15 vs. 48 days), and greater limb salvage rate (97% vs. 91%) was also reported in the free-flap group.

It is clear both from multiple reports in the literature and as a result of our own experience that the application of microvascular tissue transfer to limb-sparing surgery for extremity sarcomas is a necessary surgical adjuvant to successful performance of limb sparing (Fig. 4). Anticipating the need for free-tissue transfer prior to the onset of complications is extremely important. This is especially true in patients undergoing skeletal reconstruction with allograft or prosthetic devices. This type of approach requires the skills of a surgical "team" that actively participates in preoperative planning and communicates regularly during the limb sparing process.

IX. SURGERY WITHOUT RADIOTHERAPY

Though surgery combined with adjuvant radiotherapy has long been considered the gold standard for the management of soft-tissue sarcomas, complications are not uncommonly associated with radiotherapy (76). An attempt to define a subset of soft-tissue sarcomas that may be amenable to wide surgical resection without radiotherapy seems warranted. Very few reports have appeared in the literature regarding this approach, with the majority being based on the Scandinavian experience (52,58,59,95–100). Criteria for wide resection have been delineated with less than a 10% local recurrence rate without radiation therapy. Surgery without radiation therapy has been proposed for both intramuscular and subcutaneous sarcomas (101). The essential component of this approach is achieving a negative margin that is considered adequate, thereby negating the need for adjuvant radiotherapy. In the case of subcutaneous sarcomas, the deep fascia provides a formable barrier to deep invasion. Resection of the deep fascia is therefore considered an adequate margin in conjunction with a 3- to 5-cm cuff of surrounding subcutaneous tissue. In a study of 129 patients with subcutaneous sarcomas, epidemiologic factors and outcome were evaluated. The annual incidence was 0.6 per 100,000 persons, with subcutaneous sarcomas comprising one third of all soft-tissue sarcomas of the extremities or chest wall. The cumulative 5-year survival was 80%. Radiation therapy was not used in any patient following adequate surgical resection. There were no recurrences in 14 low-grade tumors, with only 4 of 59 of high-grade tumors recurring locally. Similar results have been reported in other series of patients with subcutaneous sarcomas, with overall survival approaching 81% (102,103). The success of local control is harder to evaluate in these studies, as a number of patients received adjuvant radiation following either marginal or wide resection. However, the use of radiation therapy did not measurably improve local control in these studies, lending further support to the success of surgical resection without adjuvant radiation. In the case of intramuscular sarcoma, advocates of a primarily surgical approach contend that an open biopsy must not be performed if adjuvant radiation is to be avoided. In a series of 24 patients with intramuscular sarcomas (20 high-grade lesions), local recurrence occurred in only 2 patients at 3.5 years of follow-up treated by surgery alone (100). The authors contend that a needle biopsy can often be performed, thereby avoiding the contamination associated with open biopsy. Though infrequently encountered, resection of a falsely malignant tumor was not felt to result in significant complications (104,105). Though these results are preliminary, there does appear to be a subset of extremity sarcomas that are amenable to wide resection without incurring the complications of adjuvant radiotherapy.

X. SARCOMAS OF THE RETROPERITONEUM

Soft-tissue sarcomas arising in the retroperitoneum compose approximately 15% of all soft-tissue sarcomas (106). The median age of diagnosis is 55 years, with men and women being equally affected. By virtue of their location, retroperitoneal sarcomas are often large and may invade adjacent organs, making them difficult to treat surgically. Because of these obstacles, retroperitoneal sarcomas are associated with a 20–40% reduction in survival rate when compared with extremity sarcomas (107). The majority of patients are asymptomatic at presentation. Symptoms include gastrointestinal bleeding, bowel obstruction, and neurologic symptoms. Urgent symptoms, such as bowel obstruction or urinary tract obstruction, occur in less than 5% of patients. Neurologic symptoms have been reported in 27% of patients with a diagnosed retroperitoneal sarcoma (108). Weight loss is an uncommon manifestation of retroperitoneal tumors (7%). Physical examination uncovers a painless abdominal mass in 75% of patients, with rectal examination leading to earlier discovery. Computed tomography (CT) and magnetic resonance imaging (MRI) are the imaging studies of choice for the identification of primary tumors and metastatic disease. The lung and liver are major sites of hematogenous metastases. Approximately 20% of patients presenting with retroperitoneal soft-tissue tumors have evidence of metastatic disease at presentation. The majority of retroperitoneal masses are malignant (80%), with at least half being sarcomas. Other retroperitoneal malignancies include lymphomas and urogenital malignancies. Following proper preoperative staging studies, biopsy is usually indicated to confirm tumor histology. To avoid abdominal contamination, laparoscopically directed and transperitoneal needle biopsy should be avoided. By performing needle biopsy from a posterior approach, the problem of uncontrolled contamination can be avoided. Another option is to perform the biopsy through a transabdominal approach and then proceed directly with surgical resection based on frozen section histologic confirmation of malignancy. Another problem of needle biopsy is inaccurate tissue sampling, especially of large tumors consisting of heterogenic tumor populations. Biopsy of necrotic areas or regions of low-grade differentiation can potentially lead to an incorrect diagnosis secondary to acquisition of nondiagnostic tissue.

Most series report that approximately 50% of retroperitoneal sarcomas can be completely resected, whereas 40% are partially resected, leaving 10% considered nonresectable. Adjuvant management utilizing radiation therapy and chemotherapy has little to offer patients who are not successfully treated with surgery. It is clear that the completeness of surgical resection is a major factor in predicting outcome (106,107,109–111). In addition to completeness of resection, histologic grade was another important prognostic factor (107). Because retroperitoneal sarcomas are often discovered late, the majority of sarcomas are greater than 5 cm at the time of diagnosis (112). The majority of retroperitoneal sarcomas are liposarcomas, malignant fibrous histiocytomas, or leiomyosarcomas (113). Liposarcoma remains the most common tumor type presenting in the retroperitoneum. Approximately 60% of the tumors are low grade and 40% high grade. Approximately 50% of patients undergoing surgery for retroperitoneal sarcomas achieve curative resections, with a 74% 5-year survival reported (114). Other reports have been less optimistic, with Jacques et al. reporting local recurrence rates as high as 50% in patients undergoing complete resection (108). Though overall survival is better with low-grade sarcomas, recurrence is a problem for both low- and high-grade sarcomas. In the report by Jacques et al., the median time to recurrence was 15 months for high-grade and 42 months for low-grade sarcomas (108). Adjacent organ resection was required in 53% of patients, with 40% requiring resection of more than one adjacent organ to accomplish a complete resection. Patient survival is reduced in the face of an incomplete resection or a palliative resection, with the 5-year survival being equivalent to the survival rate for patients with nonresectable retroperitoneal disease (15%) (114). In another study, involvement of adjacent organs was common, with up to 75% of patients requiring resection of adjacent organs to achieve local control (106). In a large series of 119 patients, complete surgical resection approached 50%, with 10 patients undergoing postoperative radiation therapy. Unfortunately, the prognosis was poor, with 2- to 5-year survival rates of 53% and 20% reported (115). These figures mirror results obtained from an earlier study of retroperitoneal liposarcoma (116). In a study of 249 patients with liposarcoma, 34 presented with retroperitoneal sarcoma. Complete excision provided the highest 5-year survival rate, longest disease-free interval, and fewest recurrence-related surgical procedures. Unfortunately, 5-year survival was only 41%. In a recent study of prognostic factors impacting local control, 80 patients with primary retroperitoneal soft-tissue sarcomas were evaluated (109). Variables studied included resectability, type of operation, surgical margins, surgical boundaries, microscopic margins, adjuvant radiotherapy, and adjuvant chemotherapy. The major factor affecting survival outcome was the ability to completely resect the lesion. When 62 patients undergoing complete resection were examined, the only independent prognostic factor for both survival and disease-free survival was grade (109). These results were supported by a recent study of 87 consecutive patients with retroperitoneal sarcomas (117). The resectability rate was 100% for primary tumors (55 patients) and 87% for locally recurrent tumors (32 patients). The 5- and 10-year survival rate for primary tumors was 66% and 57%, respectively. The overall local recurrence rate was 31%, with an improved recurrence rate of 15% for wide resection as compared with 56% after local excision. As previously reported, survival of patients with primary tumors undergoing complete resection was reflective of histologic grade, with 5-year survival rates of 88% and 44%, respectively, for grade 1 and grade 3 tumors (117,118).

While soft-tissue sarcomas of the extremities rarely invade neurovascular structures, encasement of neurovascular structures is more common in the retroperitoneum. Because a number of neurovascular structures are intimate with bony structures or associated with foramina, vessels are unable to accommodate local tumor growth. Even with complete resection, at least 90% of patients will develop recurrent retroperitoneal disease in the ensuing 10 years. Even if complete surgical resection is not feasible, some authors have promoted an approach of aggressive palliative surgical management (119). In this study, 41 patients with high-grade soft-tissue retroperitoneal sarcomas were divided into four groups based on the extent of tumor resection (119). Patients undergoing complete resection demonstrated no survival benefit in comparison with patients treated with subtotal resection. However, both groups together had a significantly longer median survival then patients undergoing either palliative or no resection. The addition of chemotherapy or radiation therapy failed to show any advantage in this series. As opposed to extremity sarcomas, adjuvant radiotherapy has not been found to improve local control for retroperitoneal sarcomas (120). Because of the proximity of adjacent organs, primarily the bowel, subtherapeutic dosing and reduced tissue tolerance is a problem. Glenn et al. reported a very high complication rate without any improvement in patient survival with a total dose of 55 Gy (121). Intraoperative radiotherapy, which can sometimes spare internal organs, has unfortunately been found to be ineffective (120).

XI. SOFT-TISSUE SARCOMAS OF THE ABDOMINAL WALL AND CHEST WALL

Soft-tissue sarcomas of the abdominal wall are extremely rare, composing approximately 15% of all soft-tissue sarcomas. Patients usually present with a palpable mass, which may be considered a benign tumor until malignancy is proven by biopsy. Weinstein and Shiu studied a total of 55 patients with soft-tissue tumors of the abdominal wall during the period 1949–1982. In this series, desmoids accounted for one third of all tumors; rhabdomyosarcoma, malignant fibrous histiocytoma, synovial sarcoma, and liposarcoma were responsible for the remainder (122). Principles of management are similar to those of extremity soft-tissue sarcomas, with wide excision being the treatment of choice. Because of underlying bowel, radiation therapy is generally reserved for recurrent desmoid tumors, large primary abdominal wall sarcomas, resections that result in positive margins, and recurrent abdominal wall sarcomas. Five-year survival was 22% in this series (122). As with extremity sarcomas, local control is often successful, with the predominant site of failure being systemic dissemination to the lungs. As opposed to retroperitoneal sarcomas, an additional independent prognostic factor in addition to surgical resectability and histologic grade for truncal sarcomas is tumor size (107). Truncal sarcomas larger than 5 cm carry a 2.5-fold greater probability of death compared with sarcomas smaller than 5 cm ($p = 0.018$) (107).

As with the abdominal wall, the chest wall is not a common location for primary sarcomas. Intrathoracic symptoms are uncommon, with the most obvious physical finding being an enlarging mass. The majority of chest wall tumors are malignant, with most being metastatic lesions such as recurrent breast cancer, lung cancer, or plasmacytoma. Malignant peripheral nerve tumors, malignant fibrous histiocytomas, fibrosarcomas, liposarcomas, and rhabdomyosarcomas account for most chest wall sarcomas (123). As with abdominal wall sarcomas, wide resection is the treatment of choice. Small defects can be repaired primarily, whereas larger defects may require chest wall reconstruction with Marlex or Gore-tex mesh reinforced with methylmethacrylate (124,125). Rigid chest wall reconstruction with methylmethacrylate, in conjunction with myocutaneous muscle flaps, has been reported to provide improved functional and cosmetic results (126). Satisfactory wound coverage without soft-tissue complications has been reported in 15 of 17

(88%) of patients undergoing resection of bone or soft-tissue sarcomas of shoulder or chest wall (127). Radiotherapy is often indicated following surgical resection. Survival and local recurrence rates are similar to those reported for abdominal wall lesions.

XII. SARCOMAS OF THE HEAD AND NECK

Soft tissue sarcomas rarely present in the head and neck, with less than 1% of all malignant neoplasms and less than 10% of all soft-tissue sarcomas being diagnosed in this region (128). Farr reported on a large series of 285 patients, with only a 32% survival rate at 5 years (129). In another study of 176 patients treated at Memorial Hospital, results of treatment were reviewed with a minimum follow-up of 2 years (130). Seventy-two patients (41%) presented with low-grade sarcomas, whereas 104 (59%) were diagnosed with high-grade sarcomas. Surgical resection was performed on 158 of these patients. In this study, combined adjuvant radiotherapy and chemotherapy was not found to impact the rate of local control. Increased risk of treatment failure was associated with large tumor size, positive surgical margins, bone involvement, local recurrence, metastatic spread, and high histologic grade. Overall survival was 75% at 2 years, 55% at 5 years, 46% at 10 years, with only 20% of patients with high-grade sarcomas being alive 10 years after treatment. A poor prognosis was associated with high-grade angiosarcoma, rhabdomyosarcoma, high-grade peripheral nerve sheath tumor, and high-grade malignant fibrous histiocytoma. In another series of 188 patients treated for soft-tissue sarcoma of the head and neck region, the results of local treatment were evaluated (131). Wide surgical excision with negative margins was the best means of local control, with negative margins being attained in only 73 patients. As with sarcomas of the extremities, tumor size and grade impacted overall outcome. These results are applicable to soft-tissue sarcomas of the shoulder region. In a study of 70 patients with primary shoulder soft-tissue sarcomas, patients were reviewed with regard to tumor size, tumor grade, histology, extent of resection, and use of adjuvant radiotherapy (132). The overall 5 and 10-year survival rates were 82% and 80% respectively, whereas the 5-year disease-free survival rate was 63%. Tumors greater than 5 cm and high-grade tumors were associated with a significantly decreased disease-free and overall survival.

XIII. SARCOMAS OF THE HAND AND FOOT

Sarcomas localized in peripheral sites, such as the hand and foot, are surgically challenging when limb sparing is an issue. Unfortunately, their peripheral location does not afford a better survival outcome. In a study of 78 patients with soft-tissue sarcoma arising in the distal extremities, the results of conservative surgery and radiotherapy were studied with respect to survival, local recurrence, functional limb preservation, complications, and distant metastases (133). With a median follow-up of 7.9 years, actuarial 5-year and 10-year survival rates were 80% and 69%, respectively, and disease-free rates were 61% and 51% for the same periods. Fifteen patients (19%) had local recurrence, but 12 of the affected extremities were salvaged. Amputation was required either to control local disease or because of complications in 21% (14 of 67 patients) of cases. Even when located in a distal site, results are comparable to those associated with more proximally located sarcomas. Small lesions (<2 cm) were found to have a low risk for metastases, intermediate-sized lesions (2–5 cm) metastasize one third of the time, whereas lesions larger than 5 cm have an incidence of metastasis in excess of 50%. Anatomical location in a distal region may be predictive for malignant neoplasm. In a study of 83 patients who had soft-tissue tumors and tumor-like lesions of the foot, 40% of the malignant lesions were located in the hindfoot (134). Unfortunately, in patients with local recurrence or positive surgical margins, amputation is the only form of surgical treatment available (135,136). In a study of 23 patients with soft-tissue sarcomas of the hand, a higher rate of metastases was reported for patients with a sarcoma of the hand than for more proximal anatomical sites (136). This may be due to the uniqueness of the sarcomas that occur in the hand. This subset of sarcomas, namely, rhabdomyosarcoma, angiosarcoma, and epithelioid sarcoma, have a greater propensity to develop lymph node metastases (137).

XIV. ATYPICAL LIPOMAS

Though wide resection followed by radiation therapy is the mainstay of treatment for most extremity soft-tissue sarcomas, low-grade liposarcomas may warrant a more conservative approach because of their relatively benign behavior. Commonly termed as low-grade or well-differentiated liposarcomas or atypical lipomas, these neoplasms have an extremely low risk for metastases (138,139). Local recurrence is the major complication and is often higher then reported for intramuscular lipomas. In a large series of 111 cases of histopathologically atypical or malignant lipomatous lesions of the extremities and retroperitoneum, local recurrence and risk for metastasis were evaluated (140). Of these cases, 48 were considered to be differentiated fatty neoplasms of low-grade potential located outside of the retroperitoneum. Among the atypical lipomatous lesions, there were no uncontrollable recurrences, distant metastases, or tumor-related deaths. The depth of the neoplasm correlated with the tendency for local recurrence. There were no recurrences of tumors originating in the subcutis, with 29% of tumors located in deep soft tissues or in the muscles recurring. None of the recurrent tumors demonstrated dedifferentiation to a higher grade sarcoma. A second group of patients (21 patients) with low-grade liposarcomas of the retroperitoneum were considered separately. Retroperitoneal liposarcomas recurred in 67% of cases, with no distant metastases. However, nine patients (43%) died of tumor-related complications. In addition, five retroperitoneal tumors dedifferentiated. The extremely low risk of metastatic dissemination with low-grade liposarcomas is demonstrated in a series of patients treated at Memorial Hospital (141). Well-differentiated liposarcomas were found to have a 5-year local recurrence rate of 30% and a survival rate of 100%. Even in the case of myxoid liposarcoma, the local recurrence rate was 25% and patient survival was 88%. In a recent series of 92 cases of well-differentiated liposarcomas of the extremity, retroperitoneum, and groin, with follow-up information of at least 2 years, tumors were studied to determine their long-term behavior (142). The tumors occurred most frequently in the muscles of the extremity (46 cases) followed by the retroperitoneum (23 cases), groin (14 cases), and miscellaneous sites (9 cases). Tumors in the retroperitoneum recurred in nearly all cases (21 of 23 cases), with 4 cases "dedifferentiating" within 8 years. Tumors of the groin behaved in a similar manner. In contrast, those in the extremity recurred less frequently (20 of 46 cases), with no disease-related mortality. As opposed to the previous study by Azumi et al., 3 of 46 patients with extremity neoplasms underwent dedifferentiation. Of the 11 patients with dedifferentiated liposarcomas, 3 died of metastatic disease. The results of this study supported the premise that dedifferentiation of recurrent well-differentiated liposarcomas is not specifically related to location (retroperitoneum) but is time-dependent. In light of these results, decisions regarding the local management of these neoplasms can be difficult. Surgery is indicated in patients with atypical lipomas or well-differentiated liposarcomas, but the aggressiveness of surgery is debatable. As discussed previously, the majority of higher grade soft-tissue sarcomas should undergo wide resection with clear or normal margins being obtained. In the case of atypical lipomas, this degree of surgical resection appears to be unwarranted given the relatively low risk of metastatic disease, especially with respect to extremity neoplasms. Wide resection of either extremity or retroperitoneal tumors predictably results in poorer functional outcomes or even amputation. For this reason, most orthopaedic oncologic surgeons prefer to manage these neoplasms with marginal resection. Though the risk of local recurrence is higher, the risk of metastases or dedifferentiation is low. However, in cases of dedifferentiation, the risk of metastases is approximately 30%. Therefore, though patients with low-grade liposarcoma are candidates for marginal resection, close follow-up is required to identify early recurrences. As opposed to the usual follow-up period of 5 years given to the majority of higher grade soft-tissue sarcomas, follow-up of at least 10 years may be indicated for this subtype of sarcoma because of its slower growth rate.

XV. PEDIATRIC SOFT-TISSUE SARCOMAS

Though rare in adults, soft-tissue sarcomas account for 4–8% of all childhood cancers in patients younger than 14 years and are the fifth most common form of cancer in this age group (143,144). This results in an age-standardized annual incidence rate of 5–9 cases per 1 million children. Rhabdomyosarcoma is the most common soft-tissue sarcoma of childhood and is diagnosed in 250 children each year, with 60–70% of series of pediatric soft-tissue sarcomas comprising rhabdomyosarcomas (145). The use of multiagent chemotherapy, radiation therapy, and surgery has led to current long-term overall survival approaching 70% (146). The surgical treatment of rhabdomyosarcoma is site-specific, with the goal being achievement of complete surgical resection while preserving extremity function. As with adult sarcomas, extremity lesions are more readily resectable than head and neck tumors. Patients with residual microscopic disease fare worse than those achieving complete excision. A series of 154 patients who underwent reexcision after an initial inadequate surgical resection before adjuvant therapy was compared with a group of patients with microscopic residual tumor (147). Surprisingly, a group of referred patients who had initially negative margins and did not undergo repeat resection also demonstrated a poorer prognosis. In review of this group, margins may have been contaminated by poor surgical resection technique. A recommendation for reexcision in patients who underwent resection prior to the diagnosis of cancer was made by the authors. In an attempt to decrease the extent of surgical resection, the Intergroup Rhabdomyosarcoma Study III protocol suggested reexploration after initial preoperative chemotherapy. In the study, 109 of 257 patients with gross residual tumor after initial surgery underwent a second-look operation (148). A complete response was documented in 88% of patients, whereas 12% of patients with a clinically complete response had residual tumor. Seventy-four percent of patients with a clinical partial or poor response were categorized as a complete response after a second-look operation. Surgical reresection was responsible for the improvement to a complete response in 28% of patients with a clinical partial response and in 43% of patients with no clinical response. Repeated surgical reevaluation has been challenged by Godzinski et al., who reported on 92 patients who had initial biopsy and then only chemotherapy for local control (149). The rates of local recurrence were not significantly different for biopsied and nonbiopsied patients (51% and 48%, respectively). This suggests that a negative biopsy may not predict risk of relapse, especially when only chemotherapy is used for local therapy.

Extremity rhabdomyosarcomas account for 20% of these tumors. As compared to an earlier surgical approach of amputation, today less than 5% of patients are treated with amputation. The experience reported in the IRS-III confirmed that complete excision with gross and microscopically negative margins is optimal in the treatment of children with extremity rhabdomyosarcomas (150). Comparison of patients who had complete resection of distal tumors with patients having an incomplete excision demonstrated significant differences in survival. Histologically negative lymph nodes were also a predictor of a favorable outcome among patients, promoting the need for histologic evaluation of lymph nodes during staging. Head and neck are the most common regions of involvement for rhabdomyosarcoma. Superficial head and neck sarcomas are more amenable to primary resection than orbital or parameningeal sarcomas, with patient survival approaching 85% (146). In a study of 32 pediatric patients with rhabdomyosarcoma, 65% (21 of 32 patients) were disease-free at most recent follow-up (151). The 5-year disease free survival was 57%. The impact of multimodality therapy, consisting of chemotherapy, surgery, and radiation, is clear as only 14% (1 of 7 patients) of patients who underwent surgery alone were cured.

Though infrequently reported, pediatric nonrhabdomyosarcomatous soft-tissue sarcomas have been evaluated in recent studies. A preexisting condition has been reported in approximately 20% of patients, with the majority being given the diagnosis of neurofibromatosis (3 patients) (152). Aside from the relationship of neurofibromatosis with malignant nerve sheath tumors, whether a preexisting condition is directly associated with the onset of the remaining soft-tissue sarcomas remains to be proven. Fibrosarcomas and other nonrhabdomyosarcomatous soft-tissue sarcomas were the next most common group. A large retrospective analysis of 75 patients was undertaken by the Pediatric Oncology Group (POG) to acquire epidemiologic statistics on nonrhabdomyosarcomatous soft-tissue sarcomas in children (153). The most common soft-tissue tumor was synovial sarcoma (42%), followed by fibrosarcoma (13%), malignant fibrous histiocytoma (12%), and malignant neurogenic tumors (10%). Sixty-five percent of all tumors presented in the extremities, with 44% in the lower extremity and 21% in the upper extremity. Tumors of the trunk and chest wall accounted for 28%, whereas head and neck tumors accounted for 7% of patients. Using the TNMG classification system, 16% presented as stage I, 21% as stage II, 33% as stage III, 30% as stage IV. Age at the time of diagnosis did not affect clinical site or stage. All upper extremity tumors presented with localized disease, whereas lower extremity tumors presented with regional nodal disease in 7% and metastatic pulmonary disease in 23% of cases. A much greater risk of metastasis was noted in patients with abdominal disease, with 78% of patients having metastatic disease at diagnosis. The majority of synovial sarcomas were identified in the lower extremity, with 84% demonstrating localized disease. Patients with neurogenic tumors presented with a much greater risk of metastasis, with only 25% having localized disease at presentation and 50% having metastasis at the time of diagnosis. In a review of 37 children with synovial sarcomas, clinical group, tumor invasiveness, and tumor grade independently predicted outcome (154). Estimated 5-year survival was 80% for patients with resectable lesions without evidence of metastatic disease, as compared with

17% for the later group. Patients with noninvasive tumors demonstrated a much better prognosis (93%) than patients with invasive tumors (39%). Higher grade was associated with a poorer prognosis, with grade III tumors being associated with an estimated 5-year survival of 40% as compared with grade II lesions (80%). In a series of 18 pediatric patients with liposarcoma, myxoid histology was prevalent, with 17 of the tumors considered low-grade (155). Five-year survival for the entire group was 65%, with patients undergoing gross tumor resection demonstrating better survival (85%). Tumor size greater than 5 cm and nonextremity location was associated with poor outcome. Four patients who developed unresectable disease died following no response to adjuvant chemotherapy. McCoy et al. reported on a mixed group (synovial sarcoma, epithelioid sarcoma, and liposarcoma) of 35 nonmyogenic sarcomas (156). At 5 years following treatment, 92% of patients were alive and 61% were disease-free. Higher grade lesions (grade 3) and larger tumors (>5 cm) carried a worse prognosis. A recent study of 67 patients with nonrhabdomyosarcomatous soft-tissue sarcomas demonstrated an actuarial 10-year period free of tumor progression or recurrence and overall survival rates of 76% and 75%, respectively (157). Of the 18 patients with gross residual disease, 9 (50%) had local progression and 6 died of local disease. By contrast, only one patient with microscopic residual disease who received postoperative radiotherapy had a local recurrence. Low histologic grade was also predictive of improved disease-free survival. Impact of tumor grade was recently reviewed in a study of 64 children with nonrhabdomyosarcomas of an extremity (158). Tumor grade was an important prognostic factor in predicting survival, with 18 of 25 (72%) patients with high-grade lesions eventually relapsing.

The key role that surgery plays in the management of these patients has been brought to light in several studies (159–162). In a large series of 62 patients, the impact of surgery and chemotherapy were evaluated. The most common soft-tissue sarcoma in this series was synovial sarcoma (18 patients). The majority of patients presented with disease either in the trunk (28 patients), extremities (24 patients), and the head and neck region (10 patients). Of the 31 patients whose tumors were completely resected, 26 (84%) survived without evidence of recurrent or distal disease. Postoperative chemotherapy was administered to half of the group without any measurable benefit. In those patients who developed metastatic disease (26 patients), only one survived. The limited impact of chemotherapy was recently reported in a randomized study of 75 patients with metastatic nonrhabdomyosarcomatous soft-tissue sarcoma (163). In patients with nonresectable regional disease (group III) and metastatic disease (group IV), the overall and event-free survival for patients at 4 years was 30.6% and 18.4%, respectively. Combination chemotherapy did not prevent recurrence or disease progression in children with high-stage nonrhabdomyosarcomatous soft-tissue sarcomas.

Nonrhabdomyosarcomatous soft-tissue sarcomas may arise in the head and neck region. In a series of 229 patients with sarcoma reported from UCLA, 33 pediatric cases of nonrhabdomyosarcomatous soft-tissue sarcoma were reported in the head and neck region (164). After salvage therapy, 5-year disease-free survival was 56% (15 of 27). Of the 16 patients treated with surgery alone, only 3 (19%) were rendered disease-free. Radiotherapy improved results of surgical treatment, with 50% of patients having no evidence of disease. In a series of 18 patients diagnosed with nonrhabdomyosarcomatous soft-tissue sarcoma of the head and neck region reported by St. Jude Children's Research Hospital, the results of surgery, postoperative chemotherapy, and irradiation were evaluated (165). Local control was achieved in 50% of patients with either surgery alone (3 patients) or in combination with radiation therapy (5 of 10 patients). The disease-free survival at 3 years was 44%. Local control was found to be difficult to achieve because of the inability to completely resect the majority of tumors. As opposed to rhabdomyosarcomas, nonrhabdomyogenic sarcomas behave much like their adult-onset counterparts. Surgery remains the mainstay of treatment for these patients, with adjuvant radiation therapy assisting local control. Chemotherapy, as in the adult population, has not been demonstrated to improve overall patient survival.

XVI. MANAGEMENT OF METASTATIC DISEASE

A. Lymph Node Metastasis

Lymph node metastases occur in only 3–5% of soft-tissue sarcomas (166,167). In a review of 374 sarcoma patients, 113 patients (30%) had histologic evaluation of their lymph nodes either as part of a major amputation or from elective lymph node dissection performed for clinically positive or high-risk nodes (168). Of these 113 patients, only 6 had involvement of the regional lymph nodes (5.3%). In addition, an extensive review was part of their study, which included more than 3000 cases of soft-tissue sarcoma. The overall incidence of regional lymph node metastasis was 9.4%. Rhabdomyosarcoma (12.2%), synovial sarcoma (17%), and hemangiopericytoma (13%) were the most common histologic subtypes. In another retrospective review of 160 patients undergoing surgical resection for soft-tissue sarcoma, the authors found only 47 patients who had undergone histologic evaluation of their lymph node status (29%) (169). Six of the 47 patients were found to have regional lymph node metastasis (12.8%). The histologic subtypes included leiomyosarcoma, rhabdomyosarcoma, synovial sarcoma, malignant fibrous histiocytoma, and anaplastic sarcoma. An additional two patients with rhabdomyosarcoma who did not undergo lymph node biopsy eventually developed lymph node metastasis for an overall incidence of 17.4%. Regardless of tumor type, an increased incidence of nodal metastasis is associated with high-grade sarcomas (170). In a study of 323 patients with soft-tissue sarcoma, 19% had low-grade lesions, 37% had moderate-grade lesions, and 44% had high-grade lesions. The overall regional lymph node metastasis rate was 5.9%, with the majority oc-

TABLE 1 Risk of Lymphnode Metastases

Histologic type	Metastases (%)
Clear cell sarcoma	27.5
Epithelioid sarcoma	20.0
Rhabdomyosarcoma	14.8
Synovial sarcoma	13.7
Alveolar soft-parts tumor	12.5
Vascular sarcomas	11.4
Malignant fibrous histiocytoma	10.2

Source: Mazeron JJ, Suit HD. Lymph nodes as sites of metastases from sarcomas of soft tissue. Cancer 60(8):1800–1808, 1987.

curring in patients with high-grade sarcomas (17 of 142 patients). An extensive review of more than 5000 patients was part of this study, with an overall incidence of lymph node metastasis of 10.8%. Patients at increased risk included several different histologic subtypes (Table 1). In a study of 183 patients with soft-tissue sarcomas, Gaakeer et al. reported that 8 patients had lymph node metastasis at initial presentation (171). The overall incidence of lymph node metastasis was 8.1%, with the onset of metastasis being correlated with the onset of disseminated disease. In a large series of 1772 patients with soft-tissue sarcoma, Fong reported that 46 (2.6%) developed lymph node metastases (172). As with the study by Mazeron et al., 98% of patients with lymph node metastases had high-grade lesions. Of the 46 patients with metastases, 25% had disseminated disease. Isolated nodal metastases were closely linked with the onset of disseminated disease in this study, with 54% of patients with isolated nodal metastases developing systemic metastases.

With an overall incidence of 3–10%, elective lymph node dissection is not necessary. In patients with high-grade neoplasms, or when presenting with a high-risk histologic subtype, evaluation of regional lymph nodes should be undertaken through careful physical examination and CT scan. Unfortunately, the presence of regional lymph node metastases is a poor prognostic indicator (173). Survival rates for patient with soft-tissue sarcomas and regional lymph node metastases vary widely from 7% to 50%. In those studies with improved patient survival, the authors support radical lymph node dissection and aggressive chemotherapy.

B. Pulmonary Metastases

Approximately 20% of patients with extremity or truncal sarcoma demonstrate pulmonary metastasis, whereas 50% of patients with recurrence demonstrate pulmonary metastasis as the only recurrence (166). In a study of 307 patients with localized high-grade soft-tissue sarcomas who underwent radical resection, only 56

(18%) developed isolated lung metastases. This represented 52% of all observed recurrences and 67% of all distant relapses (174).

Most pulmonary nodules are identified during radiographic staging, as the majority of patients are asymptomatic. In the 15–20% of patients who are symptomatic, lesions are usually adjacent to the central airways. Cough and hemoptysis are the most common symptoms. Fever, chest discomfort, and/or occasional paraneoplastic syndromes have been reported (175–182). CT of the chest can identify up to 80% of all surgically confirmed pulmonary nodules greater than 3 mm, which is 25% more than visualized on linear tomography. It is estimated that the diagnostic accuracy of radiologic staging is 40% for plain chest radiographs and 60–80% for CT scans of the chest (183–185). CT has replaced linear tomography as the radiographic modality of choice in the assessment of lung metastases (186,187).

The prognosis is extremely poor for patients who develop pulmonary metastases that are not suitable for complete resection. Even though adjuvant chemotherapy may extend the disease-free interval, the vast majority of patients die within 2 years, with no survivors after 3 years (188,189). In one study, the median survival of patients with nonresectable lung metastases was 7.4 months (166). The first reported resection of a sarcomatous pulmonary metastasis was in 1882, which was a contiguous resection along with removal of a chest wall primary tumor (190). Until recently, the majority of studies in support of pulmonary resection have been case reports (191–193). During the early 1960s, two large series reported on the results of pulmonary resection. The indications for pulmonary resection were restricted to patients exhibiting a long disease-free interval following resection of the primary tumor, and had three or fewer lesions confined to one lung (194). During this period, 221 pulmonary resections on 205 patients for metastatic disease were performed at the Mayo Clinic (195). Support for a more liberal approach to pulmonary metastasectomy came from two series of osteogenic sarcoma patients from the same institution. In this study, only 24 of 145 patients (17%) survived 5 years after resection of their primary tumor without adjuvant therapy, with the majority succumbing to pulmonary metastases (81%) (196,197). In a follow-up consecutive series of 22 patients with osteogenic sarcoma who underwent pulmonary metastasectomy, the survival rate increased to 32% (196,197).

Series dedicated specifically to the management of soft-tissue sarcoma pulmonary metastases are few. An early series of 112 patients with metastatic soft-tissue sarcoma undergoing surgery at the Mayo Clinic from 1950 to 1976 reported a 5-year survival rate of 29% (198). Survival was adversely influenced by a disease-free interval of less than 12 months and by the subsequent development of extrathoracic metastases. Gender, age, tumor histology, number of lesions full excised, and region of the lung lesions did not affect survival. Huth reported a 40% survival rate at 4 years for 43 patients who underwent resection of pulmonary metastases from soft-tissue sarcoma (199). This figure was significantly influenced by the tumor doubling time (more or less than 40 days) and by the disease-free interval (more or less than a year). Because of the relative resistance of sarcomas to chemotherapy, enthusiasm for the surgical excision of pulmonary metastases has increased.

Previous studies have reported improvement in overall 5-year survival, ranging from 25% to 45%, without the combination of other adjuvant therapy (166, 198,200–206). In one series of 136 patients with metastatic soft-tissue sarcoma who underwent surgical exploration from 1975 to 1994, 110 patients (81%) were amenable to complete macroscopic resection of all pulmonary metastases (207). The actuarial survival after complete resection was 48% at 3 years, 36% at 5 years, and 30% at 10 years, with a median survival of 35 months. Incomplete resection resulted in a reduced survival of only 16 months (207). These results are similar to those reported in a study by van Geel et al. (208). In this study of 255 patients who underwent complete resection of lung metastases from soft-tissue sarcomas, the 3- and 5-year overall postmetastasectomy survival rates were 54% and 38%, respectively. The disease-free postmetastasectomy survival rates were 42% at 3 years, 35% at 5 years, and 27% at 10 years. Favorable prognostic factors for a better outcome revealed disease-free intervals of 2.5 years or more, with microscopically free margins, age less than 40 years, and grade 1 and 2 tumors (208). A very large cooperative project established in 1991 collected clinical data from 5207 patients, with 938 patients treated by pulmonary metastasectomy for soft-tissue sarcoma. An overall 5-year survival of 30%, a 10-year survival of 22%, and a median survival of 27 months was reported for these patients (207).

As expected, the longer the disease-free interval, the better the survival. However, the cutoff ranges between 12 and 36 months (201,209). In a study of 106 cases, patients with greater than four pulmonary lesions demonstrated a median survival of 6 months after metastasectomy (201). In other studies, a favorable outcome can be identified only for patients with single lesions of less than 3 cm in diameter, with a 50% 5-year survival, in contrast to patients with multiple lesions (25%) (210). Other authors report a better survival for pulmonary metastases with a maximum diameter of less than 3 cm (211) or less than 1.5 cm (212) independent of the total number of resected lesions. In the study by van Geel et al., patients with a disease-free interval of 36 months or longer, had a significantly better survival (40% at 5 years, 24% at 10 years, median 40 months) than those with a disease-free interval of less than 12 months (19% at 5 years, 13% at 10 years, median 21 months). Patients with single metastases had a better survival (38% at 5 years, 30% at 10 years, median 37 months) than those with four or more metastases (18% at 5 years, 12% at 10 years, median 23 months).

Additional studies comparing surgery to combination of surgery and chemotherapy have failed to demonstrate differences between these two treatment approaches (213–216). Other studies have garnered some support for the multimodality management of pulmonary metastases (217–219). In a study of 24 patients with pulmonary metastases from soft-tissue sarcoma, chemotherapy was given prior to metastasectomy, with patients grouped according to response (220). Five patients had a complete response, but recurrence 5–57 months later. Seven patients had a partial response, whereas 12 patients had either no change or progression. Resectable patients had a median survival of 30 months and actuarial 5-year survival of 25%. There were no differences in postresection survival between any groups, with postthoracotomy survival not being predictive from the initial chemotherapy response (220). In any population of patients with resectable pulmonary metastases, surgery alone fails in 60–80% of all patients, with chemotherapy possibly improving these results (221). No survival benefit after metastasectomy has been demonstrated for responders, as evidenced on radiographic imaging, as compared with nonresponders to preoperative chemotherapy (222). Preliminary results of 26 patients undergoing aggressive chemotherapy followed by complete surgery are encouraging, with a relapse-free and overall survival at 2 years of 39% and 74%, respectively (222). However, one must be careful in evaluating radiologic response as compared with histologic response. In the study by Saeter et al., 11 of 26 patients demonstrated a discrepancy between evaluations of radiologic and histologic response. In conclusion, a good histologic response is rare and not predicted by radiologic response, with the histologic response being a more reliable prognostic measure of survival (222).

Though surgical resection is considered as a treatment for pulmonary metastases, patient selection criteria have remained controversial (175–181,191,194, 209,223–229) (Table 2). Casson et al. reported a 5-year survival of 26% in 58 patients who had complete resection and were followed until death or for a minimum of 5 years (204). Favorable prognostic indicators included a tumor doubling time of greater than 40 days, unilateral disease, three or fewer nodules identified on preoperative tomograms, no more than two metastases resected, and tumor histology. Using multivariate analysis, four or more nodules was the most significant prognostic indicator (204). Another study of 67 patients with histologically documented pulmonary metastases from soft-tissue sarcoma reported several predictors of enhanced survival. These included a tumor doubling time greater than 20 days, no more than four nodules on preoperative tomograms, and a disease-free interval of greater than 12 months (203,230). Even in light of these results, some studies have questioned whether the number of metastases should influence the decision for surgical intervention (231). In the study by Girard et al., complete resection of pulmonary metastases was performed in patients diagnosed with either carcinoma (230 patients) or sarcoma (151 patients). Patients were divided into three groups based on the number of metastases at the time of surgery: group 1 with one metastatic nodule, group 2 with two to four nodules, and group 3 with five or more nodules. The 5- and 10-year survival was 37% and 23%, respectively, for carcinoma patients, and 31% and 28% for sarcoma patients. Statistically the only significant difference was between the carcinoma patients in groups 1 and 2.

TABLE 2 Indications for Pulmonary Resection

Control of the primary tumor
Complete resection of metastases
Capacity to undergo surgical resection
Absence of extrathoracic metastases
Poor adjuvant therapy alternatives
Extensive disease-free interval
Long tumor doubling time of pulmonary metastases
Fewer than four pulmonary nodules

The authors concluded that the number of nodules present should not influence the decision for surgery (231). Two studies reported improved survival in patients with four or fewer nodules, a disease-free interval of more than 1 year, and a tumor doubling time more than 40 days (204,230). Repeat resection in patients with pulmonary relapse appears to be justified because the median survival for these patients has been reported to be 25 months (232,233).

Patients presenting with recurrent pulmonary metastases who undergo complete resection have been reported to demonstrate an improved postresection survival (206,232,233). Increased age and female sex have been associated with an increased risk of death from disease in resected patients with recurrent pulmonary metastases, in contrast to initially isolated pulmonary metastases (232). Patients with limited metastases demonstrated the best postresection survival (233). In a series by Rizzoni et al., 29 patients with recurrent pulmonary metastases from soft-tissue sarcomas who underwent two or more resections of pulmonary metastases were reported. Patients with a favorable prognostic outcome included those with resectable metastases, a longer tumor doubling time, fewer than three nodules, and a disease-free interval of at least 6 months. Median survival was 14.5 months and overall 5-year survival 22%. Resectable patients demonstrated a median survival of 24 months (206). A follow-up study of the same patient population reported a reduction in 5-year survival of 15%. These results were further confirmed in a study of 39 patients with soft-tissue sarcomas, whereby a 5-year survival rate of 32% was reported in patients with resectable metastases (233). The majority of relapses in patients with soft-tissue sarcomas are confined to the lung, with 37 of 71 in one series (207). In the 37 patients with intrapulmonary relapses, 20 were treated with further resections, with a survival rate of 56% at 5 years. The National Cancer Institute reported on their experience in 23 cases, with the average number of operations per patient being 1.9, with a 40% survival at 5 years (166).

The long-term outcome for patients undergoing pulmonary resection has been reported to be less favorable in a study by Gadd et al. (205). The 3-year survival rate after complete resection of all pulmonary metastases in 65 patients was only 23%. Unfortunately, only a few select patients may be candidates for pulmonary resection of their pulmonary metastases, as fewer than half of the 135 patients in this study were eligible for surgery. The remainder of patients with pulmonary metastases either demonstrated disease that was beyond pulmonary resection or were candidates for nonsurgical management. Overall, the 5-year survival rate in these series of patients ranged from 20% to 35% and represents a highly select group (199,203–205). As with localized recurrences of soft-tissue sarcomas, surgical resection of pulmonary metastases can provide the sarcoma patient with the best chance for improved survival. Unfortunately, the prognostic indicators and selection criteria justifying further surgery remain elusive. With the extremely small number of patients being treated for soft-tissue sarcomas, it has remained difficult to accrue enough data to answer these questions. Additional studies based on the collective experience of multiple centers are necessary before these criteria can be established.

REFERENCES

1. Enneking WF, Spanier SS, Goodman MA. A system for the surgical staging of musculoskeletal sarcoma. Clin Orthop 153:106–120, 1980.
2. Enneking WF. Musculoskeletal Tumor Surgery, vol. 1. New York: Churchill Livingtone, 1983, pp. 1–60.
3. Simon MA, Enneking WF. The management of soft tissue sarcomas of the extremities. J Bone Joint Surg A 58:317–327, 1976.
4. Adair FE, Pack GT, Farrier JH. Lipomas. Am J Cancer 16:1104–1120, 1932.
5. Allen PW, Enzinger FM. Hemangioma of skeletal muscle; an analysis of 89 cases. Cancer 29(1):8–22, 1972.
6. Milliken JB, Glowicki J. Hemangiomas and vascular malformation in infants and children: a classification based on endothelial characteristics. Plast Reconstr Surg 69:412–422, 1982.
7. Hajdu SI. Peripheral nerve sheath tumors. Cancer 72(12):3549–3552, 1993.
8. Pack GT, Ariel IM. Tumors of the Soft Somatic Tissues. New York: Harper and Row, 1958.
9. Myhre-Jensen O. A consecutive 7-year series of 1331 benign soft tissue tumours. Clinicopathologic data: comparison with sarcomas. Acta Orthop Scand 52(3):287–293, 1981.
10. Dahn I, Jonsson N, Lundh G. Desmoid tumors: a series of 33 cases. Acta Chir Scand 126:305–314, 1963.
11. Reitamo JJ, Hayry P, Nykyri E, Saxen E. The desmoid tumor I: Incidence, sex, age and anatomical distribution in the Finish population. Am J Clin Pathol 77(6):665–673, 1982.
12. Rock MG, Pritchard DJ, Reiman HM, Soule EH, Brewster RC. Extra-abdominal desmoid tumors. J Bone Joint Surg A 66:1369–1374, 1984.

13. Reitmano JJ, Scheinin TM, Hayry P. The desmoid syndrome. New aspects in the cause, pathogenesis and treatment of the desmoid tumour. Am J Surg 151(2):230–237, 1986.

14. Pritchard DJ. Extra-abdominal desmoid tumors. In: C McC Evarts, ed. Surgery of the Musculoskeletal System, 2nd ed., Vol. 5. New York: Churchill Livingstone, 1990, pp. 4787–4793.

15. Posner MC, Shiu MH, Newsome JL, Hajdu SI, Gaynor JJ, Brennan MF. The desmoid tumor. Not a benign disease. Arch Surg 124(2):191–196, 1989.

16. Easter DW, Halasz NA. Recent trends in the management of desmoid tumors. Summary of 19 cases and review of the literature. Ann Surg 210(6):765–769, 1989.

17. Leibel SA, Wara WM, Hill DR, Bovill EG, de Lorimier AA, Beckstead JH, Phillips TL. Desmoid tumors: local control and patterns of relapse following radiation therapy. Int J Radiat Oncol Biol Phys 9(8):1167–1171, 1983.

18. McKinnon JG, Neifeld JP, Kay S, Parker GA, Foster WC, Lawrence W Jr. Management of desmoid tumors. Surg Gynecol Obstet 169(2):104–106, 1989.

19. Miralbell R, Suit HD, Mankin HJ, Zuckerberg LR, Stracher MA, Rosenberg AE. Fibromatoses: from postsurgical surveillance to combined surgery and radiation therapy. Int J Radiat Oncol Biol Phys 18(3):535–540, 1990.

20. Sherman NE, Romsdahl M, Evans H, Zagars G, Oswald MJ. Desmoid tumors: a 20-year radiotherapy experience. Int J Radiat Oncol Biol Phys 19(1):37–40, 1990.

21. McCollough WM, Parsons JT, van der Griend R, Enneking WF, Heare T. Radiation therapy for aggressive fibromatosis. The experience at the University of Florida. J Bone Joint Surg A 73:717–725, 1991.

22. Pritchard DJ, Nascimento AG, Petersen IA. Local control of extra-abdominal desmoid tumors. J Bone Joint Surg A 78:848–854, 1996.

23. Spear MA, Jennings LC, Mankin HJ, Spiro IJ, Springfield DS, Gebhardt MC, Rosenberg AE, Efird JT, Suit HD. Individualizing management of aggressive fibromatoses. Int J Radiat Oncol Biol Phys 40(3):637–645, 1998.

24. Lopez R, Kemalyan N, Moseley HS, Dennis DD, Vetto RM. Problems in diagnosis and management of desmoid tumors. Am J Surg 159(5):450–453, 1990.

25. Kiel KD, Suit HD. Radiation therapy in the treatment of aggressive fibromatosis (desmoid tumors). Cancer 54(10):2051–2055, 1984.

26. Catton CN, O'Sullivan B, Bell R, Cummings B, Fornasier V, Panzarella T. Aggressive fibromatosis: optimisation of local management with a retrospective failure analysis. Radiother Oncol 34(1):7–22, 1995.

27. Kamath SS, Parsons JT, Marcus RB, Zlotecki RA, Scarborough MT. Radiotherapy for aggressive fibromatosis. Int J Radiat Oncol Biol Phys 36(2):325–328, 1996.

28. Markhede G, Lundrren L, Bjurstam N, Berlin O, Stener B. Extra-abdominal desmoid tumours. Acta Orthop Scand 57(1):1–7, 1986.

29. Giustra PE, White HO, Killoran PJ. Intrathoracic desmoid at previous thoracotomy site. J Can Assoc Radio 30(2):122–123, 1979.

30. Aaron AD, O'Mara JW, Legendre KE, Evans SRT, Attinger CE, Montgomery EA. Chest wall fibromatosis associated with silicone breast implants. Surg Oncol 5(2):93–99, 1996.

31. Berardi R, Canlas M. Desmoid tumor and laparotomy scars. Int Surg 58(4):254–256, 1973.

32. Strode JE. Desmoid tumors particularly as related to their surgical removal. Ann Surg 139(3):335–340, 1954.
33. Procter H, Singh L, Baum M, Brinkley D. Response of multicentric desmoid tumors to tamoxifen. Br J Surg 74(5):401, 1987.
34. Lim CL, Walker MJ, Mehta RR, Das Gupta TK. Estrogen and antiestrogen binding sites in desmoid tumors. Eur J Cancer Clin Oncol 22(5):583–587, 1986.
35. Patel SR, Evans HL, Benjamin RS. Combination chemotherapy in adult desmoid tumors. Cancer 72(11):3244–3247, 1993.
36. Waddell WR, Gerner RE, Reich MP. Non-steroidal anti-inflammatory drugs and tamoxifen for desmoid tumors and carcinoma of the stomach. J Surg Oncol 22(3):197–211, 1983.
37. Waddell WR, Kirsch WM. Testolactone, sulindac, warfarin, and vitamin K_1 for unresectable desmoid tumors. Am J Surg 161(4):416–421, 1991.
38. Gerner RE, Moore GE, Pickren JW. Soft tissue sarcomas. Ann Surg 181(6):803–808, 1975.
39. Cantin J, McNeer GP, Chu FC, Booher RJ. The problem of local recurrence after treatment of soft tissue sarcoma. Ann Surg 168(1):47–53, 1968.
40. Shiu MH, Castro EB, Hajdu SI, Fortner JG. Surgical treatment of 297 soft tissue sarcomas of the lower extremity. Ann Surg 182(5):597–602, 1975.
41. Simon MA, Spanier SS, Enneking WF. Management of adult soft tissue sarcomas of the extremities. Surg Ann 11:363–402, 1979.
42. Suit HD, Russell WO, Martin RG. Sarcoma of soft tissue: clinical and histopathologic parameters and response to treatment. Cancer 35(5):1478–1483, 1975.
43. Perry H, Chu FC. Radiation therapy in the palliative management of soft tissue sarcomas. Cancer 15:179–183, 1962.
44. Lindberg RD, Martin RG, Romsdahl MM. Surgery and postoperative radiotherapy in the treatment of soft tissue sarcomas in adults. Am J Roentgenol Ther Nucl Med 123(1):123–129, 1975.
45. Rosenberg SA, Tepper J, Glatstein E, Costa J, Baker A, Brennan M, Demoss EV, Seipp C, Sindelar WF, Sugarbaker P, Wesley R. The treatment of soft-tissue sarcomas of the extremities: prospective randomized evaluations of (1) limb sparing surgery plus radiation therapy compared with amputation and (2) the role of adjuvant chemotherapy. Ann Surg 196(3):305–315, 1982.
46. Collin C, Hadju SI, Godold J, Shiu MH, Hilaris BI, Brennan MF. Localized, operable soft tissue sarcoma of the lower extremity. Arch Surg 121(12):1425–1433, 1986.
47. Karakousis CP, Emrich LJ, Rao U, Khalil M. Limb salvage in soft tissue sarcomas with selective combination of modalities. Eur J Surg Oncol 17(1):71–80, 1991.
48. Zelefsky MJ, Nori D, Shiu MH, Brennan MF. Limb salvage in soft tissue sarcomas involving neurovascular structures using combined surgical resection and brachytherapy. Int J Radiat Oncol Biol Phys 19(4):913–918, 1990.
49. Williard WC, Hadju SI, Casper ES, Brennan MF. Comparison of amputation with limb-sparing operations for adult soft tissue sarcoma of the extremity. Ann Surg 215(3):269–275, 1992.
50. Mankin HJ, Mankin CJ, Simon MA. The hazards of the biopsy, revisited. For the members of the Musculoskeletal Tumor Society. J Bone Joint Surg A 78(5):656–663, 1996.

51. Rydholm A. Surgical margins for soft tissue sarcoma. Acta Orthop Scand (Suppl 273) 68:81–85, 1997.
52. Enneking WF, Spanier SS, Malawer MM. The effect of the anatomic setting on the results of surgical procedures for soft parts sarcoma of the thigh. Cancer 47(5):1005–1022, 1981.
53. Stener B, Stener I. Malignant tumors of the soft tissues of the thigh. Acta Chir Scand 115:457–475, 1958.
54. Stener B. Surgical treatment of soft tissue tumors. In: Canonico A, Estevez O, Chacon R, Barg S, eds. Advances in Medical Oncology, Research, and Education, Vol 10, Kumar S, ed. Clinical cancer: principal sites 1. New York: Pergamon Press, 1979, pp. 147–167.
55. Berlin O, Stener B, Angervall L, Kindblem LG, Markhede G, Oden A. Surgery for soft tissue sarcoma in the extremities. A multivariate analysis of the 6–26–year prognosis in 137 patients. Acta Orthop Scand 61(6):475–486, 1990.
56. Kawaguchi N, Matumoto S, Manabe J. New method of evaluating the surgical margin and safety margin for musculoskeletal sarcoma, analysed on the basis of 457 surgical cases. J Cancer Res Clin Oncol 121(9–10):555–563, 1995.
57. Azzarelli A. Surgery in soft tissue sarcomas. Eur J Cancer 29A(4):618–623, 1993.
58. Rydholm A, Rooser B. Surgical margins for soft-tissue sarcoma. J Bone Joint Surg A 69(7):1074–1078, 1987.
59. Karakousis CP, Proimakis C, Walsh DL. Primary soft tissue sarcoma of the extremities in adults. Br J Surg 82(9):1208–1212, 1995.
60. Pisters PWT, Leung DHY, Woodruff J, Shi W, Brennan M. Analysis of prognostic factors in 1,041 patients with localized soft tissue sarcomas of the extremities. J Clin Oncol 14(5):1679–1689, 1996.
61. Heslin MJ, Woodruff J, Brennan MF. Prognostic significance of a positive microscopic margin in high-risk extremity soft tissue sarcoma: implications for management. J Clin Oncol 14(2):473–478, 1996.
62. Tanabe KK, Pollock RE, Ellis LM, Murphy A, Sherman N, Romsdahl MM. Influence on surgical margins on outcome in patients with preoperative irrradiated extremity soft tissue sarcomas. Cancer 73(6):1652–1659, 1994.
63. Noria S, Davis A, Kandel R, Levesqu J, O'Sullivan B, Wunder J, Bell R. Residual disease following unplanned excision of a soft-tissue sarcoma of the extremity. J Bone Joint Surg A 78(5):650–655, 1996.
64. Davis AM, Kandel RA, Wunder JS, Unger R, Meer J, O'Sullivan B, Catton CN, Bell RS. The impact of residual disease on local recurrenc in patients treated by initial unplanned resection for soft tissue sarcoma of the extremity. J Surg Oncol 66(2):81–87, 1997.
65. Giuliano AE, Eilber FR. The rationale for planned reoperation after unplanned total excision of soft-tissue sarcomas. J Clin Oncol 3(10):1344–1348, 1985.
66. Goodlad JR, Fletcher CDM, Smith MA. Surgical resection of primary soft-tissue sarcoma. J Bone Joint Surg B 78(4):658–661, 1996.
67. Zornig C, Peiper M, Schroder S. Re-excision of soft tissue sarcoma after inadequate initial operation. Br J Surg 82(2):278–279, 1995.
68. Karakousis CP, Proimakis C, Rao U, Velez AF, Dirscoll DL. Local recurrence and survival in soft-tissue sarcomas. Ann Surg Oncol 3(3):255–260, 1996.

69. Ueda T, Yoshikawa, H, Mori S, Araki N, Myoui A, Kuratsu S, Uchida A. Influence of local recurrence on the prognosis of soft-tissue sarcomas. J Bone Joint Surg B 79(4): 553–557, 1997.

70. Stotter AT, A'Hern RP, Fisher C, Mott AF, Fallowfield ME, Westbury G. The influence of local recurrence of extremity soft tissue sarcoma on metastasis and survival. Cancer 65(5):1119–1129, 1990.

71. Brennan MF. Presidential address. The enigma of local recurrence. Ann Surg Oncol 4(1):1–12, 1997.

72. Pisters PWT, Harrison LB, Leung DH, Woodruff JM, Casper ES, Brennan MF. Long term results of a prospective randomized trial evaluating the role of adjuvant brachytherapy in soft tissue sarcoma. J Clin Oncol 14(3):859–868, 1996.

73. Catton C, Davis A, Bell R, O'Sullivan B, Fornasier V, Wunder J, McLean M. Soft tissue sarcoma of the extremity. Limb salvage after failure of combined conservative therapy. Radiother Oncol 41(3):209–214, 1996.

74. Skibber JM, Lotze MT, Seipp CA, Salcedo R, Rosenberg SA. Limb-sparing surgery for soft tissue sarcomas: wound related morbidity inpatients undergoing wide local excision. Surgery 102(3):447–452, 1987.

75. Lindberg RD, Martin RG, Romsdahl MM, Barkley HT Jr. Conservative surgery and postoperative radiotherapy in 300 adults with soft-tissue sarcomas. Cancer 47(10): 2391–2397, 1981.

76. Bujko K, Suit HD, Springfield DS, Convery K. Wound healing after preoperative radiation for sarcoma of soft tissues. Surg Gynecol Obstet 176(2):124–134, 1993.

77. Ormsby MV, Hilaris BS, Nori D, Brennan MF. Wound complications of adjuvant radiation therapy in patients with soft-tissue sarcomas. Ann Surg 210(1):93–99, 1989.

78. Barwick WJ, Goldberg JA, Scully SP, Harrelson JM. Vascularized tissue transfer for closure of irradiated wounds after soft tissue sarcoma resection. Ann Surg 216(5): 591–595, 1992.

79. Bell RS, Mahoney J, O'Sullivan B, Nguyen C, Langer F, Cummings B, Catton C, Czitrom A, Fornasier VL. Wound healing complications in soft tissue sarcoma management. Comparison of three treatment protocols. J Surg Oncol 46(3):190–197, 1991.

80. Peat BG, Bell RS, Davis A, O'Sullivan B, Mahoney J, Manktelow RT, Bowen V, Catton C, Fornasier VL, Langer F. Wound-healing complications after soft-tissue sarcoma surgery. Plas Reconstr Surg 93(5):980–987, 1994.

81. Chang AE, Steinberg SM, Culnane M, Lampert MH, Reggia AJ, Simpson CG, Hicks JE, White DE, Yang JJ, Glatstein E. Functional and psychosocial effects of multimodality limb-sparing therapy in patients with soft tissue sarcomas. J Clin Oncol 7(9):1217–1228, 1989.

82. Saddegh MK, Bauer HCF. Wound complication in surgery of soft tissue sarcoma. Analysis of 103 consecutive patients managed without adjuvant therapy. Clin Orthop 289:247–253, 1993.

83. Malawer MM, Price WM. Gastrocnemius transposition flap in conjuction with limb-sparing surgery for primary bone sarcomas about the knee. Plast Reconstr Surg 73(5):741–750, 1984.

84. Smith TK. Prevention of complications in orthopedic surgery secondary to nutritional depletion. Clin Orthop 222:91–97, 1987.

85. Kay SP, Moreland JR, Schmitter E. Nutrional status and wound healing in lower extremity amputations. Clin Orthop 217:253–256, 1987.

86. Wolfe BM, Phillips GJ, Hodges RE. Evaluation and management of nutritional status before surgery. Med Clin North Am 63(6):1257–1269, 1979.
87. Jensen JE, Jensen TG, Smith TK. Nutrition in orthopaedic surgery. J Bone Joint Surg A 64(9):1263–1272, 1982.
88. Chmell MJ, Schwartz HS. Analysis of variables affecting wound healing after musculoskeletal sarcoma resections. J Surg Oncol 61(3):185–189, 1996.
89. Serafin D, Sabatier RE, Morris RL, Georgiade G. Reconstruction of the lower extremity with vascularized composite tissue: improved tissue survival and specific indications. Plast Reconstr Surg 66(2):230–241, 1980.
90. Reece GP, Schusterman MA, Pollock RE, Kroll SS, Miller MJ, Baldwin BJ, Romsdahl MM, Janjan NA. Immediate versus delayed free-tissue transfer salvage of the lower extremity in soft tissue sarcoma patients. Ann Surg Oncol 1(1):11–17, 1994.
91. Karakousis CP, Emrich C, Driscoll DL. Variants of hemipelvectomy and their complications. Am J Surg 158(5):404–408, 1989.
92. Brennan MF, Casper ES, Harrison CB, Shiu MH, Gaynor J, Hajdu SI. The role of multimodality therapy in soft tissue sarcomas. Ann Surg 214(3):328–336, 1991.
93. Heiner J, Rao V, Mott W. Immediate free tissue transfer for distal musculoskeletal neoplasms. Ann Plast Surg 30(2):140–146, 1993.
94. Weinberg H, Kenan S, Lewis MM, Housman MR, Vickery CB, Bloom ND. The role of microvascular surgery in limb-sparing procedures for malignant tumors of the knee. Plast Reconstr Surg 92(4):692–698, 1993.
95. Geer RJ, Woodruff J, Casper ES, Brennan MF. Management of small soft-tissue sarcoma of the extremity in adults. Arch Surg 127(11):1285–1289, 1992.
96. Markhede G, Nistor L. Strength of plantar flexion and function after resection of various parts of the triceps surae. Act Orthop Scand 50:693–697, 1979.
97. Rydholm A. Management of patients with soft-tissue tumors. Strategy developed at a regional oncology center. Acta Orthop Scand 54 (Suppl 203):13–77, 1983.
98. Rydholm A, Rooser B, Persson BM. Primary myectomy for sarcoma. J Bone Joint Surg A 68(4):586–589, 1986.
99. Alho A, Alvegard TA, Berlin O, Ranstam J, Rydholm A, Rooser B, Stener B. Surgical margin in soft tissue sarcoma. The Scandinavian Sarcoma Group experience. Acta Orthop Scand 60(6):687–692, 1989.
100. Rydholm A, Gustafson P, Rooser B, Willen H, Akerman M, Herrlin K, Alvegard T. Limb-sparing surgery without radiotherapy based on anatomic location of soft tissue sarcoma. J Clin Oncol 9(10):1757–1765, 1991.
101. Rydholm A, Gustafson P, Rooser B, Willen H, Berg NO. Subcutaneous soft tissue sarcoma. A population-based epidemiologic and prognostic study of 129 patients. J Bone Joint Surg B 73(4):662–667, 1991.
102. Peabody TD, Monson D, Montag A, Schell MJ, Finn H, Simon MA. A comparison of the prognoses for deep and subcutaneous sarcomas of the extremities. J Bone Joint Surg A 76(8):1167–1173, 1994.
103. Gibbs CP, Peabody TD, Mundt AJ, Montag AG, Simon MA. Oncological outcomes of operative treatment of subcutaneous soft-tissue sarcomas of the extremities. J Bone Joint Surg A 79(6):888–897, 1997.
104. Markhede G, Stener B. Function after removal of various hip and thigh muscles for extirpation of tumors. Acta Orthop Scand 52(4):373–395, 1981.

105. Markhede G, Angervall L, Stener B. A multivariate analysis of the prognosis after surgical treatment of malignant soft-tissue tumors. Cancer 49(8):1721–1733, 1982.
106. Storm FK, Mahvi DM. Diagnosis and management of retroperitoneal soft-tissue sarcoma. Ann Surg 214(1):2–10, 1991.
107. Singer S, Corson JM, Gonin R, Gemetri GD, Healey EA, Marcus K, Eberlein TJ. Prognostic factors predictive of survival for truncal and retroperitoneal soft-tissue sarcoma. Ann Surg 221(2):185–195, 1995.
108. Jaques DP, Coit DG, Hajdu SI, Brennan MF. Management of primary and recurrent soft tissue sarcoma of the retroperitoneum. Ann Surg 212(1):51–59, 1990.
109. Bevilacqua RG, Rogatko A, Hajdu SI, Brennan MF. Prognostic factors in primary retroperitoneal soft-tissue sarcomas. Arch Surg 126(3):328–334, 1991.
110. Skiloni E, Szold A, White DE, Freund HR. High-grade retroperitoneal sarcomas: role of an aggressive palliative approach. J Surg Oncol 53(3):197–203, 1993.
111. Sondak VK, Econonmou JS, Eilber FR. Soft tissue sarcomas of the extremity and retroperitoneum: advances in management. Adv Surg 24:333–359, 1991.
112. Storm FK, Eilber FR, Mirra J, Morton DL. Retroperitoneal sarcomas: a reappraisal of treatment. J Surg Oncol 17(1):1–17, 1981.
113. Dalton RR, Donohue JH, Mucha PJ Jr, van Heerden JA, Reiman HM, Chen SP. Management of retroperitoneal sarcomas. Surgery 106(4):725–732, 1989.
114. Yang J, Rosenberg SA, Glatstein EJ. Sarcomas of the soft tissues. In: DeVita VT Jr, Hellman S, Rosenberg, SA, eds. Cancer: Principles and Practice of Oncology, 4th ed. Philadelphia: JB Lippincott, 1993, pp. 1436–1488.
115. Jenkins MP, Alvaranga JC, Thomas JM. The management of retroperitoneal soft tissue sarcomas. Eur J Cancer 32A(4):622–626, 1996.
116. Kinne DW, Chu FCH, Huvos AG, Yagoda A, Fortner JG. Treatment of primary and recurrent retroperitoneal liposarcoma: twenty-five-year experience at Memorial Hospital. Cancer 31(1):53–64, 1973.
117. Karakousis CP, Velez AF, Gerstenbluth R, Driscoll DL. Resectability and survival in retroperitoneal sarcomas. Ann Surg Oncol 3(2):150–158, 1996.
118. Karakousis CP, Kontzoglou K, Driscoll DL. Resectability of retroperitoneal sarcomas: a matter of surgical technique? Eur J Surg Oncol 21(6):617–622, 1995.
119. Shiloni E, Szold A, White DE, Freund HR. High-grade retroperitoneal sarcomas: role of an aggressive palliative approach. J Surg Oncol 53:197–203, 1993.
120. Willett CG, Suit HD, Tepper JE, Mankin HJ, Convery K, Rosenberg A, Wood WC. Intraoperative electron beam radiation therapy for retroperitoneal soft tissue sarcoma. Cancer 68(2):278–83, 1991.
121. Glenn J, Sindelar WF, Kinsella, Glatstein E, Tepper J, Costa J, Baker A, Sugarbaker P, Brennan MF, Seipp C. Results of multimodality therapy of resectable soft-tissue sarcomas of the retroperitoneum. Surgery 97(3):316–324, 1985.
122. Weinstein L, Shiu MH. Soft tissue sarcomas of the abdominal wall. In: Shiu MH, Brennan MF, eds. Surgical Management of Soft Tissue Sarcoma. Philadelphia: Lea and Febiger, 1989, pp. 125–136.
123. Bains MS, Pomerantz A, McCormack PM, Martini N. Soft tissue sarcomas of the chest wall. In: Shiu MH, Brennan MF, eds. Surgical Management of Soft Tissue Sarcoma. Philadephia: Lea & Febiger, 1989, pp. 137–146.
124. Faber LP, Somers J, Templeton AC. Chest wall tumors. Curr Probl Surg 32(8):661–747, 1995.

125. Perry RR, Venzon D, Roth JA, Pass HI. Survival after surgical resection for high-grade chest wall sarcomas. Ann Thorac Surg 49(3):363–368, 1990.

126. Sabanathan S, Shah R, Mearns AJ. Surgical treatment of primary malignant chest wall tumours. Eur J Cardiothorac Surg 11(6):1011–1016, 1997.

127. Capanna R, Manfrini M, Briccoli A, Gherlinzoni F, Lauri G, Caldora P. Latissimus dorsi pedicled flap applications in shoulder and chest wall reconstructions after extracompartmental sarcoma resections. Tumori 81(1):56–62, 1995.

128. Hajdu SI. Pathology of Soft Tissue Tumors. Philadelphia: Lea & Febiger, 1979.

129. Farr HW. Soft part sarcomas of the head and neck. Semin Oncol 8(2):185–189, 1981.

130. Farhood AI, Hajdu SI, Shiu MH, Strong EW. Soft tissue sarcomas of the head and neck in adults. Am J Surg 160(4):365–369, 1990.

131. Weber RS, Benjamin RS, Peters LJ, Ro JY, Achon O, Goepfert H. Soft tissue sarcomas of the head and neck in adolescents and adults. Am J Surg 152(4):386–392, 1986.

132. Meterissan SH, Rielly JA, Murphy A, Romsdahl MM, Pollock RE. Soft-tissue sarcomas of the shoulder girdle: factors influencing local recurrence, distant metastases, and survival. Ann Surg Oncol 2(6):530–536, 1995.

133. Talbert ML, Zagars GK, Sherman NE, Romsdahl MM. Conservative surgery and radiation therapy for soft tissue sarcoma of the wrist, hand, ankle, and foot. Cancer 66(12):2482–2491, 1990.

134. Kirby EJ, Shereff MJ, Lewis MM. Soft-tissue tumors and tumor-like lesions of the foot. J Bone Joint Surg A 71(4):621–626, 1989.

135. Johnstone PA, Wexler LH, Venzon DJ, Jacomson J, Yang JC, Horowitz ME, DeLaney TF. Sarcomas of the hand and foot: Analysis of local control and functional result with combined modality therapy in extremity preservation. Int J Radiat Oncol Biol Phys 29(4):735–745, 1994.

136. Brien EW, Terek RM, Geer RJ, Caldwell G, Brennan MF, Healey JH. Treatment of soft-tissue sarcomas of the hand. J Bone Joint Surg A 77(4):564–571, 1995.

137. Fong Y, Coit DB, Woodruff JM Brennan MF. Lymph node metastasis from soft tissue sarcoma in adults. Analysis of data from a prospective database of 1772 sarcoma patients. Ann Surg 217(1):72–77, 1993.

138. Kindblom LG, Angervall L, Fassina AS. Atypical lipoma. APMIS 90(1):27–36, 1982.

139. Evans HL. Classification and grading of soft-tissue sarcomas. A comment. Hematol Oncol Clin North Am 9(3):653–656, 1995.

140. Azumi N, Curtis J, Kempson RL, Hendrickson MR. Atypical and malignant neoplasms showing lipomatous differentiation. A study of 111 cases. Am J Surg Pathol 11(3):161–183, 1987.

141. Chang HR, Hajdu SI, Collin C, Brennan MF. The prognostic value of histologic subtypes in primary extremity liposarcoma. Cancer 64(7):1514–1520, 1989.

142. Weiss SW, Rao VK. Well-differentiated liposarcoma (atypical lipoma) of deep soft tissue of the extremities, retroperitoneum, and miscellaneous sites. A follow-up study of 92 cases with analysis of the incidence of "dedifferentiation." Am J Surg Pathol 16(11):1051–1058, 1992.

143. Stiller CA, Parkin DM. International variations in the incidence of childhood soft-tissue sarcomas. Paediatr Perinat Epidemiol 8(1):107–119, 1994.

144. Ross JA, Severson RK, Davis S, Brooks JJ. Trends in the incidence of soft tissue sarcomas in the United States from 1973 through 1987. Cancer 72(2):486–490, 1993.

145. Blair V, Birch HM. Patterns and temporal trends in the incidence of malignant disease in children: II. Eur J Cancer A 30(10):1498–1511, 1994.

146. Crist W, Gehan EA, Ragab AH, Dickman PS, Donaldson SS, Fryer C, Hammond D, Hays DM, Herrmann J, Heyn R. The Third Intergroup Rhabdomyosarcoma Study. J Clin Oncol 13(3):610–630, 1995.

147. Hays DM, Lawrence WJ, Wharam M, Newton W Jr, Ruymann FB, Beltangady M, Mauer HM. Primary re-excision for patients with "microscopic residual" tumor following initial excision of sarcomas of trunk and extremity sites. J Pediatr Surg 24(1):5–10, 1989.

148. Hays DM, Raney RB, Crist WM, Lawrence WW Jr, Rajab A, Wharam MD, Webber B, Gehan E, Johnson J, Maurer HM. Secondary surgical procedures to evaluate primary tumor status in patients with chemotherapy-response stage II and IV sarcomas. A report from the Intergroup Rhabdomyosarcoma Study (IRS). J Pediatr Surg 25(10):1100–1105, 1990.

149. Godzinski J, Lamant F, Rey A, Proquin MT, Martelli H. Value of postchemotherapy bioptical verification of complete clinical remission in previously incompletely resected (stage I and IipT3) malignant mesenchymal tumors in children: International Society of Pediatric Oncology 1984 Malignant Mesenchymal Tumors Study. Med Pediatr Oncol 22(1):22–26, 1994.

150. Andrassy RJ, Corpron CA, Hays DM, Raney RB, Wiener ES, Lawrence W Jr, Lobe Te, Bagwell C, Maurer HM. Extremity sarcomas: an analysis of prognostic factors from the Intergroup Rhabdomyosarcoma Study III. J Pediatr Surg 31(1):191–196, 1996.

151. Sercarz JA, Mark RJ, Nasri S, Wang MB, Tran LM. Pediatric rhabdomyosarcoma of the head and neck. Int J Pediatr Otorhinol. 31(1):15–22, 1995.

152. Hayani A, Mahoney DH Jr, Hawkins HK, Steuber CP, Hurwitz R, Fernbach DJ. Soft-tissue sarcomas other than rhabdomyosarcoma in children. Med Pediatr Oncol 20(2):114–118, 1992.

153. Dillon P, Maurer H, Jenkins J, Krummel T, Parham D, Webber B, Salzberg A. A prospective study of nonrhabdomyosarcoma soft tissue sarcomas in the pediatric age group. J Pediatr Surg 27(2):241–244, 1992.

154. Pappo AS, Fontanesi J, Luo X, Rao BN, Parham DM, Hurwitz C, Avery L, Pratt CD. Synovial sarcoma in children and adolescents: The St. Jude Children's Research Hospital experience. J Clin Oncol 12(11):2360–2366, 1994.

155. La Quaglia MP, Spiro S, Ghavimi F, Hajdu SI, Meyers P, Exelby PR. Liposarcoma in patients younger than or equal to 22 years of age. Cancer 72(10):3114–3119, 1993.

156. McCoy DM, Levine EA, Ferrer K, Dasgupta TK. Pediatric soft tissue sarcomas of nonmyogenic origin. J Surg Oncol 53(3):149–153, 1993.

157. Marcus KC, Grier HE, Shamberger RC, Gebhardt MC, Perez-Atayde A, Silver B, Tarbell NJ. Childhood soft tissue sarcoma: a 20-year experience. J Pediatr 131(4):603–607, 1997.

158. Rao BN, Santan VM, Parham D, Pratt CB, Fleming ID, Hudson M, Fontanesi J, Philippe P, Schell MJ. Pediatric nonrhabdomyosarcomas of the extremities. Influ-

ence of size, invasiveness, and grade on outcome. Arch Surg 126(12):1490–1495, 1991.

159. Horowitz ME, Pratt CB, Webber BL, Hustu HO, Etcubanas E, Miliauskas J, Rao BN, Fleming ID, Mahesh Kumar AP, Green AA. Therapy for childhood soft-tissue sarcomas other than rhabdomyosarcoma: a review of 62 cases treated at a single institution. J Clin Oncol 4(4):559–564, 1986.

160. Maurer HM, Cantor A, Salzberg PC, Thomas P, Parham D, Webber B, Marcus R, Pick T, Green D, Link M, Vietti T. Adjuvant chemotherapy vs. observation for localized non-rhabdomyosarcoma soft tissue sarcoma (NRSTS) in children. Proc Am Soc Clin Oncol 11:363, 1992 (abstract).

161. Koscielniak E, Jurgens H, Winkler K, Bunjr D, Herbst M, Keen M, Bernhard G, Trenner J. Treatment of soft tissue sarcoma in childhood and adolescence: a report of the German Cooperative Soft Tissue Sarcoma Study. Cancer 70(10):2557–2567, 1992.

162. Rao BN, Etcubanas EE, Green AA. Present day concepts in the management of sarcomas in children. Cancer Invest 7(4):349–356, 1989.

163. Pratt CB, Maurer HM, Gierser P, Salzberg A, Rao BN, Parham D, Thomas PRM, Marcus RB, Cantor A, Pick T, Green D, Neff J, Jenkins J. Treatment of unresectable or metastatic pediatric soft tissue sarcomas with surgery, irradiation, and chemotherapy: a Pediatric Oncology Group study. Med Pediatr Oncol 30(4):201–209, 1998.

164. Nasri S, Mark RJ, Sercarz JA, Tran LM, Sadeghi S. Pediatric sarcomas of the head and neck other than rhabdomyosarcoma. Am J Otolaryngol 16(3):165–171, 1995.

165. Fontanesi J, Pratt C, Kun L, Hustu O, Pao WJ, Douglass E, Fleming I, Rao B. Local-regional non-rhabdomyosarcomatous soft tissue sarcomas of the head and neck. Int J Radiat Oncol Biol Phys 19(4):995–999, 1990.

166. Potter DA, Glenn J, Kinsella T, Glatstein E, Lack EE, Restrepo C, White DE, Seipp CA, Wesley R, Rosenberg SA. Patterns of recurrence in patients with high-grade soft-tissue sarcomas. J Clin Oncol 3(3):353–366, 1985.

167. Vezeridis MP, Moore R, Karakousis CP. Metastatic patterns in soft-tissue sarcomas. Arch Surg 118(8):915–918, 1983.

168. Weingrad DN, Rosenberg SA. Early lymphatic spread of osteogenic and soft-tissue sarcomas. Surgery 84(2):231–240, 1978.

169. Lee YTN, Moore TM, Schwinn CP. Metastasis of sarcomatous lesion in regional lymph node. J Surg Oncol 20(1):53–58, 1982.

170. Mazeron JJ, Suit HD. Lymph nodes as sites of metastases from sarcomas of soft tissue. Cancer 60(8):1800–1808, 1987.

171. Gaakeer HA, Albus-Lutter CE, Gortzak E, Zoetmulder FA. Regional lymph node metastases in patients with soft tissue sarcomas of the extremities, What are the therapeutic consequences? Eur J Surg Oncol 14(2):151–156, 1988.

172. Fong Y, Coit DG, Woodruff JM, Brennan MF. Lymph node metastases from soft tissue sarcoma in adults. Analysis of data from a prospective database of 1772 sarcoma patients. Ann Surg 217(1):72–77, 1993.

173. Lawrence W Jr, Neifeld JP. Soft tissue sarcomas. Curr Probl Surg 26(11):757–827, 1989.

174. Potter DA, Kinsella T, Glatstein E, Wesley R, White DE, Seipp CA, Chang AE, Lack EE, Costa J, Rosenberg SA. High grade soft tissue sarcomas of the extremities. Cancer 58(1):190–205, 1986.

175. McCormack P. Surgical resection of pulmonary metastases. Semin Surg Oncol 6(5): 297–302, 1990.

176. Wright III JO, Brandt III B, Ehrenhaft JL. Results of pulmonary resection for metastatic lesions. J Thorac Cardiovasc Surg 83(1):94–99, 1982.

177. Wilkins Jr. EW, Head JM, Burke JF. Pulmonary resection for metastatic neoplasms in the lung: experience at the Massachusetts General Hospital. Am J Surg 135(4): 480–483, 1979.

178. Morrow CE, Vassilopoulos PP, Grage TB. Surgical resection for metastatic neoplasms of the lung: experience of the University of Minnesota hospitals. Cancer 45(12):2981–2985, 1980.

179. Takita H, Edgerton F, Karakousis C, Douglass HO, Vincent RG, Beckley S. Surgical management of metastases to the lung. Surg Gynecol Obstet 152(2):191–194, 1981.

180. Ramming KP. Surgery for pulmonary metastases. Surg Clin North Am 60(4):815–824, 1980.

181. Takita H, Merrin C, Didolkar MS, Douglass HO, Edgerton F. The surgical management of multiple lung metastses. Ann Thorac Surg 24(4):359–364, 1977.

182. Joseph WL. Criteria for resection of sarcoma metastatic to the lung. Cancer Chemother Rep 58(2):285–290, 1974.

183. Chang AE, Schaner EC, Conkle DM, et al. Surgical resection of the solitary pulmonary metastasis. In: Weiss LA, Gilbert HA, eds. Pulmonary Metastasis. Boston: GK Hall & Co, 1978, pp. 65–72.

184. Roth JA, Pass HI, Wesley MN, White D, Putnam JB, Seipp C. Comparison of median sternotomy and thoracotomy for resection of pulmonary metastases in patients with adult soft tissue sarcomas. Ann Thorac Surg 42(2):134–138, 1986.

185. Paul KP, Toomes H, Vogt-Moykopf I. Lung volumes following resection of pulmonary metastases in paediatric patients—a retrospective study. Eur J Pediatr 149(12):862–865, 1990.

186. Chang AE, Schaner EG, Conkle DM, Flyle MW, Doppmann YJL, Rosenberg SA. Evaluation of computed tomography in the detection of pulmonary metastases. Cancer 43(3):913–916, 1979.

187. Mintzer RA, Malave SR, Neiman HL, Michaelis LL, Vanecko RM, Sanders JM. Computed vs. conventional tomography in evaluation of primary and secondary pulmonary neoplasms. Radiology 132(3):653–659, 1979.

188. Eilber F, Giuliano A, Eckardt J, Patterson K, Moseley S, Goodnight J. Adjuvant chemotherapy for osteosarcoma: a randomized prospective trial. J Clin Oncol 5(1): 21–26, 1987.

189. Jaffe N, Smith E, Abelson HT, Frei E. Osteogenic sarcoma: alteration in the pattern of pulmonary metastases with adjuvant chemotherapy. J Clin Oncol 1(4):251–254, 1983.

190. Weinlecher. Aborm langer Processus styloideus als Ursache von Schlingbeschwerden Wein. Med Wchnschr 33, 1882.

191. Divis G. Ein Bertrag zur operation, behandlung der lungengeschuuilste. Acta Chir Scand 62:329–334, 1927.

192. Barney JD, Churchill EJ. Adenocarcinoma of the kidney with metastasis to the lung. J Urol 42:269, 1939.
193. Torek F. Removal of metastatic carcinoma of the lung and mediastinum: suggestions as to technic. Arch Surg 21:1416–1424, 1930.
194. McCormack PM, Martini N. The changing role of surgery for pulmonary metastases. Ann Thorac Surg 28(2):139–145, 1979.
195. Thomford NR, Woolner LB, Clagett OT. The surgical treatment of metastatic tumors in the lungs. J Thorac Cardiovasc Surg 49(3):357–363, 1965.
196. Martini N, Huvos AG, Mike V, Marcove RC, Beattie EJ. Multiple pulmonary resections in the treatment of osteogenic sarcoma. Ann Thorac Surg 12(3):271–280, 1971.
197. Shah A, Exelby PR, Rao B, Marcove R, Rosen G, Beattie EJ. Thoracotomy as adjuvant to chemotherapy in metastatic osteogenic sarcoma. J Pediatr Surg 12(6):983–990, 1977.
198. Creagan ET, Fleming TR, Edmonson JH, Pairolero PC. Pulmonary resection for metastatic nonosteogenic sarcoma. Cancer 44(5):1908–1912, 1979.
199. Huth JF, Holmes EC, Vernon SE, Callery CD, Ramming KP, Morton DL. Pulmonary resection for metastatic sarcoma. Am J Surg 140(1):9–16, 1980.
200. McCormack P. Surgical treatment of pulmonary metastases: Memorial Hospital experience. In: Weiss L, Gilbert HA, eds. Pulmonary Metastasis. Boston: GK Hall & Co, 1978, pp. 355–371.
201. Roth JA, Putnam JB Jr, Wesley MN, Rosenberg S. Differing determinants of prognosis following resection of pulmonary metastases from osteogenic and soft tissue sarcoma patients. Cancer 55(6):1361–1366, 1985.
202. Beattie EJ. Surgical treatment of pulmonary metastases. Cancer 54(11 Suppl):2729–2731, 1984.
203. Jablons D, Steinberg SM, Roth J, Pittaluga S, Rosenberg SA, Pass HI. Metastasectomy for soft tissue sarcoma. Further evidence for efficacy and prognostic indicators. J Thorac Cardiovasc Surg 97(5):695–705, 1989.
204. Casson AG, Putnam JB, Natarajan G, Johnson DA, Mountain C, McMurtrey M, Roth JA. Five-year survival after pulmonary metastasectomy for adult soft tissue sarcoma. Cancer 69(3):662–668, 1992.
205. Gadd MA, Casper ES, Woodruff JM, McCormack PM, Brennan MF. Development and treatment of pulmonary metstases in adult patients with extremity soft tissue sarcoma. Ann Surg 218(6):705–712, 1993.
206. Rizzoni WE, Pass HI, Wesley MN, Rosenberg SA, Roth JA. Resection of recurrent pulmonary metastases in patients with soft tissue sarcomas. Arch Surg 121(11):1248–1252, 1986.
207. Pastorino U. Metastasectomy for soft tissue sarcomas. Cancer Treat Res 91:65–75, 1997.
208. van Geel AN, Pastorino U, Jauch KW, Judson IR, van Coevorden F, Buesa JM, Nielsen OS, Boudinet A, Tursz T, Schmitz PT. Surgical treatment of lung metastases: the EORTC-soft tissue and bone sarcoma group study of 255 patients. Cancer 77(4):675–682, 1996.
209. Putnam JB Jr., Roth JA. Prognostic indicators in patients with pulmonary metastases. Semin Surg Oncol 6(5):291–296, 1990.

210. McCormick P. Surgical treatment of pulmonary metastases: Memorial Hospital experience. In: Weiss L, Gilbert HA, eds. Pulmonary Metastasis. Boston: GK Hall & Co, 1978.

211. Goya T, Miyazawa N, Kondo H, Tsuchiya R, Naruke T, Suemasu K. Surgical resection of pulmonary metastases from colorectal cancer: 10-year follow-up. Cancer 64(7):1418–1421, 1989.

212. Marincola FM, Mark JB. Selection factors resulting in improved survival after surgical resection of tumors metastatic of the lungs. Arch Surg 125(10):1387–1393, 1990.

213. Edmonson JH, Fleming TR, Ivins JC, Burgert EO, Soule EH, O'Connell MJ, Sim FH, Ahmann DL. Randomized study of systemic chemotherapy following complete excision of nonosseous sarcomas. J Clin Oncol 2(12):1390–1396, 1984.

214. Elias A, Ryan L, Sulkes A, Collins J, Aisner J, Antman KH. Response to mesna, doxorubicin, ifosfamide and dacarbazine in 108 patients with metastatic or unresectable sarcoma and no prior chemotherapy. J Clin Oncol 7(9):1208–1216, 1989.

215. Zalupski M, Metch B, Balcerzak S, Fletcher WS, Chapman R, Bonnet JD, Weiss GR, Ryan J, Benjamin RS, Baker LH. Phase III comparison of doxorubicin and dacarbazine given by bolus versus infusion in patients with soft tissue sarcomas: a Southwest Oncology Group study. J Natl Cancer Inst 83(13):926–932, 1991.

216. Weh HJ, Zornig C, Hoffknecht MH, et al. Metastasectomy following chemotherapy in patients with advanced soft tissue sarcomas. Onkologie 15:470–474, 1992.

217. Kawai A, Fukuma H, Beppu Y, Yokoyama R, Tsuchiya R, Kondo H, Inoue H. Pulmonary resection for metastatic soft tissue sarcomas. Clin Orthop 310:188–193, 1995.

218. Pastorino U, Valente M, Santoro A, Gasparini M, Azzarelli A, Casali P, Tavecchio L, Rayasi G. Results of salvage for metastatic sarcomas. Ann Oncol 1(4):269–273, 1990.

219. Mentzer SJ, Antman KH, Attinger C, Shermin R, Corson JM, Sugarbaker DJ. Selected benefits of thoracotomy and chemotherapy for sarcoma metastatic to the lung. J Surg Oncol 53(1):54–59, 1993.

220. Lanza LA, Putnam Jr JB, Benjamin RS, Roth JA. Response to chemotherapy does not predict survival after resection of sarcomatous pulmonary metastases. Ann Thorac Surg 51(2):219–224, 1991.

221. van Geel AN, van Coevorden F, Blankensteijn JD, Hoekstra HJ, Schuurman B, Bruggin KED, Taat CW, Theunissen EB. Surgical treatment of pulmonary metastases from soft tissue sarcomas: a retrospective study in The Nederlands. J Surg Oncol 56(3):172–177, 1994.

222. Saeter G, Alvegard TA, Monge O, et al. VIG chemotherapy in advanced soft tissue sarcoma-results of the Scandinavian Sarcoma Group SSG X trial. Acta Orthop Scand 1996; (Suppl 272): in press.

223. Morrow CE, Vassilopoulos PP, Grage TB. Surgical resection for metastatic neoplasms of the lung: experience of the University of Minnesota hospitals. Cancer 45(12):2981–2985, 1980.

224. Mountain CF, McMurtrey MJ, Hermes KE. Surgery for pulmonary metastasis: a 20-year experience. Ann Thorac Surg 38(4):323–330, 1984.

225. McCormack PM, Bains MS, Beattie EJ Jr, Martini N. Pulmonary resection in metastatic carcinoma. Chest 73(2):163–166, 1978.

226. Putnam Jr. JB, Roth JA, Wesley MN, Johnston MR, Rosenberg SA. Survival following aggressive resection of pulmonary metastases from osteogenic sarcoma: analysis of prognostic factors. Ann Thorac Surg 36(5):516–523, 1983.

227. van de Wal HJ, Verhagen A, Lecluyse A, von Lier HJ, Jongerius CM, Lacquet LK. Surgery of pulmonary metastases. Thorac Cardiovasc Surg 34(2):153–156, 1986.

228. Depadt G, Delacrois R, Mauretta J, et al. Surgical treatment of pulmonary metastasis: problems and prospects. In: Hellman K, Eccles SA, eds. Proceedings. Philadelphia: Taylor and Francis, 1985, pp. 5–8.

229. Joseph WL, Morton DL, Adkins PC. Prognostic significance of tumor doubling time in evaluating operability in pulmonary metastatic disease. J Thorac Cardiovasc Surg 61(1):23–32, 1971.

230. Putnam Jr. JB, Roth JA, Wesley MN, Johnston MR, Rosenberg SA. Analysis of prognostic factors in patients undergoing resection of pulmonary metastases from soft tissue sarcomas. J Thorac Cardiovasc Surg 87(2):260–267, 1984.

231. Girard P, Spaggiari L, Baldeyrou P, LeChevalier T, LeCesne A, Escudier B, Filaire M, Grunenwald D. Should the number of pulmonary metastases influence the surgical decision. Eur J Cardiothorac Surg 12(3):385–392, 1997.

232. Pogrebniak HW, Roth JA, Steinberg SM, Rosenberg SA, Pass HI. Reoperative pulmonary resection in patients with metastatic soft tissue sarcoma. Ann Thorac Surg 52(2):197–203, 1991.

233. Casson AG, Putnam JB, Natarajan G, Johnston DA, Mountain C, McMurtrey M, Roth JA. Efficacy of pulmonary metastasectomy for recurrent soft tissue sarcoma. J Surg Oncol 47(1):1–4, 1991.

17
Radiation Therapy for Soft-Tissue Sarcoma

Anita A. Reddy
Georgetown University Hospital
Washington, DC

Michael R. Kuettel
Roswell Park Cancer Institute
Buffalo, New York

I. INTRODUCTION

Soft-tissue sarcomas are rare, accounting for less than 1% of adult solid tumors. As discussed in earlier chapters, soft-tissue sarcomas are a very diverse family of complex and distinct diseases. This diversity, along with the lack of definitive data, has resulted in several areas of clinical controversy regarding the management of these tumors. Indeed, large prospective, randomized clinical trials have been the exception rather than the rule in treatment, resulting in great geographic variation in the management of soft-tissue sarcomas (1).

It has long been recognized that management of sarcomas is a multidisciplinary exercise. During the 1960s, multimodality management became recognized as the standard of care for sarcomas. In the 1980s, limb-sparing approaches and improved radiation delivery were developed. In the 1990s, cytogenetics, molecular insight into sarcomas, as well as new active drugs and promising technological advancements in the field of radiation oncology contributed to treatment.

The delivery of optimum treatment is best achieved by a multidisciplinary team at a cancer center where a substantial number of cases are seen. The team should include surgeons (orthopedic and general), sarcoma pathologists, bone and soft-tissue diagnostic radiologists, medical and pediatric oncologists, and radiation oncologists. Diagnostic evaluation, definition of treatment strategy, actual treatment, and follow-up are best carried out with a team approach.

The process of radiation therapy in the management of soft-tissue sarcomas is a complex one that involves many professionals and a variety of interrelated functions. If the patient has a probability of long-term survival after adequate treatment, curative therapy should be given. This may result in side effects that are undesirable but may be acceptable. In a curative setting, it is extremely important for the radiation oncologist to deliver the highest possible dose of radiation to the tumor volume for maximum tumor control while keeping the dose to surrounding normal tissue as low as possible. The prescription of irradiation is based on the following principles:

1. Evaluation of the full extent of the tumor, including preoperative examination and radiographic studies.
2. Complete pathologic review to determine the characteristics of the disease, including potential areas of spread, which may influence choice of therapy.
3. Definition of therapy goals (palliation versus curative).
4. Selection of appropriate treatment modalities: irradiation alone, versus irradiation combined with surgery, chemotherapy, or both. This decision will have a major impact on the volume treated and the total dose of radiation delivered.
5. Determination of the optimum dose of radiation and the volume to be treated. This decision is based upon the anatomical location, histologic subtype, nodal involvement, and other characteristics of the tumor, as well as normal tissue in the area.
6. Evaluation of the patient's general medical condition, periodic assessment of tolerance to treatment, tumor response, and status of the normal tissues treated.

This chapter highlights key points in the use of radiation in the management of soft-tissue sarcomas. Treatment, techniques of irradiation, modifiers of radiation, special sites, and treatment sequelae will be discussed in detail.

II. TREATMENT OF THE PRIMARY LESION

A. Combined Modality Treatment (Radiation and Surgery)

An understanding of the basic biological effects of radiation on soft-tissue sarcomas supports the clinical observation that irradiation works best in combination with surgery. This combined approach to treatment has resulted in better tumor control as well as improved retention of function and cosmesis compared with either modality alone (2). Even for small sarcomas, where irradiation alone results in reasonably good control rates, outcomes are improved by combining surgery and irradiation. Therefore, the strategy endorsed by practice guidelines is a combination of surgery and irradiation.

The rationale for combining radiation with surgery is to avoid the functional and cosmetic sequelae of a radical resection or the late consequences of high radiation doses to large volumes of normal tissue following treatment with radiation alone. Several observations support the efficacy of combined treatment. Sarcomas tend to infiltrate normal tissue adjacent to the main lesion, resulting in a high recurrence rate following a limited resection alone. A more radical resection with wide margins reduces the recurrence rate, but at the expense of function and cosmesis. Irradiation at moderate doses (60–65 Gy) is effective in sterilizing microscopic disease that extends beyond the gross lesion. Therefore, moderate doses of radiation combined with relatively conservative surgery should have similar control rates with better function and cosmesis than radical surgery alone. The efficacy of combined-modality treatment has resulted in the virtual disappearance of amputation as the initial treatment for extremity sarcomas (3,4).

It has been shown that the radiation dose needed to control microscopic tumor is less than that for gross tumor burden. Radiation can sterilize microscopic disease and decrease the rate of local recurrence in patients undergoing conservative surgery (5). If negative surgical margins are achieved with surgery, postoperative radiation doses of 60–70 Gy are recommended to decrease risk of local failure.

A randomized trial conducted by the National Cancer Institute further supports a combined-modality approach. In this study, 43 eligible patients with high-grade soft-tissue sarcomas of the extremities were treated by either amputation or limb-sparing resection plus adjuvant postoperative irradiation. The limb-sparing surgery involved wide local excision designed to remove all gross tumor with several centimeters of surrounding normal tissue. Daily radiation treatments of 1.8–2.0 Gy were delivered to a total dose of 60–70 Gy using reduced fields. After a 1-year follow-up period, 4 of 27 sarcomas recurred locally in the limb-sparing group, whereas none of the 16 patients undergoing amputation experienced recurrence. There was, however, no statistically significant difference in disease-free status or overall survival rates between the two groups. Patients with positive surgical margins were found to be at significantly higher risk of local recurrence (6). Thus, wide surgical margins are necessary to reduce rates of local recurrence. Several reports also indicate that local recurrence is significantly associated with reduced survival (7,8).

Preoperative irradiation should be considered to facilitate tumor resection. Such therapy may be beneficial for several reasons. Smaller treatment volumes are used and superior functional outcome may be achieved with combined therapy. In addition, preoperative irradiation allows delivery to a well-oxygenated tumor, reduces the viability of any tumor cells shed into the surgical wound or circulation at time of surgery, and destroys microscopic tumor foci that may lie away from the surgical site (9). Alternatively, postoperative treatment volume must include the area involved with tumor as well as all tissues manipulated during the surgical procedure.

Definitive surgery should be performed 2–4 weeks after preoperative irradiation with special attention to margins of resection. Difficulties encountered with preoperative irradiation include delay to surgery and the potential for radiation-induced delay in wound healing. In addition, it has been argued that postoperative radiation allows the opportunity to analyze the pathologic specimen with better anatomical definition of tumor extent.

The effects of irradiation, whether delivered preoperatively or postoperatively, are greatly influenced by the status of the margins and the quality of the surgical procedure. An analysis of 132 consecutive patients diagnosed with soft-tissue sarcomas of the extremities treated with preoperative irradiation revealed the importance of margins (10). In this study, the 5-year actuarial local control rates were 97% and 81% for patients with negative and positive margins, respectively. There was no difference between the various subcategories of negative margins (<1 mm, >1 mm, or not measured). In addition, local control was unrelated to tumor size if the margins were negative.

In another series of patients treated by resection and postoperative irradiation for malignant fibrous histiocytoma, local failure rates differed based on positive (39% failure) or negative (9% failure) margins (11). These reports, as well as others, have shown that positive margins are associated with a reduced local control rate and poor prognosis (12–14). Therefore, every effort should be made to obtain negative margins regardless of whether preoperative or postoperative irradiation is used. A statement that the margins are negative implies that the specimen was inked appropriately and that a skilled pathologist evaluated the margins. It is, therefore, necessary for clinicians to ensure that surgical margins have been evaluated appropriately.

B. Radiation and Chemotherapy

The role of adjuvant systemic chemotherapy remains controversial, despite several randomized clinical trials. The rationale for the use of chemotherapy (covered in more detail in a separate chapter) is based on the aggressive nature of intermediate and high-grade sarcomas. A 40–60% death rate from metastatic disease in patients with high-grade sarcomas has been shown, despite local control. Multiple trials with various agents, many of which included doxorubicin as a single agent or in combination regimens, have failed to show improvements in survival. The initial randomized trials of combination chemotherapy reported prolonged durations of disease-free survival, but not overall survival for high-grade extremity sarcomas (15,16). The largest Phase III trial of adjuvant chemotherapy used a combination of cyclophosphamide, vincristine, doxorubicin, and dacarbazine (CVADIC). This study revealed an improved local control but no increase in overall survival (17). However, a reduction in local relapses for the subgroup with head, neck, and trunk lesions was observed.

Several trials have suggested dose–response relationships for doxorubicin alone or combined with ifosfamide. Lower rates of response have been found with low doses of chemotherapy. However, complete responses remain rare, and no survival advantage has been documented with doses high enough to require hematopoietic stem cell support (18). Transplantation therapy does not yet have a role in the treatment of soft-tissue sarcomas.

C. Radiation Alone

Surgical resection has been and remains the foundation of treatment in virtually all soft-tissue sarcomas. In addition, the combination of surgery and radiation achieves better outcomes than either modality alone for nearly all sarcomas. Yet there is a subset of patients whose lesions are unresectable. In this subset of patients, a reasonable approach would be to use neoadjuvant chemotherapy with irradiation in an attempt to render the tumor potentially resectable. If the tumor shows a significant clinical response and becomes resectable, then surgery is indicated.

For those patients deemed medically inoperable and whose functional status is such that the risks of chemotherapy outweigh the benefits, radiation alone is offered. Historically, sarcomas were believed to be resistant to radiation because of slow or incomplete tumor regression following radiation therapy. For example, a 1959 *Lancet* article described a single institution's experience managing sarcomas during the preceding two decades. That article stated that "since most soft-tissue sarcomas are radioresistant, roentgen therapy as a definitive treatment or in conjunction with surgical treatment is not used" (19). By the 1980s, however, irradiation was recognized as one of the key components of multimodality therapy for this disease. Additional studies disclosed that the residual masses typically did not regrow within the irradiated volume and that microscopic evaluation revealed residual noncellular matrix elements of sterilized tumor (20).

The likelihood of tumor control following irradiation depends on the total dose, fractionation schedule (daily vs. multiple treatments per day), volume treated, and elapsed time to completion of treatment. These factors are all interdependent in the production of a biological effect within a given tissue volume. This interdependence, from a radiobiological viewpoint, is closely related to the "four R's" of ionizing radiation: repair of sublethal damage, repopulation of cells between treatments, redistribution of cells throughout the cell cycle, and reoxygenation.

Radiation sensitivity of sarcoma cell lines is similar to that of epithelial cell lines measured *in vitro*. This correlates well with the clinical observation that the dose for local control of sarcomas (to a specified probability) does not differ greatly from the dose for epithelial tumors (21). For sarcomas, the radiation dose needed to eradicate 50% of irradiated tumors (TCD_{50}) is similar to that for epithelial tumors of similar size, such as adenocarcinomas of the breast and prostate, squamous cell carcinomas of the head and neck, metastatic disease of the cervial nodes, and transitional cell carcinomas of the bladder (22).

When used without a planned surgical resection, a higher dose of radiation is required for adequate tumor control. In addition, local control has been shown to be a function of radiation dose and tumor size. Stratified by size, local control for tumors smaller than 5 cm may be expected in approximately 88% of cases, 5–10 cm in 53% of cases, and greater than 10 cm in 33% of cases (23). However, such results are less satisfactory than treatment with radical surgery or combined-modality therapy for limb preservation (24). Great care must be taken when using greater doses of radiation to improve local control, as significant long-term morbidity may result. Attention to details of the treatment and its planning can decrease morbidity and produce beneficial outcomes, although such a treatment approach should be undertaken only when a combined approach cannot be employed.

III. TECHNIQUES OF IRRADIATION

In general, fractionated irradiation prevents acute reactions related to compensatory proliferation in the epithelium of the skin or the mucosa, which accelerates at 2 or 3 weeks after initiation of therapy. A prolonged course of therapy with small daily fractions will decrease early acute reactions but will not negate the potential for serious late damage to normal tissue. In addition, prolonging treatment time may allow the continued growth of rapidly proliferating tumors. The choice of the optimal time/dose/fractionation schedule for sarcomas is individualized depending on a number of factors, including histologic subtype, status of margins and lymph nodes, and the size, grade, and location of the tumor. The muscle, compartment of origin, and anatomical boundaries must be defined. Preoperatively, these structures may be defined by physical examination along with radiographic studies. Postoperatively, additional information is available regarding the extent of resection, incision and drain sites, and operative technique.

Surgical scars should be oriented with consideration for postoperative irradiation. Extremity sarcomas are best managed with longitudinal rather than transverse incisions. This avoids circumferential irradiation and results in a better cosmetic outcome. It is recommended that the radiation oncologist evaluate patients preoperatively and discuss potential irradiation fields with the surgeon. It is also recommended that the radiation oncologist be called to the operating room at the time of resection to review orientation and to document clip placement demarcating tumor margins. Additional clips to localize close margins can be extremely helpful in assisting radiation field design.

Irradiation is generally recommended with sufficient margin around the tumor bed, with variations according to tumor grade and size. For low-grade tumors, the postoperative field traditionally extends 5–8 cm proximal and distal to the surgical scar and more than 10 cm for intermediate- to high-grade tumors (14) (see Fig. 1). To conform treatment fields as much as possible, margins should not extend much beyond the natural barriers of spread. Since nodal regions are rarely at risk in extremity sarcoma, prophylactic radiation to draining lymph nodes is generally not necessary. Efforts should be made to avoid major joint spaces when possible. The entire circumference of the extremity must not be irradiated so as to avoid chronic lymphedema.

Care should be taken in positioning the affected extremity. Tumors of the posterior compartment can be treated with the patient in the ipsilateral decubitus position. The contralateral limb is flexed at the hip, out of the radiation field. The affected extremity is placed straight on the treatment table. Alternatively, the affected extremity may be elevated off the table and treated with opposed lateral fields. In treatment of tumors of the arm, flexion and elevation of the extremity over the head separates the two compartments and allows sparing of uninvolved tissue. Forearm tumors may be treated with the patient prone or seated and with proper rotation of the hand. Immobilization in such positions is necessary. If the extremity is in a neutral position, simple reinforcements may be used. Limbs that are angled or rotated require more rigid devices. The immobilization material is placed at the proximal and distal ends of the limb, not in the treatment field. Regular port films ensure appropriate setup during the course of treatment.

High doses of radiation are generally required for local control. Depending on location of tumor, beam energies are typically chosen to avoid skin-sparing effect. A planning computed tomography (CT) scan is helpful when available, particularly for angled or non-coplanar fields. Treatment fields should be shaped with custom blocks to minimize treatment of normal tissues.

External-beam radiation therapy is typically given in a series of progressively smaller treatment volumes. This shrinking field technique is used to deliver the highest prescribed dose to the tumor bed or residual tumor while sparing surrounding normal tissue as much as possible. Postoperatively, the treatment volume is defined by radiodense surgical clips placed around the resection margins intraoperatively. All tissues handled at the time of surgery are at risk, including the scar and drain sites. Treatment begins approximately 2–3 weeks after surgery to allow for sufficient wound healing (25). For preoperative treatment, radiographic imaging with CT or magnetic resonance imaging (MRI) is used to determine the treatment volume. A course of irradiation is given, with a subsequent 2- to 3-week rest period, followed by resection. Additional therapy may be necessary, as dictated by surgical findings and extent of resection. Response is related to grade and size of the tumor.

Hyperfractionated radiation therapy has been used in the treatment of soft-tissue sarcomas. The total dose is increased, with a decrease in dose per fraction. The intent is to reduce late effects while achieving the same or better tumor con-

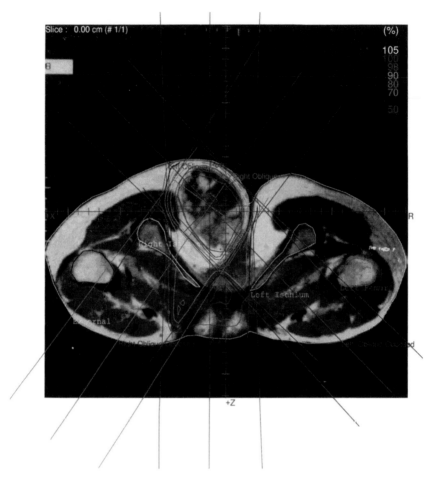

FIG. 1 Preoperative radiation therapy treatment plan for a large gluteal liposarcoma. Note the use of a CT contour and the convergence of six separate radiation fields on the tumor. This is one of many techniques used to maximize dose to the tumor while minimizing dose to the normal surrounding tissue.

trol with equal or only slightly increased early effects (26). An enhanced histologic response has been shown following hyperfractionated preoperative irradiation (27).

A. Brachytherapy

Brachytherapy (from the Greek, *brachy* meaning short and *therapy* meaning treatment) refers to the use of implantation of radionuclides directly into tissue, in proximity of the tumor bed. Brachytherapy can be divided, according to the placement of the radioactive material, into intracavitary (inside body cavities) and interstitial (within tissues). Brachytherapy can be further subdivided, according to its duration, into temporary (the radioactive material is withdrawn after a specified dose has been delivered) and permanent (the radioactive material is left to decay in the body). Brachytherapy can also be classified according to the prescribed dose rate: high-dose rate (HDR) techniques deliver more than 12 Gy/h; medium dose rate techniques deliver 2–12 Gy/h; and low-dose rate (LDR) techniques deliver less than 2 Gy/h.

Interstitial therapy has been used as the sole adjuvant therapy or, more commonly, as a boost to the tumor bed. Its advantages include shorter overall duration of treatment and patient convenience. In addition, brachytherapy has the advantage of placement of radioactive sources under direct visualization, thereby allowing a smaller volume of tissue to be encompassed in the high-dose region (28). The dose is delivered in a homogeneous distribution to areas immediately around each source.

1. Low-Dose Rate Interstitial Brachytherapy

LDR is the most common type of brachytherapy used in the treatment of soft-tissue sarcomas and is usually performed following a surgical resection. Silastic catheters are placed in the tumor bed at uniform intervals throughout the underlying soft tissues through hollow needles (29). A pair of radiographs, obtained during simulation, are used to assist with customized treatment planning. Alternatively, CT simulation can be performed to check placement and plan treatment.

Specific treatment planning is used to cover the target area of interest. The treatment volume should include the tumor bed with approximately 2 cm of surrounding normal tissue (30). Iridium-192 seeds are commonly used and are loaded into the catheters approximately one week following surgery to decrease the likelihood of wound morbidity. The patient is restricted to a shielded bed to reduce the potential radiation hazard for nursing staff. Visitor restrictions are also necessary. The length of treatment varies depending on whether brachytherapy is used alone or with external-beam irradiation.

For permanent brachytherapy, low-activity iodine–125 seeds are commonly used. These radioactive sources are embedded in Vicryl suture material and sewn directly into the tumor bed. If there is gross residual disease, the seeds can be inserted into the tumor through hollow needles. Due to the low activity of iodine–125, shielded rooms and visitor restrictions are unnecessary.

2. High-Dose Rate Interstitial Brachytherapy

The use of perioperative fractionated HDR brachytherapy for soft-tissue sarcomas has been reported to be safe, well tolerated, and useful in marginal or wide surgical margin cases (31). The short duration of therapy and small irradiated volume may allow for chemotherapy to be delivered shortly after brachytherapy. The use of HDR in conjunction with external-beam irradiation has increased in popularity in recent years. However, the use of HDR alone challenges the idea that the pre-treatment volume should include an acceptable margin.

3. Remote Afterloading Brachytherapy

The technique of remote afterloading brachytherapy is similar to interstitial brachytherapy except that the catheters are connected to a device (afterloader) for remotely controlled radioactive loading. Both HDR and LDR irradiation can be carried out with this equipment. The radioactive sources in the afterloader can be retracted back into the shielded safe during planned interruptions or in the event of an accidental entry into the treatment room. This technique thus substantially reduces the radiation exposure hazards to the medical caregivers.

Treatment is performed over a few days with LDR and over a few minutes with HDR. The short treatment time for HDR brachytherapy obviates the need for prolonged patient immobilization. Furthermore, hospitalization is not mandatory and treatment can be delivered in an outpatient setting. In most remote-controlled afterloaders, the treatment area is irradiated by a single radioactive source that moves in discrete steps (dwell positions). A customized treatment plan takes into account both the dwell positions and dwell time. The dwell times can be adjusted to minimize "hot" and "cold" spots, thus optimizing treatment.

4. Intraoperative HDR Brachytherapy

Intraoperative HDR brachytherapy is a method of delivering a single large dose of radiation to a surgically exposed area. Hollow catheters are inserted into various applicators and connected to the afterloader machine using sterile technique. The treatment is delivered using a single, high-activity (10 Ci) iridium source. Normal tissues are either displaced from the irradiated area or shielded, if clinically feasible. Due to the high activity used, treatment is confined to a shielded operating room. During treatment, all personnel must leave the room, with patient monitoring conducted remotely.

Intraoperative brachytherapy has the advantage of direct visualization of the tumor bed, thereby avoiding a geographic miss. Risk of catheter displacement is also reduced. Intraoperative HDR brachytherapy in conjunction with low-dose external-beam irradiation has been shown to be feasible with acceptable toxicity in obtaining local control and long-term disease-free survival in selected pediatric soft-tissue sarcomas (32). The major drawback is the need for a shielded operating room, which limits this treatment modality to a few centers.

5. Brachytherapy Results

Brachytherapy in the management of adult soft-tissue sarcomas has been applied with conservative surgery (with or without external-beam irradiation) as an effective alternative to more ablative procedures, such as amputation. Interstitial therapy may be used to deliver the entire radiation dose. Total doses previously studied range from 42 to 45 Gy delivered over 4–6 days (33). A trial from the Memorial Sloan-Kettering Hospital randomized patients to surgical excision of extremity soft-tissue sarcoma or superficial trunk with or without intraoperative brachytherapy (34). Two of 52 patients experienced recurrence after brachytherapy, compared with 9 of 65 undergoing surgery alone, with a follow-up period of 16 months. However, no survival differences were detected during this short follow-up period.

A report of 48 patients treated with conservative surgery and brachytherapy alone (44) or with external-beam irradiation (4) showed excellent results with small and midsize soft-tissue sarcomas located in the extremities and head and neck (35). Only two patients (4%) failed within the irradiated volume, but the marginal failure rate was unexpectedly high. In another series including 20 patients treated with brachytherapy (13 received external-beam plus brachytherapy, whereas 7 received brachytherapy alone), local control was noted in 11 of 13 and 2 of 7 in the two groups (36). When brachytherapy is used as a boost, 20–25 Gy at 0.4 Gy/h is typically prescribed.

B. Additional Radiation Modalities

The relatively poor results obtained by radiotherapy alone for nonoperable or unresectable soft-tissue sarcomas has resulted in the use of high linear energy transfer (LET) particles (neutrons, heavy ions, and pions) in an attempt to improve local control. These particles offer the advantage of a higher relative biological efficiency (RBE) and other biological properties that may theoretically enhance the effect of irradiation.

Several centers have reported improved local control using neutron therapy, compared with photons (x-rays) or electrons, for locally advanced soft-tissue sarcomas. A 66% local control rate in 221 patients treated with neutrons from 1975 to 1994 was observed. There were notable effects when evaluated in terms of tumor histology, differentiation, and amount of residual (37). Severe subcutaneous tissue fibrosis, however, was reported in 40% of patients approximately 2 years after treatment. A local control rate of 50% was reported from European neutron therapy facilities in patients with inoperable tumors or macroscopic disease after surgery. Data from 1171 patients treated at 11 centers were analyzed. There was a high incidence of late side effects observed in this review, attributed in part to poor technical conditions in which the first treatments were delivered and large treatment volumes (38).

Heavy ion beam therapy has the advantage of superior dose distribution as compared with photon beam irradiation. In addition, it provides a higher biological effective dose. The feasibility of heavy ion beam has been demonstrated, but its role in the management of soft-tissue sarcomas should be considered experimental (39). The cost of building a hospital-based facility capable of accelerating a limited number of ions does not make this a viable option at this time.

Pions offer some improvement to the depth–dose pattern and some of the advantages of high-LET radiation. A three-dimensional spot scan pion irradiation treatment technique was used for 331 patients with unresectable soft-tissue sarcomas. Results revealed this to be a successful treatment technique, with a high rate of tumor control and a low rate of severe late reactions, particularly in retroperitoneal/pelvic tumors (40). The low dose rate coupled with the high cost of building such a facility has resulted in the creation of only a few pion centers worldwide.

Proton beam therapy is similar to irradiation in terms of biological effects but is superior in terms of dose distribution. This superior dose distribution is due to a finite proton range in tissue. By comparison, absorption of photons (x-rays) is an exponential function and, hence, some dose is received along the full-beam path through the body. The potential for clinical gains is high, especially for sarcomas of the skull base or sarcomas close to the spine (41). In 1991, the Proton Radiation Oncology Group was formed to design, supervise, and coordinate clinical trials and to assist in data management (42). The number of proton treatment facilities has been steadily increasing worldwide, and this treatment is expected to play an important role in cancer management.

C. Radiation Sensitizers

Human tumor cells may be sensitized to the effects of ionizing radiation. Halogenated pyrimidine analogs represent a class of nonhypoxic cell radiosensitizers currently of renewed clinical interest (43,44). Thymidine analogs, such as 5-bromo-2'-deoxyuridine (BrdUrd) and 5-iodo-2' deoxyuridine (IdUrd), are incorporated into tumor cell DNA. This substitution results in local fragility in the DNA and, in turn, increased susceptibility to damage by γ rays or ultraviolet light (45). BrdUrd and IdUrd have been used successfully as radiosensitizers in clinical trials. The National Cancer Institute (NCI) reported results with high-dose IdUrd and twice-daily radiation therapy for patients with extensive sarcomas. Twenty of 32 patients achieved local control (46). Such results are promising in terms of tumor regression. Further study has revealed a direct relationship between percent thymidine replacement, reduction of radiation survival parameters (n, D_0), and production of DNA strand breaks in the clinically achievable dose range of BrdUrd and IdUrd (47). The use of the radiosensitizer razoxane (ICRF 159) has shown promising results in serveral uncontrolled trials. Razoxane blocks dividing cells in the G2 or the G2/M phase of the cell cycle (the most sensitive phase of the cell cycle) (48). Razoxane administration combined with irradiation seems to improve the local control in inoperable, residual, or recurrent soft-tissue sarcomas in comparison with irradiation alone (49).

D. Biological Response Modifiers/Immunomodulators

Recombinant tumor necrosis factor–α (TNF-α) is a potential highly antineoplastic agent. A unique property of TNF-α is its ability to activate and selectively destroy tumor-associated microvasculature (50). Clinically, the use of TNF-α has been hampered by severe systemic side effects, including a septic shock–like syndrome with decreased vascular resistance and hypotension. Using isolated limb perfusion (ILP), such side effects can be avoided. High-dose TNF-α with melphalan has been studied in an effort to obtain local control with limb-sparing surgery. When administered using ILP, promising results have been observed in patients with advanced soft-tissue sarcoma confined to the limb (51). However, skeptics of these studies have argued that the WHO criteria tumor response are seldom met after perfusion of sarcomas (52).

The feasibility and efficacy of external-beam irradiation after ILP with TNF-α, interferon-γ (IFN-γ), and melphalan has been reported. Eighty-five percent of patients underwent limb salvage during a 34-month follow-up period. None of the patients receiving radiation and ILP recurred locally; 26% in the ILP-alone group had local recurrences. Regional metastases occurred in 7% receiving both therapies and 14% in the ILP-alone arm. Distant metastases were observed in 27% receiving both and in 29% receiving ILP alone. It was concluded that adjuvant external-beam irradiation after ILP (with TNF-α, IFN-γ, and melphalan) with delayed tumor resection is feasible and may increase local tumor control in locally advanced soft-tissue sarcomas of the extremity (53).

However, the use of TNF-α has been associated with side effects when combined with external-beam radiotherapy. There is considerable risk of tissue necrosis and impaired healing following multimodal treatment using ILP with TNF-α, tumor resection, and postoperative high-dose irradiation (54).

IV. ANATOMICAL CONSIDERATIONS

A. Head and Neck

Soft-tissue sarcomas arising in the head and neck area are technically challenging due to the anatomical constraints of achieving wide surgical margins, frequency of rare histologic subtypes, and radiation dose limiting normal tissues. All these factors explain the high local failure rate. In a review of 188 patients treated at the M.D. Anderson Hospital with surgery combined with irradiation, chemotherapy, or both, 40% failed locally (55). The benefit of combined surgery and radiation compared to either modality alone, however, is well documented (56,57). Because cosmesis and preservation of function are of greater importance in the head and neck area, careful treatment planning and field shaping are critical. The use of CT planning can be an invaluable aid in sparing and protecting surrounding vital structures.

B. Hands and Feet

Conservative surgery and irradiation may also be feasible in sarcomas involving the hands or feet. Several institutions have published their results documenting acceptable cosmesis and function following conservative surgery and irradiation (58,59). Careful treatment planning is essential for the success of radiation therapy in this area. Radiation is a feasible alternative to amputation (60). Furthermore, in those patients who may require an amputation, the amputation is typically a minor one, involving only a toe or a digit (61). Immobilization devices and CT planning can be valuable in treating lesions in these areas.

C. Retroperitoneum

Retroperitoneal sarcomas are unique in that they are quite large at presentation, total resection with negative margins is rare, and the presence of radiation-sensitive tissues surrounding the tumor limits the use of irradiation. This has resulted in a historically high failure rate compared with sarcomas involving the extremities. Among 134 patients who had total or subtotal resection of a retroperitoneal sarcoma, 5-year disease-free survival was recorded in only 29. The majority of these 29 patients failed during the next 5 years. In those patients whose tumors returned, local recurrence was the first site of failure in 90%, demonstrating the difficulty of achieving local control (62). Additional reports confirm the low probability of disease-free survival following resection and postoperative irradiation (63,64).

Due to the high local failure rate, many centers have tested the strategy of combining surgery with intraoperative and postoperative irradiation. These published series have demonstrated that this approach is tolerable, though local failure rates remain high (65–67). In a retrospective review of 500 patients with retroperitoneal soft-tissue sarcoma, tumor mortality rate was associated with late stage at presentation, high grade, unresectable tumor, and positive margins. The authors concluded that complete surgical resection remains the most effective modality for selected primary and recurrent disease, and that aggressive attempts at complete surgical resection should be the goal. Incomplete resection should be undertaken only for symptomatic relief (68).

In an NCI Phase III trial comparing resection and postoperative irradiation (50–55 Gy) to resection plus intraoperative (10–20 Gy) and postoperative irradiation (35–40 Gy), local survival and control rates were similar (69). Newer combined-modality treatment strategies are needed to improve the prognosis in these patients.

V. PATHOLOGIC CONSIDERATIONS

A. Desmoid Tumors

Margin status is the most important predictor of local recurrence for patients with resectable, unifocal desmoid tumor. Postoperative irradiation is not indicated in patients with negative resection margins. For patients with positive margins, the role for adjuvant irradiation is more controversial. The decision should be made by weighing the potential morbidity from irradiation against the potential morbidity of another local recurrence. For example, in patients with tumor adjacent to the airway or the brachial plexus, radiation treatment may be recommended due to the potential for morbidity of another local recurrence (70).

Adjuvant irradiation is indicated in the treatment of patients with positive margins following wide excision. The local control of desmoid tumor in the adjuvant setting is excellent with a dose of 50 Gy. For patients with unresectable tumor, a dose of 56–60 Gy should be delivered, with a 75% expectation of local control (71). Field sizes should be generous to prevent marginal recurrences. In patients with extremity lesions, large-volume MRI should be used to identify patients with multifocal disease (72).

B. Dermatofibrosarcoma Protuberans

Dermatofibrosarcoma protuberans (DFSP) is a fibrohistiocytic tumor of intermediate malignancy with a strong tendency to recur locally and a low propensity for metastasis. The preferred treatment of DFSP is a wide resection beyond the evident disease with histologically negative margins. DFSP responds to irradiation (50–60 Gy), which should be considered as an adjuvant to resection if margins are positive. Combined conservative resection and postoperative irradiation should also be considered if wide local excision would result in major cosmetic or functional deficits (73–75). As with desmoid tumors, irradiation should be considered a viable therapeutic option in patients who have unresectable lesions.

VI. SEQUELAE

Complications associated with the management of soft-tissue sarcomas, including necrosis (soft tissue or bone), bone fractures, fibrosis with limited range of motion, nerve and vascular damage, and significant edema, are relatively rare if the basic principles of multimodality treatment are followed. Still, complications do occur, and the treating physician must be aware of them and know how to manage them. Complications occur more often in the lower extremity than in other sites. This may be due, in part, to the relatively large size at presentation, the extent of surgical resection, and subsequent large volume within the irradiated field. Furthermore, the physiologic effect of increased edema in the lower extremity can result in delayed wound healing or reopening of the incision site.

The process of wound healing is complex. It may be thought of in three phases—inflammatory phase, proliferative phase, and maturation phase (76). During the inflammatory phase, there is an influx of platelets and macrophages and fibrin deposition. Four to six days later, the fibroblasts undergo proliferation and synthesis of mucopolysaccharides and collagen. This is followed by wound maturation. Irradiation of tissue suppresses the proliferative phase, subsequently affecting the production of collagen. Shortly after irradiation, damage to microvasculature results.

Treatment complications from irradiation are a function of dose, volume of irradiated tissue, treatment site, surgical extent, and tumor size (77,78). Acutely, dry desquamation of the skin and erythema are often encountered but respond to conservative management following irradiation. Late complications, including impaired wound healing, lymphedema, joint stiffness, decreased range of motion, soft-tissue fibrosis, bone weakening, and decreased fertility, have been reported in 7–15% of patients treated postoperatively and 14–20% treated preoperatively (79,80). In some cases, physical therapy has been shown to help functional outcome (81).

Higher wound complications have been reported for patients treated preoperatively with radiation compared with postoperative treatment. One study reported parameters associated with significant wound healing delay, including tumor location in the lower extremity, advanced patient age, extensive blood loss during operation, accelerated irradiation regimen, and postoperative boot with an interstitial implant. The rates of wound complication have been higher with the use of brachytherapy (82). Several prior studies involved placement of brachytherapy catheters as soon as the first postoperative day, thus resulting in significant wound healing. It has been reported that afterloading of catheters with radioactive sources by at least the fifth postoperative day resulted in less difficulty with wound healing complications (83). The use of proper technique and attention to detail can help minimize treatment-related complications. Limiting the implant dose and using a combination of implant with external-beam therapy may also reduce complications.

Strategies to decrease problems with wound healing include gentler handling of tissue during the operation, attention to hemostasis prior to wound closure, avoidance of closure under tension and elimination of dead space within the wound, use of drains and compression devices perioperatively, and immobilization for approximately one week (51). The use of hyperbaric oxygen for patients with radiation-induced bone and soft-tissue complications is well known and is a potentially valuable tool in both the prevention and treatment of radiation-related complications.

VII. CONCLUSION

Soft-tissue sarcomas are a very diverse family of complex and distinct diseases. Management can vary widely, but the optimum treatment is delivered by a multi-disciplinary team. A multidisciplinary approach to the management of soft-tissue sarcomas is strongly recommended for achieving the greatest level of local control, overall survival, and optimal function and cosmesis. The team should include, but not be limited to, surgical oncologists, plastic surgeons, medical oncologists, pathologists, radiologists, and radiation oncologists. Irradiation, in various forms of delivery, has been shown to be an essential modality in the treatment of this disease. The use of irradiation must be carried out carefully, with meticulous attention to details, to maximize results and minimize complications.

REFERENCES

1. Demetri GD, Pollock, R, Baker L, Balcerzak S, Casper E, Conrad C, Fein D, Hutchinson R, Shupac K, Spiro I, Wagman L. NCCN sarcoma practice guidelines. National Comprehensive Cancer Network. Oncology 12(7A):183–218, 1998.
2. Wilson AN, Davis A, Bell RS, O'Sullivan B, Catton C, Madadi F, Kandel R, Fornasier VL. Local control of soft tissue sarcoma of the extremity: the experience of a multidisciplinary sarcoma group with definitive surgery and radiotherapy. Eur J Cancer 30A(6):746–751, 1994.
3. Willard WC, Hajdu SI, Casper ES, Brennan MF. Comparison of amputation with limb-sparing operations for adult soft tissue sarcoma of the extremity. Ann Surg 215(3):269–275, 1992.
4. LeVay J, O'Sullivan B, Catton C, Bell R, Fornasier V, Cummings B, Hao Y, Warr D, Quirt I. Outcomes and prognostic factors in soft tissue sarcoma in the adult. Int J Radiat Oncol Biol Phys 27(5):1091–1099, 1993.
5. Leibel SA, Tranbaugh RF, Wara WM, Beckstead JH, Bovill EG, Phillips TL. Soft tissue sarcomas of the extremities: survival and patterns of failure with conservative surgery and postoperative irradiation compared to surgery alone. Cancer 50(6):1076–1083, 1982.
6. Rosenberg SA, Tepper J, Glatstein E, Costa J, Baker A, Brennan M, DeMoss EV, Seipp C, Sindelar WF, Sugarbaker P, Wesley R. The treatment of soft-tissue sarcomas of the extremities: prospective randomized evaluation of (1) limb-sparing surgery plus radiation therapy compared with amputation and (2) the role of adjuvant chemotherapy. Ann Surg 196(3):305–315, 1982.
7. Emrich LJ, Ruka W, Driscoll DL, Karakousis CP. The effect of local recurrence on survival time in adult high-grade soft tissue sarcomas. J Clin Epidemiol 42(2):105–110, 1989.
8. Stotter AT, A'Hern RP, Fisher C, Mott AF, Fallowfield ME, Westbury G. The influence of local recurrence of extremity soft tissue sarcoma on metastasis and survival. Cancer 65(5):1119–1129, 1990.

9. Selch MT, Parker RG. Extremity soft-tissue sarcomas. In: Khan FM, Potish RA, eds. Treatment Planning in Radiation Oncology. Baltimore: Williams & Wilkins, 1998.

10. Sadoski C, Suit HD, Rosenberg A, Mankin H, Efird J. Preoperative radiation, surgical margins and local control of extremity sarcomas of soft tissues. J Surg Oncol 52(4):223–230, 1993.

11. Fagundes HM, Lai PP, Dehner LP, Perez CA, Garcia DM, Emami BN, Simpson JR, Kraybill WG, Kuklic NA. Postoperative radiotherapy for malignant fibrous histiocytoma. Int J Radiat Oncol Biol Phys 23(3):615–619, 1992.

12. Tanabe KK, Pollock RE, Ellis LM, Murphy A, Sherman M, Romsdahl MM. Influence of surgical margins on outcomes in patients with preoperatively irradiated extremity soft tissue sarcomas. Cancer 73(6):1652–1659, 1994.

13. Herbert SH, Corn BW, Solin LJ, Lanciano RM, Schultz DJ, McKenna WG, Coia LR. Limb-preserving treatment for soft tissue sarcomas of the extremities. The significance of surgical margins. Cancer 72(4):1230–1238, 1993.

14. Pisters PW, Leung DH, Woodruff J, Shi W, Brennan MF. Analysis of prognostic factors in 1,041 patients with localized soft tissue sarcomas of the extremities. J Clin Oncol 14(5):1679–1689, 1996.

15. Chang AE, Kinsella T, Glatstein E, Baker AR, Sindelar WF, Lotze MT, Danforth DN Fr, Sugarbaker PH, Lack EE, Steinberg SM, et al. Adjuvant chemotherapy for patients with high-grade soft-tissue sarcomas of the extremity. J Clin Oncol 6(9):1491–1500, 1988.

16. Edmonson JH, Ryan LM, Blum RH, Brooks JS, Shiraki M, Frytak S, Parkinson DR. Randomized comparison of doxorubicin alone versus ifosfamide plus doxorubicin or mitomycin, doxorubicin, and cisplatin against advanced soft tissue sarcomas. J Clin Oncol 11(7):1269–1275, 1993.

17. Bramwell V, Rouesse J, Steward W, Santoro A, Schraffordt-Koops H, Buesa J, Ruka W, Priario J, Wagener T, Burgers M, et al. Adjuvant CYVADIC chemotherapy for adult soft tissue sarcoma—reduced local recurrence but no improvement in survival: a study of the European Organization for Research and Treatment of Cancer Soft Tissue and Bone Sarcoma Group. J Clin Oncol 12(6):1137–1149, 1994.

18. Elias AD. High-dose therapy for adult soft tissue sarcoma: dose response and survival. Semin Oncol 25 (2 Suppl 4):19–23, 1998.

19. Clark RL, Martin RG, White EC. A critical review of the management of soft-tissue sarcoma. Lancet 327–331, 1959.

20. Glenn J, Sindelar WF, Kinsella T, Glatstein E, Tepper J, Costa J, Baker A, Sugerbaker P, Brennan MF, Seipp C, et al. Results of multimodality therapy of resectable soft-tissue sarcomas of the retroperitoneum. Surgery 97(3):316–325, 1985.

21. Mundt AJ, Awan A, Sibley GS, Simon M, Rubin SJ, Samuels B, Wong W, Beckett M, Vijayakumar S, Weichselbaum RR. Conservative surgery and adjuvant radiation therapy in the management of adult soft tissue sarcoma of the extremities: clinical and radiobiological results. Int J Radiat Oncol Biol Phys 32(4):977–985, 1995.

22. Suit HD, Spiro IJ. Radiation as a therapeutic modality in sarcomas of the soft tissue. Hematol Oncol Clin North Am 9(4):733–746, 1995.

23. Tepper JE, Suit HD. Radiation therapy alone for sarcoma of soft tissue. Cancer 56(3):475–479, 1985.

24. Delaney TF, Yang JC, Glatstein E. Adjuvant therapy for adult patients with soft tissue sarcomas. Oncology 5(6):105–118, 1991.

25. McGinn CJ, Lawrence TS. Soft tissue sarcomas. In: Perez CA, Brady LW, eds. Principles and Practice of Radiation Oncology, 3rd ed. Philadelphia: Lippincott-Raven Publishers, 1997.

26. Hall EJ. Radiobiology for the Radiologist, 4th ed. Philadelphia: JB Lippincott, 1994.

27. Willett CG, Schiller Al, Suit HD, Mankin HJ, Rosenberg A. The histologic response of soft tissue sarcoma to radiation therapy. Cancer 60(7):1500–1504, 1987.

28. Gemer LS, Trowbridge DR, Neff J, Reddy E, Evans RG, Hassanein R. Local recurrence of soft tissue sarcoma following brachytherapy. Int J Radiat Oncol Biol Phys 20(3):587–592, 1991.

29. Habrand JL, Gerbaulet A, Pejovic MH, Contesso G, Durand S, Haie C, Genin J, Schwaab G, Flamant F, Albano M, et al. Twenty years experience of interstitial iridium brachytherapy in the management of soft tissue sarcomas. Int J Radiat Oncol Biol Phys 20:405–411, 1991.

30. Schray MF, Gunderson LL, Sim FH, Pritchard DJ, Shives TC, Yeakel PD. Soft tissue sarcoma. Integration of brachytherapy, resection and external irradiation. Cancer 66(3):451–456, 1990.

31. Koizumi M, Inoue T, Yamazaki H, Teshima T, Tanaka E, Yoshida K, Imai A, Shiomi H, Kagawa K, Araki N, Kuratsu S, Uchida A, Inoue T. Perioperative fractionated high-dose rate brachytherapy for malignant bone and soft tissue tumors. Int J Radiat Oncol Biol Phys 43(5):989–993, 1999.

32. Nag S, Martinez-Monge R, Ruymann FB, Bauer CJ. Feasibility of intraoperative high-dose rate brachytherapy to boost low dose external beam radiation therapy to treat pediatric soft tissue sarcomas. Med Pediatr Oncol 31(2):79–85, 1998.

33. Pisters WT, Harrison LB, Woodruff JM, Gaynot JJ, Brennan MF. A prospective randomized trial of adjuvant brachytherapy in the management of the low-grade soft tissue sarcomas of the extremity and superficial trunk. J Clin Oncol 12(6):1150–1155, 1994.

34. Brennan MF, Hilaris B, Shiu MH, Lane J, Magill G, Friedrich C, Hajdu SI. Local recurrence in adult soft-tissue sarcoma. A randomized trial of brachytherapy. Arch Surg 122(11):1289–1293, 1987.

35. Habrand JL, Gerbaulet A, Pejovic MH, Contesso G, Durand S, Haie C, Genin J, Schwaab G, Flamant F, Albano M, et al. Twenty years experience of interstitial irridium brachytherapy in the management of soft tissue sarcomas. Int J Radiat Oncol Biol Phys 20(3):405–411, 1991.

36. Herskovic A, Ryan J, Han I, Lattin P, Ahmad K, Canady A, Belenky W, Phillipart A, Binns H, White B. Combined interstitial and external beam radiation therapy in soft-tissue tumors: preliminary report. Endocurie Hypertherm Oncol 4:213–217, 1988.

37. Steingraber M, Lessel A, Jahn U. Fast neutron therapy in treatment of soft tissue sarcoma—the Berlin-Buch study. Bull Cancer Radiother 83 Suppl:122s–124s, 1996.

38. Schwarz R, Krull A, Lessel A, Engenhart-Cabillic R, Favre A, Prott FJ, Auberger T, Schmidt R. European results of neutron therapy in soft tissue sarcomas. Rec Results Cancer Res 150:100–112, 1998.

39. Debus J, Jackel O, Kraft G, Wannenmacher M. Is there a role for heavy ion beam therapy? Rec Results Cancer Res 150:170–182, 1998.

40. Greiner RH, Blattmann HJ, Thum P, Coray A, Crawford JF, Kann RH, Munkel G, Pedroni E, von Essen CF, Zimmermann A. Dynamic pion irradiation of unresectable soft tissue sarcomas. Int J Radiat Oncol Biol Phys 17(5):1077–1083, 1989.

41. Isacsson U, Hagberg H, Johansson KA, Montelius A, Jung B, Glimelius B. Potential advantages of protons over conventional radiation beams for paraspinal tumours. Radiother Oncol 45(1):63–70, 1997.

42. Suit H, Urie M. Proton beams in radiation therapy. J Natl Cancer Inst 84(3):155–164, 1992.

43. Mitchell JB, Russo A, Cook JA, Straus KL, Glatstein E. Radiobiology and clinical application of halogenated pyrimidine radiosensitizers. Int J Radiat Biol 56(5):827–836, 1989.

44. Sondak VK, Robertson JM, Sussman JJ, Saran PA, Chang AE, Lawrence TS. Preoperative idoxuridine and radiation for large soft tissue sarcomas: clinical results with five-year follow-up. Ann Surg Oncol 5(2):106–112, 1998.

45. Kinsella TJ, Mitchell JB, Russo A, Morstyn G, Glatstein E. The use of halogenated thymidine analogs as clinical radiosensitizers: rationale, current status, and future prospects: non-hypoxic cell sensitizers. Int J Radiat Oncol Biol Phys 10(8):1399–1406, 1984.

46. Goffman, T, Tochner Z. Glatstein E. Primary treatment of large and massive adult sarcomas with iododexoyuridine and aggressive hyperfractionated irradiation. Cancer 67(3):572–576, 1991.

47. Kinsella TJ, Dobson PP, Mitchell JB, Fornace AJ Jr. Enhancement of Xray induced DNA damage by pretreatment with halogenated pyrimidine analogs. Int J Radiat Oncol Biol Phys 13(5):733–739, 1987.

48. Sharpe HB, Field EO, Hellmann K. The mode of action of the cytostatic agent "ICRF 159." Nature 226(245):524–526, 1970.

49. Rhomberg W, Hassenstein M, Gefeller D. Radiotherapy vs. radiotherapy and razoxane in the treatment of soft tissue sarcomas: final results of a randomized study. Int J Radiat Oncol Biol Phys 36(5):1077–1084, 1996.

50. Eggermont AM, Schraffordt Koops H, Klausner JM, Lienard D, Kroon BB, Schlag PM, Ben-Ari G, Lejeune FJ. Isolation limb perfusion with tumor necrosis factor alpha and chemotherapy for advanced extremity soft tissue sarcomas. Semin Oncol 24(5):547–555, 1997.

51. Gutman M, Inbar M, Lev-Shlush D, Abu-Abid S, Mozes M, Chaitchik S, Meller I, Klausner JM. High dose tumor necrosis factor-alpha and melphalan administered via isolated limb perfusion for advanced limb soft tissue sarcoma results in a >90% response rate and limb preservation. Cancer 79(6):1129–1137, 1997.

52. Hohenberger P, Kettelhack C. Clinical management and current research in isolated limb perfusion for sarcoma and melanoma. Oncology 55(2):89–102, 1998.

53. Olieman AF, Pras E, van Ginkel RJ, Molenaar WM, Schraffordt Koops H, Hoekstra HJ. Feasibility and efficacy of external beam radiotherapy after hyperthermic isolated limb perfusion with TNF-alpha and melphalan for limb-saving treatment in locally advance extremity soft-tissue sarcoma. Int J Radiat Oncol Biol Phys 40(4):807–814, 1998.

54. Vrouenraets BC, Keus RB, Nieweg OE, Kroon BB. Complications of combined radiotherapy and isolated limb perfusion with tumor necrosis factor alpha +/− interferon gamma and melphalan in patients with irresectable soft tissue tumors. J Surg Oncol 65(2):88–94, 1997.

55. Weber RS, Benjamin RS, Peters LJ, Ro JY, Achon O, Goepfert H. Soft tissue sarcomas of the head and neck in adolecents and adults. Am J Surg 152(4):386–392, 1986.

56. Tran LM, Mark R, Meier R, Calcaterra TC, Parker RG. Sarcomas of the head and neck. Cancer 70(1):169–177, 1992.

57. Eeles RA, Fisher D, A'Hern RP, Robinson M, Rhys-Evans P, Henk JM, Archer D, Harmer CL. Head and neck sarcomas: prognostic factors and implications for treatment. Br J Cancer 68(1):201–207, 1993.

58. Eilber FR, Huth JF, Mirra J, Rosen G. Progress in the recognition and treatment of soft tissue sarcomas. Cancer 65(3 Suppl):660–666, 1990.

59. Talbert ML, Zagars GK, Sherman NE, Romsdahl MM. Conservative surgery and radiation therapy for soft tissue sarcomas of the wrist, hand, ankle, and foot. Cancer 66(12):2482–2491, 1990.

60. Kinsella TJ, Loeffler JS, Fraass BA, Tepper J. Extremity preservation by combined modality therapy in sarcomas of the hand and foot: an analysis of local control, disease free survival and functional result. Int J Radiat Oncol Biol Phys 9(8):1115–1119, 1983.

61. Karakousis CP, De Young C, Driscoll DL. Soft tissue sarcomas of the hand and foot: management and survival. Ann Surg Oncol 5(3):238–240, 1998.

62. Heslin MJ, Lewis JJ, Nadler E, Newman E, Woodruff JM, Casper ES, Leung D, Brennan MF. Prognostic factors associated with long-term survival for retroperitoneal sarcoma: implications for management. J Clin Oncol 15(8):2832–2839, 1997.

63. Catton CN, O'Sullivan B, Kotwall C, Cummings B, Hao Y, Fornasier V. Outcomes and prognosis in retroperitoneal soft tissue sarcoma. Int J Radiat Oncol Biol Phys 29(5):1005–1010, 1994.

64. Van Doorn RC, Gallee MP, Hart AA, Gortzak E, Rutgers EJ, van Coevorden F, Keus RB, Zoetmulder FA. Resectable retroperitoneal soft tissue sarcomas. The effect of extent of resection and postoperative radiation therapy on local tumor control. Cancer 73(3):637–642, 1994.

65. Bussieres E, Stockle EP, Richaud PM, Avril AR, Kind MM, Kantor G, Coindre JM, Nguyen Bui B. Retroperitoneal soft tissue sarcomas: a pilot study of intraoperative radiation therapy. J Surg Oncol 62(1):49–56, 1996.

66. Willett CG, Suit HD, Tepper JE, Mankin HJ, Convery K, Rosenberg AL, Wood WC. Intraoperative electron beam radiation therapy for retroperitoneal soft tissue sarcoma. Cancer 68(2):278–283, 1991.

67. Gunderson LL, Nagorney DM, McIlrath DC, Fieck JM, Wieand HS, Martinez A, Pritchard DJ, Sim F, Martinson JA, Edmonson JH. External beam and intraoperative electron irradiation for locally advanced soft tissue sarcomas. Int J Radiat Oncol Biol Phys 25(4):647–656, 1993.

68. Lewis JJ, Leung D, Woodruff JM, Brennan MF. Retroperitoneal soft-tissue sarcoma: analysis of 500 patients treated and followed at a single institution. Ann Surg 228(3):355–365, 1998.

69. Kinsella TJ, Sindelar WF, Lack E, Glatstein E, Rosenberg SA. Preliminary results of a randomized study of adjuvant radiation therapy in resectable adult retroperitoneal soft tissue sarcomas. J Clin Oncol 6(1):18–25, 1988.
70. Goy BW, Lee SP, Fu YS, Selch MT, Eiber F. Treatment results of unresected or partially resected desmoid tumors. Am J Clin Oncol 21(6):584–590, 1998.
71. Ballo MT, Zagars GK, Pollack A. Radiation therapy in the management of desmoid tumors. Int J Radiat Oncol Biol Phys 42(5):1007–1014, 1998.
72. Goy BW, Lee SP, Eilber F, Dorey F, Eckardt J, Fu YS, Julliard GJ, Selch MT. The role of adjuvant radiotherapy in the treatment of resectable desmoid tumors. Int J Radiat Oncol Biol Phys 39(3):659–665, 1997.
73. Ballo MT, Zagars GK, Pisters P, Pollack A. The role of radiation therapy in the management of dermatofibrosarcoma protuberans. Int J Radiat Oncol Biol Phys. 40(4):823–827, 1998.
74. Haas RL, Keus RB, Loftus BM, Rutgers EJ, van Coevorden F, Bartelink H. The role of radiotherapy in the local management of dermatofibrosarcoma protuberans. Soft Tissue Tumours Working Group. Eur J Cancer 33(7):1055–1060, 1997.
75. Suit H, Spiro I, Mankin HJ, Efird J, Rosenberg AE. Radiation in management of patients with dermatofibrosarcoma protuberans. J Clin Oncol 14(8):2365–2369, 1996.
76. Bujko K, Suit HD, Springfield DS, Convery K. Wound healing after preoperative radiation for sarcoma of soft tissues. Surg Gynecol Obstet 176(2):124–134, 1993.
77. Stinson SF, DeLaney RF, Greenberh J, Yang JC, Lampert MH, Hicks JE, Venzon D, White DE, Rosenberg SA, Glatstein EJ. Acute and long-term effects on limb function of combined modality limb sparing therapy for extremity soft-tissue sarcoma. Int J Radiat Oncol Biol Phys 21(6):1493–1499, 1991.
78. Eilber FR, Guiliano AE, Huth J, Mirra J, Morton DL. High-grade soft-tissue sarcomas of the extremity: UCLA experience with limb salvage. Prog Clin Biol Res 201:59–74, 1985.
79. Lindberg RD, Martin RG, Romsdahl MM, Barkley HT Jr. Conservative surgery and postoperative radiotherapy in 300 adults with soft-tissue sarcomas. Cancer 47(10):2391–2397, 1981.
80. Suit HD, Mankin HJ, Wood WC, Gebhardt MC, Harmon DC, Rosenberg SA, Tepper JE, Rosenthal D. Treatment of the patient with stage M0 soft tissue sarcoma. J Clin Oncol 6(5):854–862, 1988.
81. Lampert MH, Gerber LH, Glatstein E, Rosenberg SA, Danoff JV. Soft tissue sarcoma: functional outcome after wide local excision and radiation therapy. Arch Phys Med Rehabil 65(8):477–480, 1984.
82. Arbeit JM, Hilaris BS, Brennan MF. Wound complications in the multimodality treatment of extremity and superficial truncal sarcomas. J Clin Oncol 5(3):480–488, 1987.
83. Ormsby MV, Hilaris BS, Nori D, Brennan MF. Wound complications of adjuvant radiation therapy in patients with soft-tissue sarcomas. Ann Surg 210(1):93–99, 1989.

18
Medical Management of Adult Soft-Tissue Sarcoma

Andrea D. Johnson and Kevin J. Cullen
Georgetown University Medical Center
Washington, DC

I. INTRODUCTION

A major advance in the treatment of patients with soft-tissue sarcomas has been the integration of a multidisciplinary approach involving surgical and medical oncologists and radiation therapists. In contrast to the poor local recurrence rates (40–80%) historically reported (1), refinements in surgical technique combined with advances in radiation therapy have considerably improved local control (2–4). Indeed, in referral centers with an interest in the management of sarcomas, local control may be obtained in more than 90% of patients who have extremity lesions (5–7). Despite these major advances the prognosis remains poor, particularly for high-grade lesions. Distant failure remains the principle reason for poor long-term survival because soft-tissue sarcomas often metastasize hematogenously early in the course of disease (8). This has led to substantial efforts to develop systemic chemotherapeutic regimens to better control the disease. Clearly, the integration of improved multimodality treatment is necessary to make an impact on the survival of these patients.

II. CHEMOTHERAPY IN MANAGEMENT OF THE PRIMARY TUMOR

A. Role of Surgery and Irradiation

At the time of initial diagnosis, approximately 90% of patients with soft-tissue sarcoma present with apparently localized disease and no evidence of clinical metastases (9). Historically, adequate surgical resection with or without radiation therapy has been the mainstay of treatment. In most recent series this has resulted in a limb salvage rate of approximately 90% (5–7). Nevertheless, despite initial adequate local therapy, more than half of patients with high-grade tumors subsequently develop distant metastases (10,11). This has led to substantial efforts to develop additional treatment to combat micrometastatic disease. Evidence of responses to single-agent or combination-agent chemotherapy in advanced soft-tissue sarcomas (12–14) has stimulated much interest in the use of chemotherapy as an adjunct to surgery and radiation therapy in the primary management of these tumors. The additional role of adjuvant chemotherapy has therefore been the focus of extensive investigation during the last decade.

B. Role of Systemic Adjuvant Therapy

1. Barriers to Adjuvant Chemotherapy Trials in Soft-Tissue Sarcomas

Several obstacles exist in designing and interpreting clinical trials to evaluate the efficacy of adjuvant chemotherapy in patients with soft-tissue sarcomas. First, these rare tumors account for only about 1% of all malignancies. There are about 7800 new cases per year in the United States (15). Thus, it is difficult for any single institution to accrue enough patients to perform meaningful clinical studies. Second, there is great difficulty in defining the disease. Soft-tissue sarcomas comprise a large number of histologic subsets with widely heterogeneous behavior. Several different grading systems exist, further confounding the reporting of data. Grading may be the most important prognostic indicator, but it is difficult to quantify, even by expert pathologists (16–18). Third, soft-tissue sarcomas occur in a wide range of anatomical locations. Some are more readily accessible to surgery or irradiation. The ability to obtain local control therefore varies greatly by site. Therefore, in analysis of sarcoma studies it is essential that tumors at different sites be analyzed separately. Finally, as staging criteria have changed and improvements in surgical technique and radiation therapy have evolved, the reported survival rates have also evolved (19). Indeed, independent of surgery, irradiation, or chemotherapy, for unclear reasons, recurrence and survival rates have improved (20). For these reasons, it is imperative to evaluate the efficacy of adjuvant chemotherapy for soft-tissue sarcomas by prospective randomized trials.

2. Patient Selection

Defining the prognosis of soft-tissue sarcomas is essential for considering the application of adjuvant chemotherapy. In soft-tissue sarcoma the histologic grade of the tumor is one of the most important prognostic criteria (21–23). The Surveillance, Epidemiology and End-Results (SEER) database indicates that tumor-related mortality in populations with low-grade lesions is low (24). The 5-year survival rate is 85–90%. In this group, patients are best managed with local therapies alone. In comparison, studies indicate that the prognosis of patients with high-grade lesions is considerably worse. For patients with stage II lesions, 5-year survival is approximately 50–70%. The 5-year survival for patients with stage III (grade 3) disease is below 30%. Candidates for investigative treatment with adjuvant chemotherapy should therefore be patients with high or intermediate/high-grade lesions.

3. Historically Controlled Trials

Several early trials compared results of adjuvant chemotherapy with historical controls. In many of these trials, the results suggested a survival advantage for those receiving chemotherapy (25–28). However, interpretation of these studies has raised several issues. Notably, the variability of prognostic factors and improvements in surgical management and staging techniques has made interpretation of these results difficult. Indeed, survival of patients with soft-tissue sarcoma has shown improvement irrespective of the administration of chemotherapy, thus making comparison with historical controls misleading.

4. Prospective Randomized Trials

To date, there have been 14 reported prospective randomized trials of adjuvant chemotherapy for soft-tissue sarcomas (29–42). Table 1 summarizes results from these trials. Both single-agent doxorubicin and combination chemotherapy regimens with known activity in advanced, metastatic sarcoma have been compared with control groups. Seven studies combined extremity and nonextremity tumors. Five included only patients with extremity disease and two studied only nonextremity tumors.

Initial prospective randomized trials reported by the NCI suggested benefit for adjuvant chemotherapy in the treatment of soft-tissue sarcomas in some patients. These studies included patients with grade 2–3 soft-tissue sarcomas of the extremities, head, neck, trunk, and retroperitoneum. Chemotherapy involved escalating doses of doxorubicin and cyclophosphamide and high-dose methotrexate. Reports suggested survival advantage with adjuvant chemotherapy for the subset of patients with high-grade extremity soft-tissue sarcomas (9,19). Long-term follow-up, however, failed to confirm any survival advantage (29). At a median fol-

TABLE 1 Prospective Randomized Trials of Adjuvant Chemotherapy vs. Observation in Soft-Tissue Sarcoma

Ref.	Regimen	No. of patients	Median F/U (months)	Disease-free survival (%)			Overall survival (%)		
				Chemo	Obs	p value	Chemo	Obs	p value
Alvegard et al. (38)	D	154	40	62	56	NS	75	70	NS
Gherlinzoni et al. (32,33)	D	77	68	73	45	0.02	91	70	0.04
Extremity									
Eilber et al. (40)	D	119	28	58	54	NS	84	80	NS
Extremity									
Antman et al. (36)[a]	D	168	54	67	59	NS	68	62	NS
Omura et al. (42)	D	156	NA	59	47	NS	60	52	NS
Uterine									
Edmonson et al. (39)	C,D,V,ActD,DTIC	61	64	68	65	NS	70	70	NS
Bramwell et al. (35)	C,D,V,DTIC	317	80	56	43	0.007	63	56	NS
Ravaud et al. (34)	C,D,V,DTIC	59	52	84	43	0.003	87	54	0.002
Benjamin et al. (41)	C,D,V,ActD	43	120	55	35	0.04	65	57	NS
Chang et al. (29)	D,C,M	67	85	75	54	0.037	83	60	NS
Extremity									
Glenn et al. (31)	D,C,M	15	29	84	50	NS	47	100	NS
Retroperitoneal									
Glenn et al. (30)	D,C,M	31	36	77	49	NS	68	58	NS
head, neck, trunk									

[a]Pooled data from three small studies.

Chemo, chemotherapy; Obs, observation; NS, not significant; NA, not available; D, doxorubicin; C, cyclophosphamide; V, vincristine; ActD, actinomycin D; DTIC, dacarbazine; M, methotrexate.

low-up of 7.1 years, disease-free survival was significantly higher in the chemotherapy group (75% vs. 54%, $p = 0.037$) but overall survival was almost identical in the two arms. Concerns with this study include the relatively small size as well as an unusual randomization procedure, leading to an imbalance in the total number of patients entered in each treatment arm. In addition, a higher proportion of chemotherapy-treated patients had distal extremity lesions that could have influenced the results. Unfortunately, this regimen was associated with significant morbidity related to doxorubicin-induced cardiomyopathy, with 15% of patients developing clinical evidence of heart failure (43). A subsequent trial randomized 88 patients to the same chemotherapy regimen or a lower dose regimen that eliminated methotrexate and administered doxorubicin to a cumulative dose of 350 mg/m^2 to reduce the occurrence of doxorubicin-induced cardiotoxicity (29). A control arm was not included in this study. Disease-free survival and overall survival were similar between the two arms, but the numbers in each arm were too small to detect any difference. None of the patients in either arm developed congestive heart failure.

The NCI has also conducted trials in patients with sarcomas of other sites, including one particular study of soft-tissue sarcomas of the head, neck, chest, and trunk (4). Only 31 patients were entered in this study. Local treatment consisted of resection of tumor and postoperative radiation therapy. The chemotherapy was similar to that used in the first study. Results indicated that disease-free survival was also significantly longer in the chemotherapy arm. Overall survival was again similar in both arms. Another NCI study looked at soft-tissue sarcomas of the retroperitoneum (31). Again, no statistical difference in overall survival could be demonstrated.

Overall, five studies have shown a significant improvement in disease-free survival for patients receiving adjuvant chemotherapy. In only two of these studies did disease-free survival rates demonstrate a significant correlation with overall survival rate (32–34). The first of these, from the Rizzoli Institute in Bologna, Italy (32,33) evaluated a group of 77 patients with high-grade extremity sarcomas. Patients received adjuvant single-agent doxorubicin after amputation for high-grade extremity sarcoma. One subgroup involved preoperative treatment with chemotherapy and radiation therapy. Patients with either primary or recurrent disease were included. At 86 months, improvements in disease-free survival (73% vs. 45%, $p < 0.02$) and overall survival (91% vs. 70%, $p = 0.04$) were observed in patients in the chemotherapy arm. This study has been criticized for its small size and because the randomization may not have been adequate. There was a large imbalance in the number of patients between the two arms. In addition, the control group had a large proportion of patients with proximal tumors, which portend a poorer prognosis.

The second study, from the Fondation Bergonie in Bordeaux, France (34), randomized 65 patients with high-grade extremity tumors to chemotherapy with cyclophosphamide/vincristine/doxorubicin/DTIC (CyVADIC) or observation following definitive local therapy. The results were published with only a median 4.4 years of follow-up and showed statistically significant relapse-free (84% vs. 43%, $p = 0.003$) and survival (87% vs. 54%, $p = 0.002$) benefits for the chemotherapy arm. Both local recurrence rates and the time to local recurrence were lower in the chemotherapy arm, although these failed to reach statistical significance—not surprising given the small number of patients. The quality of this study has also been questioned. The most critical defects cited are its small sample size as well as the imbalance in histologic subtypes between the two treatment arms. This study also failed to adequately randomize patients according to known prognostic variables, resulting in a higher number of patients on the chemotherapy arm with more favorable extremity tumors.

The largest study to date was carried out by the European Organization for Research and Treatment of Cancer (EORTC) (35). Included in the study were 468 patients with all histologic subtypes and all grades, with the exception of very low-grade tumors. Eight cycles of the CyVADIC regimen with a 4-week cycle interval were administered. Results demonstrated a significant improvement in relapse-free survival (56% vs. 43%, $p = 0.007$) and a lower local recurrence rate (17% vs. 31%, $p = 0.004$) for the adjuvant chemotherapy arm. No overall survival benefit was detected. Criticisms of this study include a high rate of ineligibility and the fact that only 52% of patients completed the planned chemotherapy. Accrual spanned 11.5 years, and a number of new developments and technological advances occurred during the course of the trial.

5. Meta-analyses

In an attempt to produce definitive results, meta-analyses of these adjuvant prospective randomized trials in adult soft-tissue sarcomas have been reported. Three such analyses, summarizing published data, have suggested that adjuvant chemotherapy may prolong local recurrence–free interval, recurrence–free survival, and overall survival (44–46).

The use of meta-analyses to identify common or consistent findings of related trials is useful but controversial. Particularly in the case of soft-tissue sarcomas, where inadequate sample size is one of the main deficiencies of the randomized prospective trials, combining results through meta-analyses of clinical trials is useful in overcoming the limitations of inadequate sample size in individual trials. Nevertheless, a methodologic weakness in meta-analysis is the pooling and comparison of trials with widely different eligibility criteria, treatment variable follow-up, postrandomization exclusions, and differing definitions of endpoints (47). A second caution in interpreting the findings of meta-analyses is the potential bias in the selection of trials for inclusion in the meta-analysis, either by choosing trials using nonspecified criteria or through publication bias as negative trials remain unpublished, which may confound conclusions. For all of these reasons, most meta-analysis findings should be interpreted with caution. Ultimately, validation of findings of meta-analyses concerning the size of any effect of adjuvant chemotherapy requires collection and reanalysis of individual patient data for all patients randomized in an eligible trial.

From this perspective, the most reliable findings in the last decade related to soft-tissue sarcoma are those reported in the collaborative meta-analysis from the Sarcoma Meta-Analysis Collaboration (48). This study incorporated meta-analysis of individual patient data from all available randomized prospective trials (13 published, 1 unpublished) comparing adjuvant doxorubicin-based chemotherapy with no chemotherapy. This enlarged sample comprised data from 1568 patients, representing 98% of patients from all known, eligible, and completed randomized trials. Six of the trials tested doxorubicin-based regimens only; in combination with doxorubicin, three trials added cyclophosphamide and methotrexate; two trials added dactinomycin-based regimens; two trials added cyclophosphamide, vincristine, and dacarbazine; and one trial added ifosfamide. The total doses of doxorubicin administered to the treated patients ranged from 200 to 550 mg/m^2. Results indicated a statistically significant improvement in disease-free survival of 10% at 10 years (95% CI = 5–15%) such that disease-free survival improved from 45% to 55%. For overall survival, results were not statistically significant but indicated a trend in favor of chemotherapy. The potential absolute overall survival benefit was 4% (95% CI = 1–9%) at 10 years, representing a possible survival benefit from 50% to 54%. These results confirm in the main what has been seen in most randomized trials. One of the original aims of the project was to include current re-review of pathology. At the time of publication, only 25% of tumor grades had been reviewed and only 59% of tumors had been re-reviewed for histologic subtype classification. This incomplete evaluation of pathology therefore limited the subset analyses that could have been of additional value in this evaluation.

6. Toxicities

Potential gains in local control or survival from adjuvant chemotherapy must be balanced against the substantial toxicity reported in these studies. As expected, these regimens were associated with nausea and vomiting, myelosuppression, and the possibility of neutropenic bacteremia, septicemia, hemorrhage, and death. In the EORTC study, which employed the CyVADIC regimen, 35% of patients discontinued chemotherapy early secondary to these excessive toxicities (35). In some studies, the incidence of clinical doxorubicin-associated heart failure was 4–10% (36,38). Indeed, the regimen used in the NCI studies (maximum cumulative dose of doxorubicin was 500–550 mg/m^2) resulted in congestive heart failure (CHF) in 14% of patients and subclinical deterioration in an additional 52%, as shown by radionuclide imaging (43). In contrast, no patients in the EORTC and Bologna studies developed CHF, and it is likely that the incidence of CHF will remain low as long as cumulative doses of doxorubicin can be monitored (32,35). In addition, studies show that the risk of cardiotoxicity with doxorubicin can be reduced by administration over longer infusion times (49,50).

There have been many improvements in supportive care and an increased understanding of acute and chronic toxicities. The effects of myelosuppression and the frequency of infectious complications have been ameliorated by growth factors and antibiotics. Antiemetics and prolonged infusion times have reduced the nausea and vomiting associated with doxorubicin and dacarbazine. These and other improvements in supportive care have decreased the morbidity associated with adjuvant chemotherapy and likely increase compliance with a given treatment regimen.

7. Summary

At present, the available published data from completed studies do not support the routine use of standard-dose single-agent or combination chemotherapy for the adjuvant treatment of soft-tissue sarcoma. The most cautious interpretation of these studies, including the meta-analyses, is that adjuvant doxorubicin-based chemotherapy should be reserved for selected patients with adverse prognostic factors for overall survival, ideally within the confines of a clinical trial. These factors include tumor size greater than 5 cm, deep tumor location, and high histologic grade. Patients should be offered adjuvant chemotherapy with the understanding that it is empirical therapy to treat micrometastatic disease and not based on a body of conclusive evidence documenting a survival benefit. Many patients, given data that suggest a difference in disease-free survival but only a 4% absolute difference in survival, may not wish to receive adjuvant chemotherapy (51).

This conclusion should be subjected to further evaluation based on current knowledge and practice. Patients in these studies may not have received optimal therapy for soft-tissue sarcoma. None of the studies reported a regimen that included ifosfamide, a drug with significant activity in sarcoma as a single agent and in combination; the dose intensity of cyclophosphamide/doxorubicin was often not maximized; and none of the trials incorporated routine use of growth factors, such as granulocyte colony-stimulating factor (G-CSF) to maintain dose intensity. New approaches with increased dose intensity or neoadjuvant chemotherapy may have a role in the treatment of this disease.

Several trials are currently underway in an attempt to further clarify the role of adjuvant chemotherapy for soft-tissue sarcomas. The presence of a no-treatment arm continues as the control. Unfortunately, trial accrual remains difficult because of the low incidence of these tumors. The International Soft Tissue Sarcoma Group (ISSG), attempting to produce a definitive study, initiated an adjuvant trial in soft-tissue sarcomas with an accrual goal of 450 patients in 1986. The chemotherapeutic treatment arm consisted of six cycles of doxorubicin-based chemotherapy with the MAID regimen (mesna, doxorubicin, ifosfamide, and dacarbazine). The study closed after 18 months because of insufficient accrual (20). The EORTC is currently accruing patients with high-grade soft-tissue sarcomas to a Phase III randomized study of adjuvant high-dose doxorubicin and ifosfamide with G-CSF support versus observation. The accrual goal is 340 patients. An Italian group recently published an interim analysis of another Phase III trial (52). One hundred four patients with grade 3–4 soft-tissue sarcomas were randomized to adjuvant chemotherapy with epirubicin, ifosfamide, and mesna with G-CSF support or no further treatment following definitive surgery. Preliminary results indicate a median disease-free survival of 13 months in the control group, but not in the treatment group ($p = 0.001$). The difference in survival was highly significant in favor of the chemotherapy arm with a p value of 0.007. The final results are awaited with interest.

8.　Alternative Modes of Chemotherapy Administration

a.　Neoadjuvant Chemotherapy　Neoadjuvant chemotherapy has several potential advantages over standard postoperative adjuvant therapy (53,54). In concept, drug delivery to the primary tumor may be improved because surgery and radiation therapy have not yet disturbed the tumor's vascular supply. In practice, a neoadjuvant approach would allow the patient to receive a more intense and timely chemotherapeutic regimen before the delays encountered with recovery from a large and potentially debilitating surgery. A response to preoperative chemotherapy might allow improved surgical resectability in patients who present with borderline resectable disease. In addition, the presence of evaluable tumor allows for objective determination of chemotherapeutic response, and additional postsurgical chemotherapy can be guided by the preoperative response.

　　A group at M.D. Anderson Hospital pursued this approach (55). They conducted a retrospective review in which 46 patients were treated with preoperative doxorubicin-based chemotherapy. This study yielded a 40% overall response rate for the preoperative chemotherapy arm patients. In addition, patients who responded had a significant improvement in metastasis-free survival (60 months vs. 28.5 months, $p = 0.006$) and overall survival (60 vs. 32.7 months, $p = 0.02$). Investigators concluded that preoperative chemotherapy could offer a responding subgroup of patients an improved prognosis.

　　A more recent retrospective review from M.D. Anderson Hospital examined 351 patients with large, high-grade extremity lesions (56). These patients were also treated preoperatively with doxorubicin-based combination chemotherapy. Results showed that response rates, disease-free survival, and overall survival rates were similar to those observed in the chemotherapy arm of randomized prospective adjuvant trials. Furthermore, there was no difference in local control, distant metastasis–free, disease-free, or overall survival rates between responding and nonresponding patients.

Priebat et al. recently reported their results with neoadjuvant intra-arterial cisplatin and continuous-infusion doxorubicin in 17 patients with high-grade extremity soft-tissue sarcomas that were resectable only by amputation (57). Results showed that following chemotherapy 94% of patients were able to undergo limb-sparing surgery. At 2 years follow-up there was only one local recurrence, which was reresected with no relapse in over 4 years. Although this was a small study, it does emphasize the usefulness of preoperative chemotherapy in selected patients.

The first randomized prospective trial examining this neoadjuvant approach was reported by Casper et al. (58). Patients with greater than 10 cm primary or locally recurrent high-grade sarcomas were treated with two cycles of doxorubicin-based chemotherapy prior to surgery and irradiation followed by an additional four cycles of chemotherapy. Unfortunately, only one patient met the standard criteria for partial response. Overall survival results paralleled those of historical control patients with similar high-risk features.

At this time the optimal preoperative regimen is not well defined and the definitive role of neoadjuvant chemotherapy remains unclear. The published reports have employed several different regimens, including doxorubicin as a single agent given intra-arterially or intravenously, followed by various doses of radiation, combination of doxorubicin/platinum, CyVADIC regimens, and, most recently, ifosfamide, doxorubicin, platinum, and radiation. Not enough patients have been treated with a standard protocol to determine the overall improvement utility of a specific regimen.

Further studies using the most active agents are required. A Southwest Oncology Group (SWOG) study of preoperative MAID chemotherapy is currently underway. Patients are treated with three cycles of MAID prior to surgery. Responders and those with stable disease receive an additional three cycles of MAID after surgical resection. A Phase II study is currently accruing patients with resectable soft-tissue sarcoma of the extremities for treatment with neoadjuvant chemotherapy with intra-arterial cisplatin and intravenous doxorubicin. This may add new light to the subject. At this time, the EORTC is evaluating a completed randomized trial of neoadjuvant chemotherapy in patients with soft-tissue sarcomas of the extremities, head, neck, and trunk (59). One hundred fifty poor-risk patients were treated with three cycles of doxorubicin, ifosfamide, and mesna prior to definitive surgery and irradiation.

b.   Alternative Administration Techniques   There have been several evaluations of different techniques of chemotherapy administration. The intra-arterial route has been used to administer chemotherapy to patients with localized sarcomas. Administration of drugs via the arterial supply includes intra-arterial infusion (with or without application of a tourniquet to increase the concentration in the limb), as well as isolated perfusion of a limb or organ, a technique in which the arterial supply and venous outflow are connected to an extracorporeal circulation system, isolating the organ from the systemic circulation. These approaches have been evaluated most frequently in patients with large primary or recurrent sarcoma, usually with the stated goal of permitting a limb-sparing resection in patients for whom amputation might have been necessary (60).

One particular randomized study from the UCLA series compared preoperative intra-arterial versus intravenous doxorubicin in patients with soft-tissue sarcoma (61,62). Ninety-nine patients with high-grade extremity sarcoma were randomized to receive intra-arterial or intravenous doxorubicin followed by irradiation and wide surgical resection. There was no difference in the rate of local recurrence or the rate of limb salvage, while the intra-arterial drug administration induced more toxicity. Although doxorubicin has been the most commonly used agent for intra-arterial infusion, other investigators have reported use of intra-arterial cisplatin as a single agent and in combination with intra-arterial or intravenous doxorubicin (63,64). To date, there has been no indicated role for intra-arterial therapy as similar local control and limb salvage rates can be achieved by surgical resection with irradiation with or without preoperative intravenous chemotherapy.

Other studies have examined schedule of chemotherapy administration. Eighty-seven patients with extremity sarcoma treated at Memorial Sloan-Kettering Cancer Center were randomized to receive doxorubicin 60 mg/m^2 administered by bolus or continuous 72-h infusion as adjuvant therapy (49). While the rate of cardiotoxicity as a function of the cumulative dose of doxorubicin was significantly higher in the bolus treatment arm (61% in bolus arm with median dose of 420 mg/m^2 vs. 42% in the CI arm with a median dose of 340 mg/m^2), survival status was superior for those receiving bolus doxorubicin.

c. Combination Chemotherapy and Radiation Therapy   Traditionally, limb salvage therapy for extremity sarcoma has consisted of a combination of surgery and radiotherapy. In most recent series this approach to therapy has resulted in a limb salvage rate of approximately 90%, with a local recurrence rate of less than 15% (6). For patients with tumors that are in proximity to joints or major neurovascular structures, limb salvage may not be an option owing to surgical and anatomical considerations. Therefore, in the cases of patients who are not candidates for a traditional limb salvage procedure and/or who already have distant metastatic disease, management of quality of life becomes a challenge. In an effort to obtain limb salvage in an even greater group of patients, several investigators have examined additional therapies to improve local control (65).

The UCLA School of Medicine has been conducting sequential preoperative trials in extremity sarcomas since 1974 (53). These trials were not randomized but were conducted sequentially with consecutive patients treated with a specific protocol. Using preoperative irradiation and a variety of chemotherapeutic regimens, including doxorubicin, cisplatin, and ifosfamide, results have shown an improved local control rate as well as a reduction in amputation rate. For example, in the last protocol where 62 patients were treated with high-dose ifosfamide (2 g/m^2/day for 7 days), doxorubicin (60 mg/m^2), cisplatin (120 mg/m^2), and irradiation (2800 cGy), the limb salvage rate was 98%. In addition, a complete response rate of 49% was seen, which is a marked improvement over prior neoadjuvant regimens (66). The overall survival rate is yet to be determined.

Other investigators have also used combinations of preoperative chemotherapy with doxorubicin and irradiation, or cisplatin and irradiation. A group at University of California, Davis treated 17 patients with soft-tissue sarcoma with intra-arterial doxorubicin and irradiation (67). The overall limb salvage rate was 88%. At 32 months, there were no local recurrences and overall survival was 82%. These findings are consistent with the results of the earlier UCLA study.

A pilot study from the Massachusetts General Hospital (MGH) recently reported a Phase II evaluation of the efficacy of preoperative and postoperative chemotherapy with addition of radiotherapy (68). Twenty patients with large, grade 2B or 3B extremity sarcomas were treated with three cycles of MAID combined with 44 Gy radiation. Results showed a disease-free survival of 81% compared with a matched untreated historical control group with survival of 38% at 5 years. There was considerable toxicity with bone marrow suppression, neutropenic fevers, with one case of sepsis. In addition, seven patients developed wound complications. A Radiation Therapy Oncology Group (RTOG) trial based on this pilot study, evaluating the efficacy of neoadjuvant chemotherapy plus concomitant radiotherapy, is currently in the accrual phase. The accrual goal is 60 patients. Treatment will consist of triple-drug combination chemotherapy with three cycles of the MAID regimen plus concomitant radiotherapy (44 Gy), followed by surgery and then three additional cycles of MAID.

d. Isolated Limb Perfusion   As discussed above, preoperative therapies with neoadjuvant chemotherapy and radiation have been used to improve local control. Another strategy for treating patients with soft-tissue sarcoma of the extremities is hyperthermic isolated limb perfusion (ILP). Regional perfusion for sarcomas localized in the extremity is an attractive mode of therapy because the chemotherapeutic concentrations that can be reached safely are 15–20 times higher than those in systemic administration, with minimal systemic toxicity (69). ILP may render an unresectable tumor resectable and may reduce the local recurrence rate. In cases with widespread metastases, it can also be used palliatively for alleviation of pain and to avoid further surgery (70).

ILP was first described by Creech in 1957 (71). Since then several retrospective reviews of individual institution experience with ILP for sarcoma have been published in the scientific literature (72–79). In addition, multiple studies of hyperthermic isolated limb perfusion for melanoma have included scattered sarcoma patients (80,81). The results of ILP with melphalan, as well as other drugs, have been disappointing. Kremetz et al. reported only four complete remissions (10%) and eight partial remissions (21%) in 39 patients with extremity soft-tissue sarcomas after ILP with the administration of melphalan, nitrogen mustard, and/or actinomycin D (73). Doxorubicin, an agent with known activity in soft-tissue sarcomas, has also been investigated in the ILP setting. In a series of 26 patients with grade 2–3 sarcomas treated with doxorubicin, a 0% response rate was seen with three amputations necessitated because of toxicity. When doxorubicin was combined with melphalan, only four complete remissions were observed (77). The general conclusion was that results of ILP with different chemotherapeutic agents were poor and that none of the current regimens could be considered superior to surgery plus radiotherapy.

In contrast, the results using TNF-α in combination with chemotherapy have been striking. Lienard et al. reported that a three-drug combination with TNF-α, IFN-γ, and melphalan is effective for melanoma and sarcoma (82). The initial report by Lienard included four patients with recurrent sarcoma of the extremities. The complete response rate was 89% for both tumors in this small series. TNF-α is a cytokine with multiple actions and both direct and indirect antitumor effects. Unfortunately, the maximum tolerated dose of TNF-α in the clinical trials is significantly lower than what was observed to be tumoricidal in animal models (65). In this regard, ILP of an extremity would allow high doses of TNF-α confined to the affected extremity, whereas the dose-limiting systemic toxicity could potentially be avoided. IFN-γ was added to this schedule because of its synergistic antitumor activity with TNF-α (69).

The efficacy of this TNF-α/melphalan/IFN-γ combination has been documented further. Eggermont et al. reported results from 55 patients with unresectable soft-tissue sarcomas of the extremity (83). There were 30 primary and 25 recurrent sarcomas; 48 were grade 2 and 3, and 7 were grade 1. After ILP with TNF-α, IFN-γ, and melphalan, 87% of the patients experienced a major tumor response, which rendered these large sarcomas resectable in most cases. At a median follow-up of 27 months, limb salvage was achieved in 84%, with good function in 80% of patients.

In general, it has been difficult to evaluate the actual tumor response and clinical efficacy of ILP in soft-tissue sarcomas. The reported studies have treated a variety of histologic types, stages, and grades. A variety of different chemotherapeutic agents have also been used, not only among different studies but also within the same study. Toxicity is variable. Almost all patients have local toxicity with erythema, edema, and occasionally some blistering and functional disturbance (69). About 8% of the patients have extreme epidermolysis and/or obvious damage to the deep tissues, which can cause definite functional disturbances. Transient paresthesias are reported in about 20% of patients and transient motor neuropraxia in about 3%. Most patients develop fevers and chills and a hyperdynamic cardiovascular state with a slight decrease in blood pressure. Adult respiratory distress syndrome and renal or liver toxicity have also been documented. Experience seems to have decreased the incidence and severity of the complications.

This is a promising technique, though its use is likely to be limited to patients with unresectable tumors. Local control can be achieved in most situations with irradiation and surgery in combination. To date there has not been a prospective randomized study comparing ILP with any other treatment modality using either response rate or survival as an end point. The EORTC is currently accruing high-risk patients to a large Phase III trial in which patients will be randomized to neoadjuvant chemotherapy with etoposide, ifosfamide, and doxorubicin with the addition of regional hyperthermia, or to the neoadjuvant chemotherapy alone.

III. CHEMOTHERAPY IN THE MANAGEMENT OF METASTATIC DISEASE

A. Introduction

Control of the primary site can be achieved in most patients with soft-tissue sarcoma, but ultimately close to 50% of patients develop metastatic or locally advanced disease. In these patients, systemic therapy is the most reasonable treatment option. Once metastatic disease occurs the prognosis is poor, even with the most modern therapies. Only a small fraction of patients with metastatic soft-tissue sarcoma treated with systemic chemotherapy will experience long-term disease-free survival. Even the most aggressive regimens result in a 5 year disease-free survival of less than 5% (84).

B. Chemotherapeutic Regimens

1. Activity of Single-Agent Chemotherapy

Doxorubicin is the most active single agent in soft-tissue sarcoma. Early Phase II studies demonstrated response rates between 10% and 37% (13,14,85). Clear evidence of a dose–response relationship was established by O'Bryan et al. (85). With increasing doses of doxorubicin (45, 60, 75 mg/m^2 every 3 weeks), response rates improved (18%, 20%, 37%). Various Phase III studies performed by the Eastern Cooperative Oncology Group (ECOG) and the EORTC confirmed response rates of about 25% (86–90) and optimal doses seem to be 70–80 mg/m^2 given every 3 weeks. One randomized trial confirmed that higher doses of single-agent doxorubicin (70 mg/m^2) were superior to a combination regimen that included doxorubicin at doses of 50 mg/m^2 (88). Unfortunately, cardiotoxicity, myelosuppression, and mucositis have limited dose escalation in clinical practice.

Epirubicin, a steric isomer of doxorubicin, seems to have activity similar to that of doxorubicin (89). It also appears to be less cardiotoxic for equivalent therapeutic doses (91). A large randomized study by the EORTC comparing doxorubicin 75 mg/m^2 with epirubicin 150 mg/m^2 showed an overall response rate of 18% with no difference between the arms (92). There was significantly greater myelosuppression in the epirubicin arms, and the incidence of cardiotoxicity was similar. This newer agent is being incorporated into combination chemotherapy regimens and evaluated in newer protocols.

Ifosfamide, a cyclophosphamide analog, is also an active agent in the treatment of soft-tissue sarcomas. In a randomized trial comparing ifosfamide and cyclophosphamide, higher response rates were seen with ifosfamide (18% vs. 8%) at equitoxic doses (93). In previously untreated patients, ifosfamide as a single agent led to remission rates of 22% and 47% (94,95). In various Phase II studies of patients previously treated with a doxorubicin-containing regimen, ifosfamide given as a single agent has resulted in response rates varying from 8% to 38% (96–99). As for doxorubicin, a dose–response relationship is suggested but the effect of dose or schedule has not been definitively established. A Phase II study by Benjamin et al. showed that ifosfamide 8 g/m^2 given every 3 weeks resulted in an 11% response rate, but a moderate increase to 10 g/m^2 yielded a substantially higher response rate of 25% (100). Several more recent reports have shown response rates of 43–62% with ifosfamide doses of 12–24 g/m^2 (101–105). Certain histologies, such as synovial cell sarcoma and fibrosarcoma, appear to be more responsive to ifosfamide (104). For example, Rosen et al. gave 14–18 g/m^2 in 6- to 8-day infusions to 13 patients with synovial cell sarcoma. The response rate was 100%, including four complete remissions. In addition, reports have described patients refractory to lower dose ifosfamide who have responded to higher dose ifosfamide. Le Cesne treated 40 patients with advanced soft-tissue sarcoma with ifosfamide, given by a 3-day continuous infusion for a total dose of 12 g/m^2. The overall response rate was 33%, and 11 of 12 responding patients had been treated with conventional-dose ifosfamide (105).

Dacarbazine (DTIC) is the third agent with notable activity in soft-tissue sarcomas. Remission rates are between 15% and 20% (106,107). Dose–response relationships with dacarbazine have not been investigated to any great extent. One study suggests that dacarbazine may be particularly active in leiomyosarcomas (108).

Many other chemotherapeutic agents are under investigation but few show any noteworthy response. Although actinomycin D, etoposide, and vincristine are quite active in the pediatric sarcomas, low efficacy has been observed with these agents in adult soft-tissue sarcomas. Response rates have been found only in the range of 8–17% in small Phase II trials (109). Other agents, such as methotrexate, cisplatin, and carboplatin, also have minimal activity, with response rates of less than 20%. Especially disappointing is the apparent limited activity of the taxane derivatives in light of their significant activity against other malignancies. An

EORTC study of docetaxel in pretreated patients resulted in a 17% response rate (110). Further studies have been unable to repeat these results (111,112). A study of paclitaxel by a group from Memorial Sloan-Kettering Cancer Center showed a response rate of only 4% in 28 patients (113).

2. Activity of Combination Regimens

In an attempt to improve the results of treatment of advanced soft-tissue sarcomas, several combination chemotherapy regimens have been studied. Most studies have taken doxorubicin as the most active single agent and added other active drugs.

a. *D vs. D/DTIC*   Three randomized trials have examined single-agent doxorubicin versus doxorubicin plus dacarbazine (86,108,114). These trials have revealed enhanced response rates on the order of 20–30% but found no improvement in survival rate for the combination regimen. In each of these trials, the investigators concluded that the small degree of increased response noted with the addition of dacarbazine did not justify the increased clinical toxicities. The SWOG attempted to reduce the toxicity of this regimen by comparing bolus administration with continuous infusion over 96 h. The response rate, 17%, was identical in both arms, but toxicity was significantly reduced for the infusion, particularly cardiotoxicity for doxorubicin and nausea and vomiting from DTIC (115). In view of the improved tolerance of the doxorubicin/dacarbazine combination due to current knowledge regarding mode of administration and improved support with newer antiemetics, the risk/benefit ratio of this regimen should be subjected to further examination.

b. *D vs. DC*   In contrast, the addition of cyclophosphamide to doxorubicin in randomized comparisons has not provided significant response or survival benefit (87,116,117). In one study, two treatment arms containing cyclophosphamide produced fewer responses than the single-agent doxorubicin arm, presumably because a lower dose of doxorubicin was used in the combination arms to accommodate myelosuppression caused by the combination regimen (87).

c. *CyVADIC*   The SWOG group evaluated the addition of other agents to doxorubicin and developed the CyVADIC regimen consisting of cyclophosphamide, vincristine, doxorubicin, and DTIC. In trials of variations of this four-drug combination, responses have ranged from 38% to 71% (118–120). A subsequent randomized study by the EORTC compared doxorubicin alone, doxorubicin with ifosfamide, and CyVADIC in patients with advanced soft-tissue sarcoma (88). The two combinations were associated with significantly more myelosuppression and presented no significant advantage over single-agent doxorubicin in terms of response and survival.

d. *D vs. DI*   With the identification of ifosfamide as an agent with significant antitumor activity in sarcomas, a number of investigators have combined it with doxorubicin (or epirubicin) to determine whether the combination improves response and survival in patients with advanced sarcoma (88,90,121–125). The first such study involved 24-h infusion of ifosfamide at doses of $5-8$ g/m^2 with doxorubicin $40-60$ mg/m^2 repeated every 3 weeks (121). A 30% response rate (11% complete remissions) was reported and the optimal doses appeared to be doxorubicin 50 mg/m^2 and ifosfamide 5 g/m^2. The EORTC reported a response rate of 35% (9% complete remissions) with a median time to progression for those with partial remissions of 40 weeks and for complete remissions of 67 weeks (122). Although myelosuppression was often severe (grade 3 or 4 in 73% of patients), other toxicities were less than had been seen in the EORTC trial with CyVADIC, and the activity appeared to be at least equivalent. The best remission rates, 45% and 48%, were achieved in Phase II trials by the EORTC and by Chevalier et al., respectively (124,125).

The ECOG recently performed a Phase III randomized study of doxorubicin alone, doxorubicin with ifosfamide, and doxorubicin with cisplatin and mitomycin C (90). The doxorubicin dose was 80 mg/m^2 on the single-agent arm but only 40 mg/m^2 or 60 mg/m^2 on the combination arms because of additive toxicity. In 262 patients, response rates were 20%, 34%, and 32%, respectively, in the three arms. Myelosuppression was more severe in the combination arms. No survival difference was demonstrated.

e. MAID   More recently, the focus of investigators has shifted to the use of more extensive combinations with doxorubicin and ifosfamide. The MAID regimen was developed at the Dana Farber Cancer Institute to take advantage of simultaneous administration of the three most active drugs in this disease. In an initial Phase I study, they concluded that the optimal doses were doxorubicin 60 mg/m^2, ifosfamide 7.5 g/m^2, and DTIC 900 mg/m^2 (126). The chemotherapy was given as a continuous 72-h infusion and was generally well tolerated. In a large Phase II study, this regimen resulted in a 47% response rate with 10% complete remissions (127). The substitution of epirubicin for doxorubicin provides similar activity (128,129). Of 43 patients treated in Milan with mesna, epirubicin, ifosfamide, and dacarbazine, 21 (49%) responded, with 5 pathologic complete remissions at resection (12%) (128).

In a randomized comparison of doxorubicin/DTIC versus MAID, the response to MAID was 32% compared with a 17% response to the two-drug combination ($p < 0.002$) and the time to progression was longer (6 months vs. 4 months; $p < 0.02$) (130). There were 8 toxic deaths, 7 among the 170 patients treated in the MAID arm; all treatment-related deaths occurred in patients older than 50 years. An observed survival advantage in favor of the two-drug regimen (median 13 months vs. 12 months) was not statistically significant. Nor did this increased activity for the MAID regimen translate into a statistically significant improved survival. This regimen has not yet been compared to doxorubicin alone in a randomized study. In addition, a recent study of 148 patients, randomized to MAID or an intensified MAID regimen with a 25% dose increase, showed no benefit for the intensified arm (131). Moreover, toxicity was more severe in the intensified arm, with more treatment-related deaths and early treatment discontinuation.

f. Conclusion   In summary, although some studies show that combination chemotherapy in soft-tissue sarcomas results in higher tumor response rates than single-agent chemotherapy, there is no firm evidence of a survival advantage. In situations in which the response may be important, such as in a preoperative or adjuvant setting, these additional drugs may be of value, particularly in younger patients. For the palliative management of metastatic disease, the combination regimens may offer higher response rates, but it is not clear that these translate to improved survival. Single-agent doxorubicin remains the standard against new therapeutic approaches should be compared.

3.   Dose-Intensive Chemotherapy

a. High-Dose Chemotherapy with Growth Factor Support   The importance of dose intensity is well recognized in the treatment of soft-tissue sarcomas. In order to increase the dose of chemotherapy that can be given safely, investigators are incorporating hematopoietic growth factors and support with bone marrow or peripheral blood stem cells into current regiments. Granulocyte-macrophage colony-stimulating factor (GM-CSF) has been shown to reduce the myelosuppressive effects of both the CyVADIC (132) and MAID (133) regimens. Bui et al. demonstrated that GM-CSF permits the administration of high, frequent doses of MAID and reduces the toxicity of MAID (134). The potential benefit of high-dose therapy with doxorubicin and ifosfamide has also been examined in several small pilot studies with reported response rates of 50–69% (135–139). Dose-limiting toxicity was encountered at ifosfamide 12 g/m^2 and doxorubicin 60 mg/m^2 or ifosfamide 10 g/m^2 and doxorubicin 90 mg/m^2 (138,139). The EORTC treated 104 patients with 75 mg/m^2 doxorubicin and 5 g/m^2 ifosfamide every 3 weeks. GM-CSF was given to reduce hematotoxicity (124). The remission rate was high (45% with 10% complete remissions) and median survival promising (15 months). Although all patients developed grade 3–4 leukopenia, there was only 1 death from septicemia and only 15 febrile episodes requiring hospitalization. A randomized Phase III study is now underway comparing the above regimen with standard-dose doxorubicin and ifosfamide.

b. High-Dose Chemotherapy with Autologous Bone Marrow (Peripheral Stem Cell) Support   There are few published data on high-dose chemotherapy with autologous stem cell support or bone marrow support in adult soft-tissue sarcoma. A number of nonrandomized studies have shown reasonable response rates, but also disappointingly short survival times (140–143). Blay et al. (140) treated 20 patients with advanced sarcoma with high-dose etoposide/ifosfamide, G-CSF, and autologous marrow support as consolidation after conventional therapy. A

31% objective response was achieved, with a median overall survival of 26 months and a 5-year survival rate of 21%. Dumontet et al. (141) treated 22 patients who had already received conventional-dose chemotherapy with high-dose melphalan (11 patients), ifosfamide/cisplatin/epirubicin (6 patients), or busulfan/cyclophosphamide (1 patient) with autologous bone marrow support. Twelve patients were already in complete remission at the time of transplantation. Three additional complete remissions and three partial remissions were seen among the nine evaluable patients. There was a 67% overall response rate and a 32% overall 5-year survival rate. These preliminary, uncontrolled observations lend support to the concept that high-dose chemotherapy with stem cell support may result in higher response rates; whether this translates into significant clinical benefit needs to be determined. Several trials are currently in progress to evaluate further the benefit of intensified-dose chemotherapy with peripheral blood stem cell or bone marrow support. However, more effective chemotherapy is necessary before this approach will be clinically useful in soft-tissue sarcomas, particularly because the active drugs in this disease have severe nonhematologic toxicity, which limits the dose escalation that is possible with stem cell support.

4. Future Directions

In summary, systemic therapy for soft-tissue sarcoma remains suboptimal. Only three agents—doxorubicin, dacarbazine, and ifosfamide—when used as single agents, consistently produce response rates in excess of 20% in advanced disease. Certainly no standard chemotherapeutic regimen has yet proven curative. However, there is cause for optimism as current progress in translational research produces new drugs and new treatment strategies.

Biological response modifiers, such as TNF-α, IFN-γ, or interleukin-2 IL-2), continue to be investigated in soft-tissue sarcomas. These have not been shown to have significant activity when used alone. Preliminary trials with IFN-γ and IL-2 have reported little or no activity (144,145). As discussed above, there may be benefit for TNF-α $\pm$ IFN-γ used in combination with chemotherapy for limb salvage, although further study is needed to better define what role these agents have in these effects. The preclinical data on a liposomal encapsulated synthetic muramyl tripeptide, MTP/PE, a new biological response modifier, also show promise for sarcomas. In rodents and dogs, MTP/PE causes stimulation of macrophages and results in marked antitumor activity (146). In light of these results, the EORTC Sarcoma Group treated 19 patients with metastatic disease with MTP/PE at a dose of 4 mg intravenously every week (the dose that produced biological effects in Phase I studies) (147). Apart from mild flu-like symptoms, treatment was generally well tolerated but no objective responses occurred.

Another line of intervention seeks to improve drug delivery mechanisms. Because dose-intensive therapy appears to be more effective against soft-tissue sarcomas, there is a clear reason to develop methods that will allow these drugs to be given with improved tolerability. One technique is encapsulation of drug in liposomal vehicles. This allows more tolerable and potentially tumor-selective delivery of chemotherapy. Recent studies have examined the delivery of anthracycline in liposomes. Since myelosuppression remains a significant toxicity, these trials have incorporated routine use of G-CSF support. In one study, liposomal doxorubicin was delivered every 2 weeks at doses up to 105 mg/m^2 (148). There was no cardiotoxicity noted. However, the response rate was disappointing. In 17 patients, only 2 (17%) experienced major responses.

As understanding of the molecular biology of soft-tissue sarcomas progresses, new specific antisarcoma treatments are being developed. One promising lead from translational sarcoma research involves the peroxisome proliferator-activated receptor–γ (PPAR-γ), which serves as an inducer of terminal differentiation for adipocytes. In a study of primary liposarcoma cells, levels of mRNA encoding PPAR-γ were noted to be present at high levels in the malignant cells (149). Troglitazone, a PPAR ligand, has been shown ex vivo to induce terminal differentiation in liposarcoma cells and increase mature cell characteristics (149). Based on this preclinical work there is a Phase II trial in accrual using troglitazone to treat malignant liposarcomas.

In this manner, research for the development of more effective therapies for soft-tissue sarcoma must build on advances in molecular biology and developmental pharmacology. It is hoped that improved understanding of the biology of soft-tissue sarcomas as well as the development of new approaches and discovery of new agents will enhance the ability to cure patients with this disease.

C. Clinical Decision Making in
Patients with Metastatic Disease

Studies of chemotherapeutic treatment for advanced soft-tissue sarcomas have not demonstrated statistically significant increase in patient survival rates. Yet if all detectable disease can be eliminated by chemotherapy combined with surgery or radiation, a few patients may achieve prolonged remission or even be cured. This favorable prognosis applies to less than 5% of patients with advanced disease and represents approximately one third of patients who achieve objective complete responses with chemotherapy (84,150). Despite unpromising statistical outcomes, the results of treatment may be worthwhile for the individual patient.

In recommending appropriate therapy for the individual patient with soft-tissue sarcoma, medical oncologists confront a complex array of issues. First, the risk of excess clinical toxicity must be evaluated. Although the highest response rates of standard regimens in randomized studies to date are achieved by doxorubicin-based and ifosfamide-containing combinations, the additional tumor reduction induced by aggressive chemotherapy regimens in a patient with widespread disease may not be sufficient to justify the added toxicity of such an approach over less intensive treatments. For elderly patients or patients with poor performance status who might not tolerate aggressive combination chemotherapy without disproportionate toxicity, palliation may be best achieved by single-agent doxorubicin (109). For patients with tumors potentially resectable for cure, combination chemotherapy and the anticipated high response rates might be important. For their part, younger patients with excellent performance status should be offered the opportunity of participating in aggressive clinical trials with intensification regimens.

Second, as noted above, long-term disease-free survival has been observed in a fraction of patients who show responses induced by chemotherapy. A brief trial with two cycles of aggressive combination chemotherapy might rapidly distinguish between patients with highly chemosensitive disease and those with tumors for which chemotherapy might possibly represent toxicity without benefit. Dose reduction in such a trial period should be avoided if at all possible because evidence supports a clear dose–response relationship for chemotherapy of sarcomas, and one would not wish to compromise such an effect during an initial therapeutic challenge.

Third, the decision to treat should be based on the clinical assessment of anticipated net benefit in quality of life as well as the remote possibility of complete remission or improved survival. Asymptomatic elderly patients with relatively stable disease might best be treated with watchful waiting and might enjoy months to years of survival with tumor but without toxicities of therapy. In patients with incurable soft-tissue sarcoma, there are currently few data on quality of life and the subjective clinical significance of achieving an objective tumor response. It would be useful to incorporate quality-of-life outcome measures into subsequent clinical trials, particularly those looking at combination therapy, to clarify whether the increased toxicity of such regimens is offset by measurable benefits (151).

Furthermore, as overall survival has not been impacted by standard chemotherapeutic regiments, another option for soft-tissue sarcoma patients includes participation in an investigational regimen as first-line therapy. Patients with untreated, advanced, unresectable disease or metastatic sarcoma with disease not amendable to surgical salvage are appropriate candidates for clinical trials to identify more active single agents or regimens. As there are no standard "second-line" therapies in this disease, patients relapsing after prior chemotherapy or those with refractory sarcoma may also be placed on investigational Phase I or Phase II studies. Finally, for some patients, offering supportive care as palliation with no further cytotoxic treatment is the most reasonable option.

IV. SPECIAL SITUATIONS

The above discussion focuses on patients with typical adult-type sarcoma. Two particular disease entities, Kaposi's sarcoma and desmoid tumor, deserve specific reference due to their distinct chemotherapeutic management.

A. Kaposi's Sarcoma

Kaposi's sarcoma, also known as multiple idiopathic hemorrhagic sarcoma, is a highly vascularized neoplasm. The cell of origin is still debated, although evidence suggests that it may be derived from mesenchymal cells in the vasculature (152). Before the 1980s, Kaposi's sarcoma was a rare disorder that occurred predominantly in elderly men of Mediterranean or Eastern European Jewish descent. With the advent of the acquired immunodeficiency syndrome (AIDS) epidemic, its occurrence has increased dramatically. Kaposi's sarcoma is now the most common AIDS-associated malignancy. It affects approximately 20% of patients with AIDS and is the AIDS-defining disease for approximately 15% of all cases in the United States (60).

Classic Kaposi's sarcoma usually follows an indolent and benign clinical course that rarely requires treatment. In contrast, AIDS-related Kaposi's sarcoma is often a fulminant disease that requires aggressive treatment, especially when it involves visceral organs. Despite its progressive nature, the incidence of death due to Kaposi's sarcoma is relatively low compared with other AIDS-related opportunistic infections (153). AIDS-related Kaposi's sarcoma most frequently presents as cutaneous lesions, characterized by the appearance of violaceous plaque or nodular lesions. These lesions can cause pain, bleeding, and disfigurement and impair quality of life. Visceral involvement occurs in nearly half of the cases and can cause significant morbidity and mortality. Symptomatic pulmonary involvement occurs in nearly 20% of cases and is the most life-threatening form of the disease, with median survival generally less than 6 months (154).

To date, no curative therapy for Kaposi's sarcoma exists. Prolonged survival has not been achieved with local or systematic treatment. Therefore, treatment is aimed at providing an improved performance status and effective palliation with few side effects. Local treatments, including surgical excision, radiation therapy, cryotherapy, sclerotherapy, argon laser therapy, or intralesional injections of chemotherapeutic agents, are reasonable choices for patients with tumor limited to certain anatomical sites. Systemic chemotherapy is the only treatment that produces a rapid response in progressive Kaposi's sarcoma. It should therefore be considered for patients with rapidly progressive disease or patients with documented visceral lesions or edema with associated symptoms.

IFN-α, when used alone, induces tumor responses in approximately 30% of patients with AIDS-related sarcoma, but the drug is most effective in patients with intact immune function (155,156). Combination therapy with IFN-α and antiretroviral therapy with zidovudine has been shown to produce response rates of 42–47% (157,158).

Chemotherapeutic agents active in the management of AIDS-related Kaposi's sarcoma include vinca alkaloids, bleomycin, anthracyclines, paclitaxel, and etoposide. Single-agent response rates range from 40% to 80% depending on the severity and the extent of the disease (159).

To reduce toxicity and exert synergism, various combination regimens have been studied. Two of the most commonly administered combination regimens for patients with AIDS-related Kaposi's sarcoma are doxorubicin [Adriamycin], bleomycin, and vinblastine (ABV) and bleomycin and vinctristine (BV).

In a study by Laubenstein et al., 31 patients with end-stage Kaposi's sarcoma unresponsive to other chemotherapy were administered the ABV regimen consisting of doxorubicin 40 mg/m^2 on day 1, bleomycin 15 U on days 1 and 15, and vinblastine 6 mg/m^2 on day 1 (160). The overall response rate was 84% with a 23% complete response rate. The median duration of response was 7.5 months, with median survival of 9 months. This regimen was quite toxic. Neutropenia was the most common adverse effect and led to dose reductions in 44% of patients. During follow-up, 61% of patients died from complications associated with opportunistic infections.

In an attempt to reduce the risk of myelosuppression, doxorubicin was removed from the regimen. Gill et al. treated 18 patients with advanced Kaposi's sarcoma with a median of seven cycles of bleomycin (10 U/m^2) and vincristine 1.4 mg/m^2) every 2 weeks (161). The group's median CD4 count was 58/mm^3, and 7 patients had confirmed pulmonary Kaposi's sarcoma. Thirteen patients (72%) had a complete or partial response despite the presence of poor prognostic factors. Of the patients with pulmonary Kaposi's sarcoma, 3 achieved a complete response to therapy. Opportunistic infections occurred in 16 of the 18 patients after the initiation of chemotherapy.

More intensive regimens have also been studied. Gelmann et al. used ABV alternating with dactinomycin, dacarbazine, and vincristine in 18 patients with advanced Kaposi's sarcoma (162). As expected, good responses were achieved in 72%; however, 12 of 13 (67%) responding patients subsequently died due to an infectious event.

More recently, encouraging results have been achieved with liposomal doxorubicin. Phase II trials of liposomal doxorubicin have demonstrated response rates of 67–93% (163,164). Many patients in these trials had received prior chemotherapy for Kaposi's sarcoma. These results stand in marked contrast for single-agent standard doxorubicin showing no complete response rates and only a 10% partial response rate (165).

In randomized prospective trials, liposomal doxorubicin has produced higher response rates than ABV and BV. Northfelt et al. randomized 225 patients with extensive, progressive mucocutaneous or visceral Kaposi's sarcoma and median CD4 counts of less than 14/mm^3 to treatment with liposomal doxorubicin (20 mg/m^2) or the ABV regimen. Results showed a response rate of 43% versus 25% ($p = 0.005$) in favor of liposomal doxorubicin over ABV chemotherapy (166). The median time to best response was significantly shorter in the liposomal doxorubicin-treated patients (44 vs. 64 days, $p = 0.025$). Another trial compared liposomal daunorubicin (40 mg/m^2) versus ABV in 232 patients with advanced AIDS-related Kaposi's sarcoma (167). At the interim analysis, there was no difference in response rates between the two groups, but there was a lower incidence of toxicity in the liposomal daunorubicin group. In addition, patients in the daunorubicin arm gained weight, whereas those in the ABV arm continued to lose weight throughout the study period.

These results are promising, but further studies are needed to develop an effective and better tolerated regimen. Although chemotherapy has demonstrated clinical efficacy with respect to tumor regression, these regimens are often associated with toxicities and a high rate of opportunistic infections. It remains uncertain whether the infections are related to chemotherapy or to the underlying immunodeficiency. Thus far, no chemotherapy regimen has been proven to prolong the survival of patients with AIDS-related Kaposi's sarcoma. In addition, despite the palliative nature of chemotherapy for Kaposi's sarcoma, few studies have compared the effects of different chemotherapy regimens on quality of life. As with all palliative therapy, close attention to the patient's quality of life is mandatory and is perhaps the best measure of clinical benefit from therapy.

B. Desmoid Tumors

Desmoid tumors, also known as aggressive fibromatosis, musculoaponeurotic fibromatosis, well-differentiated fibrosarcoma, or fibrosarcoma grade 1, are rare, nonmetastasizing tumors. Histologically, desmoids are well-differentiated, mature fibrous lesions composed of fibrocytes in an extensive collagen matrix (168). They are known for being locally invasive without having the potential for distant metastases and for a very high frequency of local recurrence after surgical excision (or primary resection) (169–172). By local spread, extra-abdominal desmoids can cause compression of nerves, major vessels, and trachea, whereas intra-abdominal desmoids can cause compression of intestines, ureters, bladder, and major neurovascular structures. Because of compression the spread of desmoid tumors has been fatal in rare cases (173).

The etiology of desmoid tumors remains unclear, with trauma, hormonal factors, and genetic influences suggested as possible factors (174,175). There is also a known association with familial adenomatous polyposis coli (FAP) and Gardner's syndrome (176).

Surgical resection is the standard treatment for desmoid tumors. In the rare case, control of large or recurrent extremity lesions may even require amputation. Unfortunately, due to the infiltrative nature of these tumors, resection is often incomplete and the recurrence rate is high. Recent surgical series report recurrence rates of 39–79% (177–179). In addition, patients often present with unresectable lesions secondary to mesenteric involvement, retroperitoneal location, or invasion of vital structures.

Radiotherapy has been used both in the adjuvant setting and for the treatment of inoperable disease. The role of adjuvant radiation remains controversial.

Some studies have found it to be quite effective, whereas others have reported it to be of little value (170,180,181). Radiation therapy appears to improve the control of large, bulky disease, often rendering inoperable lesions resectable (181,182). In the doses required to control desmoids, however, radiation therapy frequently causes significant local toxicity, and the morbidity of treatment may outweigh the morbidity of disease progression.

Other modes of therapy have been used, including nonsteriodal anti-inflammatory agents (NSAIDs), hormonal therapy, immunotherapy, and cytotoxic chemotherapy. These therapies have been particularly useful in patients who present with unresectable disease. A number of case reports have documented responses to tamoxifen, the antiestrogen toremifene, aromatase inhibitors, luteinizing hormone–releasing hormone (LHRH) analogs, and progestational agents (175,183–185). There also are well-documented responses to NSAIDS, in particular sulindac, and responses to combinations of NSAIDS with tamoxifen, warfarin, vitamin K, and vitamin C (174,183,186–188). In a retrospective review, Tsukada et al. showed a 50% response rate from sulindac or indomethacin in 28 patients with intra-abdominal desmoids (186). There have been no prospective randomized trials, and it has been difficult to assess the value of different drugs because of the small numbers in each study. In the various reports, most responses occurred within the first 3 months but some were observed up to 2 years after the start of therapy (189). Because these agents are sometimes effective and are relatively nontoxic, they are often used as first-line therapy in patients with unresectable tumors. On occasion, a patient in whom resection has been deemed excessively morbid will respond sufficiently to permit a less radical resection (60).

Despite treatment with these agents, there are a number of patients in whom desmoid tumors continue to progress, resulting in life-threatening complications. In these patients chemotherapy has played an important role. As desmoid tumors arise from the same tissue as fibrosarcomas, agents with activity against sarcomas have been used in the treatment of desmoids. Because unresectable desmoids are uncommon, the literature consists largely of case reports and small retrospective studies. Objective remissions of varying degrees and duration have been noted with almost all agents, including actinomycin D, cyclophosphamide, vincristine, actinomycin D, vinblastine, methotrexate, and others, but the numbers reported are small (190–195).

Patel et al. described a response to treatment with doxorubicin- and dacarbazine-based regimens in six of nine patients with desmoid tumors (190). Two patients experienced complete responses and four patients experienced partial responses. Lynch et al. described a complete response to such treatment in two FAP patients with aggressive, intra-abdominal disease who failed to respond to other forms of treatment (191). A regimen of doxorubicin and dacarbazine followed by carboplatin and dacarbazine has also shown activity in desmoid tumors. Schnitzler et al. studied five patients with symptomatic, unresectable intra-abdominal desmoid tumors unresponsive to conventional medical therapy (192). One patient had a complete response and three patients had partial responses. All patients experienced relief of pain and resolution of small-bowel obstruction symptoms. The toxicity was significant, however, with all patients experiencing nausea, vomiting, and febrile neutropenia.

In general, responses occur slowly, and it is important that treatment not be abandoned prematurely in the patient with disease that is stable. For the patient with an unresectable desmoid, a trial of hormonal therapy or NSAIDs is appropriate, but symptomatic patients who are unresponsive to such treatment should be offered chemotherapy. Lastly, as desmoids demonstrate a response to chemotherapy, such treatment should be considered before resorting to radical local therapy that is associated with significant and unacceptable morbidity.

ACKNOWLEDGMENT

The authors thank E. Gehan, Ph.D., for his comments regarding statistical analysis.

REFERENCES

1. Enneking WF, Spanier SS, Malawer MM. The effect of the anatomic setting on the results of surgical procedures for soft part sarcoma of the thigh. Cancer 1981; 47: 1005–1023.
2. Suit HD, Mankin HJ, Wood WC, Proppe KH. Preoperative, intraoperative, and postoperative radiation in the treatment of primary soft tissue sarcoma. Cancer 1985; 55: 2659–2667.
3. Leibel SA, Tranbaugh RF, Wara WM, Beckstead JH, Bovill EG, Phillips TL. Soft tissue sarcomas of the extremities: survival and patterns of failure with conservative surgery and postoperative irradiation compared to surgery alone. Cancer 1982; 50: 1076–1083.
4. Manzanet R, Antman KH. Adjuvant therapy for sarcomas. Semin Oncol 1991; 18: 603–612.
5. Romsdahl MM, Lindberg RD, Martin RG. Patterns of failure after treatment of soft tissue sarcoma. Cancer Treat Sym 1983; 2:251–258.
6. Brennan MF, Casper ES, Harrison LB, Shiu MH, Gaynor J, Hajdu SI. The role of multimodality therapy in soft tissue sarcoma. Ann Surg 1991; 214:328–337.
7. Pisters PWT, Harrison LB, Leung DHY, Woodruff JM, Casper ES, Brennan MF. Long-term results of a prospective randomized trial of adjuvant brachytherapy in soft tissue sarcoma. J Clin Oncol 1996; 14:859–868.
8. Potter DA, Kinsella T, Glatstein E, Wesley R, White DE, Seipp CA, Chang AE, Lack EE, Costa J, Rosenberg SA. High-grade soft tissue sarcomas of the extremities. Cancer 1986; 58:190–205.

9. Rosenberg SA, Tepper J, Glatstein E, Costa J, Young R, Baker A, Brennan MF, DeMoss EV, Seipp C, Sindelar WF, Sugarbaker P, Wesley R. Prospective randomized evaluation of adjuvant chemotherapy in adults with soft tissue sarcomas of the extremities. Cancer 1983; 52:424–434.

10. Potter DA, Glenn J, Kinsella T, Glatstein E, Lack EE, Restrepo C, White DE, Seipp CA, Wesley R, Rosenberg SA. Patterns of recurrence in patients with high-grade soft tissue sarcomas. J Clin Oncol 1985; 3:353–366.

11. Delaney TF, Yang JC, Glatstein E. Adjuvant therapy for adult patients with soft tissue sarcomas. Oncology 1991; 5:105–118.

12. Schable FM. Rationale for adjuvant chemotherapy. Cancer 1977;39:2875–2882.

13. Blum RH, Carter SK. Adriamycin. A new anticancer drug with significant clinical activity. Ann Intern Med 1974; 80:249–259.

14. Gottlieb JA, Baker LH, O'Bryan RM, Sinkovics JG, Hoogstraten B, Quagliana JM, Rivkin SE, Bodey GP, Rodriguez VT, Blumenschein GR, Saiki JH, Coltman C, Burgess MA, Sullivan P, Thigpen T, Bottomley R, Balcerzak S, Moon TE. Adriamycin used alone and in combination for soft tissue and bony sarcoma. Cancer Chemother Res 1975; 6:271–282.

15. Landis SH, Murray T, Bolden S, Wingo PA. Cancer statistics, 1999. CA Cancer J Clin 1999; 48:10.

16. Alvegard TA, Berg NO. Histopathology peer review of high-grade soft tissue sarcoma: The Scandinavian Sarcoma Group Experience. J Clin Oncol 1989; 7:1845–1851.

17. Coindre JM, Trojani M, Contesso G, David M, Rouesse J, Bui NB, Bodaert A, de Mascarel I, de Mascarel A, Goussot J. Reproducibility of a histopathologic grading system for adult soft tissue sarcoma. Cancer 1986; 58:306–309.

18. Presant CA, Russell WO, Alexander RW, Fu YS. Soft tissue and bone sarcoma histopathology peer review: The frequency of disagreement in diagnosis and the need for second pathology opinions. The Southeastern Cancer Study Group experience. J Clin Oncol 1986; 4:1658–1661.

19. Rosenberg SA. Prospective randomized trials demonstrating the efficacy of adjuvant chemotherapy in adult patients with soft tissue sarcomas. Cancer Treat Rep 1984; 68:1067–1078.

20. Zalupski MM, Baker LH. Systemic adjuvant chemotherapy for soft tissue sarcomas. Hematol Oncol Clin North Am 1995; 9:787–800.

21. Collin C, Godbold J, Hajdu S, Brennan M. Localized extremity soft tissue sarcoma: an analysis of factors affecting survival. J Clin Oncol 1987; 5:601–612.

22. Gaynor JJ, Tan CC, Casper ES, Collin CF, Friedrich C, Shiu M, Hajdu SI, Brennan MF. Refinement of clinicopathologic staging for localized soft tissue sarcomas of the extremities: a study of 423 adults. J Clin Oncol 1992; 10:1317–1329.

23. Russell WO, Cohen J, Enzinger F, Hajdu SI, Heise H, Martin RG, Meissner W, Miller WT, Schmitz RL, Suit HD. A clinical and pathological staging system for soft tissue sarcomas. Cancer 1977; 40:1562–1570.

24. Ries LAG, Kosary CL, Hankey BF, Miller BA, Edwards BK (eds). SEER Cancer Statistics Review, 1973–1995. Bethesda, MD: National Cancer Institute, 1998.

25. Rosenberg SA, Kent H, Costa J, Webber BL, Young R, Chabner B, Baker AR, Brennan MF, Chretien PB, Cohen MH, DeMoss EV, Sears HF, Seipp C, Simon R. Pro-

spective randomized evaluation of the role of limb-sparing surgery, radiation therapy, and adjuvant chemoimmunotherapy in the treatment of adult soft tissue sarcomas. Surgery 1978; 84:62–69.

26. Das Gupta TK, Patel MK, Chaudhuri PK, Briele HA. The role of chemotherapy as an adjuvant to surgery in the initial treatment of primary soft tissue sarcomas in adults. J Surg Oncol 1982; 19:139–144.

27. Mills EED. Adjuvant chemotherapy of adult high-grade soft tissue sarcoma. J Surg Oncol 1982; 21:170–175.

28. Sordillo PP, Magill GB, Shiu MH, Lesser M, Hajdu SI, Golbey RB. Adjuvant chemotherapy of soft-part sarcomas with ALOMAD (S4). J Surg Oncol 1981; 18:345–353.

29. Chang AE, Kinsella T, Glatstein E, Baker AR, Sindelar WF, Lotze MT, Danforth DN, Sugarbaker PH, Lack EE, Steinberg SM, White DE, Rosenberg SA. Adjuvant chemotherapy for patients with high-grade soft-tissue sarcomas of the extremity. J Clin Oncol 1988; 6:1491–1500.

30. Glenn J, Kinsella T, Glatstein E, Tepper J, Baker A, Sugarbaker P, Sindelar W, Roth J, Brennan MF, Costa J, Seipp C, Wesley R, Young RC, Rosenberg SA. A randomized, prospective trail of adjuvant chemotherapy in adults with soft-tissue sarcomas of the head and neck, breast and trunk. Cancer 1985; 55:1206–1214.

31. Glenn J, Sindelar WF, Kinsella T, Glatstein E, Tepper J, Costa J, Baker A, Sugarbaker P, Brennan MF, Seipp C, Wesley R, Young RC, Rosenberg SA. Results of multimodality therapy of resectable soft-tissue sarcomas of the retroperitoneum. Surgery 1985; 97:316–325.

32. Gherlinzoni F, Bacci G, Picci P, Capanna R, Calderoni P, Lorenzi EG, Bernini M, Emiliani E, Barbieri E, Normand A, Campanacci M. A randomized trial for the treatment of high-grade soft-tissue sarcomas of the extremities: preliminary observations. J Clin Oncol 1986; 4:552–558.

33. Picci P, Bacci G, Gherlinzoni F. Results of a randomized trial for the treatment of localized soft tissue tumors of the extremities in adult patients. In: Ryan JR, Baker LO, eds. Recent Concepts in Sarcoma Treatment. Dordrect: Kluwer Academic, 1988, pp. 144–148.

34. Ravaud A, Nguyen BB, Coindre J, Kantor G, Stockle E, Lagarde P, Becouarn Y, Chauvergne J, Bonichon F, Maree D. Adjuvant chemotherapy with CYVADIC in high-risk soft tissue sarcoma: a randomized prospective trial. In: Salmon SE, ed. Adjuvant Therapy of Cancer VI. Philadelphia: WB Saunders, 1990, pp. 556–566.

35. Bramwell V, Rouesse J, Steward W, Santoro A, Schaffordt-Koops H, Buesa J, Ruka W, Priario J, Wagener T, Burgers M, Van Unnik J, Contesso G, Thomas D, van Glabbeke M, Markham D, Pinedo H. Adjuvant CYVADIC chemotherapy for adult soft tissue sarcoma—reduced local recurrence but no improvement in survival: A study of the European Organization for Research and Treatment of Cancer Soft Tissue and Bone Sarcoma Group. J Clin Oncol 1994; 12:1137–1149.

36. Antman K, Ryan L, Borden E, Wood WC, Lerner HL, Corson JM, Carey R, Suit H, Balcerak S, Elias A, Baker L. Pooled results from three randomized adjuvant studies of doxorubicin versus observation in soft tissue sarcoma: 10-year results and review of the literature. In: Salmon S, ed. Adjuvant Therapy of Cancer VI. Philadelphia: WB Saunders, 1990, pp. 529–544.

37. Wilson RE, Wood WC, Lerner HL, Antman K, Amato D, Corson JM, Proppe K, Harmon D, Carey R, Greenberger J, Suit H. Doxorubicin chemotherapy in the treatment of soft tissue sarcoma: Combined results of two randomized trials. Arch Surg 1986; 121:1354–1359.

38. Alvegard TA, Sigurdsson H, Mouridsen H, Solheim O, Unsgaard B, Ringborg U, Dahl O, Nordentoft AM, Blomqvist C, Rydholm A, Stener B, Ranstam J. Adjuvant chemotherapy with doxorubicin in high-grade soft tissue sarcoma: a randomized trial of the Scandinavian Sarcoma Group. J Clin Oncol 1989; 7:1504–1513.

39. Edmonson JH, Fleming TR, Ivins JC, Burgert O, Soule EH, O'Connell MJ, Sim FH, Ahmann DL. Randomized study of systemic chemotherapy following complete excision of nonosseous sarcomas. J Clin Oncol 1984; 2:1390–1396.

40. Eilber FR, Giuliano AE, Huth JF, Morton DL. A randomized prospective trial using postoperative chemotherapy (Adriamycin) in high-grade extremity soft-tissue sarcoma. Am J Clin Oncol 1988:11:39–45.

41. Benjamin TO, Terjanian TO, Fenoglio CJ, Barkley HT, Evans HL, Murphy WK, Martin RG. The importance of combination chemotherapy for adjuvant treatment of high-risk patients with soft-tissue sarcomas of the extremities. In: Salmon SE, ed. Adjuvant Therapy of Cancer V. Orlando, FL: Grune and Stratton, 1987, pp. 735–744.

42. Omura GA, Blessing JA, Major F, Lifshitz S, Ehrlich CE, Mangan C, Beecham J, Park R, Silverberg S. A randomized clinical trial of adjuvant adriamycin in uterine sarcomas: a Gynecologic Oncology Group Study. J Clin Oncol 1985; 3:1240–1245.

43. Dresdale A, Bonow R, Wesley R, Palmeri ST, Barr L, Mathison D, D'Angelo T, Rosenberg SA. Prospective evaluation of doxorubicin-induced cardiomyopathy resulting from postsurgical adjuvant treatment of patients with soft tissue sarcomas. Cancer 1983; 52:51–60.

44. Jones GW, Chouinard E, Patel M. Adjuvant Adriamycin (doxorubicin) in adult patients with soft tissue sarcomas: a systematic overview and quantitative meta-analysis. Clin Invest Med 1991; 14 (Suppl 4):A772.

45. Zalupski MM, Ryan JR, Hussein MH, Baker LH. Defining the role of adjuvant chemotherapy for patients with soft tissue sarcoma of the extremities. In: Salmon SE, ed. Adjuvant Therapy of Cancer VII. Philadelphia: JB Lippincott, 1993, pp. 385–394.

46. Tierney JF, Mosseri V, Stewart LA, Souhami RL, Parmar MKB. Adjuvant chemotherapy for soft-tissue sarcoma: review and meta-analysis of the published results of randomized clinical trials. Br J Cancer 1995; 72:469–475.

47. Stewart LA, Parmar MKB. Meta-analysis of the literature or of individual patient data: is there a difference? Lancet 1993; 341:418–422.

48. Sarcoma Meta-analysis Collaboration. Adjuvant chemotherapy for localized resectable soft-tissue sarcoma of adults: meta-analysis of individual data. Lancet 1997; 350:1647–1654.

49. Casper ES, Gaynor JJ, Hajdu SI, Magill GB, Tan C, Friedrich C, Brennan MF. A prospective randomized trial of adjuvant chemotherapy with bolus versus continuous infusion of doxorubicin in patients with high-grade extremity soft tissue sarcoma and analysis of prognostic factors. Cancer 1991; 68:1221–1229.

50. Legha SS, Benjamin RS, Mackay B, Ewer M, Wallace S, Valdivieso M, Rasmussen SL, Blumenschein GR, Freireich EJ. Reduction of doxorubicin cardiomyopathy by prolonged continuous intravenous infusion. Ann Intern Med 1982; 96:133–139.

51. Antman KH. Adjuvant therapy of sarcomas of soft tissue. Semin Oncol 1997; 24: 556–560.

52. Frustaci S, Gherlinzoni F, De Paoli A, Pignatti G, Zmerly H, Azzarelli A, Comandone A, Buonadonna A, Olmi P, Ippolito V, Barbieri E, Apice G, Zakotnic B, Bacci G, Picci P. Preliminary results of an adjuvant randomized trial on high risk extremity soft tissue sarcomas. The interim analysis. Proc Am Soc Clin Oncol 1997; 16:496(abstr 1785).

53. Eilber FR, Eckardt JJ, Rosen G, Fu YS, Seeger LL, Selch MT. Neoadjuvant chemotherapy and radiotherapy in the multidisciplinary management of soft tissue sarcomas of the extremity. Surg Oncol Clin North Am 1993; 2:611–620.

54. Frei E, Clark JR, Miller D. The concept of neoadjuvant chemotherapy. In: Salmon SE, ed. Adjuvant Chemotherapy of Cancer V. Orlando, FL: Grune and Stratton, 1987, pp. 67–75.

55. Pezzi CM, Pollock RE, Evans HL, Lorigan JG, Pezzi TA, Benjamin RA, Romsdahl MM. Preoperative chemotherapy for soft-tissue sarcomas of the extremities. Ann Surg 1990; 211:476–481.

56. Pisters PWT, Patel SR, Varma DGK, Feig BW, Nguyen HTB, Chen NP, Pollack A, Pollock RE, Benjamin RS. Preoperative chemotherapy for stage IIIB extremity soft tissue sarcoma: long-term results from a single institution. Proc Am Soc Clin Oncol 1996; 15:522(abstr 1682).

57. Priebat D, Malawer M, Markan Y, Barnhill M, Shmookler B, Perry D, Jelinek J, Edwards P, Schulof R. Clinical outcome of neoadjuvant intraarterial cisplatin and continuous infusion adriamycin for large high grade unresectable/borderline soft tissue sarcomas of the extremities. Proc Am Soc Clin Oncol 1994; 13:473(abstr 1648).

58. Casper ES, Gaynor JJ, Harrison LB, Panicek DM, Hajdu SI, Brennan MF. Preoperative and postoperative adjuvant combination chemotherapy for adults with high grade soft tissue sarcoma. Cancer 1994; 73:1644–1651.

59. Verweij J, Pinedo HM. Adjuvant chemotherapy of soft tissue sarcomas. Cancer Treat Res 1997; 91:173–187.

60. Brennan MF, Casper ES, Harrison LB. Soft tissue sarcoma. In: Devita VT, Hellman S, Rosenberg SA, eds. Cancer: Principles and Practice of Oncology, 5th ed. Philadelphia: Lippincott-Raven Publishers, 1997, pp. 1738–1789.

61. Eilber FR, Giuliano AE. Intravenous vs. intraarterial Adriamycin, 2888 r radiation and surgical excision for extremity soft tissue sarcomas: a randomized prospective trial. Proc Am Soc Clin Oncol 1990; 9:309 (abstr 1194).

62. Eilber F, Giuliano A, Huth J, Mirra J. Neoadjuvant chemotherapy, radiation, and limited surgery for high grade soft tissue sarcomas of the extremity. In: Ryan JR, Baker LO, eds. Recent Concepts in Sarcoma Treatment. Dordrecht: Kluwer Academic, 1988, p. 115.

63. Kempf RA, Irwin LE, Menendez L, Chandrasoma P, Groshen S, Melbye W, Moore T, Pentecost M, Quinn M, Sapozink M, Schwinn CP, Sherrod A, Stewart M, Wolf W, Muggia FM. Limb salvage surgery for bone and soft tissue sarcoma. A phase II pathologic study of preoperative intraarterial cisplatin. Cancer 1991; 68:738–743.

64. Chawla SP, Rosen G, Eilber F, Lowenbraun S, Eckardt J, Morton DL, Selch M, Greenberg S, Mirra J. Cisplatin and adriamycin as neoadjuvant and adjuvant chemo-

therapy in the management of soft tissue sarcomas. In: Salmon SE, ed. Adjuvant Therapy of Cancer VI. Philadelphia: WB Saunders, 1990, pp. 567–573.

65. Pisters PWT, Feig BW, Leung DHY, Brennan MF. New developments in soft tissue sarcoma. Cancer Treat Res 1997; 90:91–107.

66. Eilber F, Eckardt J, Rosen G, Forscher C, Selch M, Fu YS. Improved complete response with neoadjuvant chemotherapy and radiation for high grade extremity soft tissue sarcoma. Proc Am Soc Clin Oncol 1994; 13:473(abstr 1645).

67. Goodnight J, Burger W, Voegeli T, Blaisdell FW. Limb sparing surgery for extremity sarcomas after preoperative intra-arterial doxorubicin and radiation therapy. Am J Surg 1985; 150:109–113.

68. Spiro IJ, Suit H, Gebhardt M, Springfield D, Mankin H, Jennings C, Rosenberg A, Efird J, Harmon D. Neoadjuvant chemotherapy and radiotherapy for large soft tissue sarcomas. Proc Am Soc Oncol 1996; 15:524(abstr 1689).

69. Schraffordt-Koops H, Eggermont AMM, Lienard D, Kroon BBR, Hoekstra HJ, Van Geel AN, Nieweg OE, Lejeune FJ. Hyperthermic isolated limb perfusion for treatment of soft tissue sarcomas. Sem Surg Oncol 1998; 14:210–214.

70. Eggermont AMM, Schraffordt Koops H, Klausner JM, Schlag PM, Kroon BBR, Ben-Ari G, Lejeune FJ. Isolation limb perfusion with tumor necrosis factor alpha and chemotherapy for advanced extremity soft tissue sarcomas. Cancer Treat Res 1997; 91:189–203.

71. Creech OJ, Krementz ET, Ryan RF, Winblad JN. Chemotherapy of cancer: regional perfusion utilizing an extracorporeal circuit. Ann Surg 1958; 148:616–632.

72. McBride CM. Sarcomas of the limbs. Results of adjuvant chemotherapy using isolation perfusion. Arch Surg 1974; 109:304–308.

73. Krementz ET, Carter RD, Sutherland CM, Hutton I. Chemotherapy of sarcomas of the limbs by regional perfusion. Ann Surg 1977; 185:555–564.

74. Stehlin JS, de Ipolyi PD, Giovanella BC, Gutierrez AE, Anderson RF. Soft tissue sarcomas of the extremity: multidisciplinary therapy employing hyperthermic perfusion. Am J Surg 1975; 130:643–646.

75. Hoekstra HJ, Schraffordt Koops H, Molenaar WM, Oldhoff J. Results of isolated regional perfusion in the treatment of malignant soft tissue tumors of the extremities. Cancer 1987; 60:1703–1707.

76. Lethi PM, Stephens MH, Janoff K, Stevens K, Fletcher WS. Improved survival for soft tissue sarcoma of the extremities by regional hyperthermic perfusion, local excision, and radiation therapy. Surg Gynecol Obstet 1986; 162:149–152.

77. Klasse JM, Kroon BBR, Benckhuijsen C, van Geel AN, Albus-Lutter E, Wieberdink J. Results of regional isolated perfusion with cytostatics in patients with soft tissue tumors of the extremities. Cancer 1989; 64:616–621.

78. Schraffordt-Koops H, Eibergen R, Oldhoff J, van der Ploeg E, Vermey A. Isolated regional perfusion in the treatment of soft tissue sarcomas of the extremities. Clin Oncol 1976; 2:245–252.

79. Di Filippo FD, Calabro AM, Cavallari A, Carlini S, Buttini GL, Moscarelli F, Cavaliere F, Piarulli L, Cavaliere R. The role of hyperthermic perfusion as a first step in the treatment of soft tissue sarcomas of the extremities. World J Surg 1988; 12:332–339.

80. Roseman JM. Effective management of extremity cancers using cisplatin and etoposide in isolated limb perfusions. J Surg Oncol 1987; 35:170–172.

81. Pommier RF, Stephens Moseley H, Cohen J, Huang CS, Townsend R, Fletcher WS. Pharmacokinetics, toxicity, and short-term results of cisplatin hyperthermic isolated limb perfusion for soft-tissue sarcoma and melanoma of the extremities. Am J Surg 1988; 155:667–671.

82. Lienard D, Ewalenko P, Delmotte J, Renard N, Lejeune FJ. High-dose recombinant tumor necrosis factor alpha in combination with interferon gamma and melphalan in isolation perfusion of the limbs for melanoma and sarcoma. J Clin Oncol 1992; 10: 52–60.

83. Eggermont AMM, Schraffordt-Koops H, Lienard D, Kroon BBR, van Geel AN, Hoekstra HJ, Lejeune FJ. Isolated limb perfusion with high-dose tumor necrosis factor-alpha in combination with interferon-gamma and melphalan for nonresectable extremity soft tissue sarcomas: a multicenter study. J Clin Oncol 1996; 14:2556–2565.

84. Yap BS, Sinkovics JG, Burgess MA, Benjamin RS, Bodey GP. The curability of advanced soft tissue sarcomas in adults with chemotherapy. Proc Am Soc Clin Oncol 1983; 2:239(C-937).

85. O'Bryan RM, Baker LH, Gottlieb JE, Rivkin SE, Balcerzak SP, Grumet GN, Salmon SE, Moon TE, Hoogstraten B. Dose response evaluation of adriamycin in human neoplasia. Cancer 1977; 39:1940–1948.

86. Borden EC, Amato DA, Rosenbaum C, Enterline HT, Shiraki MJ, Creech RH, Lerner HJ, Carbone PP. Randomized comparison of three adriamycin regimens for metastatic soft tissue sarcomas. J Clin Oncol 1987; 5(6):840–850.

87. Schoenfeld DA, Rosenbaum C, Horton J, Wolter JM, Falkson G, DeConti RC. A comparison of adriamycin versus vincristine and adriamycin, actinomycin-D, and cyclophosphamide for advanced sarcoma. Cancer 1982; 50:2757–2762.

88. Santoro A, Tursz T, Mouridsen H, Verweij J, Steward W, Somers R, Buesa J, Casali P, Spooner D, Rankin E, Kirkpatrick A, van Glabbeke M, van Oosterom A. Doxorubicin versus CYVADIC versus doxorubicin plus ifosfamide in first-line treatment of advanced soft tissue sarcomas: a randomized study of the European Organization for Research and Treatment of Cancer Soft Tissue and Bone Sarcoma Group. J Clin Oncol 1995; 13:1537–1545.

89. Mouridsen HT, Bastholt L, Somers R, Santoro A, Bramwell V, Mulder JH, van Oosterom AT, Buesa J, Pinedo HM, Thomas D, Sylvester R. Adriamycin versus epirubicin in advanced soft tissue sarcomas. A randomized phase II/III study of the EORTC soft tissue and bone sarcoma group. Eur J Cancer Clin Oncol 1987; 23:1477–1483.

90. Edmonson JH, Ryan LM, Brooks JSJ, Shiraki M, Frytak S, Parkinson DR. Randomized comparison of doxorubicin alone versus ifosfamide plus doxorubicin or mitomycin, doxorubicin, cisplatin against advanced soft tissue sarcomas. J Clin Oncol 1993; 11:1269–1275.

91. Robert J. Epirubicin. Clinical pharmacology and dose–effect relationship. Drugs 1993; 45 (Suppl 2):20–30.

92. Dombernowsky P, Mouridsen H, Nielsen OS, Crowther D, Verweij J, Buesa J, Steward W, van Glabbeke M, Kirkpatrick A, Tursz T. A phase III study comparing adriamycin versus two schedules of high dose epirubicin in advanced soft tissue sarcoma. Proc Am Soc Clin Oncol 1995; 14:515(abstr 1688).

93. Bramwell VH, Mouridsen HT, Santoro A, Blackledge G, Somers R, Verweij J, Dombernowsky P, Onsrud M, Thomas D, Sylvester R, van Oosterom A. Cyclophosphamide versus ifosfamide: final report of a randomized phase II trial in adult soft tissue sarcomas. Eur J Cancer Clin Oncol 1987; 23:311–321.
94. Wiltshaw E, Westbury G, Harmer C, McKinna A, Fisher C. Cancer Chemother Pharmacol 1986; 18 (Suppl 2):10–12.
95. Schutte J, Kellner R, Seeber S. Ifosfamide in the treatment of soft tissue sarcomas: experience at the West German Tumor Center. Essen Cancer Chemother Pharmacol 1993; 31 (Suppl 2):194–198.
96. Antman KH, Ryan L, Elias A, Sherman D, Grier HE. Response to ifosfamide and mesna: 124 previously treated patients with metastatic or unresectable sarcoma. J Clin Oncol 1989; 7:126–131.
97. Elias AD, Eder JP, Shea T, Begg CB, Frei E, Antman KH. High-dose ifosfamide with mesna uroprotection: a phase I study. J Clin Oncol 1990; 8:170–178.
98. Antman KH, Montella D, Rosenbaum C, Schwen M. Phase II trial of ifosfamide with mesna in previously untreated metastatic sarcoma. Cancer Treat Rep 1985; 69:499–504.
99. Stuart-Harris R, Harper PG, Kaye SB, Wiltshaw E. High dose ifosfamide by infusion with mesna in advanced soft tissue sarcoma. Cancer Treat Rev 1983; 10 (Suppl A):163–164.
100. Benjamin RS, Legha SS, Patel SR, Nicaise C. Single agent ifosfamide studies in sarcomas of soft tissue and bone: the MD Anderson experience. Cancer Chemother Pharmacol 1993; 31 (Suppl 2):174–179.
101. Jaffar Z, Blum RH, Cacavio A, Rosen G. Ifosfamide $14-24$ gm/m^2—an outpatient study in sarcomas. Proc Am Soc Clin Oncol 1998; 17:511(abstr 1968).
102. Kudawara I, Ueda T, Yoshikawa H. High-dose ifosfamide for relapsed high grade bone and soft tissue sarcomas. Proc Am Soc Clin Oncol 1998; 17:521(abstr 2004).
103. Buesa J, Lopez-Pousa A, Anton A, Martin J, Garcia del Muro J, Bellmunt J, Poveda A, Escudero P. Phase II trial of first-line high-dose ifosfamide in advanced soft tissue sarcoma patients. Proc Am Soc Clin Oncol 1997; 16:498(abstr 1793).
104. Rosen G, Forscher C, Lowenbraun S, Eilber F, Eckardt J, Holmes C, Fu YS. Synovial sarcoma: uniform response of metastases to high-dose ifosfamide. Cancer 1994; 73:2506–2511.
105. Le Cesne A, Antoine E, Spielman M, LeChevalier T, Brain E, Toussaint C, Janin N, Kayitalire L, Fontaine F, Genin J, Vanel D, Contesso G, Tursz T. High-dose ifosfamide: circumvention of resistance to standard-dose ifosfamide in advanced soft tissue sarcomas. J Clin Oncol 1995; 13:1600–1608.
106. Buesa JM, Mouridsen HT, van Oosterom AT, Verweij J, Wagener T, Steward W, Poveda A, Vestlev PM, Thomas D, Sylvester R. High dose DTIC in advanced soft tissue sarcomas in the adult. Ann Oncol 1991; 2:307–309.
107. Gottlieb JE, Benjamin RS, Baker LH, O'Bryan RM, Sinkovics JG, Hoogstraten B, Quagliana JM, Rivkin SE, Bodey GP, Rodriguez V, Blumenschein GR, Saiki JH, Coltman C, Burgess MA, Sullivan P, Thigpen T, Bottomley R, Balcerzak S, Moon TE. Role of DTIC in the chemotherapy of sarcomas. Cancer Treat Reports 1976; 60:199–203.

108. Lerner H, Amato D, Stevens C, Borden E, Enterline H. Leiomyosarcoma: the ECOG experience with 222 patients. Proc Am Assoc Cancer Res 1983; 24:142 (C-561).
109. Demetri GD. Major developments in the understanding and treatment of soft-tissue sarcomas in adults. Curr Opin Oncol 1998; 10:343–347.
110. Van Hoesel QG, Verweij J, Catimel G, Clavel M, Kerbrat P, van Oosterom AT, Kerger J, Turtsz T, van Glabbeke M, van Pottelsberghe C, le Bail N, Mouridsen H. Phase II study with docetaxel in advanced soft tissue sarcoma of the adult. Ann Oncol 1994; 5:539–542.
111. Verweij J, Judson I, Crowther D, Ruka W, Buesa J, Coleman R, di Paola E, Locci-Tonelli D, van Glabbeke M, Tursz T. Randomized study comparing docetaxel to doxorubicin in previously untreated soft tissue sarcomas. Proc Am Soc Clin Oncol 1997; 16:496(abstr 1788).
112. Amodio A, Carpano S, Vici P, Di Lauro L, Del Medico P, Manfredi C, Lopez M. Phase II trial of docetaxel in anthracycline-refractory patients with advanced soft tissue sarcomas. Proc Am Soc Clin Oncol 1998; 17:518(abstr 1995).
113. Waltzman R, Schwartz GK, Shorter S, Sugarman A, Bertino JR, Woodruff J, Fennelly D, Leung D, Casper ES. Lack of efficacy of paclitaxel in patients with advanced soft tissue sarcoma. Proc Am Soc Clin Oncol 1996; 15:526(abstr 1699).
114. Omura GA, Major FJ, Blessing JA, Sedlacek TV, Thigpen JT, Creasman WT, Zaino RJ. A randomized study of adriamycin with or without dimethyl triazenoimidazole carboxamide in advanced uterine sarcomas. Cancer 1983; 52:626–632.
115. Zalupski M, Metch B, Balcerzak SP, Fletcher WS, Chapman R, Bonnet JD, Weiss GR, Ryan J, Benjamin RS, Baker LH. Phase III comparison of doxorubicin and dacarbazine given by bolus versus infusion in patients with soft tissue sarcomas. A Southwest Oncology Group Study. J Natl Cancer Inst 1991; 83:926–932.
116. Baker LH, Frank J, Fine G, Balcerzak SP, Stephens RL, Stuckey WJ, Rivkin S, Saiki J, Ward JH. Combination chemotherapy using adriamycin, DTIC, cyclophosphamide, and actinomycin D for advanced soft tissue sarcomas: a randomized comparative trial. J Clin Oncol 1987; 5:851–861.
117. Muss HB, Bundy B, DiSaia PJ, Homesley HD, Fowler WC, Creasman W, Yordan E. Treatment of recurrent advanced uterine sarcoma. A randomized trial of doxorubicin versus doxorubicin and cyclophosphamide. Cancer 1985; 55:1648–1653.
118. Bodey GP, Rodriguez V, Murphy WK, Burgess MA, Benjamin RS. Protected environment–prophylactic antibiotic program for malignant sarcomas: randomized trial during remission induction chemotherapy. Cancer 1981; 47:2422–2429.
119. Pinedo HM, Bramwell VHC, Mouridsen HT, Somers R, Vendrik CPJ, Santoro A, Buesa J, Wagener T, van Oosterom AT, van Unnik JAM, Sylvester R, de Pauw M, Thomas D, Bonadonna G. CyVADIC in advanced soft tissue sarcoma: a randomized study comparing two schedules. Cancer 1984; 53:1825–1832.
120. Pfeffer MR, Sulkes A, Biran S. Treatment of advanced soft tissue sarcomas with modified CyVADIC protocol. Oncology 1984; 41:308–313.
121. Mansi JL, Fisher C, Wiltshaw E, Macmillan S, King M, Stuart-Harris R. A phase I-II study of ifosfamide in combination with Adriamycin in the treatment of adult soft tissue sarcoma. Eur J Cancer Clin Oncol 1988; 24:1439–1443.
122. Schutte J, Mouridsen HT, Stewart W, Santoro A, van Oosterom AT, Somers R, Blackledge G, Verweij J, Dombernowsky P, Thomas D, Sylvester R. Ifosfamide plus

doxorubicin in previously untreated patients with advanced soft tissue sarcoma. Eur J Cancer 1990; 26:558–561.

123. Weh HJ, Zugel M, Windberg D, Schwarz R, Zornig C, Dietel M, Hossfeld DK. Chemotherapy of metastatic soft tissue sarcoma with a combination of adriamycin and DTIC or adriamycin and ifosfamide. Onkologie 1990; 13:448–452.

124. Steward WP, Verweij J, Somers R, Spooncr D, Kerbat P, Clavel M, Crowther D, Rouesse J, Tursz T, Tueni E, van Oosterom AT, Warwick J, Greifenberg B, Thomas D, van Glabbeke M. Granulocyte-macrophage colony-stimulating factor allows safe escalation of dose-intensity sarcomas: a study of the European Organization for Research and Treatment of Cancer Soft Tissue and Bone Sarcoma Group. J Clin Oncol 1993; 11:15–21.

125. Chevallier B, Leyvraz S, Olivier JP, Fargeot P, Facchini T, Lo Van ML. Epirubicin and ifosfamide in advanced soft tissue sarcoma: a phase II study. Cancer Invest 1993; 11:135–139.

126. Elias A, Antman KH. Doxorubicin, ifosfamide and dacarbazine with mesna uroprotection for advanced untreated sarcoma: a phase I study. Cancer Treat Rep 1986; 70:827–833.

127. Elias A, Ryan L, Sulkes A, Collins J, Aisner J, Antman KH. Response to mesna, doxorubicin, ifosfamide, and dacarbazine in 108 patients with metastatic or unresectable sarcoma and no prior chemotherapy. J Clin Oncol 1989; 7:1208–1216.

128. Casali P, Pastorino U, Santoro A, Zucchinelli P, Azzarelli A, Quagliulo V, Bonodonna G. Epirubicin, ifosfamide, and dacarbazine in advanced soft tissue sarcomas. Proc Am Soc Clin Oncol 1991; 10:353(abstr 1255).

129. Elli A, Hernandez Moran JC, Pasccon G, Negro A, Litowska S, Mendez A, Barg S, Santos R, Koliren L, Morgenfeld E, Goldfarb A, Rivarola E, Marantz A, Gercovich F. Ifosfamide, 4 epidoxorubicin chemotherapy for advanced soft tissue sarcomas. Proc Am Soc Clin Oncol 1991; 10:350(abstr 1246).

130. Antman KH, Crowley J, Balcerzak SP, Rivkin SE, Weiss GR, Elias A, Natale RB, Cooper RM, Barlogie B, Trump DL, Doroshow JH, Aisner J, Pugh RP, Weiss RB, Cooper BA, Clamond GH, Baker LH. An intergroup phase III randomized study of doxorubicin and dacarbazine with or without ifosfamide and mesna in advanced soft tissue and bone sarcomas. J Clin Oncol 1993; 11:1276–1285.

131. Bui NB, Demaille MC, Chevreau C, Blay JY, Cupissol C, Rios M, Thyss A, Maugard C, Bastit P, Bay JO, Tanguy A, Fargeot P, Lortholary A, Bonichon F. qMAID vs. MAID 125% with G-CSF in adult soft tissue sarcoma. First results of a randomized study of the FNCLCC Sarcoma Group. Proc Am Soc Clin Oncol 1998; 17: 517(abstr 1991).

132. Vadhan-Raj S, Broxmeter HE, Hittelman WN, Papadopoulos NE, Chawla SP, Fenoglio C, Cooper S, Buescher ES, Frenck RW, Holian A, Perkins RC, Scheule RK, Gutterman JU, Salem P, Benjamin RS. Abrogating chemotherapy-induced myelosuppression by recombinant granulocyte-macrophage colony stimulating factor in patients with sarcoma: protection at the progenitor cell level. J Clin Oncol 1992; 10:1266–1277.

133. Antman KS, Griffin JD, Elias A, Socinski MA, Ryan L, Cannistra SA, Oette D, Whitley M, Frei E, Schnipper LE. Effect of recombinant human granulocyte-macrophage colony-stimulating factor on chemotherapy induced myelosuppression. N Engl J Med 1988; 319:593–598.

134. Bui BN, Chevalier B, Chevreau C, Krakowski I, Peny A, Thyss A, Maugard-Louboutin C, Cupissol D, Fargoet P, Bonichon F, Coindre JM, Gil B, Cour-Chabernaud V. Efficacy of lenograstim on hematologic tolerance to MAID chemotherapy in patients with advanced soft tissue sarcoma and consequences on treatment dose-intensity. J Clin Oncol 1995; 13:2629–2636.

135. Patel SR, Vadhan-Raj S, Burgess MA, Papadopoulos NE, Plager C, Benjamin RS. Dose-intensive chemotherapy in soft tissue sarcomas. Proc Am Soc Clin Oncol 1996; 15:522(abstr 1681).

136. Patel SR, Vadhan-Raj S, Burgess MA, Papadopoulos NE, Plager C, Jenkins J, Benjamin RS. Dose-intensive therapy does improve response rates-updated results of studies with adriamycin and ifosfamide with growth factors in patients with untreated soft tissue sarcomas. Proc Am Soc Clin Oncol 1997; 16:499(abstr 1794).

137. De Pas T, de Braud F, Zimatore M, Orlando L, Munzone E, Nole F, Fazio N, Zampino G, Aapro M. Doxorubicin and continuous infusion high-dose ifosfamide for soft tissue sarcomas. Proc Am Soc Clin Oncol 1997; 16:504(abstr 1812).

138. Leyvraz S, Bacchi M, Cerny T, Lissoni A, Sessa C, Herrmann R. A phase I trial of intensification of ifosfamide and adriamycin and GM-CSF for the treatment of sarcomas. Proc Am Soc Clin Oncol 1995; 14:515(abstr 1689).

139. Reichardt P, Lentzsch S, Hohenberger P, Doerken B. Dose intensive treatment with ifosfamide, epirubicin and filgastrim for patients with metastatic or locally advanced soft tissue sarcoma: a phase II study. Proc Am Soc Clin Oncol 1995: 14:518(abstr 1698).

140. Blay JY, Bonhour D, Brunat-Mentigny M, Rivoire J, Philip I, Philip T, Biron P. High-dose chemotherapy (VIC) and bone marrow support in advanced sarcomas. Proc Am Soc Clin Oncol 1994; 13:479(abstr 1672).

141. Dumontet C, Biron P, Bouffet E, Blay JY, Meckenstock R, Chauvin F, Philip I, Clavel M, Brunat-Mentigny M, Philip T. High dose chemotherapy with ABMT in soft tissue sarcomas. A report of 22 cases. Bone Marrow Transplant 1992; 10:405–408.

142. Kessinger A, Petersen K, Bishop M, Schmit-Pokorny K. High dose therapy with autologous hematopoetic stem cell rescue for patients with metastatic soft tissue sarcomas. Proc Am Soc Clin Oncol 1994; 13:480(abstr 1674).

143. Elias AD, Ayash LJ, Eder JP, Wheeler C, Deary J, Weissman L, Schryber S, Hunt M, Critchlow J, Schnipper L, Frei E, Antman KH. A phase I study of high-dose ifosfamide and escalating doses of carboplatin with autologous bone marrow support. J Clin Oncol 1991; 9:320–327.

144. Salem PA, Benjamin RS, Howard J, Gutterman JU. A phase II trial of recombinant interferon alpha 2-b in the treatment of advanced metastatic and refractory sarcomas. Proc Am Ass Cancer Res 1991; 32:200(abstr 1192).

145. Papadopoulos NEJ, Patel SR, Linke K, Benjamin RS. A phase II study of 5-fluorouracil infusion and interferon alpha in metastatic sarcomas. Proc Am Assoc Cancer Res 1992; 33:229.

146. Steward Chemotherapy for metastatic soft tissue sarcomas.

147. Verweij J, Judson I, Steward W, Coleman R, Woll P, van Pottelsberghe C, van Glabbeke M, Mouridsen H. Phase II study of liposomal muramyl tripeptide phosphatidylethanolamine (MTP/PE) in advanced soft tissue sarcomas of the adult. Eur J Cancer 1994; 30A:842–843.

148. Casper ES, Schwartz GK, Sugarman A, Leung D, Brennan MF. Phase I trial of dose-intense liposome encapsulated doxorubicin in patients with advanced sarcoma. J Clin Oncol 1997; 15:2111–2117.

149. Tontonoz P, Singer S, Forman BM, Sarraf B, Fletcher JA, Fletcher CDM, Brun RP, Mueller E, Altiok S, Oppenheim H, Evans RM, Spiegelman BM. Terminal differentiation of human liposarcoma cells induced by ligands for peroxisome proliferator-activated receptor gamma and the retinoid X receptor. Proc Natl Acad Sci USA 1997; 94:237–241.

150. Yap BS, Sinkovics JG, Benjamin RS, Bodey GP. Survival and relapse patterns of complete responders in adults with advanced soft tissue sarcomas. Proc Am Soc Clin Oncol 1979; 20:352(C-250).

151. Phillips K, Toner GC. Chemotherapy for soft tissue sarcomas. Indication and advances. Acta Orthop Scand 1997; 68 (Suppl 273):133–138.

152. Uccini S, Ruco LP, Monardo F, Stoppacciaro A, La Parola IL, Dejana E, La-Parola IL, Cerimele D, Baroni CD. Co-expression of endothelial cell and macrophage antigens in Kaposi's sarcoma cells. J Pathol 1994; 173:23–31.

153. Sung JCY, Louie SG, Park SY. Kaposi's sarcoma: advances in tumor biology and pharmacotherapy. Pharmacotherapy 1997; 17:670–683.

154. Gill PS, Akil B, Colleti P, Rarick M, Loureiro C, Bernstein-Singer M, Krailo M, Levine AM. Pulmonary Kaposi's sarcoma. Clinical findings and results of therapy. Am J Med 1989; 87:57–61.

155. Volm MD, Von Roenn JH. Treatment strategies for epidemic Kaposi's sarcoma. Curr Opin Oncol 1995; 7:429–436.

156. Lilenbaum RC, Ratner L. Systemic treatment of Kaposi's sarcoma: current status and future directions. AIDS 1994; 8:141–151.

157. Kovacs JA, Deyton L, Davey R, Falloon J, Zunich K, Lee D, Metcalf JA, Bigley JW, Sawyer LA, Zoon KC, Masur H, Fauci AS, Lane HC. Combined zidovudine and interferon-alpha in patients with Kaposi's sarcoma and the acquired immune deficiency syndrome. Ann Intern Med 1990; 111:280–287.

158. Krown SE, Gold JWM, Niedwiecki D, Bundow D, Flomenberg N, Gansbacher B, Brew BJ. Interferon-alpha with zidovudine: safety, tolerance and clinical and virologic effects in patients with Kaposi's sarcoma and the acquired immune deficiency syndrome. Ann Intern Med 1989; 112:812–821.

159. Volberding PA. The role of chemotherapy for epidemic Kaposi's sarcoma. Semin Oncol 1987; 14(Suppl 3):23–26.

160. Laubenstein LJ, Krigel RL, Odajnyk CM, Hymes KB, Friedman-Kien A, Wernz JC, Muggia FM. Treatment of epidemic Kaposi's sarcoma with etoposide or a combination of doxorubicin, bleomycin and vinblastine. J Clin Oncol 1984; 2:1115–1120.

161. Gill P, Rarick M, Bernstein-Singer M, Harb M, Espina BM, Shaw V, Levine A. Treatment of advanced Kaposi's sarcoma using a combination of bleomycin and vincristine. Am J Clin Oncol 1990; 13:315–319.

162. Gelmann EP, Longo D, Lane HC, Fauci AS, Masur H, Wesley M, Preble OT, Jacob J, Steis R. Combination chemotherapy of disseminated Kaposi's sarcoma in patients with the acquired immune deficiency syndrome. Am J Med 1987; 82:456–462.

163. Harrison M, Tomlinson D, Stewart S. Liposomal-entrapped doxorubicin: an active agent in AIDS-related Kaposi's sarcoma. J Clin Oncol 1995; 13:914–920.

164. Bogner JR, Kronawitter U, Rolinski B, Truebenbach K, Goebel FD. Liposomal doxorubicin in the treatment of advanced AIDS-related Kaposi's sarcoma. J Acquir Immune Defic Syndr 1994; 7:463–468.

165. Fischl MA, Krown SE, O'Boyle KP, Mitsuyasu R, Miles S, Wernz JC, Volberding PA, Kahn J, Groopman JE, Feinberg J, Woody M. Weekly doxorubicin in the treatment of patients with AIDS-related Kaposi's sarcoma. J Acq Immune Defic Syndr 1993; 6:259–264.

166. Northfelt DW, Dezube B, Miller B, Mamelok RD, DuMond CE, Henry D. Randomized comparative trial of Doxil vs. adriamycin, bleomycin, and vincristine (ABV) in the treatment of severe AIDS-related Kaposi's sarcoma. Blood 1995; 86 (Suppl 1):382a(abstr 1515).

167. Gill PS, Wernz J, Scadden DT, Cohen P, von Roenn J, Chew T, Kempin S, Silverberg I, Gonzales G, Rarick MU, Myer A, Shepherd F, Sawka C, Mukwaya G, Pike M, Ross M. A randomized trial of liposomal daunorubicin versus adriamycin, bleomycin and vincristine in 232 patients with advanced AIDS-related Kaposi's sarcoma. Proc Am Soc Clin Oncol 1995; 14:291(abstr 830).

168. Faulkner LB, Hajdu SI, Kher U, La Quaglia M, Exelby PR, Heller G, Wollner N. Pediatric desmoid tumors: retrospective analysis of 63 cases. J Clin Oncol 1995; 13: 2813–2818.

169. Masson JK, Soule EH. Desmoid tumors of the head and neck. Am J Surg 1966; 112: 615–622.

170. Posner MC, Shiu MH, Newsome JL, Hadju SI, Gaynor JJ, Brennan MF. The desmoid tumor. Not a benign disease. Arch Surg 1989; 124:191–196.

171. Das Gupta TK, Brasfield RD, O'Hara J. Extra-abdominal desmoids: a clinicopathologic study. Ann Surg 1969; 170:109–121.

172. Enzinger FM, Shiraki M. Musculo-aponeurotic fibromatosis of the shoulder girdle (extra-abdominal desmoid). Analysis of thirty cases followed up over ten or more years. Cancer 1967; 20·1131–1140.

173. Fasching MC, Saleh J, Woods JE. Desmoid tumors of the head and neck. Am J Surg 1988; 156:327–331.

174. Klein WA, Miller HH, Anderson M, DeCosse JJ. The use of indomethacin, sulindac, and tamoxifen for the treatment of desmoid tumor associated with familial polyposis. Cancer 1987; 60:2863–2868.

175. Wilcken N, Tattersall MHN. Endocrine therapy for desmoid tumors. Cancer 1991; 68:1384–1388.

176. Lofti AM, Dozois RR, Gordon H. Mesenteric fibromatosis complicating familial adenomatous polyposis: Predisposing factors and results of treatment. Int J Colorect Dis 1989; 4:30–36.

177. Easter DW, Halasz NA. Recent trends in the management of desmoid tumors. Summary of 19 cases and review of the literature. Ann Surg 1989; 210:765–769.

178. Lopez R, Kemalyan N, Mosely HS, Dennis D, Vetto RM. Problems in diagnosis and management of desmoid tumors. Am J Surg 1990; 159:450–453.

179. Plukker JT, van Oort I, Vermey A, Molenaar I, Hoekstra HJ, Panders AK, Dolsma WV, Koops HS. Aggressive fibromatosis (non familial desmoid tumor): therapeutic problems and the role of adjuvant radiotherapy. Br J Surg 1995; 82:510–514.

180. Reitamo JJ, Scheinin TM, Hayry P. The desmoid syndrome: new aspects in the cause, pathogenesis and treatment of the desmoid tumor. Am J Surg 1986; 151:230–237.

181. Ballo MT, Zagars GK, Pollack A, Pisters PWT, Pollock RA. Desmoid tumor: prognostic factors and outcome after surgery, radiation therapy, or combined surgery and radiation therapy. J Clin Oncol 1999; 17:158–167.
182. Goy BW, Lee SP, Fu YS, Selch M, Eilber F. Treatment of unresected or partially resected desmoid tumors. Am J Clin Oncol 1998; 21:584–590.
183. Waddell WR, Gerner RE, Reich MP. Nonsteroidal antiinflammatory drugs and tamoxifen for desmoid tumors and carcinoma of the stomach. J Surg Oncol 1983; 22:197–211.
184. Sportiello DJ, Hoogerland DL. A recurrent pelvic desmoid tumor successfully treated with tamoxifen. Cancer 1991; 67:1443–1446.
185. Brooks MD, Ebbs SR, Colletta AA, Baum M. Desmoid tumors treated with triphenylethylenes. Eur J Cancer 1992; 28A:1014–1018.
186. Tsukada K, Church JM, Jagelman DG, Fazio VW, McGannon E, George CR, Schroeder T, Lavery I, Oakley J. Noncytotoxic drug therapy for intra-abdominal desmoid tumor in patients with familial adenomatous polyposis. Dis Colon Rectum 1992; 35:29–33.
187. Waddell WR, Kirsch WM. Testolactone, sulindac, warfarin, and vitamin K1 for unresectable desmoid tumors. Am J Surg 1991; 161:416–421.
188. Waddell WR, Gerner RE. Indomethacin and ascorbate inhibit desmoid tumors. J Surg Oncol 1980; 15:85–90.
189. Clark SK, Phillips RKS. Desmoids in familial adenomatous polyposis. Br J Surg 1996; 83:1494–1504.
190. Patel SR, Evans HL, Benjamin RS. Combination chemotherapy in adult desmoid tumors. Cancer 1993; 72:3244–3247.
191. Lynch HT, Fitzgibbons R, Chong S, Cavalieri J, Lynch J, Wallace F, Patel S. Use of doxorubicin and dacarbazine for the management of unresectable intra-abdominal desmoid tumors in Gardner's syndrome. Dis Colon Rectum 1994; 37:260–267.
192. Schnitzler M, Cohen Z, Blackstein M, Berk T, Gallinger S, Madlensky L, McLeod R. Chemotherapy for desmoid tumors in association with familial adenomatous polyposis. Dis Colon Rectum 1997; 40:798–801.
193. Tsukada K, Church J, Jagelman DG, Fazio VW, Lavery IC. Systemic cytotoxic chemotherapy and radiation therapy for desmoid in familial adenomatous polyposis. Dis Colon Rectum 1991; 34:1090–1092.
194. Hamilton L, Blackstein M, Berk T, McLeod RS, Gallinger S, Madlensky L, Cohen Z. Chemotherapy for desmoid tumors in association with familial polyposis: a report of three cases. CJS 1996; 39:247–252.
195. Weiss AJ, Lackman RD. Low-dose chemotherapy of desmoid tumors. Cancer 1989; 64:1192–1194.

19
Soft-Tissue Sarcoma in Childhood

Jay Greenberg
Inova Fairfax Hospital for Children
Fairfax, Virginia

I. RHABDOMYOSARCOMA

Soft-tissue sarcomas are the third most common extracranial solid tumor of childhood (1). This statement does not equate to relative frequency, as the incidence of cancer in children is significantly lower than in the adult population (2). The overall incidence of all cancers for patients 0–14 years of age according to the 1995 SEER Program data is approximately 12 per 100,000 children (3). Soft-tissue sarcomas account for 9 of every 1 million cancers in children, with a slight male-to-female preponderance (9.2:7.7) and, to a lesser extent, a white-to-black predominance (8.6:8.3). This correlates to only 250 new cases of rhabdomyosarcoma (RMS) diagnosed in this age group in the United States each year. The incidence of RMS is equal to or greater than that of all other forms of nonrhabdomyosarcomatous soft-tissue sarcoma (NRSTS) combined (3,4) (Table 1).

Furthermore, as will be discussed later in this chapter, significant biological and clinical variability exists within the two larger subgroups of this pathologic entity. The rarity of these tumors further confuses the ability to diagnose, treat, and summarize the overall approach to these tumors. Most centers treat only a few varied tumors each year, often with only one or two patients presenting to any one pediatric oncology team. This underscores the importance of all patients being treated with the combined expertise of multiple specialties, including medical pediatric oncology, pediatric general and orthopedic surgery, pediatric pathology, as well as pediatric radiology and radiation oncology. In fact, as of 1995, it was estimated that 94% of all children with cancer were seen at an institution that was a member of one of the two national collaborative study groups, i.e., the Children's Cancer Group (CCG) or the Pediatric Oncology Group (POG) (5). Unfortunately,

709

TABLE 1 Age-Specific and Age-Adjusted Incidence Rates per Million of Soft-Tissue Sarcomas by ICCC Group and Subcategory, All Races, Both Sexes, SEER 1975–1995

Tumor type	ICD-O-2 codes	<5	5–9	10–14	15–19	Total[a] <15	Total[a] <20
Soft-tissue sarcoma (IX)		10.6	8.0	10.3	15.5	9.6	11.0
Rhabdomyosarcoma							
Subcategory (IXa)		6.4	4.4	3.1	3.6	4.6	4.3
Embryonal rhabdomyosarcoma	8910	4.4	2.7	1.6	1.8	3.0	2.6
Alveolar rhabdomyosarcoma	8920	0.8	0.8	0.6	0.8	0.7	0.7
Rhabdomyosarcoma NOS, pleomorphic, etc.	8900–8902, 8991	1.2	0.9	0.9	0.9	1.0	1.0
Fibrosarcoma							
Subcategory (IXb)		2.0	1.5	3.5	6.0	2.3	3.2
Fibrosarcoma	8810	0.3	0.3	0.5	1.1	0.4	0.6
Infantile fibrosarcoma	8814	0.7	0.0	0.0	0.0	0.2	0.2
Malignant fibrous histiocytoma	8830	0.4	0.4	0.7	1.7	0.5	0.8
Dermatofibrosarcoma	8832	0.2	0.5	1.2	1.9	0.7	1.0
Malignant peripheral nerve sheath tumor	9540, 9560	0.2	0.2	0.8	1.2	0.4	0.6
Kaposi's sarcoma (IXc)	9140	0	0.1	0	0.2	0	0.1
Other specified soft-tissue sarcomas							
Subcategory (IXd)		1.3	1.3	2.5	4.0	1.8	2.3
Liposarcoma	8850, 8852, 8854	0.1	0.0	0.1	0.4	0.1	0.1
Leiomyosarcoma	8890, 8891	0.1	0.2	0.2	0.7	0.2	0.3
Malignant mesenchymoma	8990	0.3	0.2	0.1	0.1	0.2	0.2
Synovial sarcoma	9040, 9041, 9043	0.1	0.3	0.8	1.4	0.4	0.7
Hemangiosarcoma & malignant hemangioendothelioma	9120, 9130, 9133	0.1	0.1	0.1	0.3	0.1	0.2
Hemangiopericytoma, malignant	9150	0.2	0.1	0.1	0.1	0.1	0.1
Alveolar soft-part sarcoma	9581	0.1	0.1	0.1	0.1	0.1	0.1
Chondrosarcoma	9231, 9240	0.0	0.0	0.2	0.0	0.1	0.1
Ewing (extraosseous) family	9364, 9260	0.2	0.3	0.4	0.6	0.3	0.4
Unspecified subcategory (IXe)	8800–8804	0.8	0.7	1.1	1.7	0.9	1.1

[a] Adjusted to the 1970 U.S. standard population.

Source: Ries LAG, Smith MA, Gurney JG, et al, eds. Cancer Incidence and Survival Among Children and Adolescents: United States SEER Program 1975–1995, National Cancer Institute, SEER Program. NIH Pub. No. 99-4649, Bethesda, MD, 1999.

although the diseases often remain the same between patients younger than 15 years and those slightly older in late adolescence and early adulthood, the incidence of referral to pediatric centers significantly decreases from 100% in the 0- to 4-year range, to 84% in the 10- to 14-year range, and only 21% in the 15- to 19-year range (6). It soon became apparent that the diversity among this group of 250 patients with complex needs for individualized surgical and therapeutic approaches was beyond the scope of even the two national collaborative efforts. This gave rise to the Intergroup Rhabdomyosarcoma Study (IRS) groups I, II, III, IV, and V. As a result, almost 12 patients per month nationally are entered into national treatment protocols with centralization of data, pathology, and radiology review, and are treated according to a relatively small number of treatment regimens designed to further our knowledge of the treatment of these rare but devastating disorders. As of the year 2000, this national collaborative effort will have led to the coordination of almost all pediatric oncology investigations under the auspices of the newly formed consolidated collaboration, the Children's Oncology Group (COG), a single entity that will direct national research and therapeutic efforts in pediatric oncology.

A. Clinical Presentation and Diagnosis

Because both RMS and NRSTS can occur anywhere throughout the body, the presenting signs and symptoms are often diverse and confusing to the clinician. Superficial lesions often present as nontender hard swellings. Frequently, the family or patient targets insignificant trauma as the cause for swelling and any associated signs and symptoms that may be present. These include pain secondary to periosteal or neurovascular impingement, red or bluish skin discoloration, and, less frequently, tenderness to palpation. Sarcomas present as palpably very hard or "woody" tumors, and can be mistaken by the clinician as a bony growth or possibly inflamed lymph nodes. Metastatic bony involvement can cause significant pain, often awakening the patient from sleep. Patients rarely present with fever.

Organ dysfunction is specific to the site of origin of the tumor. In the head and neck region, 50% of sarcomas arise in parameningeal sites including the base of the skull and sinuses; 25% arise in the orbit; and 25% arise in other head or neck locations, such as jaw, scalp, oral pharynx, and soft tissues of the neck (7). Common physical complaints and findings include headache or sinus/nasal symptoms, proptosis, and ophthalmoplegia. Truncal tumors tend to cause symptoms only after significant growth, often resulting in delays in diagnosis. They commonly infiltrate into the chest wall and retroperitoneum and are often adjacent to major neurovascular structures.

Genitourinary tumors often present in prostatic and paratesticular or scrotal locations in boys and in the vaginal region in girls. Bladder tumors are common in both sexes and tend to grow intraluminally, in or near the trigone region (8).

These tumors may cause pain on urination or present with hematuria or urinary obstruction. Less common sites for RMS include the perineum, liver and biliary tract, brain, heart, and breast. The embryonal subtype is often located in the genitourinary region. As this subtype is more responsive to chemotherapy, surgical management should be delayed to allow for tumor shrinkage prior to surgery.

In most cases, significant pain with swelling lasting several weeks leads to referral for evaluation and biopsy. Delays in diagnosis are rare as in most cases significant pain associated with swelling that lasts for several weeks leads to discovery. A delay in diagnosis of several weeks, though unfortunate, often does not affect clinical prognosis and outcome.

Initial evaluation should include the history with specific attention to exclude trauma and possibly associated conditions for genetic predisposition to tumors. The physical examination, by concentrating on the region of presentation, should include a definitive search for regional and distant lymph node involvement. Extensive examination of all areas of the body will sometimes reveal subtle superficial subcutaneous metastatic lesions.

Magnetic resonance imaging (MRI) is the modality of choice for imaging of involved regions. While utilized frequently to image the head and neck as well as the extremities, MRI has seen wider application to make visible neoplasms located in the chest wall or retroperitoneum. It is especially useful in delineating infiltration of the vertebral column adjacent to retroperitoneal neoplasms. In addition, solitary lung nodules will often enhance with gadolinium-enhanced MRI. Positron emission tomography (PET) may also prove helpful in identifying small metastatic lesions.

Preliminary studies prior to biopsies should also include basic laboratory tests. Testing should include a complete blood count, blood urea nitrogen and creatinine, liver function tests, lactic dehydrogenase, and uric acid. While infrequently abnormal in sarcomas unless organ function is compromised, laboratory testing may lead one to consider alternative diagnoses that present in a fashion similar to that of RMS. In children, the most common entities presenting in a fashion similar to that of RMS include both Hodgkin's and non-Hodgkin's lymphoma, bone sarcomas including Ewing's sarcoma and primitive neuroectodermal tumor of bone (PNET), osteosarcoma, neuroblastoma, and even leukemia. Once a malignant diagnosis is suspected, a biopsy should be undertaken as soon as possible. Definitive staging studies are often best left until diagnostic tissue has been obtained, as patterns of tumor spread are often disease- and site-specific.

B. Pathology

The common embryonal nature of many pediatric malignancies results in a primitive, undifferentiated, poorly distinguished microscopic appearance. The cells often exhibit no specific pattern of organization, have little cytoplasm containing few if any unique cytoplasmic proteins or organelles, and share the light micro-scopic description that gives rise to the entity of pediatric cancers known as small round cell tumors of childhood (9,10). This category includes PNET of bone and soft tissue, Ewing's sarcoma, neuroblastoma, rhabdomyosarcoma, as well as un-differentiated sarcomas and non-Hodgkin's lymphoma. Because of the difficulty in differentiating among these tumors, multiple nonmorphologic techniques are required to accurately differentiate between them. Immunohistochemical analy-sis, immunophenotyping, cytogenetic and molecular genetic techniques including fluorescence in situ hybridization (FISH) and polymerase chain reaction (PCR), electronmicroscopy, and biochemical analysis may be necessary. For this reason, a protocol for the amount of tissue to be acquired, the obtaining of fresh tissue for cytogenetic and tissue cultures, flow cytometry, use of frozen tissue for molecular genetics and electromicroscopy, as well as having an adequate amount of tissue in fixative for standard pathologic techniques should be understood by the surgeon and pathologist prior to biopsy. Needle biopsy, while often adequate for adult car-cinomas, usually yields inadequate material for the required extensive analysis of these tumors and rarely is useful. Open biopsy, while sometimes complicating ul-timate surgical extirpation of the tumor, is preferred. This extensive protocol of tumor analysis often takes as long as 7–10 days to complete but is necessary prior to the initiation of treatment.

The single characteristic that identifies tumors as RMS is the detection of skeletal myogenic structures. Sometimes this can be seen on initial light mi-croscopic evaluation with the identification of cross-striations typical of skeletal muscle. Not infrequently, however, these primitive muscle elements are only par-tially aligned and thus not visually obvious. In this case, immunohistochemical staining for muscle proteins, including muscle-specific actin, myosin, desmin, myoglobin, and Z-band protein, is a useful adjunct (11,12). On occasion, the diag-nosis can only be obtained using electron microscopy to identify the very small musculoskeletal elements. In difficult cases, the diagnosis can only be inferred through genetic testing.

RMSs are divided into embryonal and alveolar subtypes. Traditionally the embryonal subtype is associated with a better prognosis than the alveolar RMS in similar stage tumors at any site. The 6-year survival rate is 60% for embryonal RMS, as compared with 25% for alveolar RMS (13). Specific subtypes are char-acterized by a particular pattern of presentation at a specific site and stage. For ex-ample, metastatic tumors of the extremity almost always are of the alveolar sub-type, while localized genitourinary or orbital tumors are more commonly of the embryonal subtype. Some investigators place little importance on this histologic subtype site specificity when considering clinical prognosis and outcome (4).

Embryonal RMS tends to have a stroma-rich, less dense appearance al-though many areas may have the small round cell appearance. Groupings of spindle cells may be interspersed throughout the tumor. Cytogenetic analysis in both subtypes suggests that increased DNA content measured by flow cytometry or an increased DNA index (1.1–1.8 times the normal diploid amount of DNA) has a better prognosis for unknown reasons (14). Conversely, tumors that have normal DNA content or a DNA index equal to 1.0, while not necessarily meaning that there are no cytogenetic abnormalities such as translocations, small additions, or deletions of DNA, have a worse prognosis (15).

Molecular analysis has demonstrated a unique modification at the 11p15 locus. This region first attracted attention as a site of abnormality in the Beckwith-Wiedemann syndrome, a fetal overgrowth syndrome characterized by organomegaly, macroglossia, and unusual linear creases (16). This syndrome is associated with Wilms' tumor and hepatoblastoma (16,17). The association of the insulin-like growth factor II (*IGFII*) gene at this region suggests that this protein plays a role in the deregulation of growth in both alveolar and embryonal RMS (18,19). The common presence of a molecular abnormality at the 11p15 locus has lead to frequent use of PCR analysis for the rapid identification of changes in this region even in paraffin-embedded sections (18). A unique modification of this 11p15 terminal was identified, known as loss of heterozygosity (LOH) (20). This means that the maternal allele, which in normal cell function is turned off anyway, is replaced with two identical paternal alleles in these patients. How or why this leads to overexpression is less well understood, but the result is unregulated growth of the myoblast cells (21). Other molecular abnormalities have been identified with some frequency in fresh tumors as well as in RMS cell lines.

C. Staging

For historical reasons, a complex staging system has evolved to direct the appropriate therapy for particular RMS tumors. Initially, treatment was intensified according to the extent of surgical resection. This resulted in the Intergroup Rhabdomyosarcoma Clinical Grouping Classification (22) (Table 2). However, it soon became apparent that a pretreatment staging classification, based on biopsy and pretreatment size determined by radiographic imaging, would reduce differences in the categorization of these tumors based on the aggressiveness and skills of the treating team. Furthermore, the site of the presenting tumors often precluded complete surgical resection without a corresponding worsening of prognosis. Thus, patients began to be staged according to a second paradigm, i.e., the TNM Pretreatment Staging Classification (22). In this staging system, tumor size (≤5 cm or >5 cm), site (orbit–excluding parameningeal, bladder/prostate, GU–other, and trunk), and finally the presence of distant disease is used to characterize the patient preoperatively. Obviously, it is possible for a patient to have an extensive tumor totally resected, making him or her potentially a stage 2 or 3 group I patient.

Finally, the IRS V attempted to combine these classification systems with the biological variables that tumors at particular sites, such as orbital or genitourinary nonbladder or prostate, present regardless of extent of resection. Accord-

TABLE 2   Intergroup Rhabdomyosarcoma Clinical Grouping Classification

Group	Characteristics
I	Localized disease, completely resected
II	Total gross resection with evidence of regional spread
	(A) This includes tumors with microscopic residual, resected residual nodes positive
III	Incomplete resection with gross residual disease
	(A) After biopsy only
	(B) More than microscopic residual post attempt at resection
IV	Distant metastatic disease (excluding regional lymph nodes and adjacent organ infiltration)
	(A) Includes involvement of lung, liver, bone, bone marrow, brain, distant lymph nodes
	(B) Cellular involvement in cerebrospinal fluid, pleural effusion, or abdominal ascites with or without implants on pleural or peritoneal surfaces

Source: Lawrence W, Gehan EA, Hays DM, et al. Prognostic significance of staging factors of the UICC staging system in childhood rhabdomyosarcoma: a report from the Intergroup Rhabdomyosarcoma Study (IRS–II). J Clin Oncol 1987; 5:46–54.

ingly, this series of treatment protocols were divided according to expected outcome, with low-risk, intermediate-risk, and high-risk patients separated according to surgical stage, clinical group, histologic features, and tumor site (22) (Table 3).

D. Treatment

As stated above, the approach to treatment of these tumors has progressed in a step-wise fashion using the prospective study protocols of the IRS I–V (24–26). The use of combined modality therapy in both the adjuvant and neo-adjuvant setting has resulted in improvement of long-term survival from 25% in 1970 to approximately 70% at this time (25). Optimal treatment includes complete or wide surgical excision, with tumor-free margins of normal tissue. This may not be obtainable for a number of anatomical reasons. Depending on the site of presentation, certain lesions located in the head and neck or genitourinary regions may not be amenable to wide excision without an acceptable loss of function.

In cases where wide margins have not been achieved, surgical reexcision prior to the initiation of chemotherapy or radiotherapy treatments is necessary when possible. First, initially only a biopsy may have been undertaken in an attempt to establish the diagnosis. Second, in lesions initially thought to be benign, uncertainty as to adequacy of surgical margins often complicates the optimal postsurgical result prior to adjuvant therapies. In these situations, it is best to initiate a second procedure if a wide excision is thought possible.

TABLE 3 Intergroup Rhabdomyosarcoma Study V Classification

Risk level	
Low	All stage 1/group I patients
Intermediate	Embryonal histology—stage 2 or 3, group III
	stage 4, group IV age <10
	Alveolar or undifferentiated sarcoma
	Stage 1, group II or III (nonorbit)
	Stage 2, group II or III
	Stage 3, group I, II, or III
	Parameningeal all histology—stage 4, group IV
High	All other stage 4, group IV patients

Source: Lawrence W, Gehan EA, Hays DM, et al. Prognostic significance of staging factors of the UICC staging system in childhood rhabdomyosarcoma: a report from the Intergroup Rhabdomyosarcoma Study (IRS–II). J Clin Oncol 1987; 5:46–54.

Delayed second or even subsequent opportunities to surgically resect residual disease are part of most treatment protocols. These delayed attempts at resection are performed after an initial series of therapies if there has been good response and total excision is considered feasible. Complete excision of tumor at this time may significantly decrease or obviate the need for adjuvant radiotherapy. This is preferable because of the significant morbidity associated with irradiation in young children.

As discussed elsewhere in this chapter, specific surgical considerations in the approach to a biopsy or gross resection in this group of highly malignant tumors is very site-specific. Tumors such as orbital, nonparameningeal head and neck, or genitourinary (non-bladder or prostate) are considered to have a favorable outcome. In these, less aggressive surgical procedures are appropriate, even if total gross excision is not achieved. Unfavorable sites include extremity, trunk, parameningeal head and neck, and all other genitourinary sites. Unfortunately, total resection of these lesions often results in significant functional loss. In these patients, both radiotherapy and chemotherapy in the neoadjuvant setting often preserves the greatest function.

Finally, it should be emphasized that lymph node examination is an essential part of the staging procedure in patients with soft-tissue sarcomas. For extremity lesions, axillary dissection with preservation of the pectoral muscles in the upper extremity is suggested, and in the lower extremity inguinal node sampling is strongly recommended. Obvious clinically involved nodes should be examined proximal to distal. It must be emphasized that node examination is critical for determining therapy only and is not in itself therapeutic. In obvious stage IV patients, extensive sampling is discouraged, but knowledge of regional involvement is important for radiation therapy planning.

Pulmonary metastatic disease may exist on imaging studies through weeks 12–16 of therapy, even as other sites of involvement have responded completely. If multiple lesions persist or if this is the only site of metastatic disease at presentation, biopsy or excision of these pulmonary lesions is appropriate. Persistent disease should ultimately be resected when possible. This can be done either by unilateral staged procedures or by medial sternotomy when indicated.

While RMS is managed with adjuvant chemotherapy primarily to lessen the likelihood of later distant metastases, local recurrence has been reported in up to 75% of patients with inadequate excision (23). IRS I proved that radiation therapy was necessary for clinical group I patients (24). However, because of poor local control in successive studies, IRS III added radiation to all patients except favorable histology group I patients, with the minimum necessary dose in the range 4000–5000 cGy (25,73).

Recent advances in radiotherapy techniques include the use of three-dimensional conformal field therapy planning and the use of modified energy techniques, including proton beam therapy. While these recent advances have not been specifically addressed in the most recent IRS V protocols, they can be expected to significantly improve local control while limiting the long-term side effects of radiotherapy.

More than 2700 patients with RMS, undifferentiated sarcoma, and extraosseous Ewing's sarcoma were treated on the IRS I–III (25–27). These studies have resulted in the utilization of very exact treatment regimen for these diverse groups of tumors. Currently, as discussed under staging, IRS V protocol approaches are separated into favorable, intermediate, and unfavorable disease protocols.

Favorable patients, as defined previously, have an 80–95% disease survival (25,27,28). Therefore, it was felt appropriate to limit treatment in most of these patients to vincristine and actinomycin D. This regimen of antimetabolites excludes high–dose cyclophosphamide, which adds significantly to morbidity and mortality. The immediate hematologic toxicity of cyclophosphamide is only one concern, as the long-term morbidity also is significant (29). Radiation therapy in group I patients with embryonal histology is also considered unnecessary (73).

The intermediate disease risk study is a randomized study testing the addition of a new effective agent, topotecan, to the intensified VAC regimen (30,31). The expected outcome in these patients is for progress-free survival of 50–79% after 3 years (32). The IRS V high-risk disease treatment protocol for metastatic disease will continue to investigate new agents as they become available. This is considered essential, as progress has been limited in this group of patients, improving from 20% in IRS I to only 32% in IRS IV (26,27,32).

Despite the advances in therapy based on IRS I–V, 30% of patients will ultimately relapse, with 50–95% of these patients dying of progressive disease (74). Upon relapse the median time until progression to death was only 0.8 year. Factors impacting disease course after relapse include histology, with the alveolar subtype having only a 5% 5-year disease-free survival. Thus, new therapies, in-

cluding both newer chemotherapeutic agents and newer radiation therapy techniques, are needed if we are to continue making progress in the treatment of these
patients.

II. NONRHABDOMYOSARCOMATOUS
SOFT-TISSUE SARCOMAS

Of the 850–900 soft-tissue sarcomas diagnosed each year, approximately 350 are
RMSs (3). This subgroup tends to occur in slightly younger children, accounting
for slightly more than 50% of soft-tissue sarcomas in children less than 15 years
of age (Fig. 1). Nonrhabdomyosarcomatous soft-tissue sarcomas are considered a
group of disorders whose tissue of origin derives from connective tissue. The
group consists of numerous entities, each of which is a rare tumor with a low incidence. Since these neoplasms arise from connective tissue, they can arise anywhere in the body.

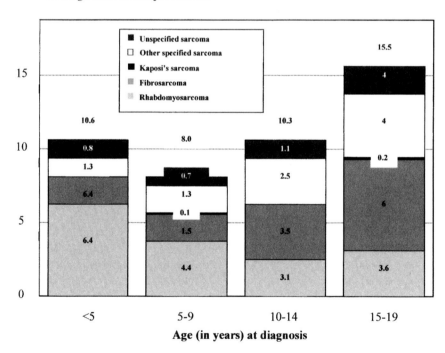

FIG. 1   Soft-tissue sarcoma age-specific incidence rates by ICCC subcategory, all races,
both sexes, SEER, 1975–1995.

The natural history is closely related to the specific histologic features, with age, site, microscopic characteristics, and degree of metastatic spread having a strong impact on the prognosis and therapy (33,34). Much of the literature and recommendations for therapy comes from the study of soft-tissue sarcoma in adults, in whom these tumors are slightly more common (35–37). The rarity of these tumors in children makes any meaningful recommendations from the literature difficult. Fortunately, the results in children seem to be more promising (38). Therefore, caution must be exercised not to merely apply the experience in adults to children with similar pathologic entities (33,34,39,40). This distinction is greatest in infants where histology and microscopic appearance often belies the frequently excellent prognosis obtained with adequate surgery as the only therapy (33,39). Unfortunately, series restricted to older children and adolescents tend to follow the results of studies in adult patients (35,41). As is the case with patients diagnosed with RMS, children with NRSTS are best treated at centers with multidisciplinary teams of pediatric general surgeons, pathologists, radiation therapists, and pediatric oncologists with experience in handling these rare tumors. Furthermore, chemotherapy when appropriate is best delivered in the context of a national collaborative therapeutic study.

A. Histology

The International Classification of Childhood Cancer (ICCC) has four subcategories of NRSTS (42). These are fibrosarcoma, malignant nerve sheath tumors (group IXb); Kaposi's sarcoma (group IXc); the other "specified" soft-tissue sarcomas (group IXd), including synovial sarcoma, tumors of blood vessels (e.g., hemangiosarcoma and malignant hemangiopericytoma), myomatous malignancies including alveolar soft-part sarcoma, and malignant mesenchymal, lipomatous cancers, extraosseous Ewing's sarcoma, and PNET; and "unspecified" soft-tissue sarcoma (group IXe). Within each subgroup are a large number of variations and mixed cellular tumors. For example, the fibrosarcoma subcategory includes dermatofibrosarcoma, malignant fibrous histiocytoma, fibrosarcoma, infantile fibrosarcoma, and malignant peripheral nerve sheath tumors. The relative rarity of these tumors and the variability of their histologic appearance leads to significant difficulty in making a definitive diagnosis. As discussed previously regarding RMS, the definitive diagnosis is often dependent on immunohistochemic stains for cellular components, electron microscopy, cytogenetic and sometimes even molecular genetic analysis. For this reason, if soft-tissue sarcoma is entertained as a diagnosis, prior pathologic consultation is essential prior to biopsy.

B. Genetics

As with RMS, NRSTS has a strong association with known genetic mechanisms of carcinogenesis. Malignant peripheral nerve sheath tumor (MPNST) and von

Recklinghausen's disease (also called neurofibromatous type 1) both have frequent abnormalities at the 17q11.2 region (43). The tumor suppressor p53 locus is very close to this region. This is similar to rhabdomyosarcoma, where the LOH of the tumor suppressor function regulated by the p53 gene seems to play a significant role in the initiation of sarcomas (19,20).

NRSTS is also frequently seen in families diagnosed with the Li-Fraumeni familial cancer syndrome (44,45). Furthermore, they have been reported as second cancers in individuals with this disorder and in others who have received radiation therapy as previous therapy for earlier cancers (46), including retinoblastoma (47).

Similarly, cytogenetic associations may help explain differences in behavior frequently seen based on age of presentation. Infantile fibrosarcomas associated with trisomy 11 are histologically similar to fibrosarcomas in adults, which rarely have this cytogenetic abnormality (48). A second genetic association common to both infantile fibrosarcoma and congenital mesoblastic nephroma, another infantile tumor with a benign natural history, is t(12;15)(p13;q25) and is associated with *ETV6-NTK3* gene fusion (49). This entity of infantile fibrosarcoma has a much more benign natural history than the adult counterpart. Even high-grade lesions under the microscope rarely metastasize. Treatment is therefore limited to complete surgical excision, resulting in a high rate of cure (50).

Synovial sarcoma is a soft-tissue sarcoma associated with fusing the *SYT* gene on chromosome 18 with the *SSX-1* or *SSX-2* gene on the X chromosome (51). PNETs have either t(11;22) or t(21;22), both involving the *EWS* gene on chromosome 22. A complete list of associated molecular associations with soft-tissue sarcomas is given in Table 4 (3).

C. Epidemiology

Most of the histologic subtypes of NRSTS in childhood occur most commonly in teenagers. Exceptions are infantile fibrosarcoma, malignant hemangiopericytoma, and malignant mesenchyoma, which are more common in the first 5 years of life. Congenital tumors in the first year of life should be considered separately with regard to epidemiology (33,34,50). The overall incidence is 15.2 cases per million children (3). Forty percent of these are RMS. While NRSTSs make up the majority of these cases, most of these comprise infantile fibrosarcoma, malignant hemangiopericytoma, and malignant mesenchymoma (3).

D. Clinical Presentation

As with RMS, NRSTS presents as a painless asymptomatic tumor. When presenting superficially, the patient often comes to medical attention quickly after a relatively short period of observation. The rate of growth of this diverse tumor type

TABLE 4 Molecular Characterization of Soft-Tissue Sarcomas

Diagnosis	Chromosomal abnormality	Genes involved
Rhabdomyosarcoma, embryonal	Hyperdiploidy, and loss of heterozygosity at 11p15	Unidentified gene at chromosome band 11p15
Rhabdomyosarcoma, alveolar	t(2;13) or t(1;13)	*FKHR* on chromosome 13 and *PAX3* (chromosome 2) or *PAX7* (chromosome 1)
Infantile fibrosarcoma	t(12;15)	*TEL* (*ETV6*) gene on chromosome 12 and *NTRK3* (*TRKC*) on chromosome 15.
Dermatofibrosarcoma protuberans	t(17;22)	Platelet-derived growth factor (*PDGFB*) gene chromosome 17 and collagen type I α1 (*COL1A1*) chromosome 22
Malignant peripheral nerve sheath tumors (also known as neurofibrosarcomas and malignant schwannomas)	Abnormalities of chromosome 17	Neurofibromatosis 1 (*NF1*)
Synovial sarcoma	t(X;18)	*SYT* on chromosome 18 and *SSX-1* or *SSX-2* on the X chromosome
Liposarcoma	t(12;16)	*FUS* gene on chromosome 16 and *CHOP* gene on chromosome 12
Chondrosarcoma, myxoid	t(9;22)	*EWS* gene on chromosome 22 (also associated with Ewing's sarcoma) and *TEC* gene chromosome 9
Extraosseous Ewing's sarcoma and peripheral primitive neuroectodermal tumor (PNET)chr 11	t(11;22)	*EWS* gene on chromosome 22 and *FLI* gene on chr 11
Alveolar soft-part sarcoma	t(X;17)	Unidentified gene at chromosome band 17q25

Source: Ries LAG, Smith MA, Gurney JG, et al, eds. Cancer Incidence and Survival Among Children and Adolescents: United States SEER Program 1975–1995, National Cancer Institute, SEER Program. NIH Pub. No. 99-4649, Bethesda, MD, 1999.

varies greatly, with some tumors presenting after much longer periods of observation. In contrast, abdominal tumors present relatively late and therefore are large and often extremely difficult to excise surgically. Symptoms are due to obstruction of the gastrointestinal or genitourinary tract or nerve impingement. Rarely, systemic symptoms, such as weight loss or fever, are seen with very large tumors.

Biological variables, such as age of presentation, tumor invasiveness, and mitotic rate, are critical in determining therapeutic approach (52). The surgical staging system proposed by the Musculoskeletal Tumor Society has historically been used in adult studies. A tumor is judged to be either low grade (grade 1) or high grade (grade 2), depending on the potential of the lesion to metastasize (53). There is some consideration as to the histologic subtype because some lesions, as synovial sarcoma, are always considered to be high grade. Metastatic disease is classified as grade 3. In one study showing a lack of benefit of chemotherapy for localized tumors, 3-year disease-free survival equaled 92% for histologic grades 2 and 1 versus 75% for grade 3 (54).

The significant variation of histologic origin of tumor has lead to a much more tissue-dependent staging system in clinical use by the POG in its current clinical study (7). Grade 1 tumors include well-differentiated fibrous tumors as well as those of fat origin. Less well-differentiated tumors of any histology showing necrosis, frequent mitoses, and nuclear atypia are considered the higher grade 2. Grade 3 tumors include pleomorphic liposarcoma, mesenchymal chondrosarcoma, extraskeletal osteogenic sarcoma, alveolar soft-part sarcoma, and any other sarcoma not included in the grade 1 grouping above, with the malignant microscopic characteristics of more than 15% necrosis and/or more than 5 mitoses per 10 high-power fields (54).

E. Therapy

Wide surgical excision is the treatment of choice in NRSTS (55,56). Surgical resection followed by radiation therapy results in local control in 80% of nonmetastatic tumors (57–59), with 5-year disease-free survival of greater than 66%. In one retrospective series at St. Jude's Hospital (55), 154 patients over three decades were analyzed according to prognostic factors. The most common histologies were synovial sarcoma ($N = 36$), malignant fibrous histiocytoma ($N = 25$), and neurofibrosarcoma ($N = 25$). Seventy percent of these tumors were in the trunk and lower extremities. The extent of disease at presentation was extremely significant in determining outcome. Almost 80% of patients with localized disease survived 5 years. Metastatic disease existed at presentation in 28% of patients. These particular patients had a very poor prognosis, with only 25% surviving at 2 years and 5% surviving at 5 years (56).

Early studies have shown no advantage to adjuvant chemotherapy after surgical excision with or without radiotherapy. The POG randomized 83 of these patients with clinical stage I and II disease, between observation alone, and treatment with vincristine, actinomycin, cyclophosphamide, and doxorubicin (53). The 3-year disease-free survival was 76% and 74%, respectively. Thus, similar to the adult experience, in resectable tumors with adequate margins no other therapy may be necessary. Similar to the discussion of RMS, if the margin is in question it is prudent, if at all possible, to reexplore the patient in an effort to ensure total excision with as wide a margin as possible.

The role of adjuvant radiation therapy in situations involving limited margins is less controversial. In the 60% of NRSTSs occurring in nonextremity sites, though surgical margin may be adequate, most centers utilize adjuvant radiation therapy (60,61). Unfortunately, the comparatively high recommended tumor dose of 50–60 Gy causes significant long-term dysfunction in younger patients. Furthermore, depending on site, surrounding radiosensitive structures may further limit the radiotherapy dose given. Studies combing intraoperative brachytherapy and reduced postoperative external-beam irradiation have so far failed to show a significant improvement in long-term disease-free control (62). It remains to be seen whether the more recent advances in radiotherapy, using three-dimensional conformal fields, with energy modulation allowing for the more adequate sparing of radiosensitive organs, will increase the role of radiation therapy in these situations.

Currently, chemotherapy is being recommended only in initially nonresectable tumors, in the hope that they can then be converted to resectable tumors. Unresectable or metastatic NRSTSs account for 20% of these cases at presentation (55). In this group, the 2-year survival rate was only 20%, whereas the 5-year survival was a dismal 5% (56). Modest single-agent activity has been shown for a number of agents. Doxorubicin produced the highest response rate of greater than 25%, with a significant dose–response effect at higher doses of 60–75 mg/m^2 every 3–4 weeks (56,63). Ifosfamide has also demonstrated extensive activity of 24% response in the initial treatment of adults with metastatic tumor (64), and 45% when combined with doxorubicin (65). Currently, the POG has an ongoing study using vincristine, ifosfamide, and doxorubicin with growth factor support, in patients with initially unresectable or metastatic lesions. The hope is that such lesions will be converted to fully resectable status after 3–6 courses of chemotherapy with or without adjuvant radiation therapy, using an aggressive surgical approach including pulmonary mestatectomy. Unfortunately, the small numbers of patients accrued so far make it unlikely that this study will definitively answer this question.

As therapy currently is practiced, there is in fact little to be done for extensive, nonresectable or metastatic tumors. It remains to be seen whether new classes of agents, such as the antiangiogenic agents, or recent advances in three-dimensional conformal field proton-beam therapy will make a difference in these patients. Again, because of the small numbers of these patients, it is imperative that all therapies be studied in collaborative research protocols with sufficient power to provide the much needed answers to these questions.

F. Posttherapy Evaluation

Long-term evaluation by an oncology team is essential after the initial therapy in these patients. The early emphasis is to screen for tumor recurrence. Knowledge of the natural history and pattern of spread is essential to screen in a meaningful way. Long-term follow-up evaluation is just as important to screen for late effects of treatment interventions, functional disabilities, and second malignancies in this population. Finally, the psychosocial impact of the therapy of childhood cancer affects almost all patients at some time in this process.

In the first posttreatment year, follow-up is recommended every 2 months, with a physical exam, complete blood count, chemistries, urinalysis, chest x-rays alternating with CT scans of the chest as screening procedures for chest recurrence. The current recommendation is to change to an every-third-month evaluation in the second and third year post therapy, with CT scans every 6 months. In years 4 and 5, CT scans are considered optional, although chest x-rays should be taken every 6–12 months.

Again, late effects are both therapy- and site-specific. A recent report of patients surviving head and neck tumors treated as part of IRS II and III reported that a number of patients had one or more problems recorded in long-term follow-up exams (66). Linear growth had decreased in 48% of patients, and 19% were actually receiving growth hormone injections. Hypoplasia and cranial asymmetry were reported in 33% of patients, with 13 children requiring reconstructive surgery. Other problems include impaired dentition, cataracts, and hearing and learning problems (67). Finally, 4 of the 213 patients followed developed second malignancies (66,68).

Functional and cosmetic consequences involving bone, muscle, and soft tissue are reported in up to one third of all childhood cancer survivors (69). These include scoliosis, atrophy, hypoplasia, avascular necrosis, and significant osteoporosis (70). The high doses of radiation employed in patients requiring this modality leads to significant long-term morbidity in affected areas.

Surveillance of cardiac function is essential in patients who have received anthracyclines and/or cardiac irradiation as part of their therapy. In a series of 200 patients treated at the Memorial Sloan-Kettering Hospital, 23% had abnormalities on echocardiogram at a median of 7 years after therapy (71). Cardiology consultation is encouraged prior to the start of vigorous exercise routines, pregnancy, or general anesthesia. Additional evaluations are recommended every 3–5 years until adulthood (72).

In summary, the therapy of soft-tissue sarcoma in childhood represents specific individualized treatments based on several significant prognostic variables.

These include histology, tumor site, extent of disease (group), and disease stage prior to attempted surgical excision. Currently, continued improvement in prognosis seems limited by the need for the development of new therapies, both chemotherapeutic and in radiation therapy. The clinical investigation of these newer approaches is hampered by the relative rarity of these tumors. Hopefully, increased collaborative effort by all clinicians caring for patients with this group of disorders will lead to significant improved outcomes in the future.

REFERENCES

1. Kramer S, Meadows AT, Jarrett P, et al. Incidence of childhood cancer: experience of a decade in a population-based registry. J Natl Cancer Inst 1983;70:49.
2. Robison LL, Courney JG, et al. Incidence of cancer in children in the United States. Sex-, race-, and 1 year age-specific rates by histologic type. Cancer 1995;75:2186.
3. Ries LAG, Smith MA, Gurney JG, et al. (eds). Cancer Incidence and Survival among Children and Adolescents: United States SEER Program 1975–1995, National Cancer Institute, SEER Program. NIH Pub. No. 99-4649. Bethesda, MD, 1999.
4. Wexler LH, Helman LJ. Rhabdomyosarcoma and the Undifferentiated sarcomas. In: Pizzo PA, Poplack DG, eds. Principles and Practice of Pediatric Oncology. Philadelphia: Lippincott-Raven, 1997, pp. 799–829.
5. Robison LL. General principles of the epidemiology of childhood cancer. In: Pizzo P, Poplack D, eds. Principles and Practice of Childhood Oncology, 3rd ed. Philadelphia: Lippincott-Raven, 1997.
6. Ross JA, Severson RK, Pollock BH, Robison LL. Childhood cancer in the United States: a geographical analysis of cases from the pediatric cooperative clinical trials groups. Cancer 1995; 77–201.
7. Month SR, Raney RB. Rhabdomyosarcoma of the head and neck in children: the experience at the Children's Hospital of Philadelphia. Med Pediatr Oncol 1986; 14:288.
8. Shapiro E, Strother D. Pediatric genitourinary rhabdomyosarcoma. J Urol 1992; 148:1761.
9. Pritchard DJ. Small round cell tumors. Orthop Clin North Am 1989;20:367.
10. Triche TJ. Diagnosis of small round cell tumors of childhood. Bull Cancer (Paris) 1988; 75:297.
11. Parham DM, Webber B, Holt H, et al. Immunohistochemical study of childhood rhabdomyosarcomas and related neoplasms. Cancer 1991; 67:3072.
12. Dodd S, Malone M, Mcculloch W. Rhabdomyosarcoma in children: a histological and immunohistological study of 59 cases. J Pathol 1989; 158:13.
13. Tsokos M, Webber BL, Parham DM, et al. Rhabdomyosarcoma: a new classification scheme related to prognosis. Arch Pathol Lab Med 1992; 116:847.
14. Shapiro DN, Parham DM, Douglas EC, et al. Relationship of tumor cell ploidy to histologic subtype and treatment outcome in children and adolescents with unresectable rhabdomyosarcoma. J Clin Oncol 1991; 9:159.
15. Pappo AS, Crist WM, Kuttesch J, et al. Tumor cell DNA content predicts outcome in children and adolescents with clinical group III embryonal rhabdomyosarcoma. The

Intergroup Rhabdomyosarcoma Study Committee of the Children's Cancer Group and the Pediatric Oncology Group. J Clin Oncol 1993; 11:1901.

16. Elliott M, Bayly R, Cole T, et al. Clinical features and natural history of the Beckwith-Wiedemann syndrome: presentation of 74 new cases. Clin Genet 1994; 46:168.

17. Bonaiti-Pellie C, Chompret A, Tournade MF, et al. Genetics and epidemiology of Wilms' tumor: the French Wilms' tumor study. Med Pediatr Oncol 1992; 20: 284.

18. Stratton MR, Fisher C, Gusterson BA, et al. Detection of point mutations in N-ras and K-ras genes of human embryonal rhabdomyosarcoma using oligonucleotide probes and the polymerase chain reaction. Cancer Res 1989; 49:6324.

19. El-Badry OM, Minniti C, Kohn EC, et al. Insulin-like growth factor II acts as an autocrine growth factor and motility factor in human rhabdomyosarcoma tumors. Cell Growth Differ 1990; 1:325.

20. Scrable H, Witte D, Shimada H, et al. Molecular differential pathology of rhabdomyosarcoma. Genes Chrom Cancer 1989; 1:23.

21. Feinberg AP. Genomic imprinting and gene activation in cancer. Nat Genet 1993; 4:110.

22. Lawrence W, Gehan EA, Hays DM. Et al. Prognostic significance of staging factors of the UICC staging system in childhood rhabdomyosarcoma: a report from the Intergroup Rhabdomyosarcoma Study (IRS-II). J Clin Oncol 1987; 5:46–54.

23. Suit HD, Russell WO, Martin RG. Management of patients with sarcoma of the soft tissue in an extremity. Cancer 1973; 31:1247.

24. Heyn RM, Holland R, Newton WA JR, et al. The role of combined chemotherapy in the treatment of rhabdomyosarcoma in children. Cancer 1974; 34:2128.

25. Crist W, Gehan EA, Ragab AH, et al. The Third Intergroup Rhabdomyosarcoma Study. J Clin Oncol 1995; 13:610.

26. Mauer HM, Beltangady M, Gehan EA, et al. The Intergroup Rhabdomyosarcoma Study—I: a final report. Cancer 1988; 61:209.

27. Mauer HM, Gehan EA, Beltangady M, et al. The Intergroup Rhabdomyosarcoma Study—II. Cancer 1993; 71:1904.

28. Donaldson SS. The value of adjuvant chemotherapy in the management of sarcomas in children. Cancer 1983; 55:2417.

29. Goldberg MH, Antin JH, Guison EC. Cyclophosphamide cardiotoxicity: an analysis of dosing as a risk factor. Blood 1986; 68:1114–1118.

30. Anderson JR, Coccia P. Is more better? Dose intensification in neuroblastoma. J Clin Oncol 1996; 9:902.

31. Houghton P, Cheshire P, Myers L, et al. Evaluation of 9-dimethylaminomethyl-10-hydroxy camptothecin against xenographs derived from adult and childhood tumors. Cancer Chemther Pharmacol 1992; 31:229.

32. Mauer H, Gehan EA, Crist W, et al. The Intergroup Rhabdomyosarcoma Study (IRS)—III: a preliminary report of over-all outcome. Proc. Am Soc Clin Oncol 1989; 8:296.

33. Salloum E, Flamant F, Caillaud JM, et al. Diagnostic and therapeutic problems of soft tissue sarcoma other than rhabdomyosarcoma in infants under 1 year of age: a clinicopathologic study of 34 cases treated at the Institut Gustave-Roussy. Med Pediatr Oncol 1990; 18:37.

34. Horowitz MD, Pratt CB, Webber BI, et al. Therapy of childhood soft tissue sarcomas other than rhabdomyosarcoma: a review of 62 cases treated at a single institution. J Clin Oncol 1986; 4:559.

35. Skene AI, Barr L, Robinson M, et al. Adult type (nonembryonal) soft tissue sarcomas in childhood. Med Pediatr Oncol 1993; 21:645.

36. Edmonson JH. Systemic chemotherapy following complete excision of non-osseous sarcomas: Mayo Clinic experience. Cancer Treat Symp 1985; 3:89.

37. Elias A, Ryan L, Sulkes A, et al. Response to mesna, doxorubicin, ifosfamide, and dacarbazine in 108 patients with metastatic or unresectable sarcoma and no prior chemotherapy. J Clin Oncol 1987; 7:1208.

38. Miser JS, Triche TJ, Kinsella TJ, Pritchard DJ. Other soft tissue sarcomas of childhood. In: Pizzo P, Poplack D, eds. Principles and Practice of Pediatric Oncology, 3rd ed. Philadelphia: Lippincott-Raven, 1997.

39. Cheung E, Enzinger FM. Infantile fibrosarcoma. Cancer 1976; 38:729.

40. Campbell AN, Chan HS, O'Brien A, et al. Malignant tumors in the neonate. Arch Dis Child 1987; 62:19.

41. Dillon P, Mauer H, Jenkins J, et al. A prospective study of non-rhabdomyosarcoma soft tissue sarcomas in the pediatric age group. J Pediatr Surg 1992; 27:241.

42. Kramarova E, Stiller CA. The international classification of childhood cancer. Int J Cancer 1996; 68:759–765.

43. Glover TW, Stein CK, Legius E, et al. Molecular and cytogenetic analysis of tumors in von Recklinghausen neurofibroatosis. Genes Chrom Cancer 1991; 3:62.

44. Li FB, Fraumeni JF Jr. Rhabdomyosarcoma in children: epidemiologic study and identification of a familial cancer syndrome. J Natl Cancer Inst 1969; 43:1365.

45. Li FB, Fraumeni JF Jr. Prospective study of a family cancer syndrome. JAMA 1982; 247:2692.

46. Laskin WB, Silverman TA, Enzinger FA. Post-radiation soft tissue sarcomas: an analysis of 53 cases. Cancer 1988; 62:2330.

47. Ruymann FB, Grufferman S. Introduction and epidemiology of soft tissue sarcomas. In: Maurer HM, Ruymann FB, Pochedly C, eds. Rhabdomyosarcoma and Related Tumors in Children and Adolescents. Boca Raton, FL: CRC Press, 1993.

48. Bernstein R, Zeltzer PM, Lin F, et al. Trisomy 11 and other non-random trisomies in congenital fibrosarcoma. Cancer Genet Cytogenet 1994; 78:82.

49. Knezevich SR, Garnett MJ, Pysher TJ, et al. ETV6-NTRK3 gene fusions and trisomy 11 establish a histologic link between mesoblastic nephroma and congenital fibrosarcoma. Cancer Res 1998; 58:5046–5048.

50. Soule EH, Prichard DJ. Fibrosarcoma of infants and children: a review of 110 cases. Cancer 1977; 40:1711.

51. Kawai A, Woodruff J, Heasley JH, et al. SYT-SSX gene fusion as a determinant of morphology and prognosis in synovial cell sarcoma. N Engl J Med 1998; 338:153–160.

52. Dillon P, Maurer H, Jenkins J, et al. Prospective study of non-rhabdomyosarcoma soft tissue sarcoma in the pediatric age group. J Pediatr Surg 1992; 27:241.

53. Parham DM, Webber BL, Jenkins JJ, et al. Nonrhabdomyosarcomatous soft tissue sarcomas of childhood: formulation of a simplified system for grading. Mod Pathol 1995; 8:705–710.

54. Jenkins JJ, Parham DM, Webber BL, et al. Prognostic value of grading in pediatric nonrhabdomyosarcomatous soft tissue sarcomas (PNRSTS). Mod Pathol 1993; 6: 126.

55. Rao BN. Nonrhabdomyosarcoma in children: prognostic factors influencing survival. Semin Surg Oncol 1993; 954.

56. Elias AD. The clinical management of soft tissue sarcomas. Semin in Oncol 1992; 19(Suppl 1):19–25.

57. Suit HD, Mankin HJ, Wood WC, et al. Treatment of patients with M0 soft tissue sarcoma. J Clin Oncol 1988; 6:854.

58. Lindberg RD, Martin RG, Romsdahl MM, et al. Conservative surgery and post operative radiotherapy in 300 adults with soft tissue sarcomas. Cancer 1981; 47:2391.

59. Sadoski C, Suit HD, Rosenberg A, et al. Preoperative radiation, surgical margins, and local control of extremity sarcomas of soft tissues. J Surg Oncol 1993; 52:223.

60. Potter DA, Glenn J, Kinsella TJ, et al. Patterns of recurrence in patients with high grade soft tissue sarcomas. J Clin Oncol 1985; 3:353.

61. Eilber FR, Eckardt JJ, Rosen G, et al. Neoadjuvant chemotherapy and radiotherapy in the multidisciplinary management of soft tissue sarcomas of the extremity. Surg Oncol Clin 1993; 2:611.

62. Sindelar WF, Kinsella TJ, Chen PW, et al. Intraoperative radiotherapy in retroperitoneal sarcomas: final results of prospectively randomized clinical trials. Arch Surg 1993; 128:402.

63. O'Bryan RM, Luce JK, Talley RW. Phase II evaluation of adriamycin in human neoplasia. Cancer 1973; 32:1–8.

64. Antman KH, Elias E, Ryan L. Ifosfamide and mesna: response and toxicity at standard- and high-dose schedules. Semin Oncol 1990; 17(4):68–73.

65. Steward WP, Verweij J, Somers R, et al. Granulocyte-macrophage colony-stimulating factor allows safe escalation of dose-intensity of chemotherapy in metastatic adult soft tissue sarcomas: a study of the European Oganization for Research and Treatment of Cancer Soft Tissue and Bone Sarcoma Group. J Clin Oncol 1993; 11(1):15–21.

66. Rainey RB, Asmar L, Vassilopoulou-Sellin R, et al. Late complications of therapy in 213 children with localized non-orbital soft tissue sarcoma of the head and neck: a descriptive report from the Intergroup Rhabdomyosarcoma Studies (IRS) –II and –III. Med Pediatr Oncol 1999; 33:362.

67. Packer RJ, Meadows AT, Rorke L, et al. Long term sequelae of cancer treatment on the central nervous system in childhood. Med Pediatr Oncol 1987; 15:241.

68. Mike V, Meadows AT, D'Angio GJ. Incidence of second malignant neoplasms in children: results of an internation study. Lancet 1982; 2:1326.

69. Meadows AT, Hobbie WL. The medical consequences of cure. Cancer 1986; 58:524.

70. Tefft M, Lattin PB, Jereb B, et al. Acute and late effects on normal tissue following combined chemo- and radiotherapy for childhood rhabdomyosarcoma and Ewing's sarcoma. Cancer 1976; 37:1201.

71. Steinherz LJ, Steinherz PG, Tan CT, Murphy ML. Cardiac toxicity 4–20 years after completing anthracycline therapy. JAMA 1991; 266:1672.

72. Blatt J, Copeland DR, Bleyer WA. Late effects of childhood cancer and its treatment. In: Pizzo P, Poplack D, eds. Principles and Practice of Pediatric Oncology, 3rd ed. Philadelphia: Lippincott-Raven, 1997.

73. Wolden SL, Anderson JR, Crist WM, et al. Indications for radiotherapy and chemotherapy after complete resection in rhabdomyosarcoma: a report from the Intergroup Rhabdomyosarcoma Studies I to III. J Clin Oncol 1999; 17:3468–3475.
74. Pappo AS, Anderson JR, Crist WM, et al. Survival after relapse in children and adolescents with rhabdomyosarcoma: a report from the Intergroup Rhabdomyosarcoma Study Group. 1999; 17:3487–3493.

20

Rehabilitation of the Cancer Patient with Soft-Tissue Sarcoma

Jeanne E. Hicks
National Institutes of Health
Bethesda, Maryland
George Washington Medical Center and
Georgetown University Medical Center
Washington, DC

I. INTRODUCTION

Soft-tissue sarcomas are rare tumors, composing 1–2% of all neoplasms. They are located most commonly in the extremities but are also seen in the trunk, head, neck, and retroperitoneal areas (1). Numerous pathologic types exist, ranging in grade from low to high (grades 1–3) (2). Multimodality treatment, determined by the type and grade of the tumor, is the accepted approach. Wide local excision (WLE), when possible, with adjunct pre- or postoperative radiotherapy (3) for moderate- to high-grade tumor is the treatment of choice. Chemotherapy is added for some high-grade tumors (4). Optimal treatment regimens are still under investigation. Amputation is recommended for large tumors when negative margins cannot be obtained and when WLE would compromise too many vital structures and result in an unacceptable functional outcome. Currently, 85–90% of patients can undergo WLE (5).

All patients undergoing WLE or amputation for soft-tissue sarcoma should have the benefit of a comprehensive rehabilitation program to ensure their reaching maximal functional potential. The rehabilitation should be delivered by an experienced multidisciplinary team of rehabilitation health care professionals working in collaboration with other surgical, medical, and radiologic professionals delivering care to the patient. The rehabilitation program should be stage-specific

731

and planned according to the treatment phase the patient is currently in: (a) initial evaluation and presurgical treatment, (b) postsurgical, early treatment, (c) long-term treatment, (d) local tumor recurrence and metastatic disease, and (e) end-of-life phases. It is believed that this multidisciplinary care is best delivered in a specialty setting (6).

II. CAUSES OF IMPAIRMENT AND FUNCTIONAL DEFICITS

A number of entities can be involved in producing impairments or functional problems associated with soft-tissue sarcoma removal. These include the tumor it-self, location of the tumor, extent of surgical resection, radiation therapy, chemo-therapy, and other medical factors. The usual impairment and functional problems include pain, lymphedema, weakness, decreased joint mobility, activity of daily living deficits, fatigue, impact on recreational activities, and vocational and sex-ual concerns.

A. Tumor

Tumor involves soft tissues (muscle, fat, skin). It is best to identify and remove soft tissue sarcomas when they are small. As tumors grow, they involve more soft tissue and may compress or involve nerve sheaths, vessels, and bony periosteum, making adequate tissue removal without serious functional deficit difficult or im-possible. Large tumors are associated with higher metastatic risk (7).

B. Tumor Location

Tumors can be located in any area of the limbs, trunk, head and neck, or retroperi-toneum. Fifty percent of tumors are in the limbs. Tumors in areas with more soft mass are easier to remove and result in less functional deficit (thigh, buttock). Tu-mors in areas such as the hand, wrist, foot, and ankle are very close to critical ten-dons and nerve structures and often cannot be removed because resultant function would be compromised to an unacceptable level. However, newer reconstructive techniques have proven useful for hand (8,9) and foot (10).

C. Surgery

Impairments, physical problems, and functional deficits often depend on the ex-tent of the soft-tissue resection and any ancillary involved structures that need re-moval. WLE is the treatment of choice and is carried out if a 2-cm gross surgical margin can be obtained while preserving adequate function for the limb. Earlier procedures, such as whole compartmental resection and origin to insertion muscle resection, have mostly become unnecessary due to pre- and postoperative adjunct radiotherapy, which allows for less tissue removal while controlling local micro-scopic tumor (11). Surgery that requires tight closure of skin proximate to joints can result in wound healing problems and decreased joint motion. Skin breakdown can occur, which requires a split-thickness skin graft (STSG). Often WLE can cause impairments of strength, joint, range of motion, edema, and pain. However, if the resected body area is still functional, despite mild to moderate physical im-pairment, WLE is acceptable. Severe impairments render unacceptable functional outcome in the areas of mobility, activities of daily living, and psychosocial and vocational pursuits.

D. Irradiation

Soft-tissue sarcoma patients with moderate- to high-grade tumors often receive one of four regimens of radiotherapy to enhance local control (12) or reduce tu-mor size. These include pre-, post-, or intraoperative radiotherapy or brachyther-apy (13). This usually commences 2 weeks postoperatively when the wound is healed and lasts 6–8 weeks. Over the past 10 years, newer fractionated and cone-down dose radiotherapy methods have reduced the adverse effects of radiother-apy (14).

     Studies indicate that such problems as skin telangiectasias, decreased strength, joint motion, and edema can still occur but are usually transient, espe-cially with doses greater than 63 Gy at 1.8 Gy per fraction (14,15). Other problems, such as skin breakdown, reduced wound healing, osteoporosis, fracture through osteoporotic bone, neuropathy, and myelopathy, can occur (16). Some side effects may occur late.

     These impairments also impact on mobility and activities of daily living as well as on psychosocial and vocational pursuits.

E. Chemotherapy

A recent research trial has shown chemotherapy (with radiotherapy) is associated with a local control benefit (17) and possibly increased survival rate in high-grade tumors (18). It can be associated with decreased wound healing, increased flexion contractures (19), infection, neuropathy, decreased cardiac function due to de-creased ejection fracture (Adriamycin), and fatigue.

F. Isolated Limb Perfusion

Isolated limb perfusion is a newer technique that is used infrequently. Its main use is when WLE is not possible and the patient refuses amputation. In many cases it is successful in reducing the size of the tumor, and it sometimes makes limb-sparing surgery possible. Even if limb sparing is not possible (Fig. 1), reduction in tumor size for cosmesis and increased ease in performing functional activities

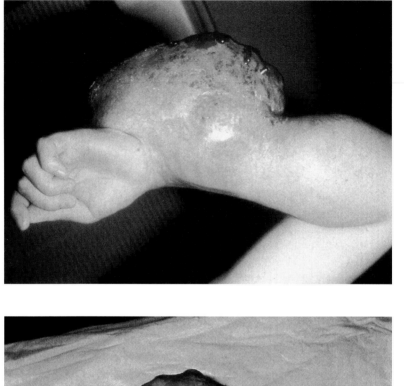

(A)

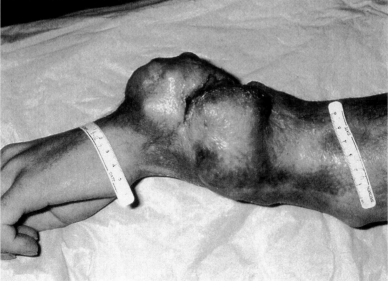

(B)

FIG. 1 (A) A large inoperable soft-tissue sarcoma of the distal exterior surface of the forearm. (B) Soft-tissue sarcoma of the distal extensor surface of the forearm (from Fig. A). Two weeks after isolated limb perfusion with tumor necrosis factor and melphalan.

is desirable. Isolated limb perfusion can cause impairment in the areas of edema, as well as skin breakdown or necrosis (20).

III. REHABILITATION

A. Team Approach

Care for soft-tissue sarcoma patients is best delivered by a cancer team (Fig. 2) consisting of multidisciplinary rehabilitation professionals (physiatrists, physical and occupational therapists, speech and language pathologists, vocational specialists, and recreation therapists). Interdisciplinary members also include social workers, surgeons, radiation and medical oncologists, psychologists, and sexual counselors. These team members are involved both during the patient's initial hospital care and throughout the long follow-up period deemed necessary for optimal health care delivery (21).

B. Goals

The general rehabilitation goal for patients with soft-tissue sarcoma, with either WLE or amputation, is to assist them in obtaining the highest functional level possible. There are three main types of goal: preventative, restorative, and maintenance. In the early and middle stages of cancer treatment, the goals are mainly to prevent functional decline and/or restore lost function. In the latter states of cancer (metastatic and hospice care levels), the main goal is to maintain function to facilitate quality of life, even during the end stage of cancer.

Besides the three overall goals of rehabilitation, specific treatment goals are developed according to the type of deficits present. These goals include increasing joint motion and muscle strength and endurance; promoting adjustment to disability; decreasing pain, anxiety, edema, fatigue, and skin breakdown; and addressing vocational, psychosocial, sexual, recreational and leisure issues. Members of the cancer team treating the patient set goals before treatment commences.

C. General Treatment Armamentarium

Rehabilitation utilizes a large nonpharmacologic treatment armamentarium in cancer patients to achieve specific goals. In some instances, the literature supports the effectiveness of these treatments, whereas others are based on the clinical judgment of experienced clinicians treating cancer patients.

1. Heat and Cold Modalities

a. Heat   Heat can be delivered by superficial and deep methods (22). Common methods to deliver superficial heat include dry and moist heat packs (the latter

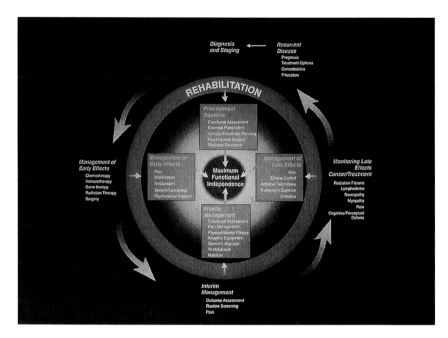

FIG. 2 Graphic of the role of rehabilitation management throughout the trajectory of cancer treatments: pretreatment phase, early, interim, late, and recurrent, disease phases. (From Gerber L, Hicks J, et al., Rehabilitation of the cancer patient. In: DeVita VT, Hellman S, and Rosenberg SA, eds. Cancer Principles and Practice, 5th ed. Philadelphia: Lippincott-Raven, 1997, pp. 2925–2956.).

penetrate tissue to a deeper level), hot tanks, tubs and showers, spas, and microwaved gel packs.

Methods to deliver deep heat involve ultrasound, microwave, and short-wave machines. The use of ultrasound at therapeutic dosages over tumors in mice has been associated with significant increases in tumor size (23). No studies on heat modalities in the management of cancer in humans are available. At this time, it is recommended that heating modalities be avoided near tumor sites.

Heat, both superficial and deep, is known to cause the following effects: analgesia, decrease in muscle spasm, and increase in tendon extensibility (24). It is used clinically over areas of painful muscle spasm and tight tendons/capsules before a stretching program to improve joint motion is implemented.

b.   Cold   Cold (22) can be delivered by ice packs, ice massage, and fluromethane spray. It causes analgesia, decrease swelling and relaxation of muscle spasm. It is also useful in areas of acute injury to decrease pain and swelling or over areas of muscle spasm. Contraindications are Raynaud's syndrome and cryoglobulinemia.

c. Transcutaneous Electrical Nerve Stimulation (TENS) TENS can be delivered by a number of machines that are either single or dual channel. They range in price from $100.00 to $800.00. They are user-friendly, and patients and/or family can be trained to operate one in a single session. Pain is thought to be reduced via the gate control mechanism wherein pain impulses through the large C-nerve fibers to the spinal cord are blocked by the electrical impulse from the TENS unit (25). These machines are useful postoperatively to reduce incisional pain. They should be used with caution over insensate skin.

2. Acupuncture

Acupuncture is delivered by small sharp needles. It can be combined with electricity to produce electroacupuncture or heated needles may also be used. Acupuncture has been proven to reduce nausea in cancer patients (26) and is clinically used to relieve pain in any soft tissue or bony area.

3. Acupressure

Acupressure implies the application of pressure to acupuncture sites. It is also used to relieve soft-tissue pain.

4. Exercise

Cancer patients participate in a variety of exercise programs: range-of-motion stretching, isometric, isotonic, and aerobic (27).

Isometric exercise implies generating a muscle force (weight) against a fixed object without the use of any adjacent joint motion. It increases strength but not muscle bulk. This is the first type of strengthening program we use postoperatively for soft-tissue sarcoma patients.

Isotonic exercise implies moving a force against gravity. Adjacent joints are actively moved. Isotonic programs increase muscle strength, endurance, and bulk. They are begun after the isometric program has been established and the surgical site is well healed (usually after 2 weeks).

Both isometric and isotonic muscle contractions are used in daily activities; therefore, it is important that both forms of exercise be instituted.

Moderate exercise enhances protein incorporation into muscle. This is important in cancer patients with muscle atrophy (28).

5. Aerobic Exercise

Aerobic conditioning occurs when large groups of muscles are used isotonically at low- or high-intensity levels for a sustained time period from 15 to 60 min, 2–3 times a week for 8–12 weeks. This can be provided in a pool, on a bicycle ergometer, treadmill, or with stair step or dance programs. In very deconditioned persons with chronic disease, low-intensity programs (50–60% Vo_2 max) for short time periods (15–20 min) and frequency (2 times a week) for 8 weeks can produce a significant increase in Vo_2 max (29).

Cancer patients are often deconditioned due to long sedentary periods during cancer treatments or from metastatic disease. Participation in an aerobic program can result in increased aerobic capacity, overall functional level, and reduction in fatigue (30). Contraindications include hematocrit under 30, abnormal electrolytes, moderate pulmonary disease, cardiac arrhythmias, significant unstable angina from valvular or coronary artery disease, and significant renal disease (27). For patients with soft-tissue sarcoma and lower limb resections with significant weakness or neurologic compromise (e.g., foot drop), a pool program is ideal.

6. Ambulation/Mobility Aids

Crutches, forearm crutches, canes, quad canes and walkers, wheelchairs, and scooters are all useful mobility aids.

In the early postoperative period, lower extremity soft-tissue sarcoma patients will be non-weight-bearing and need a wheelchair for long distances and crutches or walkers for shorter functional distances. After full weight bearing has been initiated, a cane may be needed for balance. After full rehabilitation, a mobility device is generally not needed unless there has been significant muscle or nerve sacrifice.

7. Assistive Devices

Assistive devices substitute for lost function. Many of them are needed early postoperatively, but some are needed throughout the patient's life and in the end stages of life. Generally useful items in the early postoperative period include shower chair, long-handed showerhead, and reacher. For patients with upper extremity resections, useful items may include electric can opener and vegetable peeler, large-handled eating utensils, long-handled comb, hair- and toothbrushes.

8. Orthotics

Orthotics can substitute for lost function, decrease weight over a limb segment, or relieve pain by resting a segment. They are used in soft-tissue sarcoma cancer rehabilitation according to the specific type of resection. They are custom-made to provide a good fit and thus avoid skin breakdown, pain, or nerve compression. Many upper extremity orthotics are fabricated by an occupational therapist. Shoe orthotics and modifications are often done by a physical therapist trained in foot management (pedorthopist). Orthotics made of sturdy plastic for joint support are fabricated by an orthotist.

IV. STAGES OF REHABILITATION FOR WIDE LOCAL EXCISION AND AMPUTEES

A. Wide Local Excision Rehabilitation

1. Initial Evaluation

Before the surgical staging conference is held, an initial evaluation is performed by the rehabilitation physician and the physical and occupational therapists. The medical tests and radiologic procedures are reviewed, followed by a history and physical examination. Detailed musculoskeletal, neurologic, and vascular assessment is made, particularly of the area of soft-tissue sarcoma involvement.

2. Functional Prediction

After the initial evaluation is made, the physiatrist predicts the level of function the individual would have with adequate resection. If the level of function would be adequate for performance of activities of daily living, a recommendation for WLE is made. If the physiatrist and surgeon agree that function would be significantly limited or there is no option at all for adequate tumor removal with a WLE, an amputation is recommended. The level of amputation is also recommended by the physiatrist. Postoperative WLE function or function post amputation is discussed with the patient in relation to his or her lifestyle and job (work) requirements. These issues are also discussed in staging conference. When enough data are not available to make a recommendation before staging conference, discussion with the patient is deferred until after the staging conference. In addition to magnetic resonance imaging and bone scan, arteriography may be needed before any decision concerning WLE versus amputation can be made. Occasionally, the decision cannot be made until the surgical procedure is in progress as neurologic involvement of critical nerve structures by adjacent tumor is not always easily assessed preoperatively. The deficits could be due to compression by the tumor or actual involvement of critical nerve sheaths or structures.

3. Baseline Assessments

For patients with soft-tissue sarcoma who are on research protocols, formal baseline assessments of range of motion, strength, edema, level of overall function, and quality of life are done preoperatively and at set intervals (3, 6 months to 1, 3, 5 years). A cancer-specific questionnaire is the Cancer Rehabilitation Evaluation Systems (CARES) (31). A recent questionnaire developed and validated for both soft-tissue sarcoma and osteogenic sarcoma patients is the Toronto Extremity Salvage Score (TESS) (32).

B. Staging Conference

Critical review of the soft-tissue sarcoma patient's history, examination, and all testing is done at this conference. It is attended by surgeons, a pathologist, and a physiatrist. After the patient has been brought in, other physicians who didn't see the area of involvement can do so and examine it if they wish. The patient leaves the conference and the group forms a consensus about the advisability of WLE, i.e., its extent and functional outcome acceptability, versus amputation. The opinion is discussed with the patient and family after the conference. Any additional information not discussed at initial assessment concerning functional impact of the surgery is added. The patient should have the opportunity to ask questions.

V. SPECIAL PROBLEM AREAS FOR REHABILITATION CONSIDERATIONS

A. Pain

Pain management is essential throughout the trajectory of disease. It is especially important in the early preoperative and postoperative stages. Pharmacologic management with narcotics is needed the first week postoperatively. A combination of rehabilitation procedures helps reduce pain. These include proper positioning to reduce edema and prevent contracture; immobilization of operative sites with slings, splints, or bivalved casts; and the use of heat and cold modalities, TENS, and acupuncture.

It is important not to advance a rehabilitation program too quickly during the acute management of pain phase.

B. Lymphedema

Edema is uncomfortable and can interfere with function. Some WLEs are associated with significant edema: deep adductor, hamstring, anterior compartment of the leg and breast. The use of appropriate splinting, positioning, elastic garments, or compressive nonelastic wrapping (33) is required. Long-term management is often indicated for edema.

C. Fatigue

Fatigue occurs due to many causes: inactivity, depression, chemotherapy, and the disease itself. Energy conservation techniques and assistive devices as well as appropriate posture are important in reducing fatigue. Low-intensity, low-impact aerobic programs are often prescribed for patients. Treatment for depression is important.

D. Strength and Motion Loss

Decreased strength of specific muscle groups and compromised motion of joints adjacent to the site of surgery and irradiation and after chemotherapy often occurs. Exercise programs specifically tailored to the patient's needs are important in facilitating the regaining of limb function and in maintaining it. Partial resection of muscle groups leaves residual muscles that must be strengthened by isometric and isotonic strength programs. The patient must be instructed in specific stretching programs. The intensity of these programs must take into consideration the type of resection and/or reconstructive procedure the patient has had.

Patients with soft-tissue sarcoma who receive radiotherapy of the limbs and spinal column should be evaluated for an exercise program to prevent range-of-motion deficits and preserve strength. This is particularly true if the irradiation is next to a joint or near an area of tight surgical closure. Irradiation techniques with fractionated and cone-down doses have decreased the risk of joint contracture (14) and stiffness (34). Joints next to these irradiated areas receive only scattered doses. Joints in the cone-down area receive high doses. Good functional range of motion is usually maintained with an appropriate range-of-motion program. The patient is seen by rehabilitation initially prior to irradiation and weekly during the radiotherapy program. An appropriate range-of-motion/stretching program is followed daily for joints in and surrounding the irradiated field. The exercise is performed after the radiation treatment, as exercise is a radioenhancer. Strengthening exercise is added to the treatment regimen, after the patient has completed the radiotherapy course. A long-term range-of-motion and strengthening program should be continued 3 times a week. Radiation contractures can occur years after the initial radiation program.

VI. MOBILITY AIDS AND ACTIVITIES
OF DAILY LIVING ISSUES

Soft-tissue sarcoma limb-spared patients have short- and long-term mobility problems. Immediately postoperatively, crutches and walkers are needed. By 1–2 months (depending on the procedure) they usually no longer need these devices. Likewise, assistive devices and bathroom safety equipment may be needed in the short term. When complications occur later in the disease course, devices are needed again—particularly in the end stage of life.

Orthotics are useful after some select WLE procedures. They may be functional or nonfunctional. Functional orthotics are useful in the face of weakness and may provide static support across one joint while at the same time allowing other joints to function. An example would be use of a static wrist splint to hold a weak wrist in a functional position while allowing finger motion after a wrist ex-

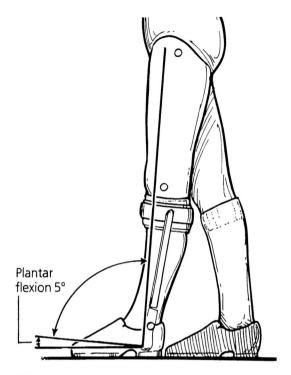

Plantar
flexion 5°

FIG. 3 Short leg brace locked in five degrees of plantar flexion to create a hyperextension movement at the knee for stabilization after quadriceps resection. (From Hicks J.
Rehabilitating patients with idiopathic inflammatory myopathy. J Musculoskel Med 12(4):
51, 1995.)

tensor resection. Dynamic functional splints are also useful. A dynamic wrist splint
(outrigger) with elastic bands and felt finger slings allows for finger extension and
wrist support if there has been a wrist and finger extensor excision.

Some orthotics are useful in maintaining the position of a joint. A simple
posterior splint for the knee may be used postoperatively to discourage knee motion while drains are still in and tissues are healing. A multipodis boot may be used
at the ankle (particularly in gastrocnemeus excisions) to prevent plantar flexion
contracture.

Orthotics with dial locks can be used in patients who have developed flexion contractures. The dial locks can be advanced 2 degrees every other day. They
are most often used for the elbow, knee, and ankle and are commercially available.
Serial casting can also be used but is more time consuming.

A brace (orthotic) metal or plastic locked in 5 degrees of plantar flexion
helps stabilize the knee after quadriceps excision (35). An extension moment is

created at the knee when the toe comes down first in plantar flexion (Fig. 3). If the anterior tibial muscle or the posterior tibial nerve has been resected, a plastic ankle–foot orthosis set at neutral will hold the ankle up (Fig. 4).

Rarely, sciatic nerve resections are performed. A short-leg metal double-upright brace with the ankle in neutral can be used. Specialized gait training is needed to help the patient use substitutive muscle patterns and walk functionally. Gait is slower with toe out. Running is not possible (36).

VII. COSMETIC ORTHOSIS

Surgical procedures for removal of soft-tissue sarcoma can cause cosmetic deficits. Some of these can be ameliorated by the use of nonfunctional cosmetic de-

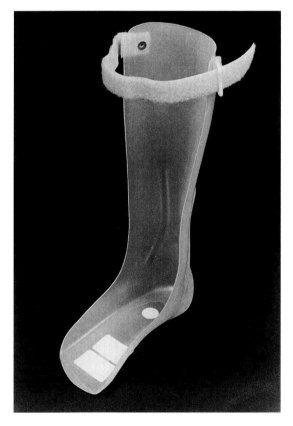

FIG. 4 Polypropylene ankle–foot orthosis is neutral at the ankle to compensate for weak ankle dorsiflexons.

vices. These are usually fabricated by an orthotist and tend to be costly. Some examples of cosmetic devices follow.

Orthotics used after WLE include hand (4th and 5th ray replacements) and toe fillers after 4th and 5th foot ray removal.

A. Shoulder Cap

Shoulder cap cosmetic devices are used after a forequarter amputation or a Tinkhoff-Lindberg procedure. After a Tinkhoff-Lindberg procedure for large soft-tissue sarcoma in the shoulder area, a significant soft-tissue deficit occurs. This causes a cosmetic problem as the deficit can easily be visualized beneath clothing. Also, wearing of a bra strap on the affected side is impossible as is carrying a purse with a strap. The fabrication of a hard plastic or softer molded shoulder cap device with the same contour as the opposite shoulder greatly enhances shoulder cosmesis (Fig. 5).

B. Buttectomy Piece

After a buttectomy for soft-tissue sarcoma, a large deficit is left in the buttock area, which creates a cosmetic problem particularly when the person is wearing snug jeans and pants. A molded buttock piece can be fashioned in the same contour as the opposite buttock. It can be held in place in a slot in panties or a stocking or retained by a strap around the waist and leg (Fig. 6).

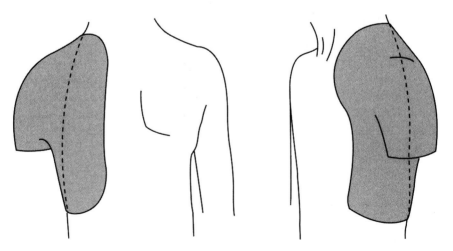

FIG. 5 Soft custom-molded cosmetic shoulder prosthesis for use after forequarter amputation to provide normal shoulder height and contour.

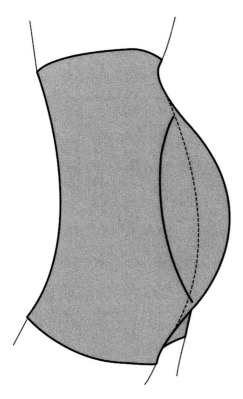

FIG. 6 Cosmetic buttectomy prosthesis utilized to restore normal buttock contour following resection of the gluteus maximus. Dotted line indicates flat resected buttock area. The prosthesis is inserted in underpants.

C. Lower Extremity Leg Pieces

Some soft-tissue surgery leaves large soft-tissue deficits that are cosmetically difficult to accept by the patient. A partial resection of the gastrocnemeus mechanism may be cosmetically distressful. The use of a molded insert contoured like the opposite calf enhances cosmesis. It can be worn under a stocking (Fig. 7).

D. Breast Prosthesis

Sarcoma of the breast is uncommon. When a breast is removed, a breast prosthesis is indicated. A temporary soft fluff is provided after mastectomy when the wound has healed. A permanent prosthesis is constructed and fitted after other treatments have been completed.

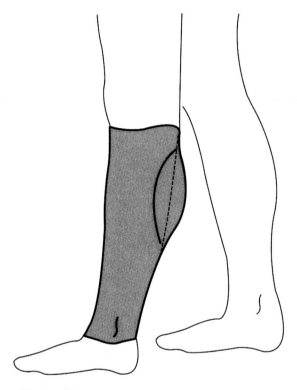

FIG. 7 Cosmetic custom-molded gastrocnemeus prosthesis utilized to restore normal contour to the calf after a gastrocnemeus or soleus calf resection. Dotted line indicates the resected gastrocnemeus area. The prosthesis is inserted in a short leg stocking.

VIII. POSTOPERATIVE CARE WIDE LOCAL EXCISION

It is important before beginning rehabilitation to review the entire operative report to ascertain the extent of the excision or any reconstructive procedures. Special note is made of large excisions, multicompartment versus single-compartment excision (more drainage may occur), tight wound closure, resections around joints with partial capsule and ligament excision (associated with joint effusion and restriction of range of motion), deep medial thigh excisions (more edema may occur), and nerve resection (corresponding muscle paralysis will occur). The early rehabilitation program is planned to take into consideration the above items. Based on these items, some programs will advance more quickly whereas others will be slower and require more caution.

IX. COMMON SPECIFIC WIDE LOCAL EXCISIONS

WLE can be done in the extremities, trunk, retroperitoneum, and head and neck. Rehabilitation programs must be individualized to the patient, but some general guidelines exist (37–39).

A. Scapulectomy

1. Indication

Scapulectomy is performed for soft-tissue sarcomas adjacent to the scapula.

2. Procedure

Depending on the exact location and size of the tumor, there are a number of different partial scapulectomies and a full scapulectomy. Partial procedures spare the glenohumoral joint and total ones sacrifice it.

3. Rehabilitation

The patient wears an arm sling until the operative site is well healed (about 3 weeks). This prevents traction on the shoulder and restricts abduction. Some arm edema occurs in the postoperative period, which is controlled with a stockinette. When the wound is healed and the drain is out (around 2 weeks), active assistive elbow exercises in the sling begin. At 3 weeks, the sling is removed, elbow exercises are advanced, and passive range of motion of the shoulder is introduced in partial abduction and flexion. Over the next month, active shoulder exercise is introduced in partial scapulectomies.

4. Function

For partial scapulectomies, there is only mild loss of shoulder range of motion. Functional elbow and wrist/hand activities can be performed for full scapulectomies, but active shoulder motion is severely restricted (0–23% of normal movement) and nonfunctional (40). Some patients experience significant pain, which may necessitate long-term management with mediation and modalities (TENS or acupuncture). Weight lifting is restricted to 20 pounds.

B. Tikhoff-Lindberg

1. Indication

The Tikhoff-Lindberg procedure is done for tumors deep to the scapula or in the proximal humoral area. The brachial plexus and axillary vessels should not be involved.

2. Procedure

Resection of the distal clavicle, upper humerus, and a partial scapulectomy are performed followed by muscle transfers and skeletal reconstruction with an endoprosthesis (Fig. 8).

3. Rehabilitation

The general rehabilitation course is similar to that for full scapulectomies (see above), with the exception that elbow and shoulder range of motion may take longer to introduce because of the extent of the reconstruction. After a month, the shoulder can usually reach passive abduction and flexion of 90 degrees.

4. Function

Full elbow, wrist, and hand function are achieved. Active motion at the shoulder is minimal and nonfunctional. A cosmetic shoulder cap or molded prosthesis is usually used (Fig. 5). Long-term edema is usually not a problem.

C. Axillary Resection

1. Indication

This procedure is done for tumors in the axillary area.

2. Procedure

The long head of the triceps and part of the latissimus dorsi muscle are resected.

3. Rehabilitation

Postoperative edema and pain from pectoral muscle spasm is common. Compressive garments or nonelastic arm wrapping are indicated. Long-term use of a compressive garment may be required, particularly if the area is irradiated. TENS is useful for pain control. Care must be taken to avoid skin breakdown from perspiration. A splint device is used in the salute position (100 degrees flexion/abduction and 75 degrees of external rotation) if radiation therapy is given.

4. Function

Function of the shoulder, elbow, and wrist/hand is preserved provided there is no nerve resection. Transient neuropraxia from stretching of the brachial plexus during surgery may occur and may last up to 6 months.

Motor Reconstruction
and Soft Tissue Coverage

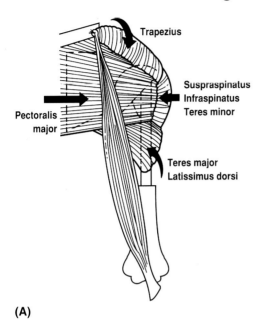

Trapezius

Suspraspinatus
Infraspinatus
Teres minor

Pectoralis
major

Teres major
Latissimus dorsi

(A)

**Static
Suspension**

**Dynamic
Suspension**

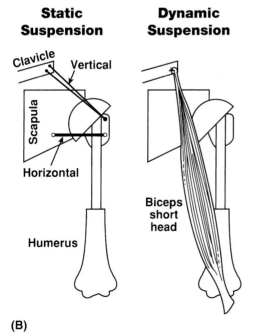

Clavicle   Vertical

Scapula

Horizontal

Biceps
short
head

Humerus

(B)

FIG. 8 (A) Graphic display of completed Tikhoff-Lindberg reconstruction with endoprosthesis in place. (B) Graphic of Tikhoff-Lindberg procedure (left resection of the distal clavicle, upper humerus, and partial scapulectomy) with vertical and horizontal static suspension of the endoprosthesis from the clavicle and scapula and right dynamic suspension with the short head of the biceps muscle tendon.

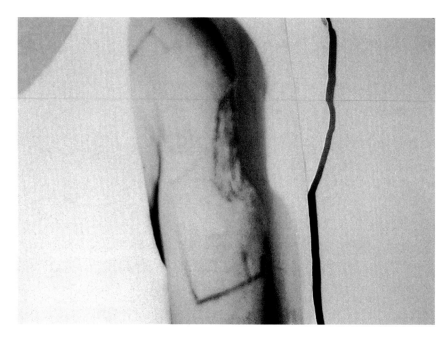

FIG. 9 Partial excision of the medial deltoid muscle.

D. Partial Deltoid / Triceps / Biceps

1. Indication

Small to medium-sized tumors of the deltoid, triceps, or biceps can be locally resected.

2. Procedure

Either the deltoid (Fig. 9), triceps, or biceps muscle is partially resected.

3. Rehabilitation

A sling is provided for 10 days until the wound is healed. In 3 or 4 days, when the drains are out, partial passive motion of the joints adjacent to the resection is done (shoulder/elbow). Active motion starts around day 10 and progresses according to extent of wound healing and tightness of the closure. Strengthening of residual muscle is started at about 2 weeks.

4. Function

There is function for daily activities. Power activities and sports may be limited depending on the extent of muscle removal. This is particularly true of the biceps and deltoid.

E. Forearm Extensors

1. Indications

Small to medium-sized tumors of the forearm extensors near the elbow may be successfully removed.

2. Procedure

This usually consists of a partial removal of some of the extensor muscle group. The procedure is more radical if the radial head and/or nerve need removal.

3. Rehabilitation

Edema control with stockinette is provided postoperatively. Passive range of muscle of the wrist and fingers is done daily. A splint is provided to keep the wrist and hand in a functional position (20 degrees of wrist extension/45 degrees of MP and PIP flexion). Active motion is started when the drains are out. Elbow range-of-motion advancement depends on the extent of the procedure. If the radial nerve was removed, the patient will need a permanent dynamic outrigger splint fixed in functional wrist extension (20 degrees) with elastic bands to facilitate finger extension. An alternative to splint use is transfer of the flexor carpi radialis tendon to facilitate wrist extension.

F. Hand Tumors

Newer reconstructive procedures and refined irradiation techniques have allowed local excision of hand tumors and/or excision and reconstruction in selected areas. Rehabilitation requires a hand therapist to maintain critical joint range of motion by stretching exercises and splinting and substitution for lost function by splinting and assistive devices.

G. Lower Extremity: Buttock Tumors

1. Indication

Most small to large tumors of the buttock muscles (gluteus maximus and minimus) are amenable to WLE.

2. Procedure

Partial excision of the buttock area is done. Significant tissue defect may be left. The sciatic nerve is left intact. Very large buttock tumors may require internal hemipelvectomy.

3. Rehabilitation

Rehabilitation is initiated with hip range of motion. Patients can generally be on crutches with toe touch on day 2 postop. Progression of weight bearing occurs with drain removal and pain control. Full weight bearing with a cane may occur by 3 weeks. Sitting is usually uncomfortable for several months, and a soft foam gel or air cushion is provided.

4. Function

Gait deviations are usually absent. There is minor difficulty in stair climbing. Radiation therapy may temporarily disrupt normal sexual function and bowel habits. Body image is affected by the flattened buttock area, which shows through jeans and pants. Usually cosmetic buttock prosthesis is prescribed (Fig. 6).

H. Internal Hemipelvectomy: Buttocks, Upper Thigh (Very Large Tumor)

1. Indication

Very large tumors of the buttock and upper thigh may not be amendable to buttectomy. An internal hemipelvectomy procedure may be needed.

2. Procedure

The procedure consists of resection of the hemipelvis and proximal femur along with transection of the sacrum through the neural foramina. Sometimes removal of the bladder, rectum, or genitalia is necessary.

3. Rehabilitation

Rehabilitation is lengthy for this extensive procedure. A prolonged period of bed rest with stabilization of the pelvis and femur by skeletal traction is needed to facilitate fusion and maintain leg length. During the period of bed rest, range of motion of the knee and ankle is done along with appropriate strengthening exercises of the thigh and distal leg muscles. A plastic splint or multipodis boot may be used to avoid Achilles tendon shortening. When the patient is allowed to stand on crutches (4–6 weeks postoperatively), a shoe lift is placed on the operated side to equalize leg length. Total union of the pelvis may take up to 6 months, during which time the patient must remain on partial weight bearing status with crutches. Since this is a complex operative procedure, with variations in the exact procedure, the rehabilitation team works closely with the surgical team in advancing the rehabilitation program and avoiding unnecessary complications.

4. Function

Independent ambulation with Lofstand crutches or a cane, depending on the resection extent, is achieved. Gait deviations include Trendelenburg and lateral trunk bending due to hip weakness. Extensive gait training is needed.

I. Abductor Excision

1. Indication

Excision of the abductor muscles is performed for medial thigh sarcomas.

2. Procedure

An excision of a portion or all of the adductor muscle group can be done. (The number of lymph nodes sacrificed with this procedure depends on the extent of the procedure.)

3. Rehabilitation

Significant leg edema usually occurs with large excisions. This is augmented after radiotherapy. Control of edema with compressive or nonelastic wrapping is needed. Long-term compressive stockings must be worn. Remeasurement should occur at yearly intervals. Initial rehabilitation is slow due to significant drainage. Exercises increase drainage and are avoided until it subsides and the drains are out. Patients are usually ambulatory with partial weight bearing at 3 weeks. At 6 weeks, weight bearing without crutches or cane is expected.

4. Function

Gait is normal. There is no functional loss.

J. Hamstring Resection

1. Indication

Soft-tissue sarcoma in the hamstring muscle group can be resected (Fig. 10). Involvement of the sciatic nerve sheath may require sciatic excision.

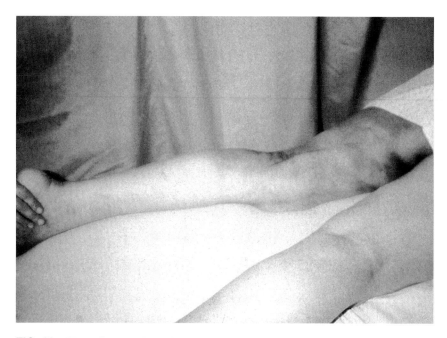

FIG. 10   Hamstring muscle excision (*left*).

2.   Procedure

A portion of the hamstring muscles or the entire group can be resected. The sciatic nerve is uncommonly sacrificed but sometimes this is necessary. The alternative procedure would be a hemipelvectomy.

3.   Rehabilitation

Drainage is usually not prolonged. Patients are able to crutch-walk with partial weight bearing when the drains are out. Range-of-motion and stretching programs are important to avoid knee and ankle flexion contractures. Patients are usually ambulating independently by 6 weeks.

4.   Function

The gait pattern is normal except for difficulty with deceleration after fast walking. Running is somewhat unsteady. If the sciatic nerve is removed, both motor and sensory problems ensue. The lower limb must be braced to correct foot drop. A double upright short leg brace locked in neutral is used. A custom-made plastic ankle–foot orthosis with good ankle control may be used in some cases. However, due to sensory loss in the foot, skin breakdown may occur with this total contact

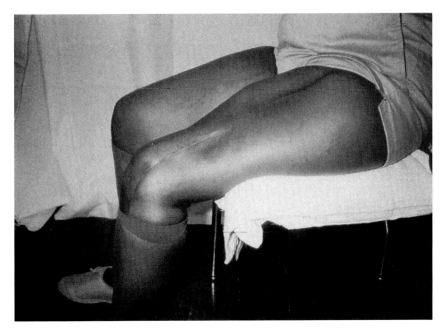

FIG. 11 Quadriceps muscle group excision (*left*).

brace. The patient needs well-fitting shoes and instructions on skin care. Gait deviations remain despite bracing and training. Gait is slow, uneven, and nonpropulsive. Fast walking and running is not possible.

K. Quadriceps Resection

1. Indication

Excision of the quadriceps is done for anterior midthigh tumors (Fig. 11).

2. Procedure

Partial or full quadriceps excision can be done for small to large tumors. Some tumors may be in the quadriceps and adductor areas and require excision of portions of both muscle groups.

3. Rehabilitation

A knee immobilizer is initially used, and active ankle motion is encouraged. When the drain is out and the wound is healing, partial weight bearing with crutches is done with the splint on. If three fourths to all of the quadriceps mechanism is re-moved, the patient is fitted with a short leg brace locked in 5 degrees plantar flex-ion to create a hyperextension moment at the knee to stabilize it (Fig. 4).

4. Function

Patients can walk independently with a cane. Some thin patients are able to de-velop compensatory gait patterns and don't need the brace. For example, they lean back, balance on the Y ligament in the groin, rotate their leg out, widen their base of support, and lock the knee in hyperextension. Gait is slow. Another mechanism is employed when they come down toe first in stance, which throws the knee into hyperextension, thus stabilizing it. Falls can occur with these substitutive patterns.

L. Gastrocnemeus Resection

1. Indication

Tumors around the post-lower leg near the gastrocnemeus can be removed.

2. Procedure

Partial removal of the gastroc–soleus complex is done. Usually the posterior tib-ial nerve is spared. If it is excised, sensory deficit of the foot occurs.

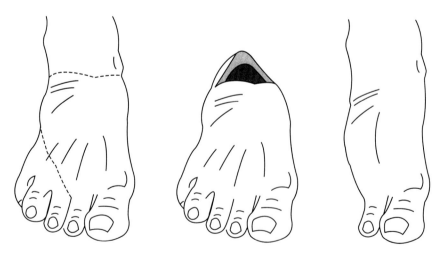

FIG. 12   Ray excision: 2–5 with molded cosmetic foot.

3. Rehabilitation

When the drains are out and the wound is healed, range of motion and stretching at the ankle to neutral is done. Care must be taken not to put too much tension on the wound while it is healing lest skin breakdown occur. A main goal of rehabilitation is to prevent contracture of the Achilles tendon. If the foot is insensate, custom inserts to provide proper foot contact are necessary. Since push-off during gait is limited, a rocker bottom on the shoe is used to make gait more propulsive.

4. Function

Patients are independent ambulators without a cane. Proper shoes improve gait and help prevent skin breakdown.

M. Foot Resection

Some small tumors can be removed from the foot. They may require partial ray excision—usually (third, fourth, and fifth). Resection of ray 1 and 2 leaves an unbalanced foot and is not recommended. Irradiation of the Achilles or sole of the foot is often associated with plantar flexion contracture and skin breakdown. Appropriate shoes, shoe fillers and cosmetic feet (Fig. 12) to substitute for lost rays, shoe modifications, stretching exercises, and skin care education are needed.

X. AMPUTATION FOR SOFT-TISSUE SARCOMA

A. Introduction

In the late 1960s, amputation was the standard treatment for many soft-tissue sarcomas of the extremities (41). Due to refined surgical techniques that preserve function and multimodality treatments, which control local recurrence and metastasis, the incidence of limb-sparing surgery has increased compared to amputation.

It would seem from a body image prospective that a limb-sparing option would always be preferable to an amputation. However, there are times when a decision to amputate is best for patient survival and functional outcome.

B. Indications for Amputation Versus Limb Sparing

The decision to amputate a limb rather than perform a limb-sparing procedure is determined by the following factors: unsatisfactory achievement of gross tumor surgical margins and tumor involvement of critical structures necessary for function that cannot be reconstructed.

Lower Extremity Amputation Levels

Front View

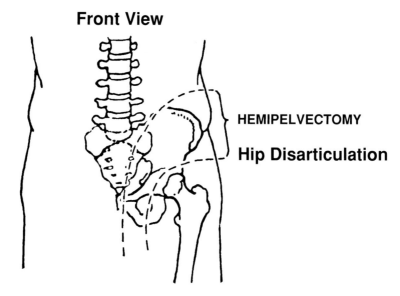

HEMIPELVECTOMY

Hip Disarticulation

FIG. 13   Graphic of hemipelvectomy and hip disarticulation amputation levels.

Advantages of amputation include low morbidity before, during, and after surgery; effective tumor control; and ability to participate in sports. Such problems as phantom sensation and pain, stump healing, prosthetic stump interface problems, bony overgrowth, and grieving for loss of a limb can occur. Spur formation on the amputated bone can be painful.

Important surgical aspects of amputation to maximize postsurgical function include sufficient preservation of stump length to assure satisfactory prosthetic fit; distribution of adequate soft-tissue closure over the residual bone; beveling of the residual bone; and avoidance of a tight closure (which is subject to skin breakdown postoperatively).

C. Types of Oncologic Amputations

In contradistinction to amputations for vascular disease and diabetes, which tend to be below-knee and above-knee amputations with mid-sized to long residual stump lengths, and Chopart's or Lisfranc's amputations, those done for soft-tissue sarcomas are often at higher limb levels: hemipelvectomy (HP) and hip disarticulation (HD) (Fig. 13), short above- (Fig. 14) and below-knee (AK, BK) amputa-

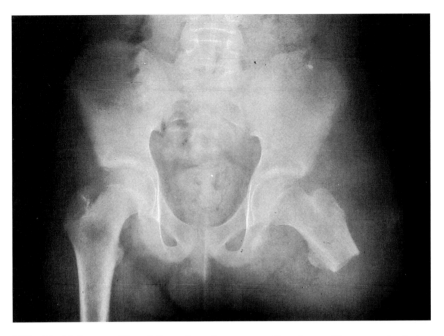

FIG. 14 Plain x-ray film of short above-knee amputation; 2 cm of bone remains below the lesser trochanter.

tion, forequarter (Fig. 15) and short above-elbow (AE) amputations. For some of these, functional prosthetics are infrequently used (forequarter, HP) due to difficulty in use and lack of patient compliance. Prosthetic fitting for short residual limb (AE/BE, AK/BK) amputations is more difficult as there is reduced biomechanical efficiency with the short residual limb in interface with the prosthetic device. The incidence of skin breakdown is often higher. Obtaining a comfortable fit due to decreased tissue over bony prominences is a greater challenge. Development of painful neuroma with high amputation (HP) is more common. Complaints of phantom pain are also more predominant with higher level amputation due to the severance, during surgery, of large major nerves and nerves trunks. High-energy requirements have been identified with HDs and HPs. Persons with HD expend 82% more energy than able-bodied individuals, and those with HP, 125% more energy. Gait is 40–50% slower (42). Midlevel AK amputations require 80% (43) and BK 35% more than the normal energy requirement (44). In some instances, a soft-tissue sarcoma that requires an HD can be converted with a short endoprosthesis to a short AK amputation with reattachment of residual muscles to metal loops on the endoprosthesis, thus allowing for excellent stump control (45) (Fig. 16).

Upper Extremity Amputation Levels

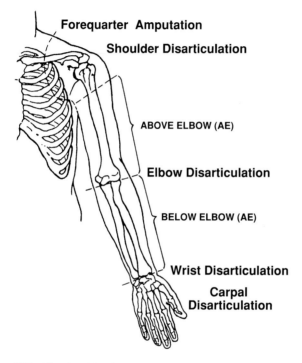

Forequarter Amputation

Shoulder Disarticulation

ABOVE ELBOW (AE)

Elbow Disarticulation

BELOW ELBOW (AE)

Wrist Disarticulation

Carpal Disarticulation

FIG. 15   Graphic of typical upper extremity amputation levels.

D.   Rehabilitation of Oncologic Amputees

1.   Preoperative Evaluation

In contradistinction to amputation in young patients due to osteogenic and Ewing's sarcoma, amputation secondary to soft-tissue sarcoma can occur at any age. Many factors are taken into consideration in the rehabilitation of amputees: age, vocation, health status, lifestyle, psychological stability, motivation, and adjunctive chemotherapy regimens. Many of these issues are addressed during a preoperative evaluation. Patients most often want to know the type of prosthesis they will be wearing, what it looks like, and how well they can function with it. Sample protheses are kept in the clinic to show patients. It is helpful to arrange for another amputee from the community to talk with the patient. Such discussion often relieves some of the patient's stress and sense of loss when thinking about losing a limb.

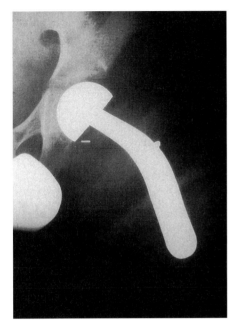

FIG. 16 Plain x-ray film of hip disarticulation. Short endoprosthesis converted condition to a short above-knee amputation.

2. Immediate Postoperative Fitting

If there are no contraindications, an immediate postoperative rigid dressing is applied in the operating room for AK, BK, AE, and BE amputations. This reduces edema, facilitates healing, and helps shape the residual limb. If a forequarter amputation is done, a plastic shoulder cap needs to be fabricated preoperatively (using another person of similar size as a model). The cap will then be ready postoperatively, and the patient can wear it after the wound has healed and the clips or sutures have been removed.

3. Temporary Prosthesis

Patients can be fitted with a temporary socket and prosthesis 10 days postoperatively if the suture line has healed. Ambulation with partial weight bearing in the lower extremities can begin. Due to fluid fluctuations from chemotherapy and weight loss, the number of stump socks used in the socket will have to be adjusted. Ace bandaging is used to control edema and shape the residual limb. Temporary limbs can be constructed by trained rehabilitation staff. Commercial temporary

Upper Extremity Prostheses

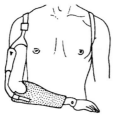

BELOW ELBOW

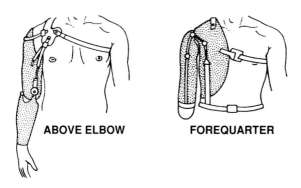

ABOVE ELBOW   **FOREQUARTER**

FIG. 17   Graphic of functional upper extremity prosthesis: below elbow, above elbow, and forequarter.

limbs are available but more expensive. They are useful if there will be a significant delay before the permanent prosthesis can be fitted.

4.   Permanent Prosthesis

When the residual limb is well healed, shaped, and stable in size for at least a week (usually 1 month to 6 weeks postoperatively), a permanent limb can be initially fitted by a prosthetist. There will be an interim fit checked by the physiatrist to ensure that the socket is properly aligned and fits well, that the other limb components are likewise well aligned, and that the patient's gait is as normal as possible. Care is taken to ensure that there are no areas of excessive compression of the skin. Some changes and adjustments are usually recommended to the prosthetist at this time, and a final checkup is done by the physiatrist after the changes have been made (Figs. 17 and 18).

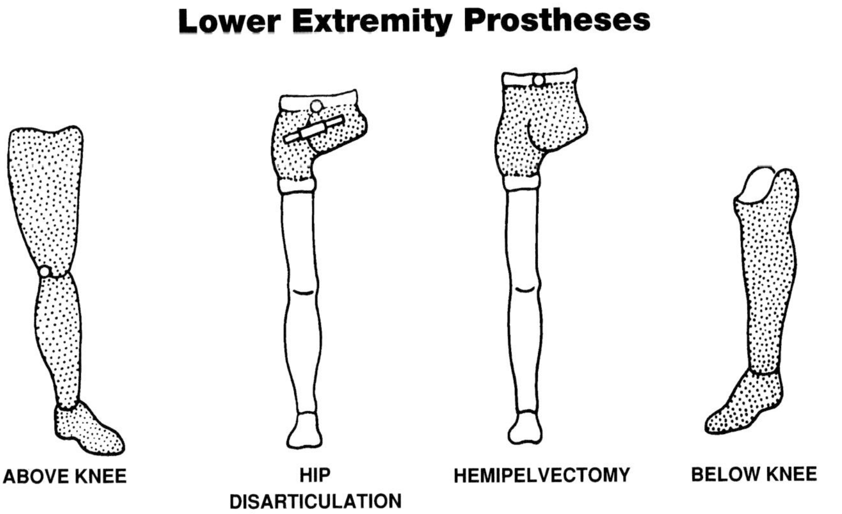

Lower Extremity Prostheses

ABOVE KNEE **HIP DISARTICULATION** **HEMIPELVECTOMY** **BELOW KNEE**

FIG. 18 Graphic of functional lower extremity prosthesis above knee, hip disarticulation, hemipelvectomy, and below knee.

5. Prosthetic Training

Both lower limb and upper limb amputees receive prosthetic training. Training for lower extremity amputees includes balance training, with or without crutches, strengthening of adjacent muscles and muscles in the uninvolved limb, stretching exercises to maintain joint motion, and education to achieve the most normal gait possible. Practice on stairs, ramps, and inclines, and entering cars is done both inside and outside. Occupational therapy ensures that the patient is safe in the home kitchen and bathroom and provides needed safety equipment. A driving assessment is done. The patient is advised about hand controls if necessary.

Usually hemipelvectomy patients need crutches or a cane. Hip disarticulations also often necessitate use of a cane. Lower level amputees achieve independence without a cane. Upper extremity amputees need training in balance, trunk and neck range of motion, and strengthening exercises. Training in terms of functional activities with the limb is provided. The activities that can be done depend on the level of the amputation and the terminal device (hand or more functional hook).

E. Prosthethic Limb Choices

The choice of whether a person should use a prosthesis and, if so, what kind is an important decision. It depends on the level of amputation as well as the patient's age, medical status, motivation, vocation, and lifestyle (46,47).

Prostheses may be functional or nonfunctional (cosmetic only) or a combination of functional and cosmetic. They may be made with a hard durable exterior shell (exoskeletal) or a rigid interior with a soft cosmetic cover (less durable). Upper extremity prothesis can have heavy-duty cable mechanisms and hook terminal device, allowing a person to pick up 50 lb, or light cable ones with cosmetic hands, allowing the person to lift only 10 lb. Different types of joints are available from simple single-axis knees to hydraulic ones that allow for easy changes in walking cadence, which are good for dancing. A number of newer prosthetic feet exist. Some have four-way motion, whereas others are more flexible and allow for a more propulsive gait and springy push-off at the toe (good for sports). The recent advent of lighter carbon components and titanium metals for joints and flexible plastic for sockets has reduced the weight of prosthesis. This is particularly advantageous for cancer amputees who may have decreased endurance from the disease, chemotherapy, or metastatic disease. Newer elastic and gel suspension cuffs and those that lock into the bottom of the socket with a metal device and have a quick release lever on the side of the socket are favored by young cancer amputees.

Myoelectric switch-regulated prostheses are available in forequarter, above-elbow, and below-elbow models but are very expensive ($20,000–$40,000). Extensive justification is needed for insurance payment.

Finally, many companies make special sports limbs and swim legs, which are also favored by young cancer amputees.

F. Prosthetic Use

Most forequarter amputees prefer a cosmetic shoulder or a long cosmetic arm rather than a functional regular forequarter prosthesis or myoelectric one. These latter prostheses are bulky, difficult to operate, and minimally functional. Some amputees prefer doing one-handed activities to wearing an above-elbow prosthesis, again because they are bulky and more difficult to use than below-elbow ones. Most below-elbow amputees use a prothesis. Functional hands and hooks are available. Hands are less functional.

Many younger people and those over 50 years prefer to use crutches rather than an HD or HP prothesis. Such prostheses require much more energy than normal gait; even then, gait is slow and altered. Prostheses also require good balance and motivation to learn to use them. Gait requires hip hiking to clear the prosthesis during swing phase. These prostheses are usually contraindicated with significant cardiac and pulmonary disease (or metastasis).

Short above-knee amputations, hip disarticulation converted to above-knee amputation, "short" below-knee or regular length below-knee amputations can all be well accommodated for by prosthesis, and patient compliance with use is high.

XI. FUNCTIONAL OUTCOME

Since a main criteria for doing limb-sparing surgery is preservation of a functional limb, it is not surprising that reports concerning functional outcome and quality of life in this patient group are generally favorable (14,19,34,48). Most of these studies have not used the same functional assessment tools, so they cannot be fully contrasted. Recent reports indicate that impairments impacting on quality of life (pain, edema, loss of range of motion and strength) tend to be mild or transient (15), generally occurring the first 12 months postoperatively.

An older report (48) indicated poorer outcome prior to 1980. A 1992 study attributed this to higher dose nonfractionated radiotherapy (14). Two (14,49) studies also note worse functional outcome with radiotherapy doses over 60 Gy. A study by Karasek (59) relates a relationship between volume of unradiated tissue to the 55+ Gy level and functional score, strength, fibrosis, and skin changes. A poorer functional outcome occurs with increased total volume of tissue irradiated. In this study, 83% of soft-tissue sarcoma patients with WLE and radiotherapy had excellent functional outcomes. A study with brachytherapy in soft-tissue sarcoma patients undergoing WLE versus no brachytherapy revealed no significant differences in strength and gait parameters; however, there was a higher level of anxiety and depression in the irradiated group (53). Two studies report that deficits and lower function are more common and greater in severity in the lower extremities (48,49). Most studies advocate that early and ongoing rehabilitation is critical in attaining and maintaining the highest functional level possible (14,15,48,50).

Although some earlier studies report no difference in quality of life of amputees versus limb-spared patients (51,52), it is the current general consensus that preservation of the extremity, if possible, is favored above amputation if general function is at least satisfactory. This is particularly true when limb sparing is done in lieu of forequarter or HP amputations. In some WLE cases, loss of function of a joint is accepted if overall function is better than would be possible with amputation (e.g., Tinkhoff-Lindberg where loss of shoulder motion is more functional than a forequarter amputation).

Because of the lifestyle of the person, even though good general function is maintained with limb-sparing procedures, some life activities must be deleted or vocational levels changed (47) (e.g., running is compromised in gastrocnemeus resections). There are also safety issues: *no contact sports should be allowed with a Tikhoff-Lindberg or with irradiation over bones (because of fracture risk).*

XII. LATE FOLLOW-UP STAGE

In the late follow-up stage, the rehabilitation team is careful to observe for late radiation effects (osteoporosis of bone, skin breakdown, loss of joint motion, fibrosis of muscle around joints, plexopathy, and myelopathy). With significant osteoporosis, the patient is instructed in appropriate exercises and precautions for activities. Adjustments or replacements are made in orthotics and prosthetic, assistive, and mobility devices and edema control garments. Advice is given about vocation and sexuality.

XIII. LOCAL/REOCCURRENCE STAGE

Local reoccurrence of tumor may happen and necessitate further surgery, chemotherapy, limb perfusion, or amputation. The patient requires a full rehabilitation assessment, and specific treatment strategies are introduced depending on the nature of the problems.

XIV. METASTATIC DISEASE

Metastasis is most commonly to the lung, occurs in about 20% of patients, and may be amenable to local lung and or chest wall resections. Studies indicate that 20–30% of patients who have a lung metastectomy are alive 5 years later (1). A new procedure that is less invasive for removal of lung metastasis has been introduced (55). Removal of metastasis has resulted in extension of survival rate (54). Rehabilitation helps with pain and stress management and adjustments to vocation. The use of assistive devices and energy conservation are required. Restoration of function after interventions is the goal.

XV. END-OF-LIFE STAGE

Maintenance of quality of life and control of pain and stress are the important goals in the end-of-life stage. Mobility and assistive devices are often needed for safety.

XVI. CONCLUSION

With multimodality treatment, satisfactory to excellent outcomes can be obtained in most limb-sparing patients. Rehabilitation, custom-tailored to the patient's needs, is considered essential pre- and postoperatively and at intervals throughout the trajectory of the patient's medical care. Taking care of problems and impairments as they arise helps patients avoid impairments, maintain the highest functional level possible, and maintain a good quality of life.

REFERENCES

1. Brennan MF, Casper EH, Harrison LB. Section II: Soft tissue sarcomas, in Chapter 38, Sarcomas of soft tissue and bone. In: DeVita VT, Hellman S, Rosenberg ST, eds. Cancer: Principles and Practice of Oncology, 5th ed. Philadelphia: Lippincott-Raven, 1997, pp. 1738–1787.
2. Enzinger FM, Weiss SW. Soft Tissue Tumors, 3rd ed. St. Louis: Mosby–Year Book, 1995.
3. Temple WJ, Temple CLF, Arthur K, et al. Prospective cohort study of neoadjuvant treatment in conservative surgery of soft tissue sarcoma. Ann Surg Oncol 4(7):586–590, 1997.
4. Eilber P, Eckardt J. Surgical management of soft tissue sarcomas. Semin Oncol 24(5):526–533, 1997.
5. Guntesbery P, Eggermont A, Ennelang WF. Current controversies in cancer: is limb amputation necessary for locally advanced soft tissue sarcomas. Eur J Cancer 33(14):2295–2301, 1997.
6. Clasby R, Tilling K, Smith MA, Fletcher CDM. Variable management of soft tissue sarcoma: regional audit with implication for specialist care. Br J Surg (84):1692–1696, 1997.
7. Pisters P, Leung D, Woodruff J. Analysis of prognostic factors in 1043 patients with localized soft tissue sarcomas of the extremities. J Clin Oncol 14:1679–1689, 1996.
8. Bray PW, Bill RS, Vaughan C, Bown A, Davis A, O'Sullivan B. Limb salvage surgery and adjuvant radiotherapy for soft tissue sarcomas of the forearm and hand. J Hand Surg 22A(3):495–503, 1997.
9. Osaka S, Hoshi M, Sanos S, Hoshi M, Nozaki M, Yamamoto M. Description of new composite tissue transfer for salvage of complex hand deficit. Clin Orthop 328:91–93, 1996.
10. Gross E, Rao BN, Bowman L, Michalkiewicz E, Pappo A, Santana V, Kaste S, Greenwald C, Pratt C. Outcome treatment for pediatric sarcoma of the foot: a retrospective review over 20 years. J Pediatr Surg 22(8):1181–1184, 1997.
11. Swit H, Spiro IJ. Soft tissue sarcomas: radiation as a therapeutic option. Ann Acad Med 25(6):855–861, 1996.
12. Liu L, Glicksman A. The role of radiation in the management of soft tissue sarcoma. Med Health 80(1):32–36, 1997.
13. Brennan MF. Long-term results of a prospective randomized trial of adjuvant brachytherapy in soft tissue sarcoma. J Clin Oncol 14(3):859–868, 1996.
14. Stinson SF, DeLaney TF, Greenberg J, Yang J, Lampert MH, Hicks JE, Vanzon D, White DE, Rosenberg SA, Glotstein E. Acute and long-term effects on limb function

of combined modality limb-sparing therapy for extremity soft tissue sarcoma. Int. J Radiat Oncol Biol Phys 21:1493–1499, 1991.

15. Yang JC, Chang AE, Baker AE, Sindelar WF, Danforth DN, Topalian SL, Delaney T, Glotstein E, Steinberg SM, Merino MJ, Rosenberg SA. Randomized prospective study of the benefit of adjuvant radiation therapy in the treatment of soft tissue sarcoma of the extremity. J Clin Oncol 16(1):197–203, 1998.

16. Hicks J. Personal communication.

17. Chang AE, Kinsella T, Glotstein E, Baker AR, Sindelar WF, Lotze MT, Danforth DN, Sugarbaker PH, Lock E, Steinberg SE, White DE, Rosenberg SA. Adjuvant chemotherapy for patients with high grade soft tissue sarcoma of the extremity. J Clin Oncol 6:1491–1500, 1988.

18. Rosenberg SA, Chang AE, Glotstein EJ. Adjuvant chemotherapy for treatment of soft tissue sarcoma: review of the National Cancer Institute Experience. Cancer Treat Symp 3:83–88, 1985.

19. Chang AE, Steinberg SM, Culnane M, Lampert M, Reggia A, Simpson C, Hicks JE, White DE, Yang JJ, Glotstein E, Rosenberg SA. Functional and psychological effects of multimodality limb spared therapy. J Clin Oncol 7(9):1217–1228, 1989.

20. Eggermont AM, Schraffond J, Koops H, Klausner JM, Kroon BR, Schlag P, Lienard D, Van Gael AN, Hoekstra HJ, Maller I, Nieweg O, Kettelhock R, Bari G, Pector JC, Lejeune F. Isolated limb perfusion with tumor necrosis factor and melphalan for limb salvage in 186 patients with locally advanced soft tissue sarcoma. The Cumulative Multicenter European Experience. Ann Surg 224(6):756–765, 1996.

21. Gerber L, Vargo M. Rehabilitation for patients with cancer diagnoses. In: DaLisa J, Gans BM, eds. Rehabilitation Medicine: Principles and Practice, 3rd ed. Philadelphia: Lippincott-Raven, 1998, pp. 1293–1319.

22. Hicks J, Nicholas JJ. Treatments utilized in rehabilitative rheumatology. In: Hicks J, Nicholas J, Swezeg R, eds. Handbook of Rehabilitative Rheumatology. Atlanta: American Rheumatism Association, 1988, pp. 32–71.

23. Rosenbaum LS, Danoff JV, Guthrie J, et al. Effects of energy-matched pulsed and continuous ultrasound on tumor growth in mice. Phys Ther 78(3):271–277, 1988.

24. Warren CG, Lehmann JF, Koblanski JN. Heat and stretch procedures: an evolution using rat tail tendon. Arch Phys Med Rehab 57:122–129, 1976.

25. Melzack R, Wall PD. Pain mechanisms: a new theory. Science 50:971, 1965.

26. Parfitt A. Nausea and vomiting. In: NIH Consensus Development Conference on Acupuncture, National Institutes of Health, Nov 1997, p. 91.

27. Hicks J. Exercise for cancer patients. In: Basmajian JV, Wolf SL, eds. Therapeutic Exercise. Baltimore: Williams & Wilkins, 1990, pp. 351–369.

28. Jensen JE, Jenson TG, Dudrick SJ, et al. Nutrition in orthopedic surgery. J. Bone Joint Surgery (AM) 64(9):1263–1272, 1984.

29. Minor M, Hewett J, Webel R, et al. Efficacy of a physical conditioning exercise program in patients with RA and OA. Arthritis Rheum 32:1396, 1989.

30. Dimeo F, Rumberger BG, Keul J. Aerobic exercise as therapy for cancer fatigue. Med SC Sports Exercise 30(4):475–478, 1998.

31. Schag CAC, Heinrich RL. Development of a comprehensive quality of life measurement tool: the CARES—a system for the functional evaluation of the surgical man-

agement of musculoskeletal tumors. In: Enneking WF, ed. Limb-Sparing Surgery for Musculoskeletal Tumors. New York: Churchill Livingstone, 1987, pp. 5–19.

32. Davis AM, Wright JG, Williams JI, et al. Development of a measure of function for patients with bone and soft tissue sarcoma. Qual Life Res 55(5):508–516, 1996.

33. Casley-Smith JR. Modern treatment of lymphadema. Mod Med Aust 35(5):70–83, 1992.

34. Temple WJ, Temple CLF, Arthur K, Schachnar N, Paterson AHG, Crabtree TS. Prospective cohort study of neoadjuvant treatment in conservative surgery of soft tissue sarcomas. Ann Surg Oncol 4(7):586–590, 1997.

35. Sugarbaker PH, Lampert MH. Excision of the quadriceps muscle group. Surgery 93:462, 1983.

36. Stanhope SJ, Siegel KL, Hicks JE. Changing adaptations in the lower extremities during gait following sciatic nerve resection. Proceedings of the East Coast Clinical Gart Laboratory Conference, Richmond, Va.

37. Lampert MH, Gahagen C. Rehabilitation of the sarcoma patient. In: McGarvey C, ed. Physical Therapy for the Cancer Patient. New York: Churchill Livingstone, 1990, pp. 111–135.

38. Lampert MH, Gerber LH, Sugarbaker PH. Rehabilitation of patients with extremity sarcoma. In: Sugarbaker PH, Nicholson TH, eds. Atlas of Extremity Sarcoma Surgery. Philadelphia: JB Lippincott, 1984, p. 97.

39. Lampert MH, Sugarbaker PH. Rehabilitation of patients with extremity sarcoma. In: Sugarbaker PH, Malower MM, eds. Musculoskeletal Surgery for Cancer: Principles and Techniques. New York: Thieme Medical Publishers, 1992, pp. 55–74.

40. Ward B, McGarvey C, Lutz M. Excellent shoulder function is attainable after partial or total scapulectomy. Arch Surg 125(4):537–542, 1990.

41. Brennan MF. The surgeon as a leader in cancer care: lessons learned from the study of soft tissue sarcoma. J Am Coll Surg 182:520, 1996.

42. Nowroozi F, Salvanelli ML, Gerber LH. Energy expenditure in hip disarticulation and hemipelvectomy amputees. Arch Phys Med Rehab 64:300–303, 1983.

43. Trough GH, Corcoran PJ, Reyes RL. Energy expenditure of ambulation in patients with above-knee amputations. Arch Phys Med Rehab 56:67–71, 1975.

44. Cummings V, March H, Steve L, Robinson KG. Energy costs of below-knee prosthesis using two types of suspension. Arch Phys Med Rehab 60:293–297, 1979.

45. Hicks J, Lampert M, Malawer M. Rehabilitation of a converted short above-knee amputation from a hip disarticulation. Arch Phys Med Rehab 68:9(S-637), 1987.

46. Leonard JA, Mercer RH. Upper and lower extremity prosthesis. In: DeLisa J, Gans M, eds. Rehabilitation Medicine: Principles and Practice. Philadelphia: Lippincott-Raven, 1998, pp. 669–696.

47. Lane JM, Knoll MA, Rossbach PG. New advances and concept in amputee management after treatment for bone and soft tissue sarcoma. Clin Orthop 256:22–28, 1990.

48. Lampert MH, Gerber LH, Glatstien I, Rosenberg S, Danoff JV. Soft tissue sarcoma: functional outcome after wide local excision and radiation therapy. Arch Phys Med Rehab 65(8):477–480, 1984.

49. Robinson MH, Spruce L, Eeles R, Fryatt I, Harmer C, Thomas JM, Westbury G. Limb

function following conservative treatment of adult soft tissue sarcoma. Eur J Cancer 27(12):1567–1574, 1991.

50. Yasko AW, Reece GP, Gills TA, Pollock RE. Limb salvage strategies to optimize quality of life: the MD Anderson Cancer Center Experience. CA Cancer Clin 47(4):226–238, 1997.

51. Karase KK, Contene LS, Rosier R. Sarcoma therapy: functional outcome and relationship to treatment parameters. Int J Radiat Oncol Biol Phys 24:651–656, 1992.

52. Sugarbaker PH, Barofsky I, Rosenberg SA, Gianola FJ. Quality of life assessment of patients in extremity sarcoma. Clinical trials. Surgery 91(17):7–23, 1982.

53. Schupek KD, Lane JM, Weilpp AE, Brennan MF. The psychofunctional handicap associated with branchytherapy in the treatment of lower extremity sarcomas. Int J Radiat Oncol Biol Phys 27:293, 1993.

54. Verazim GT, Warneke JA, Driscoll DL. Resection of lung metastases from soft tissue sarcomas: a multivariant analysis. Arch Surg 127:1407, 1992.

Index